Magic Shots

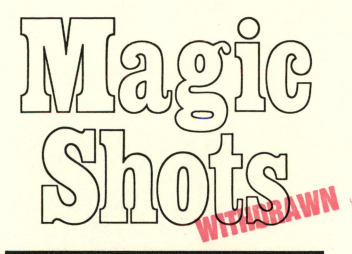

A HUMAN AND SCIENTIFIC ACCOUNT OF THE LONG AND CONTINUING STRUGGLE TO ERADICATE INFECTIOUS DISEASES BY VACCINATION

Allan Chase

William Morrow and Company, Inc. New York 1982

Library of Congress Cataloging in Publication Data

Chase, Allan, 1913–
  Magic shots.

  Includes bibliographical references and index.
  1. Communicable diseases—Prevention—History.
  2. Vaccination—History. I. Title.
RA643.C44 1982   614.4′7′09   82-12505
ISBN 0-688-00787-2

Printed in the United States of America

First Edition

1 2 3 4 5 6 7 8 9 10

BOOK DESIGN BY LINEY LI

This book is for

my wife, Martha,

and our two grandchildren,

Karen and Laurie,

with all my love

Introduction

Economists, seers, and political columnists are notorious for perceiving "the imminent dawn of new eras." New days bring yet new perceptions, and yet new dawns. Medicine has been no less lacking in prophets, too often steeped in hope and prescience. Is it hope or prescience which intimates that in medicine we are indeed at the dawn of a new era, an era whose prominent theme is prevention, and whose most powerful weapons are vaccines?

The apparent dawn of a new era in medicine—and health is neither transient perception nor wishful fantasy, but the inevitable result of increasingly evident inexorable forces. The forces are diverse and contradictory—forces generated by science and startling new revelations of the process of disease and the potential for its prevention; economic forces which escalate the appalling costs of illness and its treatment; and political forces which increasingly demand a broader equity in improved health at an affordable cost. The forces and their direction are global.

The ultimate achievement in medicine is the global eradication of a disease. This milestone has now been passed with the declaration by the World Health Assembly in May 1980 that smallpox, once the most devastating killer of all, has been consigned to history. It was achieved with a vaccine and with a program costing, in all, less than what the United States alone annually spent for smallpox control. The implications for the one billion people who lived in areas infected by smallpox little more than a decade ago are yet more profound.

The campaign demanded a global effort, and effective programs extending throughout the poorest countries and the most difficult areas. It was done. Today, vaccination programs against six major disabling and killing diseases are being implemented throughout the world as part of a global effort. The goal is to reach all children, everywhere, by 1990. The costs, by any measure, are small, and progress to date has been most dramatic. Hospital wards, indeed entire hospitals, once occupied by recuperating—or dying—children and adults are already being used for other purposes. The savings in life, in disability, in dollars, are formidable.

Recent discoveries in the biomedical sciences clearly point to the potential for development of other vaccines, of safer, less expensive vaccines, of vaccines to prevent malaria, some forms of heart disease and cancer, of venereal disease, of pregnancy. Where, in the past, developments depended heavily on many painfully slow trial-and-error methods, a newly acquired understanding of cellular biology has permitted the acceleration of research, and has revealed more insights and opportunities than we have scientists or the scientific capacity to explore.

Those concerned with medical care have been slow to perceive fully the implications of contemporary biomedical science in preventing illness. Many, more elderly legislators are often more concerned about new therapies for diseases to which they themselves are subject. Economists and lay administrators focus their energies on developing policies to restrain the costs of hospitalization and sickness care during the coming year and the year thereafter. Most fail to comprehend that an ounce of prevention applied this year and next could have an effect far more profound some years hence than could be achieved with full application of the most heroic cost-restraining economic measures. A sense of frustration prevails. Yet, immunologists now foresee many formidable new weapons that could have as decided an impact in dealing with disease as did the smallpox vaccine.

To the extent that we are willing to commit resources to the development of these powerful weapons to prevent illness, the sooner we will shift our focus from treating the sick to sustaining the healthy. This book, which so brilliantly dramatizes past achievements and the promises of the future, demands attention—and action.

—D. A. Henderson, M.D., M.P.H.

Dean, The Johns Hopkins University School
of Hygiene and Public Health
Formerly Director, World Health Organization
Smallpox Eradication, 1966–1977

Contents

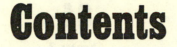

162

"The Manner of Death is Most Piteous" ... Serotherapy Rises from the Ashes of the Failed Whole-Organism Diphtheria Vaccines ... Antitoxins Reduce the Proportions of Diphtheria Deaths ... First Clinical Trials of the Diphtheria Toxoid Vaccines, 1913–1917

191

Diphtheria Vaccine Trials in Children Abandoned for the Duration ... Genesis of a Preventable Pandemic ... When the Killing Ends, the Fight for Lives Free of Diphtheria Resumes

204

Gorgas and the Forgotten Classic of Social Medicine ... Wright's Pneumonia Vaccine Fails in South African Mining Compounds, and Mineowners Call in Gorgas ... Serum Antibodies Used to Cure Selected Pneumococcal Pneumonias ... The Antiphagocytic Capsules of Pneumonia Germs ... "The Mice Did Not Die" ... Mirsky's Law and Vaccines Against Pneumonia

359

Chapter 15
The Rediscovery of
Chemical Vaccines Against Pneumonia
and Meningitis

Typing of Pneumococci Facilitates Better Antisera . . . After Antibiotics Cure Their Pneumonias, Many People Still Die of Pneumococcal Damages . . . Pneumococcal Capsular Polysaccharide Vaccines Reclaimed . . . New Pneumonia Vaccines Once Again Tested in Black South African Gold Miners . . . When Sulfa Pills Lost Their Capacity to Prevent Meningococcal Meningitis in Postwar Boot Camps . . . The Political Imperatives of Meningitis Vaccines . . . U.S. Army's New Meningitis Vaccines Rushed to Protect 130 Million People in Two Nations

386

Chapter 16
Group B Streptococcus and
Other Baby Killers—
and New Bacterial Subunits
to Block Them

Group B Strep Meningitis, an Adult Venereal Infection Passed on to Babies During Act of Birth . . . POMP, Conjugates, and Other New Vaccine Components

397

Chapter 17
The Old Gonorrhea Vaccines
and Other Doctors' Delusions

Of Gonorrhea, Penicillin, and Our So-Called "Sexual Revolution" . . . Gonorrhea Now a Major Cause of Involuntary Sterilization in Women . . . The Upward Social Mobility of Gonorrhea . . . For Centuries, Bleeding, Purgings, and Poisons Fail to Cure or Prevent Gonorrhea . . . The Biographer Boswell's Ultimately Fatal

Nineteen Bouts With Signor Gonorrhea ... Futile Heat, Shock, and Surgical Therapies Add to the Twentieth-Century Perils of Catching Gonorrhea ... Gonorrhea Vaccines Galore, 1905–1945, but Not One of Them Works ... The Dark Ages of Gonorrhea Vaccine Research End at Inuvik, 1973

Chapter 18
The New Gonorrhea Vaccines: Boon, Bust, or Time Bomb?

Hitler Rings Down the Curtain on Casper's Gonorrhea Vaccine ... Surgeon General Parran Opts for Gonorrhea Vaccine in 1941 ... Postwar Federal Grants Fund Needed Lines of Gonorrhea Research ... The Pili of the Gonorrhea Germs and Their Role in Venereal Disease ... Brinton's Purified Pili Gonorrhea Vaccine Tested in People ... New Bacterial Subunit Immunogens Bring Gonorrhea Vaccines, and Their Pandora's Box of Social Problems, Much Nearer ... Who Should Be Immunized Against America's Leading Notifiable Disease? ... If Successful Gonorrhea Vaccines Come to Be, Can Syphilis Epidemics Be Far Behind?

Chapter 19
The Future of Vaccines: Never Brighter, Never Darker

Why Major Infectious Disease Attack Rates Are Rising ... Hospital-Acquired (Nosocomial) Infections Proliferate ... Decline and Decay of Our Water Systems ... Fiscal Inflation and Its Continuum of Adverse Health Effects ... Strep Throats, Vaccines, and "Horror Autotoxicus" Heart Disease ... Otitis Media: The Extremely Common Cause of Preschool Ear Damages That Retard Mental Development ... "We'll Just Have to Develop a New Way to Fool Nature" ... New Vaccines Based on Advances in Genetics, Immunochemistry, and Basic Scientific Knowledge ... Live Vaccine Viruses and Immunogens Made From Off-the-Shelf Chemicals ... "Virtual Scientific Illiteracy" in High Places and the "Disintegration of Scientific Education" ... Vaccines Are Worthless Unless Used

Acknowledgments

Although burdened with more professional duties than any two other professors of medicine and editors of medical newspapers half his age, my good friend and erstwhile colleague, Dr. Abraham S. Jacobson, found the time to review the entire manuscript of this book before it was cut to its final length, to spot its then medical and scientific errors, and to clarify and otherwise improve the writing in various chapters. I shall never be able to thank him enough for his consideration and his great help.

It would be impossible to list all of the microbiologists, immunochemists, bacteriologists, clinical specialists in infectious diseases, and other workers who helped me assemble the materials in this book. The individuals thanked by name here represent a far greater number of people who provided information and insights and steered me to the right journal and book stacks at various medical libraries.

Some of them, most notably Drs. Austrian, Fischetti, Gotschlich, Drucker, Hirsch, Schachter, and Swanson, reviewed for accuracy of fact and interpretation various chapters dealing with their own work and/or their own fields of activity and experience. One of them, Dr. Gubner, suggested the title of the book; and (like his father) a former student under William Hallock Park at NYU-Bellevue medical school, he reviewed those chapters dealing with the diphtheria and poliomyelitis vaccines.

With profound regret I can no longer thank Dr. Wolfgang A. Casper, who opened his files to me and also shared his unwritten memories of his work on pneumococcal and gonococcal vaccines in Berlin during the last years of the Weimar Republic, and his experiences as a doctor and persistent proponent of the prevention of gonorrhea by immunization after 1934 in this country. Dr. Casper died in March 1982, at the age of eighty-one.

Again, my profound thanks to:

Dr. Michael A. Apicella, University of Nevada, Reno. Dr. Robert Austrian, University of Pennsylvania, Philadelphia. Dr. Albert Balows, Centers for Disease Control (CDC), Atlanta, Georgia. Dr. Paul A. Blake, CDC. Dr. Martin Blaser, CDC. Dr. Michael F. Barile, Bureau of Biologics (B.o.B.), Federal Food and Drug Administration (FDA), Bethesda, Maryland. Dr. Paul B. Beeson, Veterans Administration Hospital and University of Washington,

Seattle. Dr. Charles Bluestone, University of Pittsburgh, Pennsylvania. Dr. Charles C. Brinton, University of Pittsburgh. Dr. John A. Bryner, National Animal Diseases Center, Ames, Iowa. Dr. Thomas Buchanan, United States Public Health Service Hospital and University of Washington. Dr. David Bundle, Canadian National Research Council, Ottawa.

Dr. W. A. Clyde and Dr. Albert M. Collier, University of North Carolina, Chapel Hill. Dr. Lyle Conrad, CDC. Dr. Nancy Boucot Cummings, National Institute of Arthritis, Metabolism, and Digestive Diseases, Bethesda. Mr. Charles Dennison, National Center for Health Statistics, Hyattsville, Maryland. Dr. Richard E. Dixon, CDC. Dr. Ernest Drucker, Montefiore Medical Center, New York.

Dr. Gerald Fernald, University of North Carolina. Dr. Vincent A. Fischetti, Rockefeller University, New York. Dr. Carl E. Frasch, B.o.B.-FDA. Dr. David W. Fraser, CDC. Dr. Emil C. Gotschlich, Rockefeller University. Dr. Richard Gubner, Clearwater, Florida. Dr. Robert J. Haggerty, Harvard University, Cambridge. Dr. David Hanson, National Institute of Neurological and Communicative Disorders and Stroke, Bethesda. Dr. Michael Heidelberger, New York University. Dr. James Hill, National Institute for Allergy and Infectious Diseases (NIAID), Bethesda. Dr. Maurice Hilleman, Merck Institute for Therapeutic Research, West Point, Pennsylvania. Dr. Jerry Hirsch, University of Illinois, Urbana. Dr. Virgil M. Howie, Huntsville, Alabama.

Dr. John F. James, University of California, San Francisco. Dr. Walter Karakawa, Pennsylvania State University. Dr. Dennis L. Kasper, Harvard University and The National Bacteriological Laboratory, Stockholm, Sweden. Dr. Stephen J. Kraus, CDC. Dr. J. Michael Lane, CDC. Dr. Zell A. McGee, Vanderbilt University, Nashville, Tennessee. Dr. Margaret McLaren, National Heart, Lung and Blood Institute, Bethesda. Dr. Milton Markowitz, University of Connecticut, Storrs. Dr. Jack Paradise, University of Pittsburgh.

Dr. Frank J. Rauscher, Jr., American Cancer Society. Dr. John B. Robbins, B.o.B.-FDA. Dr. Richard B. Roberts, Cornell University Medical Center, New York. Dr. Jerald C. Sadoff, Walter Reed Army Institute of Research (WRAIR), Washington, D.C. Dr. E. Neil Schachter, Yale University, New Haven, Connecticut. Dr. Gary K. Schoolnik, Rockefeller University. Dr. Robert McNair Scott, WRAIR. Dr. Gordon R. B. Skinner, University of Birmingham, England. Dr. Robert Smibert, Virginia Polytechnical Institute and State University, Blacksburg, Virginia. Dr. P. F. Sparling, University of North Carolina. Dr. John Swanson, Rocky Mountain Laboratories, NIAID, Hamilton, Montana. Dr. Stephen Thacker, CDC. Dr. Joseph G. Tully, NIAID. Dr. Paul Wiesner, CDC.

My special thanks to my sponsor, Dr. Alexander Alland, Jr., Professor and Chairman, Department of Anthropology, and to the Trustees of Columbia University for the designation of Visiting Scholar. Much of the library research for this book was conducted in the university's Health Sciences, Biology, Science, Butler, Business, Law, and Social Work Libraries, and also at the New York Academy of Medicine Library.

Finally, I want to thank the individuals whose skills and enthusiasm lightened the editorial and publishing tasks, starting with Mitch Douglas, my friend and agent, Bob Bender, my first editor, and Howard Cady, who took over before the editing was completed, and Sonia Greenbaum, the copy editor.

Needless to say, whatever errors of fact or interpretation may yet be found in this book are the fault of the author alone, and should never be held against the fine scientists and clinicians whose aid is here acknowledged with such gratitude.

New York, June 1, 1982   ALLAN CHASE

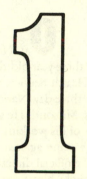

C H A P T E R

PREVENTION IS BETTER

Theoretically, it should be possible to prepare a [single] multivalent capsular polysaccharide vaccine for all common invasive bacterial organisms.

—JOHN B. ROBBINS, M.D., 1978[1]

On November 10, 1944, Wolfgang A. Casper, a trim, dapper forty-three-year-old doctor wearing the uniform of Surgeon, United States Public Health Service, was called to the speakers' podium on the second day of the three-day National Postwar Venereal Disease Control Conference in St. Louis, Missouri. He seemed a bit shaken as he organized the few typewritten sheets of his working paper on the immediate development and mass testing of a vaccine against gonorrhea. Casper had reason enough to be moved. For him the official directive from U.S. Surgeon General Thomas M. Parran that had brought him to St. Louis on this day was the beginning of the end of a quest that had begun in Berlin in 1927.

At that moment in 1944 Casper was chief of the gonorrhea section of the Service's venereal disease control program in Chicago. The last of four generations of Berlin doctors, the great-grandson of the first professor of medical jurisprudence at the University of Berlin, the youngest professor of dermatology in the history of the huge Rudolf Virchow Hospital in Berlin, Casper had committed the grievous error of having also been born to Jewish parents. In 1935 Casper and his wife, Anna, also a doctor, had escaped with their lives from Nazi Germany and arrived in New York as penniless refugees.

They might have reached New York a half dozen years earlier. In 1929 work that Casper had performed and published in German scientific journals—work involving entirely new types of vaccines against the disease-causing bacteria of pneumococcal pneumonia that were made not of whole bacteria but of polysaccharides, or sugars taken from the outer slimy capsules surrounding the bacterial cells—had led to an offer of a research post at the Rockefeller Institute in New York City. Dr. Oswald T. Avery, who had since well before World War I been investigating these three same substances, was the man who made this offer.

When the Caspers arrived in New York in 1935, Dr. Avery and his friends at Rockefeller Institute were able to find Casper a job as a urologist at New York's Bellevue Hospital. Kinsmen helped his wife, Annaliese, set up a practice in her specialty, allergy, in Manhattan.

There was a good reason for Avery's concern over Casper's welfare. During World War I, with Dr. Alphonse Raymond Dochez, Avery had shown that a material in the capsules surrounding the pneumococci—the agents of most of the pneumonia cases seen in medical practice—contributed to the virulence of these bacteria. At the time, they reported that this pneumococcal capsular material was a protein. In 1923 a young coworker of Avery's, the organic chemist Michael Heidelberger, determined that the capsular material was actually a carbohydrate in the form of polysaccharides or compounds of several types of simple sugars or saccharides.[2]

Three years later the even younger Wolfgang Casper, working in biochemist Oscar Schiemann's laboratory in Berlin, discovered that injections of purified pneumococcal capsular polysaccharides protected mice against the specific strains of virulent pneumococci from which they were taken.

When Casper and Schiemann repeated this work, and published their results with mice in 1927,[3] it caused great excitement at Rockefeller Institute and other laboratories around the world. For one thing, since the capsular polysaccharides of the pneumococci (and presumably of other encapsulated disease-causing bacteria) were germ-free, vaccines made of these carbohydrates were theoretically unable to cause pneumonia or any other disease caused by encapsulated bacteria. Secondly, vaccines made solely of these bacterial capsular polysaccharides caused mice to produce the circulating antibodies that attacked only the outer capsules of the bacteria, and thus rendered the entire bacterium nonvirulent or harmless.

The work Casper and Schiemann had performed on mice was repeated by Drs. Thomas Francis, Jr., Walter S. Tillet, and Lloyd D. Felton, using volunteers at Rockefeller Institute. Each discovered that injections of purified pneumococcal capsular polysaccharides of various strains of the bacteria found in pneumonia patients caused human volunteers to produce antibodies against the capsules of these specific strains. By 1935 when Casper arrived in New York as a refugee, Felton was in the third year of what was to become a seven-year trial of pneumococcal capsular polysaccharide vaccines in 120,000 men of the Depression-inspired Civilian Conservation Corps (CCC) in California and New England.

In 1929, when Casper's earlier work on a chemical vaccine against pneumococcal pneumonia in mice attracted Avery's offer, Casper had developed a similar vaccine against another encapsulated bacteria, *Neisseria gonorrhoeae*, the germ of gonorrhea. Unlike pneumococcal pneumonia, which can occur in most animals, gonorrhea strikes only one species—the human race. Casper had made his vaccine from polysaccharides removed from the outer capsules of fresh cultures of gonococci, purified chemically and then combined with distilled water. By 1930 he was ready to test this gonorrhea vaccine in ten men and one woman.

At the bottom of the world economic depression, the woman—a prostitute being treated in his ward for gonorrhea—and the ten jobless and homeless men in the gonorrhea vaccine experiment had been grateful for the chance it gave them to obtain free room, shelter, baths, toilets, good meals, and other hospital amenities during the weeks it took to complete Casper's first clinical trial of his gonorrhea vaccine. Until he tested it in these poor Berliners, Casper had had no way of knowing whether the capsular polysaccharide gonorrhea vaccine would protect people against gonorrhea as effectively as his earlier vaccine had protected mice against pneumococcal pneumonia. He did not even know for certain that it would not trigger violent allergic reactions in people; all he did know was that none of the many unsuccessful gonorrhea vaccines made of whole gonococci administered between 1909 and 1930 were ever reported to have caused allergic reactions. The young doctor was, however, dead sure of one thing: Since the new capsular polysaccharide vaccine was not made from whole gonorrhea organisms, or from their toxins, there was no possibility that it would cause the venereal disease it was intended to prevent.

The Casper vaccine seemed to work very well. Five of the male volunteers were inoculated with it, the other five men were not. All ten had intercourse with the gonorrheic prostitute. Four of the uninoculated men caught gonorrhea from the infected prostitute; the five inoculated men did not.

This was all very gratifying, but Casper knew that ten homeless men and one willing prostitute hardly constituted a sample population large enough really to prove anything other than that a vaccine which seems to work well in this tiny population was worth further clinical investigation.

To put this new vaccine to mass trials, it would have been necessary first to produce huge amounts of the polysaccharides Casper had isolated from the gonococci. Then and now, the only institutions with the production and engineering resources to do such jobs were the giant pharmaceutical companies. Casper took out a German patent on his vaccine, and then turned to the industry to extract and purify the polysaccharides from the gonococci in the medically required quantities. The galloping course of the world economic crisis had discouraged first Schering and then I. G. Farben—the companies to which Casper had assigned his patent for the gonorrhea vaccine—from risking the considerable costs of proving the worth or worthlessness of the vaccine.

The same economic crisis also brought Hitler to power in Germany, and speeded Casper's flight to America. If there were no jobs or funding for gonorrhea vaccine researchers in Depression-poor America, a paying job at Bellevue was still better than imprisonment and the gas chambers in the concentration camps that then awaited Jewish doctors in his native land. Frustration was more endurable than deportation to Auschwitz. If he could not actually do any work on his gonorrhea vaccine, Casper was at least living among peers who knew his worth. These were people like Thomas Francis, Jr., then chairman of microbiology at the New York University medical school, who invited Casper to teach his students about the pneumococci, and the organic chemist Michael Heidelberger, then at the Columbia University College of Physicians and Surgeons (P and S). Heidelberger in 1923 had originally demonstrated that what Avery in 1917 had termed the specific soluble substances (SSS) found in the capsules of pneumococci were chemically polysaccharides—and, in the process, had helped found the new science of immunochemistry. There was also the Surgeon General of the United States, Dr. Thomas M. Parran, who was very familiar with Casper's published work and sought the younger man out. Parran had asked many questions about Casper's work on a vaccine against gonorrhea, and promised to see if he could get the Public Health Service to sponsor the resumption of his work.

Parran kept his promise—but his request for funds was denied. Once America got into World War II, however, things seemed to change. Parran sent for Casper (by then an American citizen), told him that the time to resume his work on the gonorrhea vaccine had at last arrived, and arranged for his commission as a surgeon in the Public Health Service, a rank equivalent to major in the military service. Until arrangements could be made for a laboratory and research staff, Casper was assigned to the venereal disease division of the Service.

Wars make their own conditions, and their own medical priorities. At the outbreak of World War II in 1939, only one systemic antibacterial drug, sulfanilamide, was available to treat all fighting men. Since the ultimate function of war is the death of enemy servicemen and/or their families at home, the primary function of military medicine is to keep the soldiers and sailors who kill the enemy forces in their best fighting trim. Microbial infections in war wounds, and in human respiratory systems plagued by the contagions that hit overcrowded, undernourished, and excessively stressed troops, traditionally had always claimed as many or even more lives as had enemy weapons. In World War II, this was to change dramatically.

Seven years before the war, during Christmas week of 1932, at the medical division of the I. G. Farben drug cartel in Germany, Professor Gerhard Domagk had performed a very fruitful experiment in twenty-eight mice. All of these mice had been inoculated with live cultures of strains of streptococci lethal to mice. Half of the inoculated mice had also been injected with doses of a red dye called Prontosil. All the animals injected with the lethal bacteria plus the Prontosil lived; all the non-Prontosil-treated mice died of disseminated streptococcal infections.

For the next three years, Domagk and his collaborators tested Prontosil in people suffering from normally fatal infections caused by a variety of streptococci and other disease-causing bacteria. In nearly each clinical trial, Prontosil proved to be an effective, nontoxic, and often life-saving drug. The German workers did not know what it was in Prontosil that gave it its antibacterial functions, but they did know that it was safe and very effective; and by 1937 Prontosil was being used in Europe and America with near miraculous results against bacterial diseases for which no systemic drugs had ever existed before. In 1935 at the Pasteur Institute, a group of French scientists headed by the husband-and-wife team of Jacques and Thérèse Tréfouel showed that the antibacterial activity of the red dye came from the sulfanilamide portion of its molecule.

Like Paul Ehrlich's postulated Magic Bullets the new sulfa drugs—whether injected, or swallowed as tablets, or applied to open wounds in powdered form—swiftly spared sick and injured soldiers on both sides in World War II from what earlier would have been death from one or more of the common infectious diseases long endemic among all combat troops even before Alexander the Great. At the start of World War II, the sulfa drugs were particularly effective against the gonococci that cause gonorrhea, the spirochetes that induce syphilis, and the other venereal bacterial infections that increase exponentially in every war.

In a short time, the new sulfa drugs wiped out virtually all of the strains of sulfa-sensitive gonococci present in many localities. This left whole military posts and regiments at the mercy of those specific strains of gonococci that had always been naturally or innately resistant to the new systemic sulfa drugs. Since that time, people have mistakenly said that all strains of gonococci had "developed resistance" to the sulfas. In effect, however, since the hereditarily drug-resistant strains of gonococci were all that survived the introduction of the sulfa drugs, the sulfas became useless against gonorrhea.

At that point, penicillin came into the picture. Discovered by Dr. Alexander Fleming in 1929 in London, it was then developed at Oxford by the Autralian-born pathologist Howard Florey and the German-Jewish refugee biochemist Ernst Boris Chain. Unlike the sulfas, which inhibited the growth of bacteria by destroying their capacity to synthesize the essential vitamin folic acid, the penicillins killed germs outright. Penicillin, a compound chemically derived from the common mold *Penicillium notatum,* was used for the first time to treat a human being in London in 1941. The patient was a policeman dying of bacterial septicemia (blood poisoning). The tiny amount of experimental penicillin available to treat him reversed the disease processes, and nearly saved his life before the doctors ran out of enough of the new antibiotic drug to keep him alive.

Shortly thereafter, a group of British scientists and officials went to the United States to enlist the aid of American science and industry in developing new techniques of extracting and mass-producing penicillin, primarily for British armed forces. By 1943, when astonishingly large quantities of penicillin started to pour out of the newly built American facilities, America was also in the war.

Medically, the new antibiotic era born in times of world carnage was about to make postwar life in affluent countries safer, longer, and healthier than it had ever been. Like the sulfa drugs, the first antibiotic, penicillin, was extremely effective against venereally or sexually transmitted bacterial infections.

Throughout history, wars have always caused prostitution to proliferate. An increase in prostitution always causes massive new waves of venereal diseases. In World War II as these diseases became epidemic, the first medical priority became the treatment of members of the armed forces and the defense industries. It was at this time that Casper, as a U.S. Public Health Service medical officer, was put to work treating servicemen and service-linked civilians with venereal diseases.

Casper was kept too busy to do any further research on a vaccine against gonorrhea. By June 1944, when Casper was named chief of the gonorrhea section of the Public Health Service's venereal disease control program in Chicago, his orders from the Service made it very clear that once the clinical and educational requirements of his job were met, "research studies on gonorrhea" ranked sixth and last in the order of importance of all of his duties.[4]

As 1944 neared its close, and military victory seemed at hand, gonorrhea infections acquired overseas by hundreds of thousands of American servicemen threatened to cause outbreaks among civilians all over the country. The Public Health Service started to make itself ready to cope with the clinical and social problems of venereal diseases after the war.

By the time Parran's summons to the National Postwar Venereal Disease Control Conference in St. Louis reached Casper, he had all but abandoned his hopes of ever again being able to work on his gonorrhea vaccine. In a pessimistic letter to Professor P. S. Palouze, a urologist at the University of Pennsylvania, on March 30, 1944, Casper declared that while he still believed that "gonorrhea is a preventable disease," he was disheartened by lack of interest in his claim. He cited research which supported his belief that chemicals found on or around the cell walls of the bacteria of gonorrhea could, indeed, cause immunity to gonorrhea. He was also skeptical of the ability of penicillin and other antibiotics to eradicate the problems inherent in gonorrhea, writing, "I have never given up hope that one of these days urologists would recognize that the faster we treat gonorrhea, the faster we could get back the newly infected. Even the therapeutic results with penicillin will make no exception."

Eight months after writing this letter, Casper stood before the doctors assembled for the most important venereal disease conference of the war era, about to present his plans for making and mass testing a bacterial capsular polysaccharide vaccine against gonorrhea.

No sooner did he start to speak, however, than he was interrupted by the chief of the venereal diseases section of the Public Health Service, Dr. J. R. (Rod) Heller.

"Save your breath, Doctor," Heller said. This was not a time for blue-sky propositions, he explained. This was a very serious working conference of very busy doctors who would still be in public health when the war ended. The sulfas and the newest wonder drug, penicillin, now made only for the armed services could cure any case of gonorrhea with ease. After the war the wonder drugs would be made in vast quantities for civilians as well. Heller then turned prophet. "Once this war ends, Dr. Casper, you'll never see another gonococcus again for as long as you live."

"The gonococci," Casper retorted, "are smarter than you are!" Midway through this statement, Casper knew he had committed a gross strategic blunder: Heller had two stripes more on his uniform sleeve than he did. He knew he should stop right there, but he could not resist adding, "The gonococci will outlive both of us, Doctor."

Casper was not terribly surprised after this to be reassigned from Chicago to a gonorrhea treatment center in Jackson, Mississippi, where he worked for the duration of the war.

Frustrated, but far from disheartened, Wolfgang Casper was worldly enough to understand that when in uniform, to speak in haste is to repent in Jackson, Mississippi. He bore this self-inflicted exile in good spirits because by that time various developments in preventive medicine had given him hope about the chances of resuming his work on gonorrhea vaccines when peace came. The Public Health Service and the armed forces medical sections had now had good—even dramatic—experiences with at least two prototype bacterial capsular polysaccharide vaccines.

In 1927 in a Berlin medical journal, Casper and Oscar Schiemann had published their findings that, at least in mice, the polysaccharides of which the slimy outer capsules of the virulent strains of pneumococci are composed are complete antigens. (Most medically diagnosed bacterial pneumonias are caused by the virulent strains of encapsulated pneumococci.) Antigens are able to program the inborn immune defense systems in mammals to start producing specific antibodies or protein antagonists to themselves.

By 1916 Drs. Oswald T. Avery and Alphonse Dochez had demonstrated that specific substances present in the slimy outer capsules contributed to the virulence of encapsulated strains of pneumococci, while nonencapsulated strains of pneumococci caused no disease in people. In 1923, working in Avery's laboratory, Michael Heidelberger had shown that these capsular constituents were polysaccharides, not proteins, as had been believed.

In their 1927 research Casper and Schiemann had shown that these capsular carbohydrates could not only function as specific antigens, but also vaccines made from these purified pneumococcal capsular polysaccharides rendered mice immune to infection from the same strains of pneumococci from which the vaccine polysaccharides had been taken. Until then, biologists believed that only proteins could be antigens.

What makes the capsules of pneumococci and other encapsulated bacteria promoters of virulence is that they are, in nature, the disease germs' barriers against one of the major primary inborn host or immune defense mechanisms—phagocytosis. This is the process by which our bodies are cleared of invading pneumococci and other disease agents by phagocytes—the large array of white blood cells or leukocytes that act as guard or scavenger cells, which engulf and digest bacterial cells, dead tissues, and foreign particles. The antiphagocytic function of the pneumococcal and other bacterial outer capsules, which inhibits or prevents their destruction by the circulating phagocytes, is neutralized by attacks of antibodies specific to the capsules themselves. Once these specific antibodies attack and neutralize the bacterial capsules, the phagocytes circulating in the bloodstream engulf and (usually) destroy the bacteria formerly protected by their antiphagocytic capsules.

Unlike the virulent whole pneumococci they surround, the polysaccharide capsules themselves are incapable of causing pneumonia in people. Vaccines made of the purified polysaccharides of pneumococcal capsules act only against the capsules of virulent pneumonia bacteria, and render them subject to subsequent attack and destruction by the human body's own phagocytes. Casper's experimental mouse pneumonia vaccine of 1927 had opened the way to the development of an entirely new class of human vaccines made from noninfective cell-surface chemicals. In 1944 recurring epidemics of pneumococcal pneumonia in an army air force training base at Sioux Falls, South Dakota, led the army medical branch to ask Michael Heidelberger and various associates to make up a vaccine with the capsular polysaccharides of the principal causes of these epidemics, pneumococci Types I, II, V, and VII. This was done and the vaccine tested in 17,000 airmen at the base, with half of them being vaccinated and the others acting as controls.

The four-antigen vaccine, prepared by the pharmaceutical firm of E. R. Squibb and Sons, Inc., for the army trials, yielded three interesting results.

"Within two weeks, there were [1.] no more pneumonias caused by the four Types [of pneumococci in the vaccine] among those vaccinated," Michael Heidelberger wrote in an autobiographical memoir three decades later, when he was ninety-one and still active in his laboratory at New York University, "[2.] Even the nonvaccinated were partially protected because, as the microbiologists found, the vaccinated personnel no longer carried these pneumococci [Types I, II, V, VII] in their noses and throats. [3.] Pneumonias due to pneumococcal Types not in the vaccine remained equal in both groups, which showed the strict specificity of the protection."[5]

During the first two weeks after vaccination, pneumonias caused by pneumococci Types I, II, V, and VII had developed in four of the immunized airmen and in four of the nonimmunized controls. After that, no pneumonias due to any of these four types developed in the immunized men, while a total of twenty-three more pneumonias caused by the four types developed in the nonimmunized controls.

"The entire study, so beautifully organized and monitored under [Dr.] Colin M. MacLeod's direction, showed that epidemics of pneumococcal pneumonia in closed populations could be terminated within two weeks after vaccination with the polysaccharides of the causative types," Heidelberger wrote. The trials also showed that minute amounts of antibody triggered by the vaccine "could prevent the droplet infection by a few pneumococci that presumably initiate the disease."[6] Droplet infections are diseases caused by the few bacteria or viruses transmitted to healthy people in the sneezes or breath exhalations of infected individuals.

What encouraged Casper most about this entire triumph in mass immunization by safe, nontoxic bacterial capsular polysaccharide vaccines was not so much the clinical results—which he had anticipated—but the fact that E. R. Squibb had manufactured the thousands of doses of the four-antigen vaccine Dr. MacLeod had required for the South Dakota trials. By 1945, even before the war ended, it was common knowledge that Squibb had poured millions of dollars into building and staffing new plants to manufacture capsular polysaccharide vaccines against bacterial pneumonia, then the fifth leading cause of death in the United States. To Casper this was convincing proof that the era of the new bacterial chemical vaccines would begin in earnest with the coming of peace: Giant corporations, he knew, never gamble on risky products.

After he was demobilized and had returned to New York, Casper sought and failed to find a job in medical research. There were plenty of openings, many of them quite lucrative, for qualified dermatologists, and he did not lack for offers. There were simply no jobs open for anyone who wanted to do less-well-paid research on a vaccine against gonorrhea. Worse, most directors of university and corporate research institutions felt that the sulfas and the penicillins had made vaccines to prevent venereal diseases redundant; there was no need to spend millions on an as yet unproven vaccine against gonorrhea when the disease could be cured by a few dollars' worth of penicillin.

In January 1946 Michael Heidelberger sent Casper a reprint of an article he and MacLeod had written on the vaccine used in South Dakota. "I was sure," Heidelberger told Casper, "that you would be interested in the polysaccharide work, as you certainly 'started something' years ago. I have had no experience with gonococcus carbohydrates, but if you have a method of preparing active ones, possibly T. D. Gerlough of E. R. Squibb and Sons Biological Laboratories, New Brunswick, New Jersey, would be interested in your evidence and in extending it." Heidelberger had been one of the people Squibb consulted when they went into the pneumonia vaccine business. Now they had two capsular polysaccharide vaccines on the market, both of them six-antigen types, one for adults and the other for children.

Casper immediately phoned Squibb in New Brunswick and was invited to visit by Gerlough. He was grateful that at least one pharmaceutical company was not acting as if it believed that the new antibiotics had resolved all the problems of infectious diseases. Yes, the antibiotics could cure syphilis and gonorrhea, but gonorrhea, unlike smallpox and syphilis, was one of the many infectious diseases that did not confer immunity against themselves on their victims. Cure was fine, but prevention was better, and Squibb, thank God, understood this elementary fact of health and disease.

Gerlough acquainted Casper with a few elementary facts of economic life. The entire medical community, he told Casper, was by then so certain that the new antibiotics would soon wipe out all major bacterial diseases that Squibb could not even give their pneumonia vaccines away. There simply was no market for them, and it was only a matter of months before the corporation would decide to close down the entire vaccine operation. Unfortunately, sales resistance to the capsular polysaccharide pneumonia vaccines meant that nobody at Squibb would entertain even a modest proposal for research on a polysaccharide vaccine against gonorrhea.

At the age of forty-five, Casper found himself forced out of research, and he settled down to a practice in dermatology and cosmetic surgery in Staten Island, New York. In the years that followed, Casper's one remaining link to gonorrhea research was to show up at different medical congresses and present impassioned pleas for the resumption of active research on the capsular polysaccharides of the gonococci and their use in vaccines against gonorrhea. "For the next 33 years," he later recalled, "I became a kind of Don Quixote, tilting lances against windmills we call government and industry and university research. It was worse than shouting in the wind. Here and in Europe, whenever I was invited to a scientific congress I told everyone who would listen what I told Palouze in 1944: Fast cures with penicillin would only result in even faster jumps in the total numbers of new and repeated cases of gonorrhea. Nobody listened. Nothing happened." Then an impish grin danced over his alert face. "Correction, please. One good thing happened. After the war Rod Heller used to attend many of the same meetings. And every time we met, I'd always say the same thing to him. 'Doctor,' I'd say, 'in your lifetime you're always going to see more and more gonococci—and more people with gonorrhea.' I was right, you know. Just look at the statistics."

History was not long in bearing out Casper's predictions. In 1945, 287,181 Americans were reported to the health agencies as having had primary or repeated infections of gonorrhea, for a case rate of 155.8 per 100,000 population. By 1968 the number of reported cases of gonorrhea had climbed to 464,543, nearly double the 1945 total, for a case rate of 232.8 per 100,000 population. Ten years later in 1978, there were 1,013,436 reported cases of gonorrhea for the year, for a case rate of 468.3 per 100,000 population. Gonorrhea had climbed to first place among all reportable communicable diseases in the United States.

These figures, however, told at most only half the gonorrhea story. Although by law doctors are required to report to their local health departments all cases of gonorrhea which they treat, surveys made by the federal Centers for Disease Control (CDC) have shown that doctors in private practice report only about 15 percent of all the venereal diseases they encounter. Most of the cases reported to the health statistics agencies are treated by doctors in free hospitals and other institutional clinics. Federal health agencies estimate that the actual numbers of gonorrhea cases are at least twice as large as the total number of reported cases. In 1978 this added up to an estimate of one case of gonorrhea for every 108 Americans. The costs of treating gonorrhea and its complications are now estimated to run well over a billion dollars per year. Complications of gonorrhea in women make it the largest single cause of involuntary sterilization in the nation.

Far from having been eradicated by penicillin and other drugs as Dr. Heller predicted in St. Louis in 1944, new cases of gonorrhea today are reported every twelve seconds in the United States. Many nongovernmental venereal disease experts believe that these reported cases represent only one in every three or four actual gonococcal infections. We not only have more cases of gonorrhea than we ever had before, but it appears so frequently in sites other than the sexual organs that Dr. Richard B. Roberts, chief of the infectious disease section of the Cornell University Medical Center in New York City, recently warned doctors that in all cases of sore throat and tonsillitis in people of the most sexually active age, nose and throat smears should routinely be cultured for the presence of gonorrhea.

As with gonorrhea, so with many other bacterial infections in varying degrees since 1945. It is not that the hopes that antibiotics would be wonder drugs which would wipe out all major infectious diseases caused by bacteria have all been totally unrealized. Consider, for example, what has happened in this country since 1900. In that year the leading cause of death was pneumonia/influenza, then responsible for 11.8 percent of deaths from all causes. Of the next nine leading causes, five were bacterial diseases: Tuberculosis, diarrhea and enteritis, chronic (generally poststreptococcal) nephritis, certain respiratory and infectious diseases of early infancy, and diphtheria ranked, respectively, second, third, sixth, ninth, and tenth. As of 1980, only one of these—pneumonia/influenza—was still on the list. In 1900 when pneumonia/influenza ranked first, it killed 202 out of every 100,000 Americans. In 1978 when pneumonia/influenza was the fifth leading cause of death, it killed 20 in every 100,000 Americans, for a total of 62,000 deaths a year. This was three decades into the antibiotic era.

Until the advent of the sulfa drugs during World War II, individual medical care played a palpable but at best a minor role in the reduction of both the incidence of and the death rates from infectious diseases. Public health measures devised and implemented by or at the urging of epidemiologists and other physicians—clean water and sewage disposal systems; enforced laws and regulations governing the control of health hazards in homes and workplaces; enforced local and federal laws dealing with the cleanliness and safety of foods, drugs, and cosmetics in daily use; and, above all, rising family incomes, which resulted in better family nutrition, housing, clothing, medical and dental care, and education, were all responsible for most reductions in the numbers of and deaths from infectious diseases for roughly the first half of this century.

After 1945 antibacterial drugs played an increasingly important role in the control of and reduction of death tolls from infectious diseases caused by bacteria and other microbial organisms. Thus, where deaths from tuberculosis declined from a rate of 194 per 100,000 in 1900 to 46 per 100,000 in 1940, after the war they declined from a rate of 40 per 100,000 in 1945 to only 1.5 deaths per 100,000 in 1978. This drop in tuberculosis deaths came at a time, around 1963, when standards of living were starting to deteriorate owing to the inflation triggered by the costly Vietnam War and later exacerbated by the Arab oil boycott of 1973 and the subsequent permanently escalating fuel prices. The poor, whose health benefited most from the slow rise in real family incomes during the first half of the century, were the first to be hit, and the most traumatized, by the raging inflation that by 1978 had cut the purchasing power of the American dollar to considerably less than half of what it was exactly twenty years earlier in 1958—from one dollar to forty-four cents in two decades. Since tuberculosis is essentially a disease of urban poverty, this also suggests that the postwar antituberculosis drugs from streptomycin to isoniazid and rifampin had considerably more to do with the shrinking death rate from tuberculosis in our inflation-raped times than any improvements in the living conditions of the people at highest risk of contracting tuberculosis.

The same observations hold true of other declines in infectious disease deaths due to other bacteria since 1900. Millions of people who might have died of these diseases but for the availability of the sulfas and antibiotics are living testimony to the realization of a significant portion of the perceived early promise of the wonder drugs. However, scores of major bacterial diseases that both physicians and lay biologists expected to see eradicated by the antibiotic drugs are still very much with us; still crippling, still blinding, still deafening, still killing our children and ourselves.

In 1976, more than forty-five years after Fleming first described the antibacterial activities of penicillin, the United States government reported that "infections are the single largest group of diseases responsible for illness, represent the most frequent problem requiring professional attention and account for a large proportion of the cost of medical care. Approximately 20% of those visits are for treatment of respiratory difficulties or for kidney or bladder disease."[7]

Two years later, the National Institute of Health, which issued this report, sponsored a high-level national symposium on the impact of infections on medical care in the United States. At this symposium, Dr. Henry E. Simmons, the former deputy assistant secretary of the Department of Health, Education, and Welfare, told his medical peers what most had previously discovered for themselves: "Our problems in infectious diseases get bigger, more expensive, and more hazardous. We are at the point where thoughtful observers are not questioning whether we are in the post-infectious-disease era, but whether on balance society is much better off than we were forty years ago, despite our hundreds of new antibiotics, hundreds of millions of prescriptions, and billions of dollars of expense. In view of all the evidence, a positive answer to this question can no longer be given with confidence; it is a legitimate question."[8]

At the same meeting, Dr. John V. Bennett, of the federal Centers for Disease Control (CDC), reminded everyone that "infections [including pneumonia/influenza] and their sequelae [consequences] accounted for 123,000 deaths annually in the United States, and were the fourth commonest cause of all deaths in 1976." In short, when all reported deaths from infectious diseases are lumped into a single category, they prove to be more numerous than reported deaths from all accidents (including traffic accidents), diabetes, arteriosclerosis, and chronic obstructive pulmonary diseases like bronchitis, emphysema, and bronchiectasis. Only heart diseases, cancers, and strokes kill more Americans than infectious diseases.

The Bennnett study went beyond the death-certificate data reported to the health agencies. It has long been known that the actual numbers of notifiable infectious diseases suffered in this country actually represent only 10 percent to 20 percent of the officially reported totals. When the CDC experts converged on defined populations, such as the city of Washington, D.C., and employed more sensitive and sophisticated methods to estimate the "true incidence" of all infectious diseases, they emerged with solid evidence for estimating the total United States deaths from all infectious diseases at 311,000 annually. Of these deaths, according to Dr. Bennett, "bacterial and mycobacterial diseases and their sequelae accounted for about 86% of the total 311,000 annual deaths estimated by these methods."[9]

The currently fashionable controversies about the overuses of antibiotics, and about the relative insignificance of medical as against environmental contributions (i.e., high family incomes, which make possible better nutrition, housing, clothing, and education; and improved evironmental hygiene, from clean drinking water and sanitary sewage systems to enforced job safety laws) to the decline in gross United States death rates since 1900, take on a new dimension in the face of the approximately 311,000 reported and unreported deaths suffered from infectious diseases annually.

Today there are effective antibiotics for just about every bacterial disease. And as Dr. Stephen B. Thacker of the CDC observes, "Appropriate antibiotics are not being used by a significant segment of the population who are dying from these infectious diseases."[10] Nor for that matter is adequate use being made of the available vaccines against bacterial and viral infectious diseases.

The basic reason for this underuse and nonuse of antibiotics (and vaccines) is not medical but economic. Nearly 17 percent of the United States population lives on incomes below 125 percent of the official poverty line of $7,500 for a family of four. This adds up to 35.7 million people, 24.5 million of them white, 11 million nonwhite.[11] Combine these people with the seven million nonpoverty families with incomes between $7,500 and $10,000 who, after decades of constantly worsening inflation, no longer can afford private medical care—and who refuse to seek what they regard as "charity medicine" under Medicaid and other government programs—and you describe more than forty million Americans who cannot afford good medical care. Many of them, when gravely ill, go to free clinics; too many do not.

It is true, of course, that many of the more affluent people overdose themselves with antibiotics, often contrary to their doctors' instructions. It is also true that the environment of poverty and inflation incubates more infectious diseases than the ambience of affluence. It is painfully true, however, that for want of adequate treatment with appropriate antibiotics, and prophylaxis (prevention of infection) with available vaccines, around a quarter of a million Americans die each year of eminently curable and/or in many instances vaccine-preventable infectious diseases.

Deaths from bacterial and viral infections, serious as they are, are probably not the most damaging effects of our common and ubiquitous infectious diseases. The majority of nonusers and underusers of antibiotics and vaccines do not all die when they contract infectious disease. Millions do, however, suffer from overt to subclinical side effects—sequelae—of common infectious diseases.

These diseases include the common colds that invariably precede more serious streptococcal infections of the throat, which can then progress to rheumatic fever, ear, kidney and heart infections, and lifetime invalidism. They include childhood diseases for which good vaccines exist but which, in unvaccinated fetuses and children, can cause diphtheria, tetanus, whooping cough, polio, measles, rubella (German measles), and mumps. Each of these diseases is able to cause one or more lifetime defects—ranging from crippling and mental retardation to blindness, deafness, cerebral palsy, epilepsy or other seizures, diabetes, stunted limbs and bodies, and damaged hearts—and is responsible for a nearly endless array of causes of lifetime invalidism, reduced capacities to learn and earn, and dependency. Scores of killing and crippling bacterial and virus diseases for which no vaccines as yet exist—such as those ailments that fall in the reporting category of "streptococcal sore throat and scarlet fever," which are no longer legally notifiable, but which in 1979 were voluntarily reported by doctors in 465,430 cases in forty-one states.[12]

These diseases include bacterial meningitis, which strikes hardest at infants and children under two years old. Antibiotics can cure bacterial meningitis, but none of the available new vaccines against it are effective in children under two. Until we had antibiotics, bacterial meningitis was a major cause of death in children. Today most children with bacterial meningitis are kept alive with antibiotics, but at most only about half of them escape some of the residual effects of this infection—which today is the leading cause of acquired mental retardation.

A recent study made at Vanderbilt University School of Medicine in Nashville, Tennessee, by Dr. Sarah W. Sell and collaborators looked into the long-term effects of *Haemophilus influenzae Type b* bacterial meningitis in eighty-six children who were treated with acceptable antibiotic therapy during an acute episode that lasted from 1950 to 1964 in Nashville. What makes the findings of this study so sobering is that they are paralleled almost exactly by those of other clinical investigations of the sequelae of properly treated cases of *H. influenzae Type b* meningitis in other American and European cities. Dr. Sell and her group found that of these eighty-six children with bacterial meningitis, eleven (13 percent) were dead; twenty-six (29 percent) of the living survivors had severe handicaps; twelve (14 pecent) had possible residual damages; and thirty-seven (43 percent) were free of detectable handicaps.

The defects found in the Nashville survivors included mental retardation responsible for IQ test scores of 50 to 69; seizures requiring medication; hearing loss; partial blindness; speech and behavioral difficulties; temper tantrums; and spastic hemiplegia, or paralysis of one side of the body.

Dr. Sell and her coworkers reported, "Antibiotic therapy, while greatly reducing mortality, has not reduced the incidence of *H. influenzae* meningitis which, in fact, is reported to be on the increase in several centers in the U.S." The Nashville doctors concluded that "prevention rather than cure should now be a prime goal for the future."[13]

That future is now, according to a growing number of extremely able, and mainly young, doctors, medical microbiologists, immunochemists, microbial geneticists, experimental pathologists, and workers in other scientific disciplines now working around the world on the problems of infections and their prevention.

The old dream, nearly two centuries old by now, of preventing all infectious diseases by vaccination, rather than merely curing them, was all but killed by the historic post-World War II impact of the sulfas and antibiotics on nearly every bacterial and mycobacterial disease known to humankind. The revival of this dream is fairly recent, and when its official history is written, I am fairly sure that two events will be given primary credit for its revival.

The first event was the arrival in 1952 of a thirty-six-year-old Johns Hopkins-trained specialist in infectious diseases, Dr. Robert Austrian, at the Downstate Medical Center in Brooklyn, New York, to take up his teaching and clinical duties as an associate professor of medicine at the New York State University College of Medicine and as visiting physician at the adjacent Kings County Hospital. What Austrian saw on the wards convinced him that despite antibiotics, large numbers of people still died of pneumococcal pneumonia.

As stubborn as he was brilliant, Austrian started a long uphill fight first to get his fellow doctors at Kings County and elsewhere even to agree that pneumococcal pneumonia still existed, let along had survived into the antibiotic era. After 1963 Austrian's analysis of the experience with pneumococcal pneumonia in Brooklyn suggested what was needed, and he then set out to convince the federal health agencies that fund medical research to support new research on the redevelopment of pneumococcal capsular polysaccharide vaccines against bacterial pneumonia. That he succeeded in this initially lonely effort has put the world forever in debt to Robert Austrian.

The second event that helped stimulate the revival of the efforts to develop new vaccines against ancient bacterial and virus diseases was the emergence—in *Neisseria meningitidis,* the bacterium that causes meningococcal meningitis—of more and more strains that were genetically resistant to the sulfa drugs. For more than two decades after World War II, the American armed services had routinely used sulfa pills to protect new recruits and other servicemen at risk against meningococcal meningitis. By the mid-1960s, it became increasingly evident that the sulfa drugs could no longer be used to protect crowded training camps against outbreaks of the disease.

To find alternative ways of protection, the army set up a new unit at the Walter Reed Army Institute of Research, in Washington, D.C. This research unit was headed by a career military doctor, Major Malcolm S. Artenstein, a specialist in infectious diseases. At that time the army was still able to call up draft-eligible young researchers, and Artenstein knew just whom he needed. In short order, a recent graduate of the New York University (NYU) medical school, Dr. Emil Gotschlich, was drafted. Along with other young doctors in brand-new military uniforms, including Irving Goldschneider, Ronald Gold, Dennis Casper, John Swanson, and others, the Gotschlich group soon picked up where twenty years earlier Dr. Elvin A. Kabat of the Columbia University College of Physicians and Surgeons had abandoned his quest for a bacterial capsular polysaccharide vaccine against meningococcal meningitis—admittedly because of the resounding early successes of the antibiotics. In 1966 these young "draft-induced" researchers set out to produce and then standardize the polysaccharides present in the capsules of *N. meningitidis.* By July 1967 they had a vaccine which was injected into a handful of volunteers. By 1968 hundreds of volunteers had been injected with the new polysaccharide vaccine which produced antibodies in humans against meningococcal meningitis.

After mass trials of the new vaccine in army recruits in 1973, and in children in 1974, in 1975 the entire population of Finland—then over four million people—was immunized against group A meningococcus with one of the two vaccines developed at Walter Reed. This mass immunization was credited with preventing an epidemic. During that same year, a combined Group A and Group C meningococcal vaccine was used to immunize the entire population of Brazil, and to prevent an otherwise very probable epidemic in that nation's more than one hundred million people. Since 1971 all U.S. Army recruits have been routinely immunized with the polysaccharide vaccine against Group C meningococcal meningitis.

Obviously this revival of hopes for new vaccines also owes much to the accumulation of twentieth-century knowledge that lay dormant during the decades when many doctors and health professionals were certain that antibiotics were going to eradicate infectious diseases all by themselves. This knowledge included (1) all that Avery had learned, starting in 1913, about the role played by the specific soluble substances (SSS) in the capsules of pneumococci in the virulence of the germs of pneumonia; (2) the knowledge, published by Heidelberger and Avery in 1923 that the SSS factors that spelled greater virulence for pneumonia patients were polysaccharides; and (3) the detailed accounts published by Casper and Schiemann, starting in 1927, of how they used Heidelberger's method of extracting these polysaccharides and then used them to protect mice against pneumococcal pneumonia with vaccines made of these selfsame bacterial capsular polysaccharides.

There was a third bit of insight from the nineteenth century that had remained buried for nearly a hundred years. The father of modern microbiology, the chemist Louis Pasteur, suspected that the immune reaction in animals protected by specific bacterial vaccines was not necessarily related to the whole live organism, or attenuated live bacteria used in these vaccines, but might "be directed against certain of their constituents or products."

Pasteur had observed that in spinal cords of rabid animals that were used to make his rabies vaccine, "The heated cord which had become noninfectious was still effective as a chemical vaccine." Pasteur believed that "immunization might be due not to the living virus itself but to a nonliving substance which retained its immunizing power even after the virus had been killed by prolonged desiccation."[14]

On January 29, 1885, Pasteur informed the Académie Française in connection with its forthcoming *Dictionary*, that "I am inclined to believe that the causative virus of rabies may be accompanied by a substance which can impregnate the nervous system and render it thereby unsuitable for the growth of the virus. Hence rabies immunity. If this is the case, the theory might be a general one; it would be a stupendous discovery." It was—and it is.

Three years later, in the *Annals of the Pasteur Institute*, Pasteur wrote that "it will not be long before the chemical vaccine . . . of rabies is known and utilized."

The bacterial capsular polysaccharides—as well as other bacterial and viral constituents to be described in later chapters—are, like the nonliving substances in the rabies viruses postulated by Pasteur in 1885, the first among the groups of natural and synthetic chemicals of which the modern chemical vaccines are made.

Since young Wolfgang Casper made the first of these chemical vaccines in 1927, a veritable torrent of new information on the biology and chemistry of immunity has poured out of the world's laboratories. This vast and ever-growing body of solid scientific data has created a dream in the minds of some current researchers that could not possibly have occurred to Pasteur and Koch, Metchnikoff and Ehrlich, Cohn and Cohnheim, Pacini and Davaine, Villemin and Leeuwenhoek—the founders and precursors of modern microbiology and immunology. The dream of some modern investigators, simply stated, is the development of a single vaccine, made of immunologically active and interacting polysaccharides and other constituents of the cells of pathogenic bacteria, that will protect people against all of the common invasive bacteria.

Far-fetched as this "supervaccine" might sound, there are today far more scientific grounds for believing that this is an attainable goal in our era than there would have been in 1796, when a British country doctor named Edward Jenner developed his safe and effective vaccine against smallpox. Probably not even Jenner dreamed that this first modern immunizing agent against a killing and deforming contagious disease would in time be followed by other vaccines against many other diseases.

As a matter of fact, nearly a century was to pass before Jenner's vaccine against the smallpox virus was followed by Pasteur's rabies vaccine of 1884.

The dream of a single vaccine against all invasive bacterial organisms is possibly closer to being realized right now. It has already led, among other things, to the immunization of two entire nations, Brazil and Finland—over 130 million people—against meningococcal meningitis using safe, efficient, noninfective vaccines made from nonliving immunizing chemicals extracted from the cell surfaces of those meningitis bacteria. That these nationwide vaccinations were undertaken and carried out in the face of threatening epidemics they succeeded in preventing adds to the drama of the story. More exciting, however, is the pace at which talented and determined men and women are trying to make their dream of a supervaccine come true in our times.

While it is tempting to see this as happening soon, the entire history of vaccinations and their adequate and/or inadequate utilization since 1796 offers grounds for caution. Before we start cooling the champagne and ordering the gold medals, it might be well to remember that in the nearly two centuries since Jenner, and in the century since Pasteur, the world's microbiologists have given us less than a dozen safe and universally effective vaccines—those against diphtheria, whooping cough, tetanus, measles, polio, mumps, rubella, and yellow fever; one vaccine against pneumococcal pneumonia; two against meningococcal meningitis that work well in people over two years old, but fail to protect infants and younger children; two very promising sophisticated new vaccines against serum hepatitis and typhoid; a brace of fair to poor vaccines now in use against influenza, cholera, and typhoid; and one still highly controversial one against tuberculosis. The grand total of less than twenty good to not so good vaccines is, at least quantitatively, not much to rave about after two centuries of medical research.

Yet the same history that provides us with such cautionary markers is far from lacking in good evidence that one or more Pasteurian "chemical vaccines," each acting against large groups of common bacterial and viral diseases, are quite possibly not nearly as utopian as they sound. Given adequate and prudent support by intellectually mature and morally responsible governments, the world's younger and more adventuresome investigators now working on sophisticated new vaccines synthesized wholly of off-the-shelf chemicals might, in this century, well enable us to rid humankind of many of the most common killing, crippling, and mind-deforming infections and postinfection disorders to which we are all at lifelong risk.

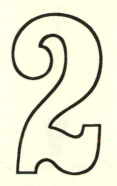

C H A P T E R

"SOMETHING CURIOUS IN THE MEDICAL LINE": AN ANIMAL DISTEMPER THAT PREVENTS SMALLPOX IN PEOPLE

It now becomes too manifest to admit of controversy that the anihilation of the Smallpox, the most dreadful scourge of the human species, must be the result of this practice [vaccination]

—EDWARD JENNER, M.D., in *The Origin of the Vaccine Inoculation,* London, 1801

... in the populous parts of the Metropolis, where the abundance of children exceeds the means of providing food and raiment for them, this pestilential disease, i.e. smallpox, is considered as a merciful provision on the part of Providence to lessen the burthen of a poor man's family.

—Mr. JOHN BIRCH, Surgeon to St. Thomas's Hospital, in *Serious Reasons for Uniformly Opposing Vaccination,* 2nd Ed., London, 1807

41

Vaccination, the prevention of infectious diseases with reasonably safe preparation made from whole live or killed microbial disease agents, or from chemical components of bacteria or viruses, or from toxins (poisons) produced by such microbial pathogens, as well as immunology—the medical science dealing with the various biological and chemical processes of resistance or the impairment of resistance to infectious agents and other foreign bodies and conditions—were both created in 1796 by a forty-seven-year-old general practitioner, Edward Jenner, in the English rural town of Berkeley, Gloucestershire.

The knowledge that certain contagious diseases, such as variola (from the Latin for spotted) or smallpox, confer on their survivors long-lasting or permanent immunity to reinfection with these select diseases—and that, at least in the instance of smallpox, such immunity could be transferred to healthy people by inoculations of biological matter from people suffering from smallpox—was well established in many parts of this planet for more than two millennia before Jenner was born.

Centuries prior to the Christian era, Chinese doctors regularly dried and pulverized the crusts of smallpox scabs and blew them into the noses of healthy patients through special bone inoculation tubes. In many but not all instances, these intranasal doses of smallpox-virus-laden materials induced mild cases that nevertheless immunized inoculated individuals against subsequent infections of the disease. The Chinese doctors also collected pus and lymph from the skin eruptions of people with active cases of smallpox, smeared these infectious materials inside children's nightshirts, and made the children sleep in the contaminated garments in quest of the same mild but immunizing cases of smallpox.

In Asia Minor, Asia, and Africa, people of various cultures swallowed smallpox scabs and/or had the crusts or lymphs implanted in their veins by skilled inoculators or variolators, who opened the veins with sharp needles. In Russia, where saunas or steam baths were followed by vigorous pounding massages with birch-twig brooms, smallpox pus or lymph was smeared over these brooms and pounded into the body through the steam-widened pores. In Africa, as in Greece and Turkey, variolation involved scratching smallpox lymphs into the skins of healthy people.

The witch-hunting Boston clergyman, Cotton Mather, learned of this technique from his African slave, Onesimos. When a ship in the West Indian trade imported enough cases of smallpox to cause a serious outbreak in Boston in 1721, the Reverend Mather induced the physician Zabdiel Boylston to try the African method of smallpox inoculation on two of his own African slaves, his six-year-old son, and thirty-five healthy Bostonians. This was the introduction of smallpox variolation to Colonial America, but smallpox cases and deaths caused by these inoculations forced Virginia and other colonies to outlaw such uses of live viruses.

During the American Revolution, smallpox decimated the rebel Colonial troops besieging Quebec, and was "the main cause of the preservation of Canada to the British Empire."[1] After General George Washington ordered the variolation of the entire Continental Army, this act of medical intervention played a major role in the ultimate victory of the Colonial forces, albeit at the high cost of one soldier killed by smallpox in every three hundred inoculated with lymphs bearing active smallpox viruses. Historically, variolation was only too often deadlier than the average smallpox infection.

In 1722, soon after Mather and Boylston introduced smallpox inoculations to Boston, Lady Mary Wortley Montagu, wife of the British Ambassador to Constantinople, succeeded in getting the royal family in London to variolate some of their grandchildren. Royal acceptance soon turned smallpox inoculations into procedures that were routinely administered to noble and upper-class families. Thus it came to pass that in 1757, when the wellborn eight-year-old Edward Jenner, son of the late Anglican rector of Berkeley, and brother of the new rector, the Reverend Stephen Jenner, Jr., was packed off to a school run by the Reverend Clissold at Wotton-under-Edge, he joined a group of affluent boarding-school boys being prepared for inoculation against smallpox.

This preparation, Jenner told his biographer, Barron, was a most unpleasant ordeal for children and adults alike. "There was," Jenner recalled, "bleeding till the blood was thin; purging till the body was wasted to a skeleton; and starving on a vegetable diet to keep it so."[2]

Decades later, Jenner could still recall, vividly, every moment of his own rites of body purification and variolation. "For six weeks I was bled and purged," he told Barron, "kept on a low diet, dosed with medicine, and was then removed to one of the so-called inoculation stables and haltered up with others in a terrible state of disease." These abuses were not among the famous cruelties practiced solely upon English boarding-school boys; the standard medical practice in those days was to put all candidates for smallpox inoculations through a course of intermittent bleedings, purges, and constant starvation to "purify" their blood prior to being inoculated with pustular matter from people with smallpox. It was not punishment for young Jenner and his schoolmates but, curiously, one of the privileges of wealth.

The inoculation stable to which Jenner and his peers were taken in

1757 was the barn of a local apothecary, a Mr. Holbrow. There, the apothecary himself performed the variolation operation by scratching the skin on the arms of each boy with a knife tip, and then bandaging the dried scabs of smallpox victims into these fresh scratches. After being inoculated with smallpox virus, young Edward and the other children were kept in the foul-smelling barn for the week or so required for the inoculations to take—that is, until they each developed a mild case of the disease, complete with high fevers and nausea associated as much with the stable environment as with their inoculation-induced smallpox.

During the next ten days or so, until the fevers subsided and the infected inoculation wound formed a scab, each of the boys was kept inside the stinking barn. Not until the scabs dried and fell off the boys' bodies by themselves were Jenner and his schoolmates allowed to leave that stable.

There were sound public health reasons, derived from decades of clinical experiences, for the by then established medical custom of isolating children and adults for weeks after they were inoculated with smallpox virus. Like most infections that are spread by close contact between infected and healthy people, smallpox is in large measure a disease of crowding. People inoculated with virus-bearing smallpox matter can transmit the smallpox viruses to healthy people during the entire time that their inoculation wounds are still raw and infective and their scabs have not yet formed, dried, and fallen away. When entire groups of young children were boarded with their inoculators until, during their own spell of artificially induced but generally mild infection, they could no longer pass the causal viruses on to nonimmune children and adults, this enforced isolation made their variolations less dangerous to their schools, families, and communities.

Similarly, when adult gentry could pass contagious postinoculation periods in splendid isolation on their country estates, or in the expensive private inoculation hospitals that sprang up in London and elsewhere, until they could no longer transmit smallpox to their peers, variolation was fairly safe. Fairly but not completely safe, because at times the inoculation-induced disease proved as severe as naturally acquired smallpox; and at other times the donors of the smallpox viruses also happened to be suffering from other concurrent infections, such as syphilis, hepatitis, and tuberculosis. In such cases, the microbial agents of the concurrent infections were transmitted to inoculated individuals along with the stuff that immunized them against smallpox. Purchasing protection from smallpox at the price of acquiring syphilis or tuberculosis was hardly a bargain worth seeking.

Even in the absence of such unwanted side infections 3 percent to 5 percent of all those variolated with live viruses developed fatal cases of smallpox. A somewhat greater number of inoculated patients developed "mild" cases of smallpox that were, nevertheless, severe enough to scar and blind them. At times, the outbreaks of severe smallpox infections caused by nonisolated people shortly after their own inoculations became so devastating that various communities, from the city of Paris in 1763 to the Crown Colony of Virginia on the eve of the American Revolution, passed and enforced laws that either flatly banned smallpox inoculations or mandated enforced isolation in smallpox hospitals or private institutions until inoculated people no longer menaced every nonimmune individual they encountered. After Jenner developed his infinitely safer cowpox vaccine against smallpox, most European countries were quick to outlaw smallpox inoculations. England waited until 1840 before ultimately banning them.

Except for a nasty fever, a lingering nausea, and harrowing memories that would haunt him for the rest of his days, Edward Jenner came through the experience of variolation against smallpox otherwise unharmed. As a country doctor in his native Berkeley, however, the adult Jenner was ever less than enthusiastic about variolation, and he was notorious among his professional peers for paying more attention than most other physicians to the folklore about smallpox never attacking milkmaids who had contracted the humanly benign disease of cowpox from the pustules on infected cows' udders. At one point, fellow members of the county medical society threatened to have Jenner expelled from its ranks unless he agreed to stop constantly bringing up the subject of cowpox and its possible uses in the prevention of smallpox.

Jenner was keenly aware that some countryfolk were said to follow the custom of deliberately acquiring cowpox from infected cows in order to protect themselves against the far less benign smallpox. Some farmers in Gloucestershire were known to have, like the cattle dealer Benjamin Jesty in 1774, used the lymph in cowpox pustules to inoculate themselves and their families. It is quite probable that Jenner, who had earlier made some false starts on an antismallpox inoculation based on a horse infection called grease, and another one on a disease of pigs called swine pox—with which he had inoculated his ten-month-old son and namesake in 1790—was aware of the local uses of cowpox virus as an immunizing agent against smallpox well before 1796.

As every bright English schoolchild knows, on May 14, 1796, at his private clinic in Berkeley, Jenner treated a Gloucestershire dairymaid, Sarah Nelmes, for cowpox. This disease, which causes fever and skin pustules similar to but less disseminated than those caused by smallpox, neither killed nor scarred nor blinded people who contracted it from infected cows. When people milked cows with one or more cowpox pustules or vesicles on their udders, and when the pustules broke and a few drops of the watery lymph inside these skin eruptions got into cracks or cuts in the skin of a milker's hands, then cowpox usually developed.

Once this happened, and the cowpox pustules turned into scabs and fell off the milkmaids' or dairymen's skins, the men and women who milked cows never again got cowpox. Nor, if rural farmers, milkmaids, apothecaries, doctors, naturalists, and mothers of many farm children could be believed, did any person who had ever had cowpox catch smallpox. Women who had recovered from cowpox were, as a matter of fact, in great demand as nurses for smallpox patients for just this reason.

Jenner, who had been a doctor for twenty-four of his forty-seven years, had heard these tales often enough, and had at least confirmed to his own satisfaction the fact that smallpox never seemed to develop in people who had ever had cowpox. Why, on this late spring day in 1796, Jenner chose to draw some lymph from Sarah Nelmes's cowpox pustules, and carefully set it aside before he applied a soothing unguent to the cowpox sores on her hands, was something he never made clear in any of his writings on his inoculation, which he named vaccination (from the Latin word *vaccinus,* "relating to cows,") in deference to its bovine source.

Later that day, since his own variolation had left him immune to smallpox and therefore unable to test the immunizing power of cowpox on himself, Jenner inoculated the cowpox lymph into a needle scratch on the arm of an eight-year-old boy named James Phipps. As the doctor fully expected, young Jamie developed a mild and very transient case of benign cowpox—in marked contrast to Jenner's own terrifying experiences in Holbrow's inoculation stable when he was Jamie's age.

Jamie had not had to be kept in Jenner's clinic, or otherwise isolated, during the period of his cowpox incubation and infection; it was, with good reason, considered a blessing in those times to be able to "catch the pox" from another person.

On July 1, after his cowpox vaccination took, young Phipps was inoculated by Jenner with matter taken from the pustules of a person with true smallpox. There was no reaction of any sort in the boy. A few weeks later, Jenner inoculated Jamie with a second dose of smallpox virus taken from another patient. Again the boy developed no infection of any sort. Clearly, cowpox virus had rendered eight-year-old Jamie Phipps immune to smallpox virus.

With this act, and with the various vaccinations Jenner soon performed on local people using lymphs taken from inoculation-induced cowpox pustules of other vaccinated individuals, Jenner produced more than the first safe immunizing agent against smallpox or any other infectious disease.

Jenner not only unwittingly started the science of immunology, but he also scored an historic precedent: In the act of immunizing James Phipps against the then and still medically untreatable disorder of smallpox, Jenner had become the first person in history to transform a clinical disease into a wholly social or societal disorder. That is, he turned smallpox into the first major disease to be made completely preventable by massive societal intervention whether or not—as was true of smallpox—the disease was caused in the first instance by biological rather than social or environmental factors.

That the development of the safe vaccine against smallpox did not lead to its nearly instant control and eradication in Jenner's native England, and in other nations in Europe and elsewhere, was not due to uncorrectable flaws in the vaccine. Rather, it was due to social causes and governmental decisions (or lack of them) beyond the influence of the country doctor who created the vaccine. Since these social causes included the changes that made possible the Industrial Revolution in which all subsequent patterns of living, health, and disease were to emerge in all industrial nations—including our own—we should now take a brief look at how smallpox came to Europe and America, and at what happened to smallpox in the land where the Industrial Revolution, and our own ways of life, were born.

Changing conditions have always altered the geography and the prevalence or endemicity of killing infectious diseases. Smallpox, for example, is a disease whose causal agent—the variola or smallpox virus—has only one host in nature: the human race. In the presence of people who are not immune to the smallpox virus, the infection flourishes. Without enough people to infect—and in whose infected cells millions of replicas of the viruses are synthesized and then passed on to other susceptible people—smallpox is eradicated.

Smallpox "spreads in a continuing chain of infection between a patient and a susceptible person," writes Dr. Donald K. Henderson. "Usually, the patient does not infect more than two to five additional persons. Smallpox, when introduced to a remote village, for example, will die out after a few generations of disease, even if nothing is done. This may also occur over extensive, sparsely populated areas."[3]

Although smallpox was an ancient scourge of humankind in China, India, and Africa before the birth of Christ, there are only a few scattered and clinically undocumented accounts of what might have indeed been outbreaks in Greece, Rome, and other sites in continental Europe, as well as in Ireland, between roughly 500 and 1100 A.D. Some authors suggest that most of these outbreaks might actually have been measles or leprosy, whose superficial symptoms resemble those of smallpox. On the other hand, equally competent authorities feel that in the majority of cases, smallpox came, conquered, and was then in turn eradicated for want of more people to infect.

It was not until a Holy Crusade was launched in 1096 to recapture Jerusalem from the Moslems—the first of four expeditions to the Holy Land that peaked with the sack of Constantinople, which ended the Fourth Crusade in 1204—that the conditions conducive to the introduction and dissemination of smallpox began to prevail in Europe and the British Isles. For over a century, the four Holy Crusades saw men, women, and children of Christendom mounting very slow-moving invasions of the Levant. Moving on foot,

47

on horse, and by sail, the crusaders brought with them the infectious diseases then more common in Europe than in the Middle East, bringing home in exchange the then rare smallpox viruses.

Many of the crusaders died of smallpox in the Levant. Many more were still infected and, shedding smallpox viruses, they returned to their native hearths, fiefdoms, villages, towns, and cities as carriers of the ancient plague. With this mass importation, the nature of smallpox itself changed in Europe and England—from a rarely seen or remembered disease to a common and endemic killer, blinder, and crippler of infants, children, and adults.

Europe, too, was changing. As the expansion of world commerce that followed Marco Polo and the later explorers and discoverers, then the Agricultural Revolution of circa 1700, and finally the Industrial Revolution, which followed it a half-century or so later, swelled the population of older towns and cities and created crowded new factory towns and cities, smallpox became as much a product of rapid urbanization and domiciliary overcrowding as of the virus itself.

Cortés, Narváez, and the other Spanish conquistadores who conquered Mexico and Peru a generation after the voyages of Columbus brought smallpox to South America, where it had never been known before. This clinical by-product of empire building swept "over the land like fire over the prairies," wrote Prescott, "smiting down prince and peasant, and adding another to the long train of woes that followed the march of the white men." African slaves and the sailors who manned the ships of the slave trade brought smallpox to the future southern and New England states of this country, where it became endemic before the American Revolution.

By the sixteenth century, few people in Europe or the British Isles ever escaped having smallpox at least once. In 1593 Dr. Simon Kellwaye, author of the first treatise on smallpox written in English, *A Defensitive Against the Plague,* wrote, "I need not greatly stand upon the description of the disease because it is a thing well known to people." Two centuries later in 1747, the British physician Richard Mead wrote that "scarce one in a thousand escaped having smallpox once."

In eighteenth-century England one out of every ten deaths was caused by smallpox. Throughout Europe at that time, smallpox was the chief cause of all deaths in children under ten years old. Fully one third of all child deaths in Glasgow, between 1783 and 1802, were caused by smallpox. In Germany the very name for the disease, *kinderpocken,* was eloquent testament to the fact that 90 percent of all smallpox cases reported in Prussia, Bavaria, and other Germanic states were suffered by children under ten.

It would be a mistake, however, to judge the severity of a disease solely by the number of deaths that it causes. In 1871, at a time when "two out of every three persons applying for relief to the Hospital for the Indigent Blind in Liverpool owed their loss of sight to smallpox," the Manchester physician William Henry Barlow underscored this point in his subsequently published lecture on the history of smallpox and vaccination. The death rate of smallpox, he noted, deals only with "the measure of its fatality [in] those of its victims, though perhaps the happiest portion, who had succumbed entirely to its force; and we but guess at that vast amount of misery, permanent injury, blindness, lameness, ruin of mind as well as body, deafness and disfigurement, which formed the signs by which its track was marked—results happily so rare in modern times."

Dr. William Buchan, a busy general practitioner in Edinburgh and London, in each of the many English and foreign-language editions of his popular textbook *Domestic Medicine* (published between 1769 and 1815), wrote the following passage in his chapter on smallpox: "This disease, which originally came from Arabia, is now become so general that very few escape it at one time or another. It is a most common malady, and for many years proved the scourge of Europe. . . . Children are most liable to this disease, and those whose food is unwholesome, who want proper exercise, and abound with gross humors, run the greatest hazard from it. . . . The disease is so generally known that a minute description of it is unneccessary." (Buchan's spelling)

A few pages later, he wrote, "Such as have not had the small-pox in the early period of life are not only rendered unhappy, but likewise in a great measure unfit for sustaining many of the most useful and important offices. Few people would choose to even hire a servant who had not had the small-pox, far less purchase a slave who had the chance of dying of this disease. How could a physician or a surgeon who had never had the small-pox himself attend to others under that malady? How deplorable is the situation of females who arrive at mature age without having had the small-pox! A woman with child seldom survives this disease; and if an infant happen to be seized with the small-pox upon the mother's breast, who had not had the disease herself, the scene must be distressing. If she continue to suckle the child herself it is at the peril of her own life; and if she weans it, in all probability it will perish. How often is the affectionate mother forced to leave her house and abandon her children at the very time when her care is most necessary? Yet should parental affection get the better of her fears, the consequences would often prove fatal."

In Russia, prior to Jenner's vaccine, the disease caused two million deaths a year; one out of every seven children born in the Russian Empire in the seventeenth and eighteenth centuries died of smallpox. In Sweden between 1774 and 1800, the average annual death rate for smallpox was 2,049 deaths per million population. The great eighteenth-century Swiss physician, professor of anatomy at Basel, Switzerland, and mathematician Daniel Bernoulli (1700–1782) estimated that in his era fifteen million Europeans alone died of smallpox every twenty-five years. This put the European smallpox death toll at sixty million fatalities during the eighteenth century.

This enormous death toll was exclusive of smallpox deaths in Asia, Africa, and the Americas. In North America alone, the artist and historian

George Catlin (1796–1872) wrote, "Thirty millions of white men are now scuffling for the goods and luxuries of life over the bones and ashes of twelve millions of red men, six millions of whom had fallen victims to the small-pox, and the remainder to the sword, bayonet or whisky."

Catlin, who lived with and painted the Native American tribes for many years, added this about smallpox, "I would venture the assertion from books that I have searched, and from other evidence, that of the numerous tribes which have already disappeared and of those that have been traded with quite to the Rocky Mountains, each one had had this exotic disease in their turn, and in a few months have lost one-half or more of their numbers."

These tragedies were compounded by the fact that at no point in human history, including our own times, did anything even resembling a medical cure for smallpox ever exist. Some of the cures physicians trusted and used were poisons as dangerous as the smallpox virus itself. The noted eighteenth-century Dutch physician Hermann Boerhaave, for example, developed a compound of antimony and mercury which he claimed would not only cure smallpox but also act against the peculiar contagion he described as being exhaled or "thrown out from the bodies" of people with active cases.

Less toxic than mercury was the cure described in the first known medical book on smallpox, written during the seventh century A.D. by Ahrun, or Aaron, of Alexandria, who was variously described as having been either a Catholic priest or a Jewish physician. Whatever he was, Ahrun/Aaron did not believe that smallpox was either contagious or not medically curable. His written cure for smallpox directed that "when the smallpox pustules are suppurated [producing pus], the patient is to lie upon a flour of rice, and be fumigated with myrtle and leaves, which will dry them." The nineteenth-century British physician Henry George, inspired by this harmless "cure," improved upon it around 1840 by coating the entire body and face of every smallpox patient with soothing layers of powdered calamine. At the very least, this cure was nontoxic and relieved the constant itching that caused smallpox sufferers to scratch pus-filled skin eruptions and spread the smallpox viruses to other parts of the body.

When serotherapy against tetanus and diphtheria was introduced at the close of the nineteenth century, it was not long before some doctors started to isolate the bacteria they were certain were "smallpox germs" found in the blood of smallpox patients. These mislabeled bacteria were then cultured, injected by the millions into the bodies of animals to "immunize" them against smallpox, and the blood serums of these so-called immunized animals were then injected into smallpox patients to "cure" them of their infections. Similarly, when Sir Almroth Wright developed his opsonic therapy based on the use of autogenous vaccines—that is, vaccines made from the bacteria isolated from the patients' own circulatory systems, cultured and multiplied, then heat-killed and shot into the very same patients to cure their bacterial infections of all kinds—such autogenous bacterial vaccines were widely recommended to cure smallpox.

Smallpox being a virus disease and not the product of any bacteria, administering these autogenous bacterial vaccines was as useless as attempting to cure smallpox patients by bathing them in the rays of different-colored electric lights, as was widely practiced by many doctors who took up this popular late nineteenth- and early twentieth-century health fad.

Since more than 75 percent of all people who got smallpox survived, if not always quite as intact as before, whenever many of these medically treated survivors—including physicians themselves—returned to their homes, jobs, and careers, they became walking testimonials to the sedatives (which did, in fact, keep them sedated and less likely to scratch their itching pustules), the immune sera, the autogenous vaccines, the colored lights, the secret nostrums of the Kickapoo Indians, and other highly touted but clinically useless "cures." There was rarely any way of convincing these recovered smallpox patients, or their families, that their "cures" were quite coincidental to their recovery from smallpox.

All things being equal, in terms of the sheer numbers of people killed, blinded, crippled, pitted, and scarred by smallpox for at least two thousand years of oral and written history, this disease was most probably the worst pestilence ever to afflict humankind.

Societal diseases and their management are each the product of major social changes. After the four Crusades to the Holy Land brought back enough smallpox viruses to enable the disease to find a permanent home in Europe, England became the birthplace of many of the social changes that would on the one hand cause the wide dissemination of smallpox, and on the other hand impede all efforts to turn Jenner's vaccination into the irrevocable birthright of every child born in England and everywhere else.

The first of these social changes was the wood famine that developed in the British Isles around 1550. The British and the Scots were forced to seek alternatives to wood for heating homes, cooking, making bricks, extracting salt from seawater, forging ships' anchors, refining sugar, and boiling laundry. It was fortunate that as they began to run out of trees, they still had ample reserves of coal. What the British and the Scots, and all the other nations, then lacked was an adequate knowledge of how properly to burn coal.

The forced development of this technology in England led to the creation of crude steam engines to pump water out of the coal mines. As England switched over from being a wood-burning nation to the world's first coal-burning country, the early steam engines of Thomas Savery (patented in 1698) and Thomas Newcomen, developed a dozen years later, evolved in swift stages into the Watt rotary steam engine of 1775. The rotary engine enabled the use of the fossil-fuel energy in coal to power the steam-driven ships and trains that were built to haul coal to the new factories, whose steam engines turned the wheels and lathes of their machines—and to carry manufactured goods from these steam-powered factories to new markets around the world.

The wood famine and its resolution were to lead directly to the crucial second phase of the Industrial Revolution, the era based on the exploitation of fossil-fuel energy. Between both of these social changes, however, two equally significant developments were to alter the developing patterns of health and disease for better and for worse.

The first event was the Agricultural Revolution, "the greatest move forward in agriculture since neolithic times,"[4] which began around 1700 or earlier in Europe. Within a century the Agricultural Revolution was to increase the yields per acre of foods, fibers, and food animals by over 50 percent in England alone, and by even greater proportions in the Lowlands, the Scandinavian countries, and the German states. This revolution was based largely on the introduction of new crops from the Americas and Asia, such as potatoes, rice, maize, peanuts, squashes, pumpkins, tomatoes, pineapples, manioc, and sweet potatoes. (The Agricultural Revolution was global; today, for example, native American maize and manioc are staple foods in much of Africa, while China is the world's largest producer of America-originating sweet potatoes. Most of the staple foods consumed in the United States, including beef cattle, wheat, pigs, rice, melons, onions, apples, bananas, oranges, chickens, and sheep were not native to the Americas, and had to be imported by European explorers, traders, and settlers.)

The Agricultural Revolution also developed new uses for turnips and other root crops as winter fodder, which vastly increased the production of animals raised for meat and wool. Finally, it introduced new techniques of farm husbandry, based in part on those devised in the Lowlands to make the best uses of limited land and water resources, and also in some measure on the new labor-saving human- and horse-powered agricultural machines that, in due time, were eventually to be powered by fossil fuels like coal and oil.

Woolen cloth, England's major export, was a cottage industry at the start of the Agricultural Revolution, with the wool being raised, sheared, spun, carded, woven, shrunk, and dyed in rural villages. The people in the trade made the textiles on their own equipment in their own cottages, and grew much of their own food on the commons lands in their villages.

Even before Richard Arkwright and Edmund Cartwright invented the power-driven spinning machines and looms that rendered obsolete the hand-powered tools of the cottagers before the close of the eighteenth century, the economic bounties of the Agricultural Revolution had started to convert yeoman agriculture to large-scale agribusiness; and events themselves combined to change textile handcrafts from a cottage-based to a centralized and soon a water-powered industry.

First, textile merchants who traditionally went to the villages to buy yarn and textiles from the cottagers set up new factories to hand spin and loom textiles under one roof. These were soon followed by water-powered factories in which the manufacture of woolen and American cotton cloth was all done on power-driven spinning jennies and looms under one roof in locations as close as possible to the major domestic and trading markets. At the same time, as increased farm yields plus the Napoleonic wars made farming much more profitable, Parliament passed various Enclosure Acts, which drove the cottage artisans off the lands of the village commons and led to bountiful, large-scale commercial agriculture. Now, as the nation's production of sheep and wool increased, the wool was sent to the new factories to be turned into yarn and textiles, and Cottage England passed into history.

These changes led very quickly to the next major social change that altered the national patterns of human health—industrial urbanization. Industrialization, with its inevitable dense concentrations of miners, mill, and factory workers within walking distance of their work places, was to transform older cities, such as London, and to create grievously overcrowded new industrial centers, like Manchester. The new instant slums, their families packed into humanly inadequate spaces in buildings without running water, in cities without sewage or other sanitary waste disposal systems, became the natural breeding grounds for smallpox and many other infectious diseases.

The impacts of these social changes on human health and preventable infectious diseases had become apparent long before the perfection of Watt's steam engine in 1775.

In older cities, when rivers like the Thames and the Seine were converted by changes in technology and population density into festering sewers, doctors and nonmedical people alike did not need the insights of germ theory to tell them that the greater the fecal and garbage pollution of their drinking water, and the more densely crowded the average living quarters of their city, then the higher the incidence of typhoid, pneumonia, smallpox, bronchitis, measles, diphtheria, rheumatism, dysentery, and other communicable diseases rendered endemic by the new industrial-era urbanization. People merely had to sample the smells of a city's streets and rivers to estimate its levels of what were already being called the "filth diseases."

Florence Nightingale, one of the greatest achievers in the history of public health, never did outgrow her lifelong conviction that it was the smells of filth, rather than the bacteria that produce noxious gases when they decompose organic matter, that were the real causes of most contagious diseases. Nor did she believe that there was more than one infectious disease, but only a single one that worsened and added newer and nastier symptoms as crowding (a prime source of ambient filth) and fever increased. "I have seen, for instance," she wrote in her best-selling *Notes on Nursing* in 1859, "with a little overcrowding, continued fever grow up; and with a little more, typhoid fever; and with a little more, typhus, and all in the same ward or hut."

Smallpox, in Nightingale's thinking, was caused by foul smells, and the filth in which foul smells were generated. In the same book she wrote that she had been brought up "by scientific men and ignorant women to believe that small-pox was a thing of which there was once a first specimen in the world, which went on propagating itself . . . and that small-pox would not begin itself [arise *de novo*] any more than a new dog would begin without there having been a parent dog. Since then I have seen with my own eyes and smelt with my own nose small-pox growing up in first specimens, either in close rooms, or in overcrowded wards, where it could not by any possibility have been 'caught', but must have begun."[5]

The biological impacts of industrialization and its haphazard styles of urbanization led to another major social change: the development of two opposing schools of what we could now term sociology.

The first of these schools included physicians, nurses, Christian ministers, and lay thinkers who were convinced that the growing outbreaks of contagious and deficiency diseases were due to impure drinking water; the absence of sewage and other sanitary means of waste disposal; foul air, resulting from overcrowding in the industrial warrens; unsafe workplaces; and wages too low to provide adequate food, clothing, and shelter for the families of the new working classes, and that these diseases were all social in both origin and solution. These people were by and large the most vociferous supporters of universal compulsory vaccination laws aimed at the total eradication of smallpox. They felt that the other newly significant contagious diseases of towns and cities were public health problems that could be resolved by building better homes for the poor, by municipal and county pure water and other hygienic systems, by job safety legislation, and by laws mandating adequate minimum wages and maximum working hours for the physical producers of the vast new wealth of the Industrial Revolution.

These educated, and for the most part wellborn, reformers were not of course aware of the biological mechanisms that make hungry people living in overcrowded filthy lodgings, drinking and washing with microbially contaminated water, and suffering environmentally acquired chronic respiratory infections, less resistant to deficiency and contagious diseases than well-fed people who enjoy adequate and uncrowded living quarters, and who are born and live out their lives in hygienic environments. All that the humanly concerned medical and civic reformers knew—or, for that matter, really had to know—was what they observed in two broad classes of people: their own, and the new working poor and the marginal "midling classes," like the Admiralty clerk's family into which Charles Dickens had been born in 1812.

The opposing school of sociology (and/or political science) that developed in England and other rapidly industrializing states during the second half of the eighteenth century and all of the nineteenth century included doctors, political and economic leaders, Christian philosophers, and academic and lay philosophers who believed that the swiftly widening gap between increasing wealth and increasing poverty was inevitable and even just, because it was ordained by God and maintained by nature, which they saw as God's mechanism for expressing His divine will. The misfortunes of the working poor were therefore the will of God, and such plague diseases as smallpox, malaria, tuberculosis, and cholera were created by our Heavenly Father to keep a wholesome balance between birthrates of the blessed and the damned. Since such pestilences were divinely or naturally ordained, they therefore could not—and, at the peril of invoking God's wrath, should not—be prevented by mere mortal men.

As early as 1786, in his *Dissertation on the Poor Laws,* one of the prime English movers of this school, the Reverend Joseph Townsend, wrote, "Wretchedness has increased in proportion to the efforts made to relieve it." Far from agreeing with those few members of Parliament who even then were talking of the need for higher wages, Townsend maintained that "hope and fear are the springs of industry. It is the part of a good politician to strengthen these: but our laws weaken the one and destroy the other." The poor, said this Christian philosopher, "know little of the motives which stimulate the higher ranks to action—pride, honour, and ambition. In general it is only hunger which can spur and goad them on to labour." Since the poor were little higher than animals in God's scheme of things, it behooved Parliament to remember that "hunger will tame the fiercest animals, it will teach decency and civility, obedience and subjection, to the most brutish, the most obstinate, and the more perverse."

In the midst of the Agricultural Revolution, Townsend blandly conceded, "It is indeed possible to banish hunger," but he hastened to warn that to "increase the quantity of food" would be to cause reckless breeding among the least worthy elements of the population. The only remedy for the evils of society was to let hunger and all of the plagues in God's armory regulate the population.

In 1798 when Jenner published at his own expense his little monograph, *An Inquiry into the Causes and Effects of the Variolae Vaccinae,* in which he described his work with the antismallpox vaccine, a somewhat longer book was published by the foremost disciple of the Reverend Joseph Townsend. Its name was *An Essay on the Principle of Population,* and its author was a clergyman and political economist, the Reverend Thomas Robert Malthus.

Whereas Jenner urged the universal uses of his cowpox vaccine to rid humankind of the scourge of smallpox, Malthus—whose book described catastrophes like war, famine, and smallpox as divinely created natural checks to the reckless breeding of the Undeserving Poor—had a very different view of the social worth of Jenner's vaccine.

Jenner saw the prevention of smallpox as the moral obligation of science and society. After he tested the smallpox-preventing efficacy of his cowpox vaccine in people, and made his results and methods known publicly, Jenner viewed people who caught, suffered, and in considerable numbers died of smallpox as victims of societal neglect born of stupidity, venality, or the combination of both. Malthus saw the problem of the cause, social functions, and prevention of smallpox and other mass diseases somewhat differently.

Malthus, the first professor of political economy in British university history, was not a fool. He was as aware as were the sanitary and civic reformers that, as he himself wrote in *Population,* "In the history of every epidemic it has invariably been observed that the lower classes of people, whose food was insufficient, and who lived crowded together in small and dirty houses, were the principal victims."

In his very next sentence, however, Malthus blamed not the prevailing low wages of the times but the victims of poverty themselves for the epidemic diseases of poverty: "In what other manner can Nature point out to us that, if we increase too fast for the means of subsistence [this was written at the end of the century during which the Agricultural Revolution more than doubled food production in England alone] so as to render it necessary for a considerable part of society to live in this miserable manner, we have offended against one of her laws?" In 1798 this was not only a gross libel against the responsibility of poor working people who married and had children before, as Malthus warned them to, they invested their wages wisely and grew rich enough to afford to have children. It was also a blasphemy against the God of love the Reverend Malthus professed to serve. In our own times this Pecksniffian blame-the-victims posture persists as an integral portion of the legacy of Malthus to all too many people in the corridors of governmental power in the United States, England, and elsewhere.

Far from hailing Jenner as a benefactor of humanity, Malthus called for the censure of "those benevolent, but mistaken men, who have thought they were doing a service to mankind by projecting schemes for the total extirpation of particular disorders." As the battle between the followers of Jenner and Malthus raged over the next few years, Malthus sharpened his attack on the doctor who gave the world the gift of vaccination.

In the 1806 edition of *Population,* Malthus warned, "Nature will not, nor cannot be defeated in her purposes. The necessary mortality must come, in some form or other; and the extirpation of one disease will only be the signal for the birth of another perhaps more fatal. . . . If we stop up any of these channels, it is most perfectly clear that the stream of mortality must run with greater force through some of the other channels. . . . The small-pox is certainly one of these channels, and a very broad one, which Nature has opened for the last thousand years, to keep the population down to the level of the means of subsistence; but had this been closed, others would have become wider or new ones had been formed." Then Malthus lowered the boom directly on Jenner's cowpox vaccine. "For my own part," he continued, "I feel not the slightest doubt, that if the introduction of the cow-pox should extirpate the small-pox, and yet the number of marriages continues, we shall find a very perceptible difference in the increased mortality of other diseases."

In the plainer-spoken world of parliamentary politics, these jeremiads by Malthus and the new Malthusian subprophets were translated into more direct acts by members of the dominant social faction Malthus served as mentor and spokesman. These acts centered about first opposing and usually managing to kill any legislation providing for vaccination and then, if such bills had to be passed in response to public clamor, weakening their structure, or denying or limiting the funding of any vaccination bills Parliament found it more expedient not to enact.

In other countries legislators with similar moral views indulged in like acts of opposition and sabotage. The results are now a matter of history. The industrial world's opponents of free and compulsory universal vaccination against smallpox were to win most of their battles more than a century after Jenner developed the means of eradicating smallpox from the human experience.

While he lived, Jenner was not without his supporters at home and abroad. In 1800, when an epidemic of smallpox erupted in Vienna, Dr. Johann Peter Frank, a pioneer of modern preventive medicine, was the director of the Austrian capital's general hospital. He was aware of Jenner's work, and followed events very closely when a few Viennese physicians used the Jenner vaccine successfully to protect their patients and themselves from smallpox during that epidemic. Shortly after this Frank inoculated a number of children with the Jenner cowpox vaccine. When it took in these children and immunized them against subsequent challenges with smallpox virus, Frank prevailed upon the government to issue an official circular recommending the Jenner cowpox vaccine as an agent to prevent smallpox.

No sooner did the Jenner vaccine prove itself against the smallpox virus in a handful of London patients than the British Army, still smarting from the lessons it had absorbed about the military functions of smallpox and its prevention during its defeat in the American Revolution, began to vaccinate whole regiments at home and abroad. Like other European countries, such as Prussia, England lost little time in vaccinating its military population against smallpox, regardless of what Parliament did or did not do about protecting the far more numerous civilian population.

By 1801 the Admiralty had the entire British fleet vaccinated, and, to mark the occasion, presented Jenner with a special gold medal struck in honor of this episode in military medicine. Napoleon, England's mortal foe, also had a medal struck in honor of Jenner's vaccine in 1804, and a year later the entire French Army was vaccinated against smallpox.

Jenner's English supporters included the unjustly forgotten Tortuga-born Quaker physician John Coakley Lettsom, who is remembered today almost solely for a bit of contemporary verse:

When any sick to me apply,
I physics, bleeds and sweats 'em,
If after that they choose to die,
Why Verily! I Lettsom.

Actually, Lettsom was one of the few physicians at that time who had little faith in such standard modalities as bleeding, purging, and heating. A prominent variolator in London, he was one of the first British physicians to abandon inoculation with smallpox virus in favor of the far safer Jenner cowpox vaccine.

When he was still in his twenties, Lettsom founded the Medical Society of London for the swifter dissemination of new medical developments to practicing physicians. In 1798, shortly after Jenner's book on his vaccine was published, Lettsom sent many copies to doctors in England and other countries, among them Dr. Benjamin Waterhouse (1738–1846), then professor of physic at Harvard College in Cambridge, Massachusetts.

Waterhouse was an outsider at Cambridge for two glaring reasons: He was a Rhode Island-born Quaker in a community that still revered the fairly recent ancestors who had forbidden the Quakers to live in the Massachusetts Bay Colony; and he was not a Harvard graduate. After learning medicine as an apprentice to Dr. John Halliburton of Newport, Rhode Island, and practicing for over a decade, Waterhouse went to Europe in 1775 to study and live with the noted Quaker physician, and a relative on his mother's side, Dr. John Fothergill. Halsey writes that "while living and studying with Dr. Fothergill, it is probable that he met John Hunter [Jenner's postapprenticeship teacher], John C. Lettsom, Edward Jenner and many others who were intimate with the doctor and prominent in medical circles."[6] Waterhouse studied at the medical school of the University of Edinburgh in 1775, and after two years of study with Fothergill, he entered the medical school of the University of Leyden, Holland, where he took his diploma in 1780.

Waterhouse was quick to grasp the clinical implications of Jenner's work. He immediately wrote an article about the cowpox vaccine for the *Columbian Sentinel,* where it appeared in the issue of March 12, 1799, under the headline "Something Curious in the Medical Line." Waterhouse described cowpox as a newly discovered disease, and wrote, *"No person was ever known to die of this distemper,* but what makes this newly discovered disease so very curious, and so extremely important, is that every person thus affected, is EVER AFTER SECURED FROM THE ORDINARY SMALLPOX, *let him be ever so much exposed to the effluvium of it, or let ever so much ripe matter be inserted into the skin by inoculation.* In other words—a person who has undergone the *local* disease and *specific fever* occasioned by the cow-pox infection, is *thereby rendered ever after* unsusceptible of the small-pox."

Waterhouse added, "It is worthy of remark that the infection of the cow-pox can be conveyed to the human species by the ordinary mode of inoculation," and that there was "no difference in the effects of the matter taken from the cow, and of the matter generated successively in the second, third, fourth or fifth human creature.

"SUCH are the outlines of a mild disease, the knowledge of which may lead to consequences of the utmost importance to the whole human race, no less indeed that of superceding, if not extinguishing, that terrible scourge, the small-pox."

Like Jenner, this American Quaker doctor saw no logical reason why the new cowpox vaccine should not be used immediately, starting in the young United States of America, to make the entire world at last free of smallpox, and he expanded on this idea in a hastily written pamphlet, *A Prospect of Extinguishing the Small-Pox.*

Waterhouse sent his pamphlet to the second President of the new republic, John Adams, whom he had known in England when the older man was minister to the Court of St. James's. Adams responded in the mellifluous clichés most American Presidents were to use for the next two centuries to bury carefully with gracious but noncommittal praise most good ideas for preventing major diseases.

The third President of the nation was, fortunately, an exception to this wordy tradition.

On December 1, 1800, four months before Thomas Jefferson's inauguration, Waterhouse mailed the then Vice-President a copy of his pamphlet on the global eradication of smallpox. On December 25, Jefferson answered from his home, Monticello, in Virginia, and assured Waterhouse, "I had before attended to your publications on the subject in the newspapers, and took much interest in the result of the experiments you were making."

These experiments consisted of the vaccinations of Waterhouse's children and friends with samples of Jenner's vaccine, some of them mailed to him on impregnated threads by Jenner, who whimsically observed that he had suddenly been turned into the "Vaccine clerk of the World." Now Jefferson added a sentence all present and future American Presidents and public policymakers would do well to memorize: "Every friend of humanity must look with pleasure on this discovery, by which one evil more is withdrawn from the condition of man; and must contemplate the possibility that future improvements and discoveries may still more and more lessen the catalogue of evils." Jefferson quite obviously sensed that smallpox would not remain the only vaccine-preventable major disease.

In July 1800, six months before he wrote to Jefferson, Waterhouse vaccinated his five-year-old son, Daniel, by inserting a small section of cowpox-lymph-impregnated thread (furnished by Dr. John Haygarth of Bath, England) into a small incision on the boy's arm, and covered it with sticking plaster. Waterhouse subsequently inoculated three of his other children, and

"3 others of my family." One thing, he wrote, then remained to be done, "and that was to prove that it absolutely secured the system from the small-pox, and this was accomplished the month following, by placing them in the small-pox hospital, where they were inoculated [with smallpox virus] by Dr. *Aspinwall,* and they all came out at the end of 10 days, without any signs of [smallpox] infections and thus my leading assertions passed the test of *demonstration."*

By 1801, when Jefferson was President, Waterhouse had vaccinated enough people in and outside of his family to convince himself of the Jenner vaccine's worth and safety, and he was in good conscience able to honor Jefferson's request that he send a supply of the original "vaccine matter," as well as a batch of Jennerian vaccine Waterhouse had made up from the lymphs of American cows, to Jefferson's estate in Monticello. Jefferson, who had been inoculated with smallpox at the age of twenty-three by Dr. Richard Shippen of Philadelphia, was himself immune to the disease, but most of the members of his household were still subject to smallpox.

In November 1801, in a letter to Dr. John Vaughan, Jefferson told of how "I inoculated about seventy or eighty of my family; my sons-in-law about as many of theirs, and including our neighbors who wished to avail themselves of the opportunity, our whole experiment extended to about two hundred persons." Jefferson observed that the Jenner vaccine "generally gives no more of disease than a blister as large as a coffee-bean produced by burning would occasion. Sucking children did not take the disease from the inoculated mother." The President regretted that "in my neighborhood we had no opportunity of obtaining Variolous matter [smallpox virus], to try to test the genuineness of our Vaccine [cowpox] matter," and asked Vaughan to send him some "fresh Variolous matter" so that he could test the immunizing powers of the Jenner vaccine.

This was but one of various important letters Jefferson wrote on the subject of vaccination against smallpox. Historically, one of the most significant was the letter Jefferson sent to Edward Jenner in 1801. Like Malthus, Jefferson also observed that Jenner's vaccine had the potential to totally extirpate the ancient pestilence of smallpox from the legacy of humankind; unlike Malthus, Jefferson did not see this as a reason to brand Jenner as an enemy of humanity, God, or nature. Jefferson congratulated Jenner because "medicine has never produced any single improvement of such utility" as the vaccine against smallpox. "You have," Jefferson wrote, "erased from the calendar of human afflictions one of its greatest. Yours is the comfortable reflection that Mankind can never forget that you have lived; future generations will know by history only that the loathsome smallpox has existed, and by you had been extirpated."

The completely opposite views of Malthus and Jefferson on the general subject of remedies and vaccines to cure or prevent contagious diseases reflected their different personal obligations. When Malthus, in his *Population,* asserted that "above all, we should reprobate specific remedies for ravaging diseases, and those benevolent but mistaken men who have thought they were doing a service to mankind by projecting schemes for the total extirpation of particular disorders," and then went on to attack Jenner's cowpox vaccine as the ill-conceived cause of worse diseases, he was about to leave his church post as curate in Surrey and to embark upon a lifelong career as professor of political economy at the East India Company's staff college. There Malthus's job from 1805 to the year he died, 1834, was to help increase the flow of profits from the Company's main asset: the royal monopoly of the entire commerce of the subcontinent of India.

When Jefferson praised Jenner for having "erased from the calendar of human afflictions one of its greatest," he was the chief executive of a very young republic whose Constitution's preamble dedicated it to "promote the general welfare" rather than only the economic and political interests of the royal monopoly that was one of the most lucrative organs of British imperialism. Jefferson understood that without universal good health no nation could ever seriously undertake to provide the "unalienable Rights" defined in his Declaration of Independence as "Life, Liberty and the Pursuit of Happiness."

Although variolation, or inoculation with true smallpox virus, had by 1798 become a very lucrative medical specialty in England, with many doctor-owned inoculation hospitals doing a brisk business, this did not stop many variolators, such as Lettsom and Haygarth, from switching to the less lucrative Jenner vaccine. In 1799 the director of the London Smallpox Hospital, M. Woodville, announced that he had made a large clinical trial of the Jenner vaccine and found it to be safe and effective. By 1807 when the Royal College of Physicians, after studying the Jenner vaccine in people, pronounced it to be safer than variolation, well over 100,000 people had already been vaccinated in England.

Many doctors with vested emotional and economic stakes in smallpox variolations united in attacking Jenner's cowpox vaccine. There were however some notable exceptions, such as Dr. William Buchan. In most editions of his book, *Domestic Medicine,* he had reminded readers that "by a well-laid plan for extending smallpox inoculation, more lives might be saved at a small expense than are at present preserved by all the hospitals in England, which cost the public such an amazing sum." As soon as Jenner published his findings in 1798, Buchan realized the cowpox vaccine was a superior and infinitely safer method of achieving immunity against smallpox. He immediately stopped inoculating his patients with virulent smallpox matter, and switched over to vaccinating them with cowpox lymph.

Buchan's enthusiasm for Jenner's discovery extended even to the farm animal from whom the vaccine flowed. He concluded his new chapter on cowpox vaccination in the next editions of *Domestic Medicine* with this charming tribute: "From the beginning of the world, the cow had, in all countries, been esteemed a valuable animal. Besides cultivating the ground, which her species performs, she supplies us with an aliment of her own preparing, the most wholesome as well as nourishing in nature; but never before was it known, except, as appears, in some particular districts in England, that, even from a disease to which she is liable, she can likewise be further useful, in preserving us from one of the most fatal calamities that ever infested human kind."

For every Thomas Malthus who excoriated Jenner for the crime of making smallpox vaccine-preventable, there were a dozen of his peers who agreed with Matthew Baillie, the prominent physician and anatomist. Baillie in 1802 reported to the parliamentary commission studying the matter of awarding a cash grant to Jenner that the smallpox vaccine was, in his professional opinion, "the most important discovery ever made in medicine." In the same statement, he told Parliament, "If Dr. Jenner had not chosen openly and honourably to explain to the public all he knew about the subject, he might have acquired a considerable fortune." Parliament twice, in 1802 and 1807, awarded Jenner grants totaling thirty thousand pounds.

Nevertheless, in 1808 the same Parliament voted down a proposed Bill to Prevent the Spreading of the Infection of the Small-pox by providing free smallpox vaccinations to everyone. Nor would any law mandating either free or compulsory vaccinations be passed by Parliament before Jenner died in 1823, bitter in the knowledge that other countries had by then made much wider uses of his vaccine.

In lieu of government vaccination programs, the British societal establishment set up privately endowed and supported voluntary organizations to provide free vaccinations to respectful members of the Deserving Poor who humbly sought them. The East India Company, for which Malthus, the archenemy of vaccinations, toiled for many years, was a prominent contributor to one of these societies. For all the good faith of many of the decent people who contributed to them, the underlying function of these societies—whether planned or coincidental—was to block the enactment of government-funded and administered universal compulsory vaccination programs, and in this they succeeded in England for the better part of the nineteenth century.

The Germanic state of Bavaria had made vaccination compulsory as early as 1807. It was soon to be joined by Denmark in 1810, and Sweden and Wurtemberg in 1818; and, after Jenner died, by Prussia in 1835 (but enforced only for the Prussian military population), Roumania in 1874, Hungary in 1876, and Serbia in 1881. Not all of these smallpox vaccination laws were equally well administered.

The actual worth of the compulsory vaccination laws of two great countries, France and Prussia, was tested by fire during the Franco-Prussian

War of 1870–1871. Neither country had had very good vaccination laws to start with, but patriots in both nations were assured that their respective armies were not sent forth to battle the foes of righteousness and Christian civilization until they were duly vaccinated against smallpox. Certainly the respective fiscal agencies of both warring nations appropriated the funds needed to pay for these military vaccines.

The great smallpox pandemic of 1870–1875 broke out almost at the very moment that the Franco-Prussian War started. This subjected both armies to a much higher than normal risk of smallpox. The Prussian soldiers, most of whom had been vaccinated and revaccinated before they went into combat, suffered only 8,360 cases and 297 deaths from the disease, primarily among the civilians drafted into the Prussian army when war broke out. The French soldiers, who on paper had been equally well vaccinated and revaccinated, suffered 280,470 cases of smallpox, 23,470 of them fatal, during the six months that the war was fought.

Thousands of French soldiers who were taken prisoner by the Prussian victors proved to be suffering from smallpox. The Prussian military leaders and civilian superpatriots naturally concluded that this was part of a nefarious French plot to infect Prussia's civilian population with smallpox, and complained to all who would listen. Fortunately, wiser heads among German doctors and scientists prevailed. It was not, they reminded Bismarck, French duplicity but the absence of good and well-enforced universal compulsory vaccination and revaccination (booster) legislation that put the civilian population at constant risk of smallpox. Under the guidance of these physicians, Prussia enacted and proceeded properly to enforce compulsory vaccination and revaccination laws under which every German child at the ages of two and twelve was given primary and secondary vaccinations against smallpox.

Prior to Jenner's vaccine, the Prussians had a rate of about four thousand cases of smallpox per million population. By the eve of the Franco-Prussian War, the total rate had, thanks to the Jenner vaccine, been reduced to about 225 smallpox cases per million population, and to considerably less for the military forces. After the passage of the improved compulsory vaccination laws in 1874, their honest administration caused the Prussian smallpox attack rate to fall to only two cases in the entire nation during the decade 1889–1898, or virtually zero. "In the year 1899 not a single death from smallpox occurred in any large town of the whole German Empire, numbering 54 millions. There were 28 smallpox deaths in all, giving a rate of 0.5 per million population. These 28 deaths occurred chiefly near the frontiers; and lastly, the 28 deaths occurred in 21 separate districts and yet no local epidemic was started. This," observed the London doctor E. J. Edwardes in the July 5, 1902, special smallpox isssue of the *British Medical Journal*, "is very significant."

In England after Jenner died, a series of vaccination acts were ultimately passed by Parliament. One, passed in 1835, made the vaccination of infants compulsory in England and Wales; a companion act, passed in 1845, made such vaccination equally mandatory in Scotland and Ireland. Another act of Parliament in 1840 provided free vaccinations to anyone who requested them, and also, at long last, made variolation, or the inoculation of true smallpox matter, illegal. In 1853 Parliament passed the Act to Extend and Make Compulsory the Practice of Vaccination, under which the government undertook to provide vaccinations to the entire population of England, Ireland, Scotland, and Wales.

There was only one weakness in each of these parliamentary measures: Not one of them was, until the great smallpox pandemic of 1870–1875, ever adequately funded or seriously implemented. At best, their enforcement was left to the local governing bodies, and this in most instances, as everyone in Parliament knew, was the equivalent of nonenforcement.

Racism also limited the honest administration of Britain's vaccination laws. In August 1872, at the Birmingham meeting of the very conservative British Medical Association, a Professor Houghton delivered an address before its section on public medicine. He noted that "for the present year, 10,500 pounds was voted [by Parliament] for the National Vaccination Institution of England; in addition to which, nearly as much has been paid out of the public funds in payment for the services made by medical men in vaccination. Thus, nearly 20,000 pounds has been properly spent in providing the people of England with gratuitous vaccination. In Ireland, only 400 pounds per year is spent on the same object."

Houghton's data on the vaccine appropriations for Ireland were widely challenged, and he was forced to document them. Five years later the Association's organ, the British Medical Journal, wrote in its issue of February 24, 1877, "The statement, however, was perfectly true in 1872, and it is still true in spite of the experience of the small-pox epidemic of 1871, 1872, and 1873. Ireland has been again attacked by small-pox, and the disease is stealthily spreading. In spite of these warnings, no steps were taken by either the late or the present Government to increase the supply of [cowpox] lymph or improve the character of vaccination in Ireland . . ." As noted above, since Jenner's vaccine was introduced in 1798, smallpox has been as much the product of government policy as of the smallpox virus.

From the moment Jenner's vaccine was announced at the close of the eighteenth century, those who opposed it ranged from physicians and publicists to England's major employers and taxpayers. The reasons why physicians attacked the vaccine ranged from the commercial to the scientific to just plain envy. Since cowpox vaccination did not turn people into smallpox carriers during their vaccine-induced cases of mild cowpox, there was no need to board them in private inoculation hospitals until it was safe to return to normal life.

Various of Jenner's British medical peers, such as the surgeon of London's St. Thomas's Hospital, Mr. John Birch, attacked Jennerian vaccination for Malthusian reasons. A fervent advocate of variolation to prevent, and friction electricity to cure, smallpox, John Birch kept as many people from being vaccinated as did the fashionable variolators, Drs. Benjamin Mosely and William Rowley, who claimed that Jenner's cowpox vaccine would cause people to develop bovine features. After Jenner and his contemporary medical enemies were all dead, a popular British versifier, William Wadd, published this mock epitaph in 1827:

MOSELEY AND ROWLEY
Here lies as queer a pair as ever
Were by their peers accounted clever;
They kicked Vaccinia out of town,
And pulled poor Doctor Jenner down.

The powerful segments of British economic and political life who from the very start opposed all vaccination legislation, the main pillars of the ruling Establishment whose representatives in Parliament for nearly a century saw to it that such vaccination acts that they could not stop were, once passed, deprived of both funds and powers to administer those laws, were in their personal lives not opposed to the Jenner vaccine. As individuals, they were among the first to be vaccinated, and to have their families, servants, clerks, and secretaries vaccinated. They also followed all the sanitary rules that the doctors in the sanitary reform movement urged for the entire population.

As a social class, these opponents of universal compulsory vaccination were among the world's first and leading customers for new inside plumbing systems for their town and country homes, and certainly they were among the first to have inside baths, toilets, and clean drinking water on tap. They had no quarrel with their doctors, and had no doubt at all that as the reform and the conservative doctors all agreed, filthy rivers, unclean and crowded living conditions, and inadequate family nutrition made poor people far more prone to the infectious diseases of urban life than people of more affluent classes.

It was not the medical judgments of the public health and sanitary reformers that the major opponents of government-funded compulsory vaccination programs rejected. What they abhorred was the moral posture of the Health of Towns Association (whose leaders ranged from the physicians John Simon, Joseph Toynbee, and R. D. Grainger, to bishops, vicars, and rising young Tory politicians like Benjamin Disraeli), let alone affiliated sanitary and social reform groups, which included the Association for Promoting Cleanliness among the Poor, the Society for the Improvement of the Conditions of the Labouring Classes, and the Social Science Association. These and related reform bodies were organized not to overthrow the sociopolitical Establishment but to preserve it by making it work better for greater numbers of people.

However, this simple truth was overlooked by the less intelligent leaders of the Establishment. Free vaccinations for all at the expense of the nation's few prudent taxpayers was, they complained, the least of the demands of the sanitary and public health reformers. Smallpox was only one among many contagious diseases the big spenders-of-other-people's-money proposed to control with all sorts of costly measures—from free vaccinations for every tart and guttersnipe, to new water and sewage systems, to whole armies of official inspectors hired to enforce the reformers' proposed compulsory mine and factory safety regulations—let alone the economically ruinous hygienic and fire-prevention regulations in the tenement warrens of every town and city.

Whether or not they believed, as their first spokesmen Townsend and Malthus had written, that the working poor and the equally impoverished "midling classes" together constituted a race apart, doomed to suffer plagues and pestilences because God willed it so, is quite irrelevant. The probability is that they certainly knew that these theological claims were as fraudulent as were the Malthusian ratios on the proliferation of food versus people, which some educated people believe to be true to this very day. The Establishment leaders did know that, when needed, a strong army and navy were the best things for a flourishing imperialist power to have, and they really did not need either Townsend or Malthus to remind them that poverty and its anxieties forced thousands of able-bodied poor men to enlist in the nation's armed forces in the interests of plain survival.

There was one thing that the most influential members of the Establishment had always understood: The entire production cost and pricing structures of the Industrial Revolution were based on the prevalence and institutionalization of extremely low wages, and on the preservation of chronic and hereditary poverty so acute that it produced endless supplies of workers willing to work for any wages, as well as ample supplies of essential but even less expensive child labor. Although such Establishment propagandists as Malthus raised false alarms about nonexistent nineteenth-century population explosions as rationales for not having state public health and therapeutic medical programs, universal compulsory vaccination programs, and minimum wage and maximum working hour laws, he was quick to attack the attempts of Francis Place, Richard Carlile, and other British civic reformers to instruct working people and married people of all social classes in some simple and inexpensive birth-control techniques to "avoid having more children than they wish to have and can easily maintain," as well as to spare themselves the need to send their young children "to different employments, to Mills and Manufactories, at a very early age."

In his 1823 broadside, *To the Married of Both Sexes of the Working People,* the Benthamite reformer Francis Place, himself a merchant tailor, observed that "the misery of these poor children cannot be described, and need not be described to you, who witness and deplore them every day of your lives."

To Malthus, such efforts to impede the flow of child labor into the mines and factories of rapidly industrializing England constituted a blend of heresy and treason. To this clergyman-turned-political economist, children packed off to work in the coal mines and textile mills at the age of six or seven were merely "a necessary stimulus to industry." Little children were paid even lower wages than their parents; they competed successfully against adults, and thus kept all wage scales down; and in the absence of any available birth-control technologies, they were in constantly replenished supply when mine and mill labor were needed.

During Malthus's years with the East India Company, Parliament in 1813 and 1833 passed the acts that modified and ultimately terminated its India trade monopoly. After 1813 many of the Company's major shareholders began to invest in England's new mining, manufacturing, and mercantile enterprises. This gave Malthus and the other Company economists a vested interest in the preservation of low wages and low taxes. National vaccination programs would, of course, have had to be funded by national tax revenues.

As Malthus and his righteous contemporaries passed on to higher or lower firmaments, their successors in later generations dropped scriptural pieties for more rationalistic simplisms, derived from the lexicon of the sciences, in order to preserve the role of poverty as the wellstream of cheap labor. In place of Malthus, there arose the equally cruel and insensitive Victorian sages Sir Francis Galton, the founder of the pseudoscientific cult of eugenics, and Herbert Spencer, founder of the equally pseudoscientific cult of social Darwinism.[7] Both leaders discovered in their scientistic perversions of biology, evolution, and sociology far better rationales for the preservation of low wages and governmental inaction concerning vaccination and health, housing, hygiene, wages, and hours than Townsend and Malthus had ever been able to torture out of the Holy Bible.

It was Herbert Spencer, who was not a biologist, and not Charles Darwin, the quintessential biologist, who coined the phrase "survival of the fittest." Spencer then proceeded to teach the opponents of universal compulsory vaccination and all other public health and environmental safety measures how to pervert the revolutionary new Darwinian theory of natural evolution to justify the continuation of the pre-Darwinian law of the jungle.

The poor were poor, Spencer wrote, simply because they were innately unfit. "The whole effort of nature," the nonnaturalist Spencer wrote in his *Social Statics* (1864 edition), "is to get rid of such, to clear the world of them, and make room for the better." Nature made its own wise natural selection: "If they are sufficiently complete to live," Spencer added, "they *do* live, and it is well that they should live. If they are not sufficiently complete to live, they die, and it is best they should die."

In his *The Study of Sociology,* which was serialized in the American *Popular Science Monthly* before coming out as a book in 1874, Spencer wrote that it was time that all governments started to act according to the "general truths of biology." Furthermore, he wrote, they should stop ignoring the great "biological law" that those who interfere with natural selection by making life safer and more livable for the working poor thus become responsible for what Spencer termed "the artificial preservation of those least able to take care of themselves." Small wonder the humanitarian Darwin had such profound contempt for Spencer's preachments.

Spencer's 1884 essay "The New Toryism" listed all of what he considered to be the unwonted acts of government interference with everything that had made England and America great. Vaccination was prominent in Spencer's 1884 hit list: "Power was given [by Parliament] to poor-law guardians, etc. to enforce vaccination"; and before that, "In 1863 came the extension of compulsory vaccination to Scotland, and also to Ireland"; and in 1864, there was passed "an Act for compulsory testing of cables and anchors, an Act extending the Public Works Act of 1863; and the Contagious Diseases Act: which last gave the police, in specified places, powers which, in respect of certain classes of women, abolished sundry of these safeguards to individual freedom established in past times." Spencer was referring here to the freedom of every good Briton to contract any venereal disease of his choice from any whore of his fancy.

There were other horrible examples in Spencer's long list, and it would be impossible to cite them all. However, it is difficult to overlook what he described in the same essay as "an Act making compulsory regulations for extinguishing fires in London. Then, under the Ministry of Lord John Russell, in 1866, have to be named an Act to regulate cattle-sheds etc. in Scotland, giving local authorities powers to inspect sanitary conditions ... ; a Public Health Act, under which there is a registration of lodging-houses and limitations of occupants, with inspections and directions for lime-washing, etc; and a Public Libraries Act, giving local powers by which a majority can tax a minority for their books." Finally, Spencer lamented, "there is the 'endowment of research,' of late energetically urged. Already the Government gives every year the sum of 4000 pounds for this purpose, to be distributed through the Royal Society ..." This sum, Spencer felt, was already too much to waste on such things as vaccines against other potentially preventable diseases of humankind.

Spencer, and other apostles of his New Toryism, were as widely published and as highly regarded in the United States as in England. The influence of his thinking, and that of his ideological precursors and successors, can be seen in the smallpox mortality data for the United States since 1801, when Jefferson vaccinated two hundred relatives and friends at Monticello.

Jefferson's early efforts to have individual physicians take charge of introducing smallpox vaccination into the still sparsely settled young American republic were soon followed by attempts in the state and national legislatures to extend this protection from smallpox to all Americans. In 1809 the Maryland Assembly set up a $30,000 lottery to fund a state vaccination agency, but this effort raised less than half of that amount. In 1813 Congress empowered President James Madison "to appoint an agent to preserve the genuine vaccine matter, and to furnish the same to any citizen of the United States." Inadequate funding, the lack of state and local health departments, and the absence of communications and transportation networks equal to the task of serving every citizen of the rural and frontier settlements of the new republic, turned this congressional initiative into a dead letter on the law books.

Lemuel Shattuck, the Boston bookdealer who was inspired by the publications of the British Health of Towns Association to found the American sanitary reform movement, served as chairman of the three-man board of commissioners appointed by the state to make a sanitary survey of Massachusetts. In 1850 the board isssued what has since been known as the Shattuck Report. This landmark document dealt with recommendations for filling many as yet unmet health needs. These included creating and extending, in towns and villages, "ample provision ... for a supply, in purity and abundance, of light, air, and water; for drainage and sewerage, for paving and cleanliness ..."

The Shattuck Report also recommended that "local Boards of Health endeavor to prevent or mitigate the sanitary evils arising from over-crowded lodging houses and cellar dwellings," and that "measures be adopted for preventing or mitigating the sanitary evils arising from foreign emigration." Recommendation number XXVII in the section of the report dealing with "Legal Measures" opened with these words: "We recommend that every city and town in the State be REQUIRED to provide means for the periodical vaccination of the inhabitants."

No other recommendation in the Shattuck Report was made with this degree of emphasis. The reference to "periodical" vaccination recognized that by 1850 the world's doctors had learned that secondary or booster vaccinations were required to provide truly lifelong protection against smallpox.[8]

This excellent suggestion was not to be implemented in Shattuck's century. For American urban dwellers, the poor and the affluent alike, it was a dangerous century. Smallpox, like all other infectious diseases of overcrowding and environmental degradation—tuberculosis, cholera, pneumonia, typhoid, typhus, malaria, yellow fever, and microbial enteritis—continued to be endemic and frequently flared into raging epidemics in America's industrial towns and major cities.

The urban overcrowding caused by industrialization and the related expansion of mercantilism was further aggravated by the influx of refugees from European poverty and famines. American industry and city building needed all the labor they could get. Immigrant labor became as essential to America as domestic child labor had been to Europe at the dawn of the Industrial Revolution. Jobs in American industry, as well as the free land for landless European farmers, attracted millions of refugees of various skills from the Scandinavian, German, British, and other Old World countries.

The Irish potato famines of midcentury, exacerbated by British racial policies dealing with nearly every aspect of daily life in Ireland, contributed more than a million Irish poor to the American labor pool. Companies organized or encouraged by the railroads, the shipping companies, and the major employers of mine, factory, and construction labor sent agents abroad to encourage the restless poor and near-poor of Europe to emigrate to America. They even sold them the steamship and railroad tickets to reach the promised free land or jobs in the new utopia of unlimited opportunities.

When such voluntary emigration lagged, there were the entrepreneurs who imported bonded Chinese coolies to work on the hardest menial tasks of building railroads and cities for the new industrial colossus. There was also the considerable internal migration of black people born into slavery in the South, who had achieved freedom by manumission or by the much more common method of fleeing to the sanctuary of cities in the North, where they were henceforth to be paid even less for the same amount of work than the pittances given the native and immigrant white poor.

To the owners of lodging houses and tenements, these waves of new urban poor were recurring bonanzas. Now the numbers of human beings paying rent for lodging in such buildings could be trebled and quadrupled—and quite legally. In the absence of any laws that for health and/or safety reasons limited the number of paying tenants who could be crowded into a single poorly ventilated room, the landlords themselves were constantly amazed at how profitably crowded the abodes of the poor could become.

In Boston, Shattuck observed, writes the American historian of medicine and public health John Duffy, that "whereas the average single dwelling held eleven persons in 1845, by 1850 there were parts of town in which the average had jumped to thirty-seven. Only two or three cities had any decent kind of water system, and even in these the best that the lower-income groups could hope for was one hydrant for every fifteen families. No city had a sewerage system worthy of the name, and the reek of overflowing privies in the impoverished sections must have been beyond imagination. Adding to the foul atmosphere were the dairies, stables, manure piles, and heaps of garbage scattered through the towns. Butchers and slaughterers frequently let blood flow into the gutters and simply piled offal and hides next to their places of business. Tanners and fat- and bone-boilers gathered hides and offal in open wagons, thus adding further to the already pungent aromas. Rivers, creeks, streams, and brooks flowing through the cities had all become open sewers by midcentury. Shallow wells, which still supplied most city-dwellers with water, were polluted beyond redemption. The wonder is not that mortality rates were soaring but that so many of the poor survived."[9]

In America and Europe the poor were not the only victims of urban infections born of overcrowding, ambient filth, and malnutrition. They were merely the first to be infected. Infectious diseases spread from town to country, from hovel to palace; microbial disease agents are not class-conscious. From plague and typhus to cholera and smallpox, the world's infectious diseases killed more monarchs than all the fiercest wars and the most regicidal revolutions in history. Kings killed by smallpox have included Pharaoh Ramses V of Egypt, who died in 1132 B.C., Louis XV of France, William II of Orange, Peter II of Russia, and Emperor Joseph I of Germany. England's Queen Elizabeth I in 1562, when she was twenty-nine, survived a smallpox infection that left her bald and her face blemished with lifelong scars. The poor might predominate on the death rolls of smallpox and other preventable urban diseases, but they are never there alone for very long.

Between 1820 and 1875, all America's leading cities were hit by great and recurring epidemics of smallpox, cholera, and typhoid fever, although "the important causes of death were tuberculosis, and diarrhea and enteritis of babies."[10] Between the Civil War and the Spanish-American War, Philadelphia was the healthiest city in the United States. Philadelphia had a total death rate that was half or less than half the death rates of New York, Chicago, New Orleans, and other American cities. For the five years between 1868 and 1872, Philadelphia had a smallpox death rate of 132.5 per 100,000 population. This was high, but not quite as high as the death rates in Philadelphia for three other preventable diseases of poverty, crowding, and environmental degradation. During those same years, the death rate for pulmonary tuberculosis in Philadelphia was 320.7 per 100,000 population. The death rate for infant diarrhea and enteritis—intestinal disorders caused by microbes and viruses in contaminated water and food, and exacerbated by chronic malnutrition—was 235.4 per 100,000 population, or not quite twice the smallpox mortality toll. The death rate for pneumonia, a not very common disease prior to the Industrial Revolution, was 153 per 100,000 population in the healthy Philadelphia of 1868–1872.

Even in the twentieth century, after most American communities adopted—at least on paper—Shattuck's recommendations for universal smallpox vaccinations, 48,907 cases of smallpox were reported in the United States in 1930. On the eve of World War II in 1939, 9,875 cases were reported by physicians in the United States.

These figures did not compare very favorably with those of France, Germany, England, Sweden, and Switzerland. Germany, Sweden, and Switzerland reported zero cases of smallpox in 1939. France reported five cases of smallpox in metropolitan France and 4,772 smallpox cases in French Indo-china (now Vietnam, Laos, and Cambodia), and England reported a total of only one case in England and Wales combined in 1939, but 133,616 cases (an obvious undercount) in British India (now India and Pakistan).[11]

The vast differences between the smallpox attack rates of such imperialist countries as France and England and what were then their Asian colonies again underscore the fact that after Jenner made the disease vaccine-preventable in 1796, smallpox has been largely the product of the social values and political decisions of the world's great nations. Obviously, the vaccine prevention of smallpox had a far higher priority in the French and British motherlands than in their colonies, where human lives were patently held in lesser value than at home.

As we know, from the moment Jenner published his account of the smallpox vaccine, various spontaneous and/or highly organized antivaccination movements acted to impede all efforts to eradicate smallpox by using this vaccine. These movements were inspired by different real and imaginary causes.

Some doctors with vested interests in the smallpox variolations that Jenner's vaccine had rendered obsolete spread the cynical but widely accepted claims that cowpox inoculations would transmit bovine features to human faces. Other doctors and laymen opposed vaccinations because of honest fears of the adverse and even rare fatal consequences of inoculations with contaminated materials.

Some sincere sanitarians and public health workers believed that better urban sanitation in industrialized towns and cities, rather than the widespread use of Jenner's vaccine, had reduced the smallpox attack and fatality rates in Europe and America since 1800.

Finally, there was the messianic and/or lunatic fringe, the nonbiologists and nonphysicians whose archetypal members included the playwright, eugenicist, and Fabian socialist Bernard Shaw (1856–1950) and the Scottish-born Pennsylvania oil, railroad, and plate-glass magnate John Pitcairn (1841–1916), president of the Anti-Vaccination League of America, who was appointed in 1911 by Governor Tener to be a member of the Pennsylvania State Vaccination Commission. For the last decade of his life, Pitcairn was the guiding spirit of the Anti-Vaccination League, according to Charles M. Higgins, author of *Horrors of Vaccination Exposed and Illustrated: Petition to the President to Abolish Compulsory Vaccination in the Army and Navy*, which held that "medical compulsion, like religious compulsion, is Un-American and must be abolished" (published by the author in Brooklyn, New York, 1921).

These otherwise highly competent laymen had very different reasons for opposing vaccination, but they shared two beliefs. They were convinced (1) that they knew more about infection and immunity than any doctors and life scientists who had ever lived, and (2) that Jenner's vaccine could only cause harm to and kill people, and had never prevented a single case of smallpox.

The sanitation-versus-vaccination controversy raged during the last third of the nineteenth century. Oddly enough, this controversy peaked in Gloucester, the principal town in Jenner's native Gloucestershire, in 1896, the hundredth anniversary of his first use of arm-to-arm cowpox inoculations in people. A few years earlier, the Gloucester Anti-Vaccination Society had "formally presented Gloucester to the Royal Commissioners on Vaccination as a sample of how a well-ordered town could defy smallpox unaided by vaccination."

Now, on the centennial of Jenner's vaccine, a massive smallpox epidemic broke out in this well-sanitized town. Immediately, the London Anti-Vaccination Society and the London Society for the Abolition of Compulsory Vaccination dispatched activists to Gloucester. There they staged meetings at which Jenner was denounced as a charlatan. They also spread the charge that "the epidemic was a veritable judgment on the city for its insanitary and even filthy condition, and that vaccination had no more to do with the matter than Registration [of births, deaths, and the causes of these deaths] had."[12]

Thanks to this national Registration Act of 1834, more objective observers were able to determine that while the reduction of overcrowding in dwelling places had probably helped reduce the smallpox attack and death rates to some degree, other general sanitation measures dealing with water, sewage, and pollution had little or no effect on smallpox. Glasgow, for example, was one of the least sanitary cities in all the British Isles; the Glasgow stinks made the endemic London stench seem quite bearable. Prior to the large-scale smallpox vaccinations of infants and young children, nineteen out of every one hundred deaths from all causes in Glasgow were due to smallpox alone—close to 20 percent of the city's entire death toll. "Under vaccination, the 19 were reduced in six years to less than 9, and in the next six years to less than 4. At the same time, whooping cough became more prevalent and measles increased enormously."[13]

Dr. E. J. Edwardes, secretary of the Imperial Vaccination League, made a study of the documented effects of compulsory and voluntary smallpox vaccinations in eight northern and central European countries during the smallpox pandemic of 1870–1875. During that pandemic, the 1871 smallpox deaths reached 2,432 per million population in London; 6,326 per million population in Berlin; and 10,750 per million population in Hamburg. At that time, England had a fairly good but poorly enforced set of laws for the compulsory infant vaccination; Prussia was not to have a viable compulsory vaccination law for children until after 1874.

Edwardes's carefully assembled data showed that in countries with moderately to really well-enforced compulsory vaccination programs for all infants—England, Scotland, Bavaria, and Sweden—the combined average smallpox death rate for the pandemic years 1871–1875 was 338 deaths per million population.

In contrast to these rates were those reported by the health ministries of four European countries without any compulsory vaccination programs for infants: Prussia, Austria, Belgium, and Holland. In the pandemic years 1870–1875, these four countries had a combined average smallpox death rate of 1,141 per million population, or three times the smallpox mortality rates of the countries with compulsory smallpox vaccination for infants and young children.[14]

Despite these convincing proofs that universal compulsory vaccination laws prevented and, as demonstrated in Prussia between 1874 and 1879, were thoroughly capable of completely eradicating domestic smallpox in any nation that cared really to make the effort, the clinical reality persisted that, in some individuals, smallpox vaccination induced serious and at times fatal side effects.

Nearly all these adverse and killing consequences were due to contaminants in the vaccines themselves. It took a few decades for it to become evident that, exactly as had happened with smallpox virus inoculations before they were finally outlawed, human arm-to-arm transmission of cowpox virus could and at times actually did also transfer the microbial agents of hepatitis, syphilis, leprosy, and other infections present in the bodies of human lymph donors. This danger was eliminated by switching from arm-to-arm transfers of cowpox virus back to calf-to-human routes of transmission.

In New York City, where postvaccinal complications forced the abandonment of compulsory vaccinations in the city's public elementary schools in 1867, the city's three-year-old Board of Health concluded that the only way to guarantee the safety and effectiveness of all cowpox vaccines was not only to go back to the calf-to-arm route of transmission but also to make the vaccines themselves. Their initial efforts were not very promising, but the Board's doctors and veterinarians persisted. A vaccine farm was opened in 1876 at Lakeview, New Jersey, by the Board of Health. This successful vaccine operation was moved to New York City in 1884, and continued to produce good vaccine from clean calves.

In 1875, the last year of the world smallpox pandemic, there had been 4,648 reported cases of smallpox, 484 of them fatal, in New York City. A year earlier the state legislature authorized the New York City Board of Health to establish, at municipal expense, a "permanent corps of vaccinators" who would, according to the Board's fourth annual report to the people of the city, "visit your house twice each year, and offer free vaccination." These vaccinators—eight doctors constituting the permanent corps of vaccinators with the rank of inspector, and fifteen to fifty other physicians who were hired as temporary vaccinators during the year—visited schools, orphanages, neighborhood dispensaries, and hospitals, as well as factories, banks, stores, and horse-car railroads where people in need of primary and secondary revaccinations worked.

During 1893, for example, the vaccinators performed 36,994 primary vaccinations and 175,197 secondary, or booster, vaccinations, for a total of 212,191 smallpox immunizations. The Board noted in its annual report for that year that "the large number of adult cases of smallpox removed to the hospital during the latter part of August and September made it evident that revaccination, as well as primary vaccination, was necessary in order to protect the public from this disease." This effort brought results. "During the year 1895 there were only ten reported deaths from smallpox in the entire city of New York, a city which, according to the census of April 1895, had a total population of 1,851,060."[15]

Before American and European health services established national agencies—such as the Bureau of Biologics, now part of the Food and Drug Administration (FDA)—to test all vaccines for safety and effectiveness, many inferior (and often criminally negligent) manufacturing procedures used to turn out commercial vaccines often caused tragic disasters. Not only were a large percentage of the available products sold as vaccines unable to prevent smallpox, but they were also frequently contaminated with wide arrays of microbial disease agents. Of these vaccine contaminants, the most fatal were the bacilli that caused the incurable disease tetanus (lockjaw). In the United States, most of the deaths that followed smallpox vaccinations were caused by tetanus.

Prior to the advent of germ theory and the isolation of the tetanus bacilli, many doctors believed that postvaccinal lockjaw was caused by the cowpox vaccine itself. After germ theory, it was demonstrated, principally by Robert Koch in Germany and S. Monckton Copeman in England, that glycerin inhibited the growth and proliferation of all pathogenic bacteria. The addition of this bacteriostatic substance to cowpox vaccines helped reduce the instances of bacterial contaminants in commercial vaccines.

Glycerinated lymphs could not, however, completely eliminate the dangers of fatal tetanus infections following some vaccinations against smallpox. Many women chose to be vaccinated in the legs, near the ankles, which in the Victorian and Edwardian eras left their scars all but invisible. In the days before electric trolley cars and private automobiles, the streets of most European and American cities bore liberal accretions of horse manure, one of the favorite nutrients of the tetanus bacilli. Various epidemiological studies in Philadelphia, Glasgow, Camden, New Jersey, and London made in 1902 showed that "as we can never be certain that street dust may not contain tetanus spores, women who insist upon being vaccinated on the leg run a slight risk that, in the apparently unavoidable road sweeping process which their skirts sometimes perform, they may inoculate themselves with that disease [tetanus]."[16]

Finally, in the absence of microbial contaminants in the vaccines, and of tetanus spores on city streets, there were still adverse and even fatal complications following the vaccination of certain children and adults with perfectly good vaccines that could be given without causing harm to all but one in a few million individuals.

At times, children and adults would scratch at an itching and still infectious cowpox sore, and this would spread the cowpox viruses and their pustules to other parts of the body. More rarely, disseminated cowpox virus (vaccinia) sores would spread without scratching and cover a child's entire face and body. In perhaps one case in every ten or twenty million children vaccinated, the cowpox vaccine would cause systemic infections that could result in encephalitis—inflammation of the brain—with its attendant risks of permanent brain damage and even death.

For the better part of two centuries after Jenner, none of the known adverse effects of cowpox vaccinations against smallpox occurred in numbers great enough even to come near equalling the calculable risks of not vaccinating all children in any given country.

There would eventually come a time, particularly in the United States, the Soviet Union, and other giant industrial states, when the risks of continuing vaccinations in countries where mass immunization programs had eradicated domestic smallpox would prove too costly to be tolerated.

That time was to begin shortly after World War II.

Despite the fact that Jenner's vaccine was widely used in many countries for well over a century, by the end of World War I, smallpox was still endemic in most affluent countries, and it was both endemic and frequently epidemic in most poor nations where the major portion of the human race lived and still lives.

In 1920, for example, 401,318 cases of smallpox (98,684 of them in the United States) were reported by that very tiny percentage of the world's nations that collected and released such data at that time. Smallpox was not then a notifiable disease in most of the world. The cases reported to local and national health agencies were far outnumbered by the cases of smallpox in those poor countries that then suffered the most outbreaks: the majority of the African, Asian, Middle Eastern, and Latin American countries, which neither registered nor reported data on any diseases at all.

In most countries that did report cases and deaths from smallpox and other diseases, all infectious diseases were as a general rule grievously underreported (as they still are in the United States). A caveat printed on the table prepared by the World Health Organization (WHO) on the numbers of smallpox cases reported around the world between 1920 and 1980 warns that "these numbers must be interpreted with extreme caution, due to underreporting of cases. Except where endemic transmission of smallpox was close to being interrupted, it is generally safe to assume that no more than 1% of the actual number of cases was reported." This caveat applies to most of the smallpox numbers cited below, particularly from nations other than the economically advanced ones in Europe, North America, the Antipodes, and Asia (primarily Japan).

Smallpox was not an internationally notifiable disease until 1926. In that year the Japanese delegation to the Thirteenth International Sanitary Conference proposed that smallpox be made notifiable to this world health agency. With such mandatory registration, epidemiologists and health agencies worldwide would at least know where smallpox was still infecting people and threatening to cross national frontiers.

A Doctor Carrière, speaking for the Swiss delegation, rose to attack the Japanese proposal on the grounds that smallpox "had, in reality, no place in an international convention. It is not a pestilential disease in the proper sense of the term; it is," said this Swiss doctor, "in effect a disease that exists everywhere. There is probably not a single country of which it can be said that there are no cases of smallpox."[17]

The reason for the Swiss government's opposition to reporting national smallpox data to international health conventions was hardly a secret to any of the sophisticated health workers from many nations gathered at that meeting. Squeaky-clean, tourism-dependent Switzerland was just then emerging from a six-year epidemic of smallpox, the end product of the rise in the world's smallpox attack rates that marked World War I and its chaotic postwar effects. In 1920 Switzerland had reported exactly two cases of smallpox. During 1921 she suffered 596 cases of smallpox, most of them probably imported by native and foreign travelers. One year later the smallpox incidence reached 1,153 cases, to be followed by 2,146 smallpox cases in 1923; 1,234 cases in 1924; 325 cases in 1925; and 54 cases in 1926, when the Swiss delegate suggested that no nation would ever be completely free of smallpox. (He was wrong, of course, on two counts. By the next year (1927) Switzerland itself would be down to zero smallpox cases, and for most years after that would remain free of the disease to the present day; between 1926 and 1980, a grand total of nine smallpox cases were reported during eight of these years, the last one in 1963.)

Smallpox epidemiological data, particularly in terms of the average annual number of cases—918—reported in tiny Switzerland during the half dozen years of the postwar smallpox pandemic, were hardly conducive to tourism.

Other nations backed the Swiss opposition to revealing their smallpox cases, and for very similar reasons. In the end a compromise was struck "between the Japanese and the Swiss points of view," writes Dr. Norman Howard-Jones. "The disease became notifiable under the International Sanitary Regulations of 1926, but only in the case of epidemics, and not, as with

77

the three traditionally international diseases [cholera, plague, and yellow fever], on the appearance of a first case." In short, smallpox cases that became so numerous as to become front-page news the world over were henceforth made officially notifiable.

Smallpox was reported in ninety-five countries in 1945, at the close of World War II. The numbers of cases reported, which were of course far fewer than the actual numbers in most countries, ranged from 287,074 in India; 17,800 in Japan; 12,283 in what is now Tanzania; 1,355 (down from a reported 11,194 cases the year before) in Egypt; 1,055 in the United States; forty-seven in France; and precisely one case in Sweden.

By that time, doctors agreed that smallpox was one human disease that could be eradicated from this earth. To begin with, there was Jenner's vaccine, which was effective and generally safe for nearly all people. Then there was the fact that smallpox is a virus infection for which there are no nonhuman reservoirs of the causal virus. Finally, there are no asymptomatic human carriers of the smallpox virus: Because of the pus-filled eruptions (pustules) that break out all over their faces and bodies, the victims are easy to find and isolate, and all their recent human contacts can be found and vaccinated. Even without such post-World War II technological advances as Collier's freeze-dried vaccine of 1954 and the Wyeth bifurcated vaccinating needle of 1966, there were countries (like Switzerland and Sweden) where domestic endemic smallpox was completely eradicated by effective vaccination and revaccination policies.

Sweden, where universal vaccination had been made compulsory in 1814 and compulsory revaccination mandated before 1850, wiped out domestic endemic smallpox by the end of the nineteenth century. France and England, which had good but palpably unenforced universal compulsory vaccination laws on their books, did not start to implement them seriously until after the pandemic of 1870–1875—and they took over a half century to catch up with medically more prudent nations such as Sweden, Denmark, and Bavaria.

After World War II, one of the first goals of the United Nations' World Health Organization (WHO) became the global eradication of smallpox. The first of the WHO smallpox programs, proposed by the Soviet Union and aimed at vaccinating 80 percent of the world's population, failed. The second WHO program raised the goal to vaccinating 100 percent of the world's people. It too failed. In 1966 the WHO appropriated $2.5 million to start up its third attempt to eradicate smallpox by mass vaccinations. This effort finally succeeded.

It is a matter of record that in 1967, the year in which the third WHO smallpox eradication program got under way, ten million smallpox cases—two million of them fatal—were reported by forty-two nations. In thirty-four of these reporting nations, smallpox was endemic. In the eight other reporting nations, most of the fatal and nonfatal cases were imported into the more or less smallpox-free countries from near or distant lands having endemic smallpox.

A little more than ten years later, on October 22, 1977—a disgracefully long 181 years after Edward Jenner vaccinated the first human being with his new vaccine—the world's last known case of naturally acquired smallpox was reported in Somalia.

Officially, the world is now completely free of smallpox. For safety's sake, supplies of sufficient freeze-dried smallpox to immunize 200 million people are now maintained by the WHO in two refrigerated depots on two continents. Experts are certain that these reserve vaccines will never have to be used.

These are the well-known facts about the program that eventually rid the world of smallpox once the most powerful nations decided it was time to heed Jenner's plea to use his vaccine for "the annihilation of the Smallpox, the most dreadful scourge of the human species."

Less well known are the circumstances surrounding the development of the political and economic considerations, and the epidemiological and clinical immunological findings, which all combined to make this WHO smallpox eradication program succeed where its immediate postwar precursors had failed.

No smallpox cases were reported by physicians in the United States after 1949. The nation whose third President, Thomas Jefferson, had played such a valiant role in introducing Jenner's vaccine was now at last smallpox-free (even if more than a century after the time Jefferson believed this would happen).

Nevertheless, for more than two decades after 1949 the real and present danger of smallpox infections imported from smallpox-endemic nations caused millions of children and thousands of high-risk adults (primarily military servicemen) to undergo routine vaccinations and revaccinations as before.

Not until the early 1960s when University of Colorado professor of pediatrics, Dr. C. Henry Kempe started writing about the continuing risks of adverse side effects of vaccinations in children now that the United States was smallpox-free did American public health officials begin to take a hard look at the level of the clinical complications of the disease and at the overall dollar costs of routine vaccinations against it. Until then, the known fatal and maiming effects of smallpox itself overshadowed the well-known if very rare adverse effects of antismallpox vaccinations.[18]

After Kempe raised the clinical problems that had resulted from a few vaccinations, epidemiologists began to consider what steps would have to be taken before it would be safe to end the routine primary and secondary vaccinations of children and military personnel. Obviously, with smallpox still endemic and even epidemic in scores of other countries around the world, there remained the ever-present danger of imported cases causing domestic smallpox outbreaks, particularly in America's most densely populated cities.

A new Bureau of Smallpox Eradication was established in 1966 at the federal Centers for Disease Control (CDC) in Atlanta, Georgia. Its basic function was to make it possible to safely end routine smallpox vaccinations in the United States. There was only one way this could be accomplished, and that, of course, was by helping to eradicate smallpox the world over.

A study made by Dr. J. Michael Lane and Norman W. Axnick of the new Bureau showed that in 1968 an estimated 14.2 million people in the United States were vaccinated against smallpox, 5.6 million of them for the first time. These vaccinations produced 8,024 complications, but only 153 were major ones.

These 153 major complications occurred at the rate of 0.08 per 100,000 Americans, which made them statistically insignificant. Human beings, however, are not statistics. Of these major complications, nine had caused death. Another sixteen vaccinees suffered postvaccinal encephalitis. Of these sixteen patients with inflammation of the brain caused by smallpox vaccinations, three developed permanent mental damage, and one had to be institutionalized for life.

The economic costs of vaccinating children and adult civilians in 1968 had come to $135.6 million. The total dollar cost of the control of smallpox—vaccinations, hospitalization for postvaccinal complications, and public health inspection and quarantine measures to protect the United States against imported smallpox viruses—came to over $159 million in 1968, when the purchasing power of the dollar was more than twice its current levels. (For reasons apparent only to their editors, this study was rejected by every American medical journal to which Lane and Axnick had submitted it for publication.)

The U.S. Public Health Service, of which the CDC is part, actually got into the world smallpox eradication picture in 1963 by a very indirect route. In that year Dr. Harry Myers of the Bureau of Biologics conducted the first large-scale trials of the new Edmonston B strain of the live virus measles vaccine in Upper Volta. The trials were successful, and seven neighboring African countries then asked the United States ambassadors to their nations to help them eradicate measles as had been done in Upper Volta.

The State Department's U.S. Agency for International Development (AID) asked the CDC to send some physicians and other public health professionals to train local vaccinators and set up national immunization programs in these West African nations. The CDC agreed to do so on condition that smallpox eradication be added to the original measles program, and the AID officials acquiesced.

By 1966 the dual measles-smallpox eradication program, with the assistance of a $47 million grant from AID (of which only $30 million eventually had to be spent), had been expanded to include twenty nations in West Africa.

Toward the end of 1966, CDC units directed by Dr. William Foege in Eastern Nigeria and Dr. J. Michael Lane in Sierra Leone and Guinea had discovered that rather than attempting the mass vaccinations of entire populations, the technique of surveillance containment could make villages, regions, and entire nations completely smallpox-free. Surveillance containment meant simply training local laymen to find everyone in a specific area with active cases of smallpox, to question them carefully, and then to search out and vaccinate every one of their human contacts still at risk of contracting the disease and transmitting its viruses to other people. This technique was ultimately to play a major role around the world.

In 1967, when the third global WHO smallpox eradication program was launched, the field-experienced CDC doctors and laboratory workers in West Africa were available to enter the United Nations program. They were soon able to convince their international peers of the clinical effectiveness of surveillance containment. Dr. Donald A. Henderson, chief of the surveillance section of the CDC Bureau of Epidemiology, was seconded to the WHO to direct its program for the next decade. In 1971, the WHO program officially adopted the surveillance-containment strategy.

During the same year, thanks to the measurable results of the WHO program, the CDC was at last able to recommend that compulsory and routine voluntary smallpox vaccinations be ended in the United States. The CDC recommendations are not mandatory, but they are regarded seriously by state and local health officials and by nongovernment medical practitioners throughout the nation. Within a year, smallpox vaccinations in the United States dropped from sixteen million to eight million annually. Then, by slower stages, they dropped to about 600,000 routine and what the CDC terms "inappropriate" vaccinations by 1980.

In just over ten years of the WHO's planned cooperative efforts, 200,000 people in forty countries—most of them nondoctors trained by seven hundred doctors and health professionals from over seventy participating countries—spent $300 million, and used forty million bifurcated vaccinating needles to administer 24,000 million (2.4 billion) doses of smallpox vaccine. The Soviet Union donated 140 million doses of smallpox vaccine; the United States forty million doses; twenty other nations combined to donate another 220 million doses.

The remaining two billion—i.e. two thousand million—doses of vaccine used to eradicate smallpox from the human experience were made in new laboratories, set up with the help of visiting WHO specialists in India, Iran, Pakistan, Brazil, Kenya, Guinea, and Argentina, which were staffed and operated by WHO-trained nonprofessional nationals of these poor countries. Before the program ended, large amounts of smallpox vaccines made by newly trained people in new facilities were donated to the smallpox eradication workers in even poorer countries.

The total cost to all the world's nations of the WHO smallpox eradication program came to only $300 million, or far less than the going price of a half dozen F-16 or equivalent fighter-bombers. Economically, by far the greatest gainers of the planetary eradication of smallpox were, of course, the richest nations, starting with the United States. As early as 1979, only two years into this smallpox-free age, the WHO was able to estimate that "over a billion dollars is the amount being saved by the industrially advanced countries as a direct result of the eradication of smallpox."

It would be nice to believe that sheer altruism was the primary or even a significant inspiration for launching the successful global smallpox eradication program of 1966–1977. It would also be nice to believe in the corporeal existence of Santa Claus and the Tooth Fairy, and that the Peter Pans who soar over the heads of delightedly screaming children in packed theaters at Christmastime are actually real, flying, and eternally young boys and not frightened actresses dangling from piano wires manipulated by bored stagehands. The truth is that the empathy and compassion of the powerful, industrialized, and, as of 1967, smallpox-free superstates—starting with the United States, the Soviet Union, England, and France—had very little if anything at all to do with the mounting of this astoundingly inexpensive effort to stamp out smallpox in bone-poor countries where vaccinations of all sorts were largely unknown and smallpox still the "dreadful scourge of the human species" it had been in Jenner's day.

Doctors, starting with Jenner, Lettsom, Haygarth and Waterhouse, and insightful laymen, such as Jefferson, who each strove for the better part of two centuries for the universal vaccine-eradication of smallpox, had very little to do with the ultimate political and economic decisions to launch the third WHO smallpox eradication program.

The WHO program owed its political origins, its adequate funding, and its epidemiologically rational execution to the painful truth that until smallpox was eradicated everywhere in the world, no nation—no matter how effective its domestic smallpox eradication program was, or however efficient its international smallpox surveillance and quarantine machinery—would ever be truly free of the clinical and economic costs of defending itself against the existence of the disease anywhere else in the world. As long as smallpox persisted among the impoverished people, who constitute most of the human race, the richer and domestically smallpox-free nations would have to continue to vaccinate their children and subject them to the statistically rare but humanly tragic risks of minor and major postvaccinal complications.

In the United States, in order to rid ourselves of the risks of both smallpox and vaccinations against smallpox, we first had to invest our skills and dollars in the international effort to help scores of less fortunate nations rid their entire populations of the same risks. In the end the cost of eradicating smallpox proved to be considerably more modest than the infinitely greater human and economic costs of permitting this vaccine-preventable pestilence to continue to prey upon humankind.

The same lesson has yet to be learned, starting in the United States, about other fatal and damaging infectious diseases for which good vaccines now exist, or for which good vaccines can be developed. Great nations must recognize and live up to what, when this century was young, an activist president of the American Medical Association called their moral obligation to be intelligent.

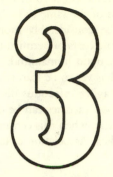

ON THE EVE OF GERM THEORY, SANITARY REFORMS HELP REDUCE SOME CONTAGIONS

Our children perish out of our homes ... because there is ... a want of sanitary discipline and a want of medical knowledge.... We fail to prevent disease, and in the case of our children we fail to cure it. Think of it again. Of all the coffins that are made in London, more than one in every three is made for a little child: a child that has not yet two figures to its age. Although science has advanced, although vaccination has been discovered and brought into general use, although medical knowledge is tenfold greater than it was fifty years ago, we still do not gain more than a diminution of two per cent in the terrible mortality among children.

—CHARLES DICKENS AND
HENRY MORLEY, M.D., 1852[1]

Early in the Industrial Revolution, only thirty-four years after Watt's rotary steam engine harnessed the energy locked in coal to the Satanic Wheels[2] of the new mills, mines, and factories of England, Europe, and even the United States, there was a fleeting moment—the year was 1819, the setting Padua, Italy—when the germ theory nearly came of age, thanks to the demonstrably life-saving discovery of three men. They were Abbot Dr. Pietro Melo, director of the Vigodarzere Botanical Gardens at Savonara; Dr. Bartholomeo Bizio, then a young pharmacist and student at the University of Padua, where he was later to be a professor; and Dr. Vicenzo Sette, physician and district health officer in the town of Piove di Sacco, near Padua.

Prior to the thoroughly forgotten but seminal discovery of these Italian investigators, other men in other times had advanced what might be called pregerm theories of contagion.

Marcus Terentius Varro (116–26 B.C.), a friend of Cicero and a writer on agriculture, warned against building a villa near marshes, since invisible animalcules—microscopic animals—that he claimed breed in swamps and cannot be seen by human eyes could get into the human body through the nose and mouth and cause "obstinate diseases," of which malaria was probably the chief disorder. Varro deduced the existence of such disease-causing animalcules but never actually saw them. It would be nearly two millenia before the microscopic creatures were finally seen.

Girolamo Fracastoro (1478–1553), better remembered by his Latin name of Hieronymus Fracastorius, was lecturer on logic at the University of Padua until bloody political upheavals forced the closing of the school in 1507. Fracastorius subsequently lived through a great plague epidemic in Verona, and made other observations which led to his seventy-seven-page book on contagions in 1546. In this book he wrote of the *seminaria* of disease, which the historian of bacteriology, William Bulloch, remarked "may be translated as the 'seeds' or 'germs' of disease, remembering, however, that he knew nothing about germs as we understand them today."

In 1675 Anton van Leeuwenhoek of Delft, Holland, started using a primitive handheld microscope to find what he too called animalcules, which he drew and described for the Royal Society in London. Leeuwenhoek found these "little animals" in the scrapings of his teeth, in rainwater, well water, seawater, pepper water, river water, spittle and tongue scrapings from people, and other biological sources. He kept at these observations for many years, and as late as 1716 when he was eighty-four, the Delft burgher was still sending descriptions of his microscopic findings to the Dutch doctor Hermann Boerhaave and other scientists.

Although Leeuwenhoek found more animalcules—some of which, to judge from his drawings, were clearly not little animals but full-sized bacteria—in the mouths of people "who don't ever clean their teeth, whereby such a stench comes from the mouth of many of 'em, that you can scarce bear to talk to them" than he found in the mouths of more fastidious people, all his samples of human bacteria came from the mouths of healthy persons. Leeuwenhoek never associated his microbial animalcules with any human disorder other than bad breath.

Athanasius Kircher (1602–1680), a Jesuit who studied Classical and Oriental languages and taught at various German universities, published many books on many subjects. In two of them, written in 1646 and 1650, Kircher wrote that human effluvia—foul-smelling exhalations or air—were alive with invisible living bodies, which penetrated linen sheets and porous surfaces and "found new hot-beds of contagion."

In 1720 a London physician, Benjamin Marten, published *A New Theory of Consumption; more especially of phtisis or consumption of the lungs.* This book offered a theory to explain why people in close contact with tuberculosis patients often contract the disease themselves. The cause of consumption, Marten suggested, "may possibly be some certain species of animalcula or wonderfully minute living creatures that by their peculiar shape or disagreeable parts are inimicable to our nature," and find their way to our lungs.

Four decades later the Viennese physician Antonius Plenciz (1705–1786) wrote that specific microbes caused specific infectious diseases. "Plenciz believed, moreover, that these organisms were capable of multiplication in the body, and suggested the possibility of their being conveyed from place to place through the air."[3] Plenciz was unable, however, to prove these ultimately correct suppositions clinically.

None of these early concepts of microscopic disease agents had ever been tested in people nor employed in nonmedical efforts to save human lives. In 1819, however, the prehistory of germ theory took a dramatic and demonstrably life-preserving step forward.

Early in July 1819, Abbot Pietro Melo was called to the house of "a certain Borgato (known as Culata)" in Savonara, Italy, where he was shown a sick child and a potful of polenta (corn mush) discolored with what looked like spots of blood. These red spots, which appeared from time to time in different places on foods, church wafers, and in other materials, were not unknown in the countryside. Indeed, to this very day, in the United States and elsewhere, they materialize on cottage cheese, cereals, and other common foods.[4]

The Borgato family blamed the red spots on the polenta for their child's sickness, and assured the abbot that the red spots were caused by witchcraft. They wanted the abbot to bless their house and expel the evil spirits. He managed, he wrote later, to convince the family that the red spots were a natural occurrence and of no harm to their child or to anyone else.

The appearance of bloodlike spots on foods was not a new phenomenon. Before the Christian Era, they had been considered omens of either good or bad fortune in the armies of Alexander the Great, the Etruscans, the Romans, and other Mediterranean nations. In 1290 A.D. when the red spots appeared on a sacramental wafer in a Paris church, they were identified as the Blood of the Lord, which had been caused to materialize by the sins of the Jews of Paris. This led to a pogrom in which thousands of Jews were burned or hacked to death. This was the first of a long series of historically recorded large-scale massacres of Jews to be caused by the appearance of red spots on holy wafers and other edibles during the next three centuries in France, Germany, Italy, Belgium and Poland, and there was probably a considerably larger number of historically unrecorded smaller pogroms.

On August 2, 1819 the red spots appeared on polenta in the home of a family named Pittarello in Legnaro, a village near Padua. A priest came to bless this house, but the next day more red spots materialized on rice soup and a boiled hen in the family's kitchen. It became a local sensation, known so widely that Dr. Sette went to look into the matter. As he was to write later, the road from Padua to Legnaro was crowded with "persons of every category, every age, from our province or from others" who flocked to see what was happening. "Speeches, deductions, interpretations and even furious arguments reigned, while the unhappy family, already upset and mortified by the mysterious visitation, trembled for fear of future extermination, as predicted by the crowds. The predominating fanaticism was so great as to cause the populace to believe that the red color was pure blood, which had been caused to spring from the polenta by a supernatural power . . ."

Melo studied the phenomenon and concluded that the red color was caused by a spontaneous fermentation of the polenta. Dr. Bizio, however, reproduced the red spots on polenta in his laboratory. As the American microbiologist Eugene Gaughran wrote, his study "may be considered the first recorded use of a solid culture medium (corn meal mush) in the culture of a bacterium, and antedates the work of Fresenius and Ehrenberg with potato by more than 30 years." Bizio found the reddening was caused by small masses of microscopic fungi unlike any ever seen before. He named the fungus *Serratia* (after the Italian inventor Serafino Serrati) *marcescens* (meaning putrifying or decaying).

Sette also produced the red spots on polenta in his laboratory, and also isolated the fungi that caused them, which he named *Zaogalactina imetrofa.* Under either name the organisms were subsequently classified as bacteria, and through succeeding years were given over twenty names. Finally, in our own times, they again came to be called *Serratia marcescens*—rodlike bacilli of a type originally described by Leeuwenhoek.

Unfortunately, once the natural causes of the red spots were resolved and the results published by Bizio and Sette, they each abandoned further studies of the natural history of *S. marcescens.*

With the work of these pioneer investigators, a venerable rationale for massacring Jews was eradicated from the cultural fabric of Western civilization. Of course, this did not end anti-Semitism, and bigots went on planning and executing pogroms and holocausts for over a century, but never again was *S. marcescens* to trigger another major massacre of Jews. Early in the germ theory era in 1894, Professor E. Schurlen of the University of Strasbourg made a study of pogroms initiated by red-pigmented colonies of this bacterium, and he concluded that starting in the year 1290, *S. marcescens* had caused more human deaths than many of the infection-causing bacteria then known to science.

In the absence of germ theory, doctors and nonmedical people concerned with human health in the industrializing nations concentrated their main efforts on the prevention of the contagious diseases that proliferated in the degraded environments of the new technological stage of civilization. The land of the birth of the Industrial Revolution was quite inevitably also the nation that produced the earliest efforts to mitigate the degradations of the human environment—the crowding, the poverty, the rising rates of job-associated diseases and injuries, and the burgeoning and now endemic levels of pneumonia, fatal diarrheas and other enteric diseases, tuberculosis, rheumatic fever, measles, smallpox, ague (malaria), scarlatina (scarlet fever), typhus, typhoid, and other infections so clearly linked with crowding, poverty, and the lack of hygiene. Then in 1830 a new affliction was visited on the overcrowded cities of Europe—Asiatic cholera, an unwelcome dividend of the vastly increased and highly profitable trade with India and the Orient made possible by the explosive productivity of the new industrial age.

People did not need a medical degree—merely a good nose, a pair of seeing eyes, and some memories or knowledge of the state of public health before the Thames turned into a stinking cesspool—to recognize the chronological relationships between the degradation of the environment and the proliferation of contagions. A little experience in the practice of medicine, however, helped sharpen one's insights, as the London general practitioner Dr. Charles Hall (1745–1825) wrote, since "the principal effect of civilization [industrialization] is the reduction of the mass of people in civilized [industrialized] societies to their present condition. Of this condition, i.e. the manner in which people live, who has more opportunities of acquiring the knowledge than a Physician? He is admitted into the dwelling of all ranks of people, and into the innermost parts of them: he sees them by the fire-side, at their tables, and in their beds: he sees them at work, and at their recreations: he sees them in health, in sickness, and in the article of death: . . . . The physician therefore is put in possession of more facts with respect to the condition of the people than any other person . . ."[5]

Concerned physicians, because of their experiences with the diseases of "civilization," predictably were in the forefront of all individual and organized efforts to make daily life safer for "the mass of people." For similar reasons, clergymen, in the established and in dissident churches, often went to extraordinary lengths to make life safer and healthier for the men, women, and children whose labor produced the new wealth.

It was not even necessary to have the existential empathy of a physician or the Christian love of all people to join in the broad social efforts to eradicate the filth and crowding and poverty so many doctors and clergymen perceived as the real causes of killing and crippling contagious diseases. Sincere adherence to the social philosophy of Jeremy Bentham, which held that preventable diseases and deaths, ignorance, and poverty interfered with the goal of the greatest good for the greatest number of people, turned as unsentimental and cold a human being as the barrister and journalist Edwin Chadwick into one of the principal leaders of the great sanitary movement. In the Benthamite philosophy, the waste of human resources (i.e., the failure to make the most capital out of human potentials) was the greatest offense. That Chadwick despised such waste far more than he ever loved people is of less importance than the Herculean roles he would play in the Augean stables that constituted England in most of the nineteenth century.

In 1794, early in the rise of the factory system in England, an outbreak of persistent fever in the children and adults working in textile factories seriously affected production in some Radcliffe mills, in Lancashire. The mill-owners sought help from the doctors of Manchester, where Dr. Thomas Percival, a fifty-four-year-old physician, volunteered to investigate the outbreak. What Percival found in Radcliffe was exactly what prevailed in Manchester and the even newer industrial towns in the Manchester area—the two most preventable of all contemporary causes of fevers, child labor and overcrowding.

When in 1795 Percival and other Manchester physicians accepted the task of organizing and running the new Manchester Board of Health, they spelled out its very specific functions. These were: "To prevent the generation of diseases; to obviate the spreading of them by contagion, and to shorten the duration of those which exist, by affording the necessary aids and comfort to the sick." To make it plain that they were not talking about the planet Mars, but about the dangers to public health particularly apparent in "the large cotton factories established in the town and neighborhood of Manchester," Percival summed up for the town fathers the results of the investigations he and other local doctors had made. This read, in part:

"1. It appears that the children and others who work in the huge factories are peculiarly disposed to be affected by the contagion of fever, and that when such infection is received, it is rapidly propagated, not only amongst those who are crowded together in the same apartments, but in the families and neighborhoods to which they belong. . . .

"4. It appears that the children employed in factories are generally debarred from all opportunities of education, and from moral or religious instruction.

"5. From the excellent regulations which subsist in several cotton factories, it appears that many of these evils may in a considerable degree be obviated; we are therefore warranted by experience, and are assured we shall have the support of the liberal proprietors of these factories, in proposing an application for parliamentary aid . . . to establish a general system of laws for the wise, humane and equal government of all such works."[6]

In 1805, two years after the second edition of Malthus's *Population,* the London physician Charles Hall published a book, *The Effects of Civilization on the People in European States,* as well as a pamphlet, *Observations on the Principal Conclusion in Mr. Malthus' Essay on Population,* which was also reprinted and bound into the book as the appendix.

Hall saw the structure of the new industrialized society as one divided into two basic classes, the rich and the poor, with the poor "being by far the greatest number of the people" in most industrial countries. "Therefore, whatever regards them should be deemed of the greater importance."

To begin with, "The poor are not sufficiently supplied with the necessaries of life," which Dr. Hall defined as adequate proper food, adequate shelter, adequate education, and workplaces and jobs safe for human beings.

What he wrote about food could only have been written by an experienced family doctor. The food of man "is of a mixed nature, partly animal, and partly vegetable. A certain proportion of the former is necessary to the health, strength, and growth of the human species [this was long before proteins found largely in animal foods were known and their role in nutrition understood], and without it those things cannot be obtained. It would be difficult to discover whether the poor have a sufficiency of animal and vegetable food, or by any other method than by considering the quantity of each sort which their nature requires; and their means of obtaining that quantity; or, in other words, what their earnings are, and what quantity of food such earnings could procure." After nearly two centuries, family income remains the best instant gauge of family nutritional status.

Hall argued that if the people who worked for a living, and who produced food and goods worth eight to ten times more money than the total sums of their wages, were more equitably paid, then they, like the rich, would also be able to afford the "necessaries of life" and enjoy equally good health.

Malthus, in a famous passage in each edition of his *Population,* proposed a law "declaring that no child born from any marriage taking place after the expiration of a year from the date of the law . . . should ever be entitled to parish assistance [tax-supported welfare relief]." Of any man who could not find work, Malthus elsewhere in his *Essay* had strongly recommended that "to the punishment of nature should he be left; the punishment of severe want: all parish assistance should be rigidly denied him. He should be taught that the laws of nature had doomed him and his family to starve; that he had no claim on society for the smallest portion of food."

Now, in 1805 Hall answered Malthus. "The treatment of this labouring man, I cannot help saying, appears to me not only inhuman to the last degree, but unjust and iniquitous. I will ask, why is he thus treated? Because, it will be answered, he does not produce by his labour sufficient to maintain his family. But I say he produces six or eight times as much as his family consumes or requires, but which is taken from him by those who produce nothing. What he is entitled to is all that his hands have made or produced, the whole fruits of his labour, not that pittance his wages enable him to purchase."

There was more. "It is not true" that the poor laborer who finds himself in need of parish assistance "has *doomed himself,* or that nature has doomed *him, and his family, to starve* [Hall's emphases]; that cruel doom is brought on him by the rich. If any are to be treated in this cruel manner, it is those who have been rich, and who have never produced any part of all they have consumed. But none ought to receive such hard usage." Hall, who lacked Malthus's cruelty, sought simple equity, not revenge.

Where Malthus, the clergyman turned economist, attacked Jenner's cowpox vaccine as being undue and even dangerous interference with such natural checks on "overpopulation" as smallpox, Hall, the physician, noted that the "destructive disease the small-pox is made milder by inoculation," and that it was shocking to think of Malthus's natural checks as divinely ordained or acceptable to decent people. It was simply not true, Hall wrote, that the only way to keep population down was "by keeping the mass of the people down . . . by bringing scarcity, want, and disease on them," or that the quality of life for the mass of people "must always be a miserable one, and admitting of no mitigation" lest they be tempted to breed more of their kind.

In a chapter titled "The Employments of the Poor Injurious to Health," Hall showed how the physiological, ventilatory, and chemical conditions of jobs in mines, mills, and factories caused diseases, deformities, and deaths. One observation—that in the "great multiplicity of trades in which mercury is made use of," mercury poisoning becomes endemic and that in people with this industrial disease "after suffering excruciating torments they die, with great punctuality, in a year and a half"—is a medical judgment that has stood the test of time.

If Hall lived in an England where "we see half of the children born die before they are two years and a half old; and a very great part of the remainder drop off before they are seven," he also knew how socially skewed these child mortality statistics really were. In a remarkable passage in his book, this London doctor looked beyond these data.

"It has frequently happened to me, and to all other physicians, that, after being called to a child of a man of fortune, ill of this disease [diarrhea or dysentery], whom I have found in a large lofty room, well ventilated, clean and sweet; bed soft, undisturbed by noise, anxiously attended by people relieving each other; furnished with everything the cellars, the kitchen, the garden, the druggist, can furnish; in short, everything the four quarters of the world can supply: after, I say, being with such a patient, we are frequently entreated to visit a child or children of a poor man, in the same illness; several of them generally lying in the same bed; heated by and heating one another, in a small room, corrupted by the exhalations of the whole family; disturbed by one another's cries; their wakefulness and restlessness, the effects of the disorder, increased by vermin and hard beds, covered by filthy clothes; having nothing proper to use from the cellar, the kitchen, the garden, the apothecary's shop; no attendants but the poor mother, worn out by watchings, anxiety, &c.; the father from home, obliged to leave it to get their daily bread.

"That these things happen unavoidably in almost all cases, in poor families, all medical people must bear testimony; and also to the ill effects of them on the sufferers. I have said unavoidably, which is true; for, though single instances by charitable assistance may in some things be relieved, it is impossible that in general the poor can be better supplied; unless you alter the condition of the whole, by giving them good houses, containing more and better rooms; better furniture; better linen; better supplies; in short, making their condition nearer to the first described; that is, wholly altering the condition of that whole order of people."

If Hall was physician enough to be able to state that "this greater mortality among the poor can only be owing to the difference in the manner in which they are supplied with the necessaries of life," he was also aware that there were enough exceptions to give the lie to the Malthusian rule that the killing diseases of poverty were heavenly punishment for the crime of having been born poor. Hall cited a letter from James Neel to Dr. Lettsom as the source of his statement that "there are, at the cotton-mills belonging to Mr. Dale, of Lanark, in Scotland, three thousand children; these children are said to be treated in a proper manner, in most respects; the consequence is, that during a term of twelve years, viz. from 1785 to 1797, only fourteen have died."

Hall's solutions for the problems of low family incomes and diseases caused by industrialization were unique, at the very least. As a doctor, Hall recommended that most factories and mills be shut down forever. As an educated layman in the second century of the great Agricultural Revolution, he knew that the soil of England was more than capable of producing enough food to feed every inhabitant of the British Isles three times over. As a religious man, Hall found in Scripture the key to his overall solution to the problem of ending poverty and its diseases in England: "In Deuteronomy chap. xv. Leviticus chap. xxv verse 10. Joshua chap. xxii. verse 8; it may be seen that the debts contracted by the individuals of the Jewish nation were remitted, and ceased to be recoverable, every seven years; and that all landed estates, if alienated, returned to their former possessors, every Jubilee, which was every fiftieth year." From this, Hall derived his plan to redistribute the land to every family in England, so that each could grow its own food, and thus be free of the need to toil in mines or mills. The people then would restore the necessary cottage industries, and be assured by a Parliamentary Act of Jubilee that their lands would remain in their families to the end of time.

It was not Charles Hall's visions of a factory-free utopia that offended his solvent readers; it was his very precise social and medical diagnoses of the origins of the contagious and enteric diseases and deformities of the new industrial era that earned for him the enmity of the comfortable. Hall had paid for the printing of his book with his own money. Shortly after it was published, he was thrown into debtors' jail, where he died around 1825 when he was over eighty years old.

Child labor, an early target of the medical and civic reformers, was one of the first issues dealing with the prevention of infectious and industrial diseases on which the British Parliament, in response to the data and the arguments generated by the reformers, took some legislative action. What made child labor in the new mills, mines, and factories particularly offensive to the decent people of the country was the indenture system under which parish workhouses, and impoverished parents, sold their wards and natural children into what amounted to chattel slavery for the duration of childhood. The indentured children, in return for a fixed fee, were handed over to the mill- and mineowners, who undertook to shelter, feed, and train the "apprentices" until they were of age. The indenture system not only brought in a little cash, but it also enabled the workhouses and orphanages, as well as the poor parents, to be spared the costs of rearing the indentured children.

Robert Owen, the son-in-law and successor to David Dale in the operation of the cotton mills at Lanark, was one of the early opponents of this indenture system. The mills, operated by water power from the falls in that Scottish town, were dependent upon child labor from the beginning. "The directors of the public charities," Owen wrote, "from mistaken economy, would not consent to send their children under their care to the cotton mills unless the children were received by the proprietors at the ages of six, seven, and eight. And Mr. Dale was under the necessity of accepting them at these ages, or of stopping the manufactory which he had commenced."[7]

Dale was one of the kinder millowners, and conditions for the indentured child apprentices at his mills were far better than at most other mills in the British Isles. Nevertheless, even though Dale voluntarily undertook to provide these children with an education, "it was absolutely necessary that the children should be employed within the mills from six o'clock in the morning till seven in the evening, summer and winter; and after these hours their education commenced." They naturally learned very little from these lessons after a thirteen-hour workday, and, as Owen recorded, "many of them became dwarfs in body and mind, and some of them were deformed. Almost all looked forward with impatience and anxiety to the expiration of their apprenticeship of seven, eight or nine years," and then the boys and girls fled to Glasgow or Edinburgh and their "innumerable temptations ... to which many of them fell sacrifices."

Owen felt that the chief fault of the apprentice system "proceeded from children being sent from the workhouses at an age much too young for employment. They ought to have been detained four years longer, and educated; and then some of the evils which followed would have been prevented."

Owen, who ran a much more humane mill than his competitors, turned out fine products that earned millions. He established a health fund to which his employees voluntarily contributed one sixtieth of their pay, and which provided medical care when they needed it. When unwanted pregnancies caused tragedies among the married and unmarried women at Lanark, Owen went to France to investigate the rumors of a safe new method of preventing unwanted pregnancies. It proved to be the simple use of ordinary sponges as barriers to conception, and he promptly passed on the information to all his employees.

When in 1802 Parliament debated the wisdom of passing an Act for the Preservation of the Health and Morals of Apprentices and others, employed in Cotton and other Mills, and Cotton and other Factories, Owen was one of the few millowners who testified most vigorously for it. He was very instrumental in the final passage of this first factory act in England. The basic provisions of the act, over the next seventy years, would be refined and expanded in the factory acts that followed. Many of them were supported by employers as kindly as Owen—the millowner John Fielden, a Tory M.P., the importer of Irish linens, and also a Tory M.P., Michael Thomas Sadler, for example—but most of the factory acts were fought tooth and nail by the mill- and mineowning community and their literary spokesmen as instruments guaranteeing bankruptcy and unemployment.

The first act, passed in 1802, ordered that "all and every Rooms and Apartments in or belonging to any such Mill or Factory shall, Twice at least in every Year, be well and sufficiently washed with Quick Lime and Water over every part of the Walls and Ceiling thereof; and that due Care and Attention shall be paid by the Master or Mistress of such Mills or Factories, to provide a sufficient Number of Windows and Openings in such Rooms and Apartments, to insure a proper Supply of fresh Air in and through the same."

Other provisions of this 1802 Children's Magna Carta ordered the masters and mistresses to deliver to each apprentice at least one new complete suit every year. They "further enacted, That no Apprentice shall be employed or compelled to work for more than Twelve Hours in any One Day . . . exclusive of the Time that may be occupied by such Apprentice in eating the necessary Meals." In response to the advice of Robert Owen and other reformers, Article VI mandated that "in some Part of every working Day" every apprentice should be instructed in "Reading, Writing, and Arithmetick" . . . "by some discreet and proper Person . . . in some Room or Place in such Mill or Factory to be set apart for that Purpose."

Article VII decreed that the sleeping accommodations of both sexes had to be separate, and "that not more than Two Apprentices shall in any Case sleep in the same Bed."

Another provision ruled that every apprentice "shall, for the Space of One Hour at least every Sunday, be instructed and examined in the Principles of the Christian Religion, by some proper person to be provided and paid by the Master or Mistress of such Apprentice."

The act called for each community to appoint two visitors of such mills or factories, one the justice of the peace, and "the other shall be a Clergyman of the Established Church of England or Scotland, as the Case may be." The visitors were to visit the factories from time to time, and to report "any infectious Disorder [that] appears to prevail," and all infractions of the articles of the act. Failure to willingly comply with any provision of this act subjected the millowners and factory owners to "forfeit and pay any Sum not exceeding Five Pounds nor less than Forty Shillings, at the Discretion of the Justices before whom such Offender shall be convicted."

The cut-rate enforcement provision patently constituted a license to violate all the other provisions of this well-intended law "for the wise, humane, and equal goverment" of factories run by child labor. The same pattern was to prevail in all the succeeding factory acts and other labor acts until the closing decades of the century. The legal minimum working ages climbed, and the legal working hours declined, even after the indentured apprentice system ended. The visitors were replaced by civil-service factory inspectors. The penalties for violation of the provisions of the many succeeding acts became, at least on paper, more severe than a forty-shilling fine. The acts changed very little in the health and welfare of the children who had to work in the mines and mills.[8]

Child labor remained a linchpin of the British mine and factory systems. In 1823, when the Benthamite reformer and merchant tailor Francis Place published a broadside, *To the Married of Both Sexes of the Working People,* in which he described the birth-control method Robert Owen had brought back from France, it declared that "when wages have been reduced to a very small sum, working people can no longer maintain their children as all good and respectable people wish to maintain their children, but are compelled to neglect them; to send them to different employments; to Mills and Manufactories, at a very early age. The Misery of these poor children cannot be described, and need not be described to you, who witness and deplore them every day of your lives."

This was more than a plea for better working conditions for children in the mines and factories. It was, rather, a direct attack on not only the institution of child labor itself, but also on its roots: the poverty of the parents. Such heresy could not be ignored by Malthus, who in the 1817 edition of *Population* wrote, "I should always particularly reprobate any artificial and unnatural modes of checking population, both on account of their immorality [Malthus was a one-time clergyman] and their tendency to remove a necessary stimulus to industry." This stimulus was a plentiful supply of child labor. Malthus was after all an Establishment economist.

Malthus and his circle mounted a successful attack on both the wisdom and, more important, on the legality of Place's advocacy of birth control for the working poor. The flow of child labor continued unabated through factory act after factory act. Testimony in favor of ever stricter legislation poured forth from generations of doctors in the tradition of Percival and Hall, and from social reformers in the tradition of Owen and Place. But not all doctors were like Hall. One of the formidable defenders of the institution of child labor was Sir Gilbert Blane, who, as a Royal Navy doctor, in 1796, convinced the Admiralty that (as James Lind had written nearly a half-century earlier) regular rations of citrus juice would protect the entire British fleet from scurvy. In 1816 Dr. Blane—then physician to the family of the Prince of Wales—told a parliamentary commission on child labor that "loco-motive exercise is particularly salutary to young people," and that "in children under ten" if the workday "was limited to five or six hours, that would not only not be pernicious, but salutary." In 1835 Andrew Ure, M.D. and Member of the Royal Society, testified before a later parliamentary inquiry that in Manchester's factories "the scene of industry, so far from exciting sad emotions in my mind was always exhilarating ... The work of these lively elves seemed to resemble a sport, in which habit gave them a pleasing dexterity." Nor did child millworkers seem, to this eyewitness, ever to be exhausted at the end of a day's work.

Dr. Ure also testified that "so much nonsense has been uttered about the deformities and diseases of factory children" that he did not expect to be believed when he declared he had never seen such "pleasing countenances and handsome figures as I saw at Mr. Ashton's nine power-weaving galleries. Their light labor and erect posture in tending the looms, and the habit which many of them have of exercising their arms and shoulders, as if with dumb-bells, by resting their hands on the lay or shuttle-bearer, as it oscillates alternately backwards and forwards with the machinery, opens their chest, and gives them generally a graceful carriage."

Such testimony, and the prevalence of toothless enforcement provisions, made the many factory acts less than useless, since they convinced many decent citizens that they were indeed bringing about long-needed reforms. The truth remained otherwise, as was made plain in the testimony of parliamentary investigator J. E. White in 1865. White told about what he learned from the owners of the huge Cyclops Steel and Iron Works in Sheffield, which employed between two and three thousand persons: "The answer of question 7 of the [parliamentary commission's] Tabular Form asking for an opinion as to the prohibition of night work by children and young persons is, 'It is impossible for us to do so; it would be tantamount to stopping our works.' "[9]

To be sure, each new impotent law dealing with working conditions continued to enrage major employers and some of their spokesmen, like Herbert Spencer.

What Spencer called the freedom-from-government-regulation philosophy of his New Toryism nevertheless reigned supreme. Not all mill- and factory- and mineowners were men with the humanity of Robert Owen, John Fielden, and Michael Thomas Sadler. Not all statesmen had the empathy of Old Tories such as the Earl of Shaftsbury and Benjamin Disraeli. In the absence of both the political parliamentary franchise of working people, and of a strong trade union movement legally empowered to use the strike weapon to enforce all the consistently violated and ignored Factory Acts passed by Parliament between 1802 and 1870, the fine protections written into these acts remained all but worthless.

The children who toiled from dawn to dark in the mines and mills remained victims of the benign neglect of a Parliament in which, for most of the century, the mature voices of the violators spoke far louder than the young voices of the violated. And the infectious diseases, crippling and killing mine and factory accidents, and other preventable diseases and disorders of the "necessary stimulus to industry" Malthus termed child labor remained endemic in British life.

When it came to the preventable diseases and disorders of urbanized societies, those of the new times were usually identical to those of the preindustrial era, but the proportions of populations attacked and/or killed by them differed. Not only the times but also the places showed differences. Where on the average hundreds of people, many of them children, died in outbreaks of dysentery, diphtheria, pneumonia, and cerebrospinal meningitis in the dormitories and family warrens of the mill and mining villages, thousands of people soon suffered the same contagions in the towns and cities nearest the sites of these local epidemics.

Not until after 1836, when the parliamentary sanitary reformers pushed through their Registration Act for the official registry of all births, marriages, deaths, and the ages and causes of these deaths, was it possible even to roughly estimate the actual numbers of deaths from specific causes (such as the diseases of child labor). It was to be many years before doctors and health statisticians could estimate with any degree of certainty that every reported death from any specific infectious disease represented at least five to twenty cases in which the patients survived.

In the cities, as in the factory and mining enclaves, the social causes of contagious diseases were painfully obvious to doctors and concerned laymen alike. The first cause was filth, endemic in all areas where no practical provisions were ever made for the sanitary disposal of body wastes and garbage, and where human excrement accumulated in primitive privies and cesspools and more often in open piles in alleys between houses, in streets, and in backyards. Commercial scavengers, from time to time—and never very often—were hired to empty the privies and cesspools and cart their stinking messes away to the nearest rivers or to farmers who used them as fertilizers.

Inside plumbing was a rarity for nearly all the first half of the nineteenth century, and only slightly less unique until the start of the twentieth century. Drinking water, and water used for washing, laundry, and cooking, came from contaminated rivers, from wells in ground polluted by cesspools and privies, and, for those who could afford it, from water companies that transported somewhat cleaner water from less dangerous sources to city customers.

The second basic cause of infectious diseases was malnutrition. It was already well known that infectious diseases were more common and more deadly in the families of the working poor of the overcrowded tenements and rural hovels. Not only did the poor lack the incomes sufficient to pay for the foods rich in the nutrients required for the maintenance of health, but much of what they could afford to purchase was polluted by environmental filth or adulterated by unscrupulous purveyors. Milk was diluted with water (the water was often fecally contaminated), thickened with flour to hide the dilutants, flavored with sugar to hide the taste of the contaminated water, and then stored in unrefrigerated vessels. Bread, cereals, tea, coffee, flour were combined with cheaper and less nutritive materials to make them more profitable.

The steam engines of industry, mining, and the new networks of railways that contributed to the burgeoning wealth of the nation also polluted the air and the waters with hydrocarbon wastes—already known since 1775 to be the cause of at least one form of cancer,[10] and long since implicated in the etiology of emphysema, bronchitis, and other pulmonary diseases. Alexis de Tocqueville, visiting Manchester in 1835, observed that "a sort of black smoke covers the city. The sun is seen through it as a disc without rays. Under this half daylight 300,000 human beings are ceaselessly at work." He noted that "below some of their miserable dwellings is a row of cellars to which a sunken corridor leads," and that in the "damp, repulsive holes" in these basements "twelve to fifteen human beings are crowded pell-mell." The huge sprawling factories of the new prototypical industrial center "keep air and light out of the human habitations which they dominate; they envelop them in perpetual fog; here is the slave, there the master; there the heath of some, here the poverty of most; there the organized effort of thousands produce, to the profit of one man, what society has not yet learnt to give. Here the weakness of the individual seems more feeble and helpless even than in the middle of a wilderness; here the effects, there the causes."

To this French aristocrat, for whom history was the key to understanding, Manchester symbolized the best and the worst of the Industrial Revolution. "From this foul drain the greatest stream of humanity flows out to fertilize the world. From this filthy sewer pure gold flows. Here humanity attains its most complete development and its most brutish; here civilization works its miracles, and civilized man is turned back almost into a savage."[11]

A decade later, as shown so deftly by Charles Dickens in *Hard Times,* the same steam engines that befogged the skies were also daily hauling the more affluent Manchester millowners and merchants to and from the new family estates they had built far enough from Manchester to be relatively free of its noxious wastes, but near enough to permit them to run their prosperous enterprises. For those who had to live as well as work in Manchester, Liverpool, Birmingham, London, and the smaller industrial and mining centers of England, contagious diseases born of filth and exacerbated by crowding and poverty grew worse from year to year as the Satanic Mills so dreaded by Blake at the dawn of the century became the "huge palaces of industry" that loomed so monstrously before Alexis de Tocqueville in 1835.

Visitors like de Tocqueville, and novelists like Dickens, have left their own insightful descriptions of the impact of industrialization on the daily lives and the health of the people. None of them, however, have given us the masses of unvarnished data on the effects on human health that were to be collected and broadcast to the world by generations of sanitary reformers who, for the five decades prior to the birth of germ theory, sought to make industrial nations healthier for those who had to inhabit them. Elsewhere the records of who they were, what they accomplished, and where they worked has been amply documented. Here we shall only consider, and very briefly, a few of the founders of the great sanitary movement which, starting in London, would spread throughout the world.

Many of the pioneers of this movement were physicians. There was

William Buchan of Scotland (1729–1805), whose *Domestic Medicine: or a Treatise on the Prevention and Cure of Disease* was first published in 1789. Dr. Buchan warned that "many things are necessary for the sick beside medicine," and, as Dr. Charles Hall was to reiterate sixteen years later, that disease in the poor would be unavoidable unless that had "the necessaries of life." Dr. Buchan included decent and uncrowded housing as one of these "necessaries." Society, he wrote, had a major role in the preservation of life: "Many things injurious to the public health are practiced with impunity, while others, absolutely necessary for its preservation, are entirely neglected.

"Some of the public means of preserving health are mentioned in the general prophylaxis, as the inspection of provisions, widening the streets of the great towns, keeping them clean, supplying the inhabitants with wholesome water, &c; but they are passed over in a very cursory manner."[12]

There were the observant British and Scottish doctors, starting with Dr. Gordon of Aberdeen in 1795, who alerted their peers to the fact that puerperal fever—the dread childbirth fever—was an infectious disease that "seized such women only as were visited or delivered by a practitioner, or taken care of by a nurse, who had previously attended patients affected with the disease." Fifty-two years before Ignaz Semmelweis made the same basic observations in Vienna, Gordon wrote that this "infection was as readily communicated as that of smallpox or measles," and confessed that "although it is a disagreeable declaration for me to mention, I myself was the means of carrying the infection to a great number of women." Moreover, Gordon reported that puerperal fever "was a specific contagion, or infection, altogether unconnected with a noxious constitution of the atmosphere."

There were Dr. Thomas Percival and Dr. James Philip Kay (later Sir James Kay-Shuttleworth), who was born in 1804, two years after Dr. Percival's efforts helped bring about the first Factory Act of 1802. Kay's pamphlet *The Moral and Physical Condition of the Working Classes Employed in the Cotton Manufacture in Manchester,* written in 1832, was based on his observations of the families he treated both for the ordinary diseases of poverty and crowding as well as for Asiatic cholera, which first hit England in 1831.

There was the surgeon Peter Gaskell of Cheshire, whose book *The Manufacturing Population of England* published in 1833, compared the health of the textile workers before and after the cottage industries were swallowed up by the new factory towns. The housing arrangements of the people of the Industrial Revolution typified these changes for Gaskell. Of the houses of the millworkers, Gaskell wrote that whole blocks of "these houses are either totally undrained, or only very partially. The whole of the washings and filth from these consequently are thrown into the front or back street, which being often unpaved and cut up into deep ruts, allows them to collect into stinking and stagnant pools; while fifty, or more even than that number, having only a single convenience common to them all, it is in a very short time completely choked up with excrementitious matter."

Gaskell's observations on crowding were equally as sharp. "Five, six, seven beds are arranged on the floor—there being in the generality of cases no bedsteads, or any substitutes for them; these are covered with clothing of the most scanty and filthy descriptions. They are occupied indiscriminately by persons of both sexes, strangers perhaps to each other, except a few of the regular occupants. Young men and young women; men, wives, and their children—all lying in a noisome atmosphere, and often intoxicated." In such towns, smoking and drinking became vices common, he wrote, to both sexes.

There was the physician Charles Turner Thackrah, one of the principal founders of the Leeds Medical School in 1831, who was born in that industrial town in 1795 and died there of tuberculosis in 1833, when he was still two years short of forty. An early British specialist in occupational diseases, Thackrah studied the health effects of over two hundred different trades and occupations in Leeds. The title of his 1831 treatise pretty well sums up his life's work: "The Effects of the Principal Arts, Trades and Professions, and of Civic States and Habits of Living, on Health and Longevity with Suggestions for the Removal of many of the Agents, which produce Disease, and shorten the Duration of Life."

Few doctors were personally more clinically aware of what jobs in industry and commerce did to the physical and mental well-being of children. Thackrah did not believe that any new parliamentary Factory Acts regulating hours or working conditions or wages could ever make child labor biologically and psychologically safe for children. "The employment of children in *any* labour is wrong," this observant young doctor wrote in 1831. "No man of humanity can reflect without distress on the state of thousands of children, many from six to seven years of age, roused from their beds at an early hour, hurried to the mills, and kept there, with the interval of only forty minutes, till a late hour at night;—kept, moreover, in an atmosphere impure, not only as the air of a town, not only as defective in ventilation, but as loaded also with noxious dust. Health! Cleanliness! Mental improvement! How are they regarded?"[13]

Two young Benthamite doctors in London, Neil Arnott and Southwood Smith, were both members of the personal circle of the wealthy Jeremy Bentham, prophet of the utilitarian philosophy of achieving the greatest good for the greatest number of people. Smith, who started professional life as a Unitarian minister, had seen too much misery to continue to offer only moral aid to the families whose lives were most drastically changed by the new industrialization. He obtained training as a physician, and then dedicated himself to doing whatever he could to help people survive these historic changes in life-style. Very early in his new medical career, Smith came to the conclusion that filth was the primary cause of most of the new, or newly important, diseases and disorders of urban life.

There was the physician and mathematician William Farr. For forty years, Farr—starting in 1839 when he was, with the aid of the Benthamites in public health, appointed compiler of abstracts for the new Registrar-

General—worked with great success to turn health statistics into a useful tool of epidemiology and public policy. There was Farr's colleague and friend, the anatomist and health officer Dr. John Simon, who in 1867—after a lifetime in public health—succeeded in making universal vaccination against smallpox legally (albeit not actually) compulsory in the British Isles.

Finally, there was the most influential sanitary reformer of them all, the dogmatic, opinionated, ruthless, impatient, and at times brillant barrister-journalist-civil servant Edwin Chadwick. A child of the century, Chadwick was born near Manchester in January 1800. His father, James, a multi-talented musician and natural philosopher—he taught the Quaker John Dalton botany and music—was a devoted partisan of the French Revolution, and when Edwin was very young, James started a permanent career as a successful newspaper editor. James and private tutors provided Edwin's education until at eighteen he became a clerk and apprentice to a London lawyer. At twenty-three Chadwick started a new seven-year apprenticeship as a barrister.

Chadwick helped earn his keep during his apprentice years by writing about the life of London's poor for various newspapers. By 1824 he included as his close personal friends Drs. Arnott and Smith, and through them became a member of Jeremy Bentham's inner circle. When Bentham died in 1832, he left Chadwick a small legacy, which helped the young man maintain for life the prickly independence and arrogance that were to terrify generations of his associates.

In 1828, in response to an invitation from John Bowring, editor of the *Westminster Review,* for an article about the life of London's poor, Chadwick wrote an essay titled "The Means of Insurance Against Accidents, etc.," which embodied the core of what he later termed "the sanitary idea." According to his brilliant biographer, Professor S. E. Finer, this article showed "that the duration of life had steadily improved, but concluded that by appropriate measures of hygiene and sanitation it might well be improved still more. It concluded by ... reviewing the administrative arrangements by which one could remove the causes of poverty, dissipation, crime, and disease which he had observed so closely."[14]

For the next half-century, Chadwick would lead physicians and lay social and civic reformers in the crusades to make the Industrial Revolution safe for human life, which were to become known as the great sanitary movement. It was intended to make the new social order work, not to overthrow it. In a letter written in 1837, Chadwick spelled out the political convictions he retained for life.

"I am a zealous advocate for all social improvements and I am therefore an ally of any people by whom improvements would be made. I am therefore a supporter of the existing [Whig] governmennt. . . . If, however, I were driven to choose between two extremes: between the Tories and the Radicals of the Cobbettite school; I should certainly choose the Tories."[15]

Unlike most contemporary reformers, who were appalled by the meager incomes of factory workers, miners and other foot soldiers of the Industrial Revolution, Chadwick believed that the prevailing English wage scales would be more than adequate for their human needs once clean water and sewage systems and other urgent sanitary reforms spared them the soaring costs of preventable contagious diseases. For this reason, and because he believed in the freedom of capital, Chadwick was a zealous and lifelong enemy of the new trade unions that sought to improve the qualities of British family life by working for increases in family incomes.

The chief aims of the sanitary movement were clean towns, clean drinking water in the living quarters of the cleaned-up towns, sanitary sewerage systems, and waste disposal systems. Chadwick and his colleagues truly believed that such measures would reduce all prevailing infectious disease levels to one third of their current levels, and that their "great preventives" would also end pauperism in England. As parliamentary investigators, they produced mountains of evidence suggesting that filth, a preventable environmental affliction, was responsible for most of the morbidities and mortalities in the factories, the factory towns, and the great cities. Their efforts included such effective instruments as Chadwick's parliamentary *Report on the Sanitary Conditions of the Labouring Population* of 1842, and the 1845 *Report of the Health of Towns Commission,* which confirmed in England's fifty largest towns what the Chadwick report of 1842 first proved: The Industrial Revolution had turned urban England into a network of loci of multiple infections.

The investigations, generally led or inspired by Chadwick, resulted in local, then regional, and, ultimately (in 1875), national health agencies responsible for improving and maintaining the public health. They led to new agencies for sewers, garbage removal, and the inspection of food plants, as well as to erratically enforced laws governing vaccination, working conditions, housing safety, and child welfare.

In the years that followed his admission to the inner Benthamite circles, Chadwick was to hold many civil-service jobs connected with health, welfare, and sanitation. *Ex officio,* he was also one of the principal leaders of the internationally effective Health of Towns Association, founded as a coalition of other national and local voluntary health societies primarily to convince Parliament to enact legislation that would eliminate "the physical and moral evils that result from the present defective sewerage, drainage, supply of water, air, and light, and construction of dwelling houses."

Health of Towns Association publications, dealing with specific proposals for sanitary improvements and with specific bills before Parliament, went out by the thousands to concerned physicians and lay people in England and elsewhere. In Munich, they were used by Dr. Max von Pettenkofer, the great hygienist, as arguments to get the city's leaders to adopt what he described as "the English reforms." In America they played a significant role in the improvement of the structures and the operations of local and regional health agencies, as well as stimulating the interests of influential citizens in sanitary reform.

One of the first Americans to be profoundly influenced by the publications of the Health of Towns Association was Lemuel Shattuck (1793–1859), a former itinerant Yankee schoolteacher who kept a bookshop in Boston. Shattuck was one of the active founders of the public health movement in the United States and, in 1839, of the American Statistical Association. Shattuck devoted most of his lifetime to working for the social and governmental prevention of diseases caused by domiciliary overcrowding, environmental pollution, and the widespread failure to make available vaccinations universally compulsory.

The Health of Towns Association, like its leaders, strongly advocated vaccination against smallpox. However, this was only one of many major infectious diseases they tried to eradicate. As Dr. William Farr wrote, "It is, however, by no means proved that the general mortality under favourable sanitary conditions is much reduced by rendering a child insusceptible of one type [of infection], while he remains exposed to all other types of zymotic [infectious] diseases." Given the endemic and often epidemic conditions of all major killing and crippling infectious diseases in England during the nineteenth century, Farr had a very good point. The conquest of smallpox by vaccination could not be sought at the expense of the main effort against all infections too.

The guiding scientific principles of the Health of Towns Association were spelled out in 1846 by Dr. Southwood Smith, a leading member of its central committee, in an Association report. "The ultimate end of sewerage, drainage, and a supply of water adequate to the cleansing of sewers, drains and streets, is to maintain the air, wherever human beings take up their abode, in a fit state for respiration. . . . Wherever animal and vegetable substances are undergoing the process of decomposition, poisonous matters are evolved which, mixing with the air, corrupt it, and render it injurious to health and fatal to life." Unless removed, these poisonous by-products of organic decomposition cause the "slow deterioration and corruption of the whole mass of blood; a consequent disorganization of the solid structures of the body, and the excitement of those violent commotions of the system which constitute fevers, choleras, dysenteries and other mortal epidemics."

His friend Chadwick, soon to be appointed a metropolitan commissioner of sewers, stated Smith's thesis much more bluntly. "All smell is, if it be intense, immediate acute disease," Chadwick told Parliament, "and eventually we may say that, by depressing the system and rendering it susceptible to the action of other causes, *all* [Chadwick's emphasis] smell is disease."

A fervent convert to the dogma that all smells are or produce disease, and the fouler the stench the more acute the disorder, was the wellborn, well-educated, mystically religious Florence Nightingale. A society belle, she chose to remain unwed, and in 1851, at the age of thirty-one, took herself to Germany, where she went through a three-month *practicum* at the Kaiserswerth Institute for Deaconesses. She learned nothing, she wrote, because "the nursing was *nil*. The hygiene terrible ... I took all the training there was to be had—there was none to be had in England—but Kaiserswerth was far from having trained me."

She was right about Kaiserswerth, and for good reasons. Nursing as a paramedical health profession did not exist until Florence Nightingale invented it. The invention took place in three laboratories. The first was the Institution for the Care of Sick Gentlewomen in Distressed Circumstances, at 1 Harley Street in London, of which she became superintendent in 1853. The second was a festering death house misnamed a British military hospital in Scutari, a backward Turkish village on the Asian side of the Bosphorus. The third setting was St. Thomas's Hospital in London, where the Nightingale School and Home for training nurses—created and directed by Miss Nightingale—took in its first class of fifteen trainees in June 1860.

When the Crimean War casualties began to die like flies in the army's field and base hospitals, the British Secretary of War, Sidney Herbert, a social friend of Miss Nightingale's, accepted her offer to recruit and take to the war zone a staff of thirty-eight nurses. From the moment she arrived at the Barracks Hospital in Scutari, where most of the principal cemeteries of Constantinople were also quite providentially located, in November 1854, Nightingale was confronted with the classic mix of chaos, corruption, and cynicism that made the infective and nutritional disorders of modern wars infinitely more deadly than enemy bullets. From the very start of her mission to hell, Nightingale found shabbily clad, unwashed, poorly fed, and severely traumatized soldiers dying of fevers, cholera, dysentery, erysipelas, gangrene, rheumatic fever and other infections—in overcrowded, unventilated, filthy wards filled with too many dirty beds and pallets. Monies appropriated by the war ministries for the soldiers' food, linens, beds, and medical supplies—from bandages to medicines—were so scandalously misappropriated that were it not for funds raised by the London *Times* from its readers and administered by Florence Nightingale, as well as frequent expenditures of her considerable personal wealth, the death toll would have been even greater than it was.

Nightingale and her nurses, and such military personnel as she could cajole from a most reluctant military medical establishment, fell to with amazing vigor in the wholesale application of the practices and principles of the sanitary movement as well as the elements of basic nutrition. Soap, water, brushes, mops, chlorine, lime, and other basic tools of sanitation were applied constantly. Threats and political wire-pulling were employed to rid hospitals and barracks at Scutari and elsewhere of overcrowding and filth. Human body wastes, and barracks and hospital garbage were disposed of sanitarily. Decent food, hygienically prepared and served, helped bring dying soldiers back to life. Proper laundry services were established to provide sanitary, clean-smelling bed and body linens.

It was hard and often thankless work, which when done well was always performed at the risk of contracting the soldiers' infections. In May 1855, while inspecting the military hospitals at Balaclava, Nightingale collapsed and was hospitalized for "Crimean fever," which could have been anything from influenza or lobar pneumonia to bacterial septicemia. For two weeks she suffered delirium in addition to her fever, and at the height of her illness all her hair was cut off. She was luckier than those of her nurses who died of their fevers. The results, however, justified the risks. As one of her friends and biographers, Sir Edward Cook, noted, "In the first seven months of the war the mortality among the troops had been at the rate of 60 percent per annum—*from disease alone* [Sir Edward's emphasis]—a rate of mortality which exceeds that of the great plague of London." Within six months at Scutari, Nightingale and her nurses had reduced the death rate from 42 percent to 22 percent per thousand among hospitalized soldiers.

After the war ended, Nightingale continued work on improving the treatment of military traumatic and disease patients by organizing the routine administration of the hygienic reforms of the great sanitary movement in tandem with adequate portions of clean, nutritious food. In only three years, between 1859 and 1861, the military death rates were halved, bringing them down to parity with the civilian death rates from the primarily infectious and deficiency diseases of daily life. During this postwar period, Nightingale not only started her training school for nurses, but also turned her attention to two important areas of civil health.

She designed what were known for a half-century and more as Florence Nightingale Architecture hospitals, in which her principles of hygiene and sanitation dictated the forms and structures of most hospitals built anywhere until well into the mid-twentieth century. In 1859 Florence Nightingale also wrote a best-selling little book, *Notes on Nursing: What it Is, and What it Is Not*. It was addressed not to the professional nurses, but, rather, to every woman in England who has "at one time or another of her life, charge of the personal health of somebody, whether child or invalid." This also meant that "in other words, every woman is a nurse."

Every woman in England, then, Nightingale wrote, had to have "every day sanitary knowledge, or the knowledge of nursing, or in other words, of how to put the constitution in such a state as that it will have no disease, or that it can recover from disease, takes a higher place. It is recognized as the knowledge that everyone ought to have—distinct from medical knowledge, which only a profession can have."

This little book, simply written, became the standard handbook of millions of British families, who used, or sought to use, it as a guide to the proper ventilation, warming, and hygienic management of their home environments during and between health crises. Civic reformers also used *Notes on Nursing* as arguments for legislation to assure healthy standards of living space, ventilation, warming, sanitation, and facilities for food preparation and storage. Trade union spokesmen used *Notes on Nursing,* and its catalog of the necessities of family health, to argue effectively for wages adequate to purchase or rent such basic needs as uncrowded bed chambers with healthy air.

Florence Nightingale's contributions to the public health did not end there. In 1892, at the age of seventy-two, she created the new profession of lady health visitors, who were trained to visit wives and mothers and teach them the principles of hygienic home management. The work of these later products of her fertile imagination led to a new profession, the health visitor, whose function in England today is to make certain that every family in the nation makes full use of the medical care that is now part of the heritage of every newborn child.[16] The fact that Florence Nightingale also refused ever to concede that infectious diseases were caused by microbial agents (which incidentally breed in filth), or that there was more than one kind of infectious disease, should in no way blind us to her enormous contributions to the sanitary and hygienic concepts of the public-health movements of the nineteenth and twentieth centuries. The ideas of the sanitary reformers merit the honors paid them even if their slavish devotion to the belief that it was the stench of human body wastes, and nothing else in them, that caused infections would prove so costly in their own times.

Thanks to great improvements in cleanliness of the drinking water piped into ever-increasing numbers of British homes, and to the steadily growing numbers of sewage and garbage disposal systems, the sanitary reformers were able to make vast improvements in the health of towns. The cholera epidemic of 1866 would be, in fact, the last one in England, although cholera and the Asian trade that brought it to England and the rest of Europe were still very much alive. Of course, the new water and sewage disposal systems that had made cholera, typhoid, and other water-borne infections far less common in Victorian England could not prevent all deaths from these disorders. In 1861 the Royal Consort, Prince Albert, died of typhoid at the age of only forty-two; it was a mark of the times that, as Professor Peter B. Medawar recently reminded us, "when he died of typhoid, the twenty cesspools in Windsor Castle were found to be full to overflowing."[17]

The efforts of the sanitary reformers were given a great assist by bacteria which, in decomposing the organic wastes of the Thames River, produced the noxious gases associated with putrefaction. From time to time, when the smell became particularly unbearable on a summer's day, the heavens would mercifully unburden themselves of torrents of rain, which helped wash away these microbial gas factories. In June 1858, however, nature failed to cooperate, and the unusually hot summer was marked by an untoward drought. The combination of great heat and little or no rain produced what soon became known as London's Great Stink.

"Parliament was in a good position to appreciate the nuisance," wrote the British social historians Mitchell and Leys, "for the windows at Westminster had to be draped with curtains soaked in chloride of lime so that members could breathe. To cross Westminster Bridge it was necessary to hold a handkerchief firmly over one's nose and mouth and those who travelled on the river steamers suffered greatly when the paddles churned the water into stinking eddies. . . . There was talk of moving the Law Courts to Oxford or St. Albans, and a Select Committee was set up [by Parliament] to report on the Stink and to find means of abatement." A Mr. Gurney proposed to the Select Committee that 369 of the Thames sewers be sealed and their gases led away and dissipated by being ignited, a solution that would have blown up a good chunk of London. "A more conventional remedy, the use of slaked lime in large quantities, and the coming of rain cured The Great Stink, but it had served its purpose in awakening Londoners to the realities of their position," and to their now taking seriously the sanitary proposals of the Health of Towns Association.[18]

Not every disaster of the environment assisted the sanitary reformers in improving the health of urban England. During the great cholera epidemic of 1848–1849, which peaked in January 1849 and began slowly to reappear in the spring of that year, Chadwick, then London's commissioner of sewers, ordered that his sewers be kept scoured and flushed. London's filth, he ordered, should be kept from the sewers, where it would only create what he called "pestilential exhalations," and should therefore be deposited directly in the river. This, he maintained, was better than letting it accumulate in his sewers, since it would only pollute the Thames to the ratio of one part of human excrement to every five thousands parts of river water.

Throughout the spring and summer, Chadwick's sewer department kept flushing sewage directly into the Thames, instead of, as *The Times* thundered, sending his cartloads of human manure "to fertilize the fields of Kent or Essex." London's "hoarded refuse, including the fresh infected faeces of the cholera victims, was flushed into the Thames at a point opposite the main intake of London's water supply." The consequences added up to nothing less than a series of acts of biological warfare against the people of London. By July "the epidemic had become water-borne, and the monthly mortality shot up from 246 [deaths] in June to 1852 in July, to 4,251 in August, until it reached a peak of 6644 in September."[19]

Clearly there was something other than the smell in the excrement of cholera victims that caused the deaths of 53,293 people during the London epidemic. Chadwick's successful effort to keep his sewers from accumulating undue levels of "pestilential exhalations" had doomed thousands of Londoners, who drank Thames water and washed with it, to die of preventable cholera infections.

Usually the sanitary reforms the Chadwicks and the Nightingales accomplished in England did more good than harm. In towns where their efforts forced the municipalities to set up local health agencies and hire municipal or country health officers—generally but not always physicians—some striking reductions in the death rates of various diseases were accomplished. In other localities the new health departments were moribund and their inspectors little more than political hacks. The sanitary reformers pressed for a national public health act that would set enforced health standards for all communities, for which they were accused by self-styled "anticentralizers" of conspiring against traditional British freedoms. These accusations were painfully prescient of the complaints heard in the United States a century later, when the federal government set up some astoundingly toothless agencies to make the environment and the workplace somewhat less dangerous to human life.

One of the leaders of the campaign for an effective national health act was Dr. Alexander P. Stewart, a London physician trained in Glasgow. Despite a very busy clinical practice, Stewart found time to make a study of the differing roles of local health officers in varied sections of the British Isles. In 1866 Stewart described the work of many of these local health officers and nuisance inspectors in a long paper read in Manchester before a national congress of the then new National Association for the Promotion of Social Science. He made the point that the successes of the better health officers in improving the public health in their towns were probably the exceptions to the national mode, and he used them as examples of the types of benefits to be expected if and when a proper national health act were promulgated.

The significant aspect of the gains achieved by these health officers was that so much of their work consisted of removing nuisances ranging from live pigs in tenement cellars to "obstructions from drains, defective traps, &c.," and serving "lime-washing notices" on owners of "dirty houses," ordering the evacuation of tenants illegally housed in the cellars of dwelling houses, forcing tenement owners to comply with local laws against overcrowding, ordering the draining of stagnant pits of water, converting illegal privies into legal water closets, and hauling offenders before the magistrates for offenses against the prevailing sanitary laws. This was sanitary reform in action, and its results were often very gratifying.

In Liverpool, to cite one of Stewart's examples, the Health Committee, acting under "their intelligent medical officer of health," Dr. W. S. Trench, achieved massive reductions in the annual death rates from five common leading infectious diseases between 1864 and 1865—smallpox (from 121 cases in 1864 to only thirty-seven in 1865); scarlatina, or scarlet fever (from eighty-one to thirty-seven cases); measles (from seventy-six to twenty-one cases); and typhus [and/or typhoid fever] down from seventy-one cases in 1864 to sixty-eight in 1865. These reductions in infectious disease rates were accomplished solely by the enforcement of sanitary not medical regulations. Stewart was also aware that in 1865, nearly seventy years after Jenner immunized Jamie Phipps against smallpox, vaccination should long since have been made universal and compulsory, and that by 1864 there should have been literally no cases of smallpox in Liverpool or anywhere else in England.

Less than two years after Stewart presented this success tale of sanitary reform in Liverpool, the city was hit by a typhus epidemic. Agnes Jones, trained by Florence Nightingale and chief of nursing in the Liverpool Workhouse Infirmary, came down with typhus. A close friend of Nightingale's, she was terribly overworked. On the eve of the typhus epidemic, Nightingale had written in a letter to a friend that Nurse Jones "has had 1350 patients and to fight for every necessary of life for them. She has never been in bed until 1:30 A.M. and always up at 5:30 A.M." A few days after this letter was written, Nurse Jones caught typhus and quickly died.

What was true in the case of Agnes Jones was, alas, true of most people who worked equally hard for their livelihoods in England throughout the years of the sanitary movement's greatest triumphs. The health gains of the sanitary reforms barely affected the total health of those who had to struggle, generally without complete success, for the "necessaries" of family life.

The British health ministry's accurate statistics told a grim story. Then, as now, the two most sensitive indices of a nation's health were the total and the infant death rates. During the five years ending in 1845, the years of the great initial parliamentary reports on the health of the nation, the standardized death rate per thousand living in England and Wales was 20.6; during the same years, the deaths of infants under one year old averaged 148 per 1,000 live births. During the next five years, ending in 1850, the total death rate rose to 22.4, and the infant mortality rate climbed to 157. By 1861–1865, when Stewart made his report, the infant death rate stood at 151 per 1,000 live births and the standardized death rate was 21.2 deaths per 1,000 living.

In sharp contrast to the death rates in England's military populations, which had been cut in half by Florence Nightingale's successes in making adequate diets, decent living quarters, and standard sanitary reforms routine in the armed services, the civilian death rates were even higher in 1865 than in 1842, when Chadwick's *Report on the Sanitary Conditions of the Labouring Population* was issued. The reasons for this apparent paradox had been well defined by Charles Hall in 1805: In the absence of adequate levels of food, clothing, shelter, and related "necessaries of life," the health of "the poor, they being by far the greater number of the people in most civilized countries" could never be improved.

Clean drinking water and sanitary waste disposal systems were calculated to prevent the water-borne infections, such as cholera, typhoid, dysentery, and certain other enteric disorders like paratyphoid fevers. These diseases are all spread by microbial parasites in the feces of infected people and animals. They are transmitted to people in drinking water, by eating or handling contaminated foods and eating utensils, and by washing in contaminated water. Environmental sanitary improvements often worked very well against such infections, as demonstrated by the elimination of epidemic cholera in England after 1866 by the construction of new clean water systems.

However, most contagions are caused by crowding and by exhalation droplet transmission of infectious agents, fecally contaminated water, and direct (including venereal) contact. The lack or absence of clean running water and soap makes domiciliary crowding more dangerous. The diseases caused by exhalation include the major killers of industrial nations: pneumococcal and other bacterial pneumonias, streptococcal and staphylococcal infections, diphtheria, tuberculosis, meningococcal and other bacterial meningitis, the common cold, influenza, and other common viral respiratory diseases. Industrial accidents cause wound infections like tetanus and gas gangrene. Human body and head lice carry the microorganisms of epidemic typhus and relapsing fever; fleas, ticks, and mosquitoes as well as rats, mice, and people transmit the germs and viruses of plague and yellow fever; mosquitoes carry the parasites of malaria; and dogs and other infected animals transmit the rabies virus.

In these and other microbial and protozoan infections, chronic malnutrition diminishes people's inborn host defenses against microscopic invaders, so that the malnourished populations of the world become more prone to contagious disorders—and far less able to cope with infections and protozoan infections when they occur. To this day, for example, in all industrialized nations where such records are kept, the children of poor families miss far more school days because of infections and parasitic diseases than do the children of more affluent families.

Sanitary reforms, per se, also had little effect on the human infectious diseases that were transmitted by direct contact. These ranged from severe and often fatal infectious diseases transmitted from animals to people, such as anthrax, brucellosis, and tularemia, to such ubiquitous venereal diseases as gonorrhea, syphilis, nongonococcal urethritis, and lymphogranuloma venereum. The venereal diseases were and are, to a great extent, as socioeconomic in origin as were the infectious diseases causally associated with child labor, crowding, work injuries, and malnutrition. However, while it was and still is poverty that drives most prostitutes into the sale of their bodies, it was as true in 1865 as it is now that it was not poverty that produced most of their customers, nor defined all victims of venereal diseases endemic in the practitioners and purchasers of prostitution.

Outside of the military populations, whose health needs were provided by the government, the first to benefit physically from the massive efforts of the English sanitary reformers were that lucky minority who were well housed, well fed, well clothed, and well insulated from the sources of infectious diseases and their carriers. The high morbidity and mortality rates for infectious diseases in the first century of the Industrial Revolution—when there was only one vaccine against a common contagion, and there were no systemic antibacterial drugs—were as much the products of socioeconomics as of microbial agents.

"Infant mortality, due largely to gastrointestinal and respiratory infections, was at the rate of several hundred [infant deaths] per 1000 births during the nineteenth century, at a time when in royalty the rate was 12 per 1000 births," observes Professor Edward H. Kass. "That is, before antibiotics and before contemporary methods of control, the infant mortality rate in royal families was lower than that which is found in the best national rates now being recorded in any country of the world. Clearly, rich is better."[20]

For the significant hygienic and environmental gains of the great sanitary movement to have any real impact on the overall health statistics of the industrialized British Isles, it would first be necessary for various impending social and scientific goals to be won.

The first of these gains was achieved in 1868, when the right to vote was won by the nation's workingmen and other nonpropertied males. Only after generations of bitter struggle was the equal right extended to their wives, sisters, and daughters in 1928.

In 1870 Parliament finally mandated compulsory free education. This helped reduce the considerable exploitation of child labor, as well as give some few very fortunate children a rudimentary tool of upward social mobility.

In 1871, by now aware that men who worked in the mines and factories had the vote, and the political power to turn unfriendly officials out of office, Parliament in its new wisdom passed the Trade Union Act, which at long last made unions legal and protected union funds. In 1875 a second act legalized peaceful picketing. Like the sanitary reformers, the leaders of the new trade union movement were not out to destroy the social order, but to make it work for the greater benefit of the greatest number of people, primarily by winning higher wage scales, shorter workdays, and safer workplaces.

Finally, the long-sought passage of the Public Health Act of 1875, which made national and meaningful and, above everything, enforced the new codes of public health—that is, the institutionalization of sanitary reform—put the might of the government behind the programs of the doctors and laymen who sought to make the environment safer for human health.

All these developments, particularly the higher wages that stemmed from the two trade union acts and helped the working poor get more of life's biological necessities, starting with more adequate food and shelter, helped improve British health statistics. Between 1875 and 1900, for example, the standardized death rates in England and Wales fell from 20.9 to 17.6 deaths per 1,000 living, but the infant mortality rate rose from 153 to 156 deaths per 1,000 live births. By 1939 on the eve of World War II (and just before antibiotics), the standardized death rate was down to only 8.5 deaths per 1,000 living, and the infant mortality rate was down to 50 deaths per 1,000 live births—less than one third of what it had been in 1900.

While higher family incomes and other social, environmental, and clinical advances reduced the total and infant death rates in England and Wales, the live birthrate—despite the Cassandran prophecies of the Reverends Townsend and Malthus—also continued to fall. In 1875 the live birthrate in England and Wales stood at 35.5 births per 1,000 population of all ages. By the five-year period 1896–1900, live births in England and Wales averaged 29.3 per 1,000 per year. In 1939 the live birthrate stood at 14.9 per 1,000, or just about one half the 1900 rate. Far from causing a population explosion (and encouraging sin and idleness, as predicted by Townsend and Malthus) raising wages and otherwise improving the total quality of life for the majority of any population invariably triggers what demographers term the Demographic Transition, in which declining death rates are always followed (but never preceded) by falling birthrates.[21]

By 1875 many scientific workers, most notably Louis Pasteur and Robert Koch, were actively bringing into being the single advance that was to take up where the sanitary movement left off. Had it occurred before the cholera epidemic of 1848–1849, it most certainly would have prevented the ghastly slaughter of thousands of Londoners because of the incorrect hypothesis about the actual mechanism of infection. This scientific advance, germ theory, would soon show what really causes infections, and why people deprived of adequate food, shelter, clothing, and sanitation would always suffer more contagions than their more fortunate contemporaries. Germ theory would also save lives by demonstrating new ways of preventing and treating the infectious disorders of our species, starting with the method originally employed against smallpox by Edward Jenner in 1796, but now, thanks to the newborn germ theory, about to be extended to the prevention of other killing diseases.

CHAPTER

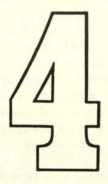

A VACCINE FOR EVERY INFECTION

He that thoroughly understands the nature of ferments and fermentations, shall probably be much better able than he that ignores them, to give a fair account of divers phenomena of several diseases (as well fevers as others) which will perhaps be never thoroughly understood, without an insight into the doctrines of fermentation.

—ROBERT BOYLE, 1663

The theory that infectious diseases are caused by pathogenic microbial entities, such as bacteria and fungi, was first demonstrated in 1835 in Italy in the work of Agostino Bassi (1733–1856). Trained as a lawyer, Bassi also studied the natural sciences at Pavia. When illness and failing vision, which was ultimately to leave him sightless, forced him to quit the civil service, Bassi tried farming for a living. It was not very successful, but a small inheritance came in time to meet his modest needs. Bassi started to study various natural systems and disorders, from the natural history of potatoes, other plants, and cheeses to pellagra, cholera, and one of the economically ruinous diseases of silkworms—muscardine, or *mal de segno calcinaccio.*

Bassi discovered that this silkworm disease is caused by a microscopic fungus (*Botrytis bassiana*). He was able to show how this fungus infected its silkworm hosts by invasion, by contact, and via food contaminated with the microorganism. Once the cause of this infection and its mechanisms were understood, Bassi proceeded to work out the logical sanitary measures for the prevention of muscardine in commercial silkworm nurseries.

He then took a historic intellectual stride forward. What was true of this infectious disease in silkworms, Bassi wrote in 1838, would be proven true of the as yet unisolated microbial agents of cholera, plague, syphilis, smallpox, typhoid fever, and other known infectious diseases. So compelling were his scientific work and his analytical logic that other serious investigators began to seek the postulated microscopic pathogens. These investigators included the codiscoverer of the cell theory, Theodor Schwann, who in 1837 had discovered that the yeasts which caused alcoholic fermentation were living microscopic organisms; and Schwann's lifelong friend and colleague, the anatomist and pathologist Jakob Henle.

William Farr (1807–83), the physician and medical statistician, observed in his Second Annual Report of the Registrar-General in 1840, "The hypothesis that the causes of epidemics are generations of minute insects transmitted from one individual to another, through the medium of the atmosphere, has been ingeniously put by Dr. [Henry] Holland in his *Medical Notes and Reflections.* Henle, of Berlin, has supported the theory by new facts and analogies."

In that same year Henle, in his essay *On Miasms and Contagions,* had put forward the hypothesis that "the material of contagion is not only organic but living, endowed with individual life and standing to the diseased body in the relation of a parasitic organism." Henle at the same time spelled out the conditions under which this hypothesis could be tested for its validity (and, if confirmed, promoted from the status of an unproven working hypothesis to an experimentally validated theory). These conditions, or postulates, called for the unknown agent of any specific infection to be isolated from the body of an individual animal or person suffering from a specific infectious disease; then for the agent to be able to cause the same disease in a second host; and then for the same agent to appear in the body of the second host, to be isolated by the experimenter, and then to be used to produce the same disease in a third host.

Fourteen years later in 1854, two physicians, one in Florence, Italy, and the other in London, discovered, in the intestines of cholera victims, the germs of cholera. The Florentine, Filippo Pacini, recognized that this agent, which he called the vibrio cholera, was an "organic, living substance of a parasitic nature, which can communicate itself, reproduce itself, and thereby produce a specific disease" called cholera. The Londoner, Arthur Hill Hassall, notified the Medical Council of the General Board of Health that he had found "myriads of vibriones . . . in every drop of every sample of rice-water discharges—i.e., the loose stools of cholera victims. As Norman Howard-Jones comments, "Neither [Hassall] nor the General Board of Health appreciated, as did Pacini, the etiological significance of the vibrios."[1]

What made this all the more curious was that in the same year an equally important finding had been made on the mechanism of transmission of what in due time would be identified as this very microbial agent of cholera. This was the demonstration, at the well of the Broad Street pump in London, of what Sir John Snow (1813–1858) had written as early as 1849 and had argued since then—that cholera was transmitted by a specific contaminant in drinking water.

At that time, many London families obtained their water from large neighborhood wells, and disposed of their body wastes in adjacent neighborhood cesspools. The more affluent families bought their water from private companies, which obtained it from their own commercial wells, from various locations along the Thames, and from more rural streams. In August and September 1854, when an outbreak of cholera killed 616 people in an area within 250 yards of the pump at the Broad Street well, Snow showed that each of these people drew his or her drinking water from this pump.

The Broad Street well was less than a block away from a workhouse sheltering 535 homeless poor people. The workhouse had its own well and drew no water from the Broad Street pump. Also nearby was a brewery, which relied on its own well to make its beer and ale, and to supply the drinking water consumed by its seventy employees. While the epidemic raged, only five of the 535 workhouse inmates died of cholera. Not a single brewery employee came down with cholera, nor were there any reports of its products serving as conduits for the spread of the disease. Curiously, a woman who had formerly lived in the area and become fond of water from the Broad Street well, hired a carter to deliver supplies of it to her when she moved to Hampstead. On September 6, 1854, she proved to be the only person in Hampstead to catch and die of cholera during this localized outbreak.

At Snow's direction, an investigation of conditions below the surface of the Broad Street pump revealed that the contents of a large neighborhood cesspool had been seeping into the well for some time. Not only was the well itself contaminated with fecal matter from the adjacent cesspool, but the Broad Street pump was contaminated with highly visible organic debris from the well water. Despite the published reports of Pacini and Hassall, nobody, including Snow, seemed interested in applying Henle's postulates to the organic matter found in the Broad Street well pump during the cholera outbreak in 1854.

Neither Pacini nor Snow were unknowns. Pacini, professor of histology at Florence, at the age of twenty-three had discovered the tactile corpuscles since named after him. Snow, a prominent anesthetist, soon would include Queen Victoria among his patients. Although Dr. John Simon, England's senior medical officer and a lifetime leader in the sanitary reform movement, did not mention Pacini's cholera vibrios in any of his papers, in an 1858 report to the General Board of Health he did refer to Snow's "peculiar doctrine (first advanced in 1849) as to the contagiousness of cholera." Snow, in Simon's mind, had failed to prove his concept or to answer many of the arguments raised against it by other doctors. Simon conceded, however, that Snow's data were "valuable evidence of the danger of drinking fecalized water during the epidemic prevalence of cholera."

Neither Snow nor Pacini during their lifetimes—Snow died in 1858, Pacini lived until 1883—were able to win any support for their findings and their views on the natural history of cholera. Prior to 1858, for example, both men submitted papers on their work to the Paris Academy of Sciences in a competition for a hundred-thousand-franc prize offered for original work on the causes and cure of cholera. The scientists who judge the 153 submissions included men as acute as Dr. Claude Bernard, one of the fathers of experimental medicine. No prizes were awarded for any of the papers, but the Academy of Sciences' judges did in 1858 single out for high praise a paper by the chief physician of Smolensk, Russia, who suggested that smallpox pus be inoculated into cholera patients, since he claimed that the virus of smallpox also produced typhoid fever, typhus, and cholera. The judges had fine words too for the presentation of an English physician who claimed to get excellent results by having his cholera patients swallow one grain of calomel (mercurous chloride) every five minutes.

Only one major figure in the world of medicine took the work of

Snow and Pacini seriously. He was Dr. William Farr, the Registrar-General of England. In 1867, while attending a statistical conference in Florence, Farr made a point of visiting Pacini in his pathology laboratory, and later included nine very complimentary pages on his work in the 1868 annual report of the Registrar-General.[2]

For three decades after Pacini started to present his elegant proofs of the role of the cholera vibrio in the infection and its major symptoms, the one opposing concept which defeated him was that of the Munich hygienist, Max von Pettenkofer (1818–1901). It was not that Pettenkofer's entirely wrong hypothesis of cholera as an infection caused by poisons in spoiled groundwater made more sense than Pacini's microbes. Pettenkofer's cholera hypothesis was far less impressive than the public health results he achieved during these years by forcing Munich to institute the sanitary disposal of wastes, the provision of clean drinking water, and the rigid enforcement of his new "English" housing sanitation regulations. Pettenkofer's accomplishments as a municipal sanitarian were so spectacular that their sheen rubbed off on his totally inane groundwater hypothesis for cholera.

It would take the scientific work of a great many investigators, in fields ranging from crystallography to botany, chemistry, and medicine, to help establish the basic principles of germ theory, and to make them palatable to leaders in medicine and public health. The ranks of these scientific workers included five whose shared interests and discoveries symbolize some of the main currents of inquiry responsible for the establishment of germ theory. They were: the chemist Louis Pasteur (1822–1895), the botanist Ferdinand Julius Cohn (1828–1898), and the physicians Casimir Joseph Davaine (1812–1882), Jean Antoine Villemin (1827–1892), and Robert Koch (1843–1910).

Davaine, a general practitioner in Paris, never had a laboratory. He did all his research on sheep, rabbits, and other experimental animals kept in the backyard of a friend in Paris. It was there in 1850, on time stolen from his clinical practice, that Davaine inoculated healthy sheep with the blood of sheep who had died of anthrax, then as now a very costly disease of farm animals and a deadly infection in people who handled animals. Under a microscope a few days later, the blood of the inoculated healthy sheep was found to contain some unusual microscopic rods. Davaine published a short account of his finding and then lost interest in this line of inquiry.

A dozen years later, after Pasteur had reported finding similar rods in his studies of lactic-acid fermentation, rods which Pasteur described as "specific butyric acid ferments," Davaine again began to wonder about the rods found in association with anthrax. In his article Pasteur had called these "small cylindrical rods" by various names, such as vibrios, infusoria, and animalcules. He described them as living without "free oxygen gas," and reported that they reproduced "by simple fission," which led to the "segmented chainlike arrangement" in which they were found. Pasteur's work suggested to Davaine—as indeed to Pasteur himself—that these microbial bodies might be pathogens, or causes of disease.

There were a number of reasons for this concept. One of them was what had long appeared to sanitarians as the causal links between putrefaction—the rotting or decomposition of organic matter, and its malodorous by-products like hydrogen sulfide—and the onset of infectious diseases. As a matter of fact, in the nineteenth century infectious diseases were called zymotic diseases (from the Greek word *zymotikos*, "causing fermentation"). No one had yet learned that putrefaction is caused by bacteria, but when Pasteur showed that these microbial organisms caused fermentations, many people joined Pasteur and Davaine in suspecting that there might be causal links between bacteria and infectious diseases in people.

Davaine went back to his studies of the anthrax rods, which he first described as bacteria and subsequently as bacteridia. Davaine showed that these microbes seemed to be present whenever there was anthrax; that anthrax could be transmitted to healthy animals by inoculating them with blood containing these bacteria; and that when these organisms were not present, there was no anthrax. His papers were carefully read by Pasteur and, in Germany, by Robert Koch, who was a twenty-year-old medical student (studying with Jakob Henle, among other professors) when Davaine's series of reports on anthrax rods appeared in 1863.

By then, much of what we know now about the forms and nature of bacteria had been explored and described by the botanist Ferdinand Julius Cohn, one of the major founders of bacteriology. Born in the Prussian city of Breslau (now Wroclaw, Poland) and educated at the Universities of Breslau and Berlin, Cohn studied under a number of great teachers, including the anatomist and physiologist Johannes Müller (whose students included Jakob Henle, Rudolf Virchow, and other giants), and Christian Ehrenberg, who had been one of the first scientific workers in Europe to become interested in the blood-red pigmented *Serratia marcescens* following the work of Bizio and Sette in 1823. It was Ehrenberg who interested Cohn in the natural history of life forms too tiny to be seen except under the microscope. In 1850 Cohn published a landmark monograph on *Serratia marcescens*, (then known as *Monas prodigiosa*). The different types of bacteria were already Cohn's major research interest by 1859 when he returned as professor of botany to Breslau, where he would remain for the rest of his life.

Cohn realized that although bacteria were the smallest of all living organisms, they were not animals or bugs but closer to the plant family, closely related to blue-green algae. He divided them into different genera and species by form and by function, and showed that not all bacteria cause diseases. "Bacteria certainly develop in every fermentation, and where there is any putrefaction, without exerting the least influence on health," he wrote in

About Bacteria: The Smallest Forms of Life (1872). "We already know that the bacteria of contagion are of a different kind from those that cause putrefaction; the former are distinguished from the latter under the microscope mostly through their form; they exist under entirely different circumstances of life; they often battle for existence with the bacteria of putrefaction, and are by them exterminated if they are conquered."

These conclusions were based on direct observations made under the microscope, and by techniques of growth and measurement that Cohn had to develop by himself. He devised one of the first standard liquid growth media for culturing bacteria. Cohn's discoveries included bacterial spores, and the heat-resisting properties of *Bacillus subtilis* spores. His contributions to the development of bacteriology and germ theory did not end in the laboratory: As a teacher, and as the founder and editor of the scientific journal *Beiträge zür Biologie der Pflanzen,* (Contributions to the Biology of Plants), Cohn provided inspiration, information, and a forum for generations of aspiring young life scientists.

When Pasteur, still an outsider, became embroiled with prominent members of the French Establishment in his battle over spontaneous versus biological generation, Cohn supported him with a vigor that belied his extremely gentle personality. Although Pasteur was one of those indomitable fighters who always deliver more telling blows than they receive, Cohn's support proved most helpful when Pasteur was not yet himself a member of the Academy of Sciences.

Louis Pasteur was, by any scale of measurement, a man unique for any time. Throughout his life, Pasteur made a point of repeating to friends and foes that "in the field of experimentation, chance favors the prepared mind." It was only hard work and not hereditary brilliance that prepared the human mind. The son of a poor ex-sergeant in Napoleon's army who eked out a precarious living as a tanner in Dôle, Louis Pasteur grew up with few illusions about making his way in life except by hard work.

The only son among the family's four children, Pasteur had a sister who, in his words, "suffered at the age of three from a cerebral fever which completely interrupted the development of her intelligence," and left her "mentally a child although an adult in body." This early experience with the lifelong effects of childhood diseases was to be compounded more tragically for Pasteur as a father: Between 1859, when his first-born child, Jeanne, died at nine, and 1866, childhood diseases and typhoid were to kill three of his five children. In 1868, when Pasteur was forty-four and professor of chemistry at the Sorbonne, he suffered a stroke that permanently paralyzed his left arm and leg. This handicap, however, did not keep him from resuming his work on silkworm diseases begun at Alais in 1865; undertaking his studies of the diseases of beer and wine between 1871 and 1877; running unsuccessfully for the

French Senate in 1876; starting his studies of anthrax and, a little later, of puerperal fever, septicemia, and gangrene; publishing, in 1878, his monograph *The Germ Theory and Its Applications to Medicine and Surgery;* and, a year later, developing and testing the first vaccine made since Jenner's against smallpox, Pasteur's vaccine against fowl cholera. Pasteur's lifelong respect for the killing and crippling disorders of humankind was matched by the unblinking realism with which he viewed his place in the France of the Industrial Revolution. If he was a humorless, intense, and fanatically hard-working individual for all of his student and adult life, the reasons were evident in his background.

As a youth, Pasteur showed great talent and took great pleasure in the graphic arts. When, however, the time came to prepare for making a living, Pasteur abandoned art for the economically more sensible goal of a career as a secondary-school science teacher. Born in 1822, in an era when the early Industrial Revolution created a well-perceived social need for scientific and technological skills, Pasteur devoted himself to his school studies with all the grim determination of a poor youth who fully understood that success in his academic examinations spelled the only difference between a secure life as a teacher in the schools of the Ministry of Education and the less attractive prospects of an uneducated tanner's son.

The choice of the two doctoral theses Pasteur prepared and defended at the École Normale in 1847 also reflected his very practical goals. One thesis was in chemistry, on the nature of arsenous oxide. The other thesis, in physics, dealt with the optical rotation of tartrate crystals. The twenty-five-year-old doctoral candidate demonstrated that in these crystals "the ability of certain molecules to deviate the plane of polarized light is due to, or at least linked most intimately to the dissymmetry of these molecules," in which what seemed to be structurally identical crystals deviate polarized light either to the left or to the right.

For discovering molecular dissymmetry, Pasteur won the admiration and lifelong support of the academicians whose "errors" this work had corrected, Jean Baptiste Biot and Eilhardt Mitscherlich.

Pasteur's studies of molecular dissymmetry were done with tartaric-acid crystals derived from the tartar in wine fermentation vats, and with racemic-acid crystals derived from grapes. It was only in crystals derived from living organisms, rather than from substances of nonliving origin such as quartz crystals, that he could find molecular dissymmetries. Pasteur found, under the microscope, that some molds, which feed and proliferate on tartrates, "destroy by their nutrition one of the categories of molecules to the exclusion of the other, and finally leave an active solution either to the right or left." This finding was of obvious and immediate interest to distillers of industrial alcohol because of other and possibly adverse effects such molds might have on fermentation.

Once the young doctoral candidate discovered molecular dissymmetry in crystals derived from one organic component of fermentation, the logic of scientific inquiry would impel him to do further work on the nature of fermentation itself. Medically the basic inquiry into fermentation—and the analogous putrefaction—were long overdue.

As early as 1663 the great British chemist Robert Boyle (1627–1691) had written, "He that thoroughly understands the nature of ferments and fermentations, shall probably be much better able than he that ignores them, to give a fair account of divers phenomena of several diseases (as well as fevers as others) which will perhaps be never thoroughly understood, without an insight into the doctrines of fermentation." Now, nearly two centuries later, Pasteur took his first giant stride on his way to demonstrating the roles of microbial organisms in both fermentation and putrefaction. In the coming decades, this work on fermentation would help Pasteur and other fine European scientists develop and apply the germ theory of infectious diseases and revolutionize private and public health medicine.

In 1848, two months after Pasteur was appointed professor of physics at the Lycée in Dijon, Biot's influence at the Ministry of Education succeeded in having Pasteur transferred to the University of Strasbourg as professor of chemistry, where he met and married Marie Laurent, the daughter of the university's rector.

In 1854, when Pasteur was appointed professor of chemistry and dean of sciences at the University of Lille, he did not resist when the Ministry suggested that he focus his teaching and research on the needs of local industries. To Pasteur, the quintessential pragmatist, there was nothing improper or anti-intellectual in this request. He believed there was no vast distinction between what gentlemen scholars revered as the pure sciences and what they denigrated as the applied sciences. Pasteur told the students in his inaugural address, "Without theory, practice is but routine born of habit. Theory alone can bring forth and develop the spirit of invention." Routine medical practice alone could at best make three-year-old children stricken with cerebral meningitis more comfortable; but only through discoveries that led to new theories could improved medical care prevent meningitis and other infections from killing the minds and bodies of children like his little sister.

Pasteur's respect for theory had very practical roots. Much as it represented a love of truth for its own sake, it also reflected his fear of the damage caused when false hypotheses were accepted as valid theories. Both feelings were apparent in his lifelong crusade to demolish the concept of spontaneous generation of life and natural processes.

Pasteur's effort to refute the idea that life forms and processes arise spontaneously from diverse internal and external vitalist causes came to a dramatic and triumphant conclusion in 1864. His elegant demonstrations in arrays of glass flasks presented the members of the Academy of Sciences with the irrefutable proofs that life derives only from life and not from some mysterious "vital force" as maintained by Félix Pouchet and other scientific spokesmen. For Pasteur the debate was far from a mere intellectual exercise; in his mind the idea of spontaneous generation directly threatened acceptance of the germ theories of fermentation and disease.

For as long as die-hard advocates persisted in advancing the ideas of spontaneous generation, Pasteur remained on the attack. On July 9, 1878, for example, while presenting a report to the Academy of Medicine on the bacterial transmission of anthrax, Pasteur's lecture included a continuing critique of spontaneous generation. "I can tell you my program in only two words: I have sought for twenty years, and I am still seeking, spontaneous generation properly so called," he said. "If God permit, I shall seek for twenty years and more the spontaneous generation of transmissible diseases."

Even before he began to study fermentation at Lille in 1855, Pasteur was acutely aware of how mistaken concepts, particularly when held and advocated by well-regarded authorities, acted as barriers to both understanding and investigating natural laws and processes.

A year after Pasteur settled in at Lille, he began his studies on fermentation, in this instance on the fermentation of beet sugar. The use of locally grown beet sugar in the production of alcohol had made distilling one of the major industries in and around Lille. What Pasteur learned from these studies would lead him directly to the germ theory of infectious diseases.

During the two decades since Cagniard de Latour, Theodor Schwann, and Friedrich Kutzing demonstrated that the yeasts used in fermentation were living organisms and not, as previously believed, chemicals, a spirited and often caustic controversy had raged in Europe on the nature of fermentation and ferments. The opposition to the theory that ferments were living organisms was led by three of the world's most towering figures in chemistry, Baron Justus von Liebig, one of the founders of biochemistry; the Swedish master Baron Berzelius; and his former student, Friedrich Wohler, who in 1828 became the first to synthesize organic or "living" matter (urea) from inorganic materials (potassium cyanate treated with ammonium sulfate). In an age when scientific controversies could produce bizarre literary broadsides, Liebig and Wohler were quite in accord with their times when they collaborated in 1839 on an anonymous burlesque of a scientific article in Liebig's journal, *Annals of Chemistry*, entitled "The Riddle of Vinous Fermentation Solved."

In this tongue-in-cheek "scientific" report, yeasts were described as eggs that grew into microscopic animals made up of limbs and organs modeled on the parts of a laboratory distilling apparatus. These animalcules, according to Liebig and Wohler, could be observed under the microscope to ingest sugar, digest it, and then excrete its waste products as alcohol through their rectums, and as carbonic acid from their genitalia. When satire failed them, Liebig and his supporters fell back on their well-earned scientific authority. As Pasteur observed in 1860, in his own memoir on alcoholic fermentation, "M. Liebig has expressed his ideas in most of his publications with such persistence and conviction that they have gradually been accepted" by most of the world's scientists.

By then, Pasteur had entered upon his own studies of the nature and mechanisms of fermentation. The mountains of incontrovertible scientific evidence these studies generated, plus Pasteur's relish in offering abundant experimental proofs to counter Liebig's brilliant but unsubstantiated rhetoric, would completely alter most accepted notions. This, however, was not to happen until Pasteur had put in five solid years of study and preparation. Pasteur not only proved that some bacteria cause fermentation and other microbes cause putrefaction; in his own mind, he was already convinced that similar germs cause infectious diseases. As early as 1863, when Pasteur's friend, the chemist and senator Jean Baptiste Dumas, presented him to the emperor Louis Napoleon, Pasteur declared that his "ambition was to arrive at the knowledge of putrid and contagious disease."

The period between 1865, when Pasteur began his studies on the infectious diseases of silkworms, and 1879, when he developed and tested his vaccine (the term vaccine was chosen in honor of Jenner) against fowl cholera, would be one of the most amazing eras in the history of biology and medicine.

Toward the end of the American Civil War, a French army doctor, Jean Antoine Villemin, was intrigued by the similarities between *morve* (glanders), an infectious disease of horses, and tuberculosis. Villemin, who later became one of the physicians who attended Pasteur, began to suspect that human tuberculosis was an infectious disease. He started a series of experiments, in which sputum and materials from the lesions of tuberculosis patients were inoculated into the bodies of rabbits, guinea pigs, dogs, and other animals. Some of these inoculations were made directly, by needle scratch and syringe. Others were made using more indirect routes. In the people-to-guinea-pig inoculations, for example, Villemin "took the sputum of tuberculosis patients, spread it on cotton wool, dried it, then made the cotton wool into a bed for little guinea-pigs, who became tuberculous."[3]

By 1865 Villemin was able to use inocula from people with tuberculosis to infect animals with the disease; to use sputum and other tuberculous materials from these animals to produce tuberculosis in animals of the same or other species; and to repeat the infection-and-transmission processes between animals of the same and different species again and again. In his book *Studies on Tuberculosis,* published in 1868, Villemin described tuberculosis as a contagious disease, like glanders. He made a point of writing, however, that the "visible, tangible" sputum and other tuberculous materials used in the infective inocula were not in themselves the agents of tuberculosis, but contained "a more subtle principle which escapes our senses." The organism into which tuberculous materials are inoculated, Villemin wrote, "Plays only the role of a medium in which the virus multiplies as a parasite." He pointed out that although the smallpox virus "is contained in the pus of the [smallpox] pustule ... the pus is not the virus."

Villemin had proved, to those who would study his evidence objectively and repeat his experiments, that tuberculosis is an infectious, inoculable, and therefore transmissible disease, most probably caused by a subtle "principle" carried in the sputum and tuberculous lesions of infected people and other animals. In the face of the commonly accepted belief that, as the prominent French physician Pidoux maintained, "tuberculosis ... is the common result of a quantity of divers external and internal causes, not the product of a specific agent ever the same," Villemin had to contend with the regressive effects of the conventional wisdom of the educated classes. His failure to produce, along with his demonstration of the transmissibility of tuberculosis, the invisible active "principle" of infection carried in the tuberculous materials of consumptive people did not help his case in most scientific quarters.

There were exceptions, of course. For example, there was the pathologist Julius Cohnheim (1839–1884), who had trained under Virchow and was a colleague of Cohn's at Breslau. Cohnheim verified Villemin's work by inoculating tuberculous matter into the anterior eye of a rabbit, and he reported on how he watched the tuberculosis lesion gradually form there. Another German physician who took Villemin very seriously was Robert Koch, who ultimately isolated and described the active principle of tuberculosis. In 1868 when Villemin's book appeared, Koch was two years out of medical school, the father of a newborn daughter, and scrambling for a living after the abolition of his job as house physician in an institution for mentally ill children in Langenhagen.

By 1870, shortly after a few months of service as a field physician in the Franco-Prussian War, the twenty-seven-year-old Koch successfully applied for a job as district health officer in the town of Wollstein, in the province of Posen. The job had many responsibilities, including the supervision of a small hospital and the monitoring of diseases of farm animals. It provided a decent house for the young doctor and his family which was also large enough to hold an office for his private medical practice. Without his private practice, which included frequent night calls to the farms of the vicinity, Koch would have been hard-pressed to meet his family's minimal needs.

Trained under teachers like Wohler and Henle, and coming of age during the years when the work of Pasteur, Davaine, Lister, and Lemaire resulted in frequent mention of a new germ theory of contagious diseases, Koch was passionately interested in studying the newly developed concepts of infection. He set up his own laboratory in a small room next to his medical office, and started to cultivate bacteria on slices of cooked potato, as described by Cohn. He kept guinea pigs, rabbits, and even apes at the hospital, but experimented with them and autopsied them both at home and the hospital. With only the journal literature of France and Germany as his guides, Koch embarked on years of self-training and self-development of the principles and techniques of medical microbiology.

An enthusiastic amateur photographer, he was one of the first to photograph bacteria through the microscope. Because Koch had to work alone, he was spared the mistakes of other people, and often had to improvise new techniques of making certain observations and measurements. One of the products of these efforts was a superior method of obtaining pure cultures of bacteria suspected of being pathogens, and of maintaining these cultures in nutrient media free of other bacteria. In 1873 a particularly costly outbreak of anthrax in the farms around Wollstein made necessary an investigation of Davaine's earlier work on the microbial rods (*Bacillus anthracis*) found in the blood of infected animals part of Koch's official duties. For the first time he was able to do bacteriological research on official time rather than at his own expense.

Koch was eager, but he was not going to be rushed. It was to be three years before the district medical officer, after working doggedly on the problem, had anything to publish on anthrax. Prior to submitting his findings for publication, Koch sent a letter off to Cohn at Breslau. "Esteemed Professor," he wrote, "stimulated by your bacterial investigations which were published in *Contributions to the Biology of Plants* [Cohn's scientific journal], and having ample access to the necessary source material [i.e., infected farm animals], I have been investigating the etiology of anthrax for a considerable time. After many failures, I have finally succeeded in completely elucidating the development cycle of *Bacillus anthracis*. I believe I have amply confirmed my results. Nevertheless, esteemed Professor, I would be most grateful if you ... would give me your criticism of my work before I submit it for publication. Since my demonstration material cannot be preserved, I seek your kind permission to demonstrate the critical experiments for you over a period of several days at the Institute of Plant Physiology."

A man of exquisite courtesy, Cohn invited young Koch to Breslau even though, as he would write later, he "anticipated little of value of this request from a completely unknown physician from a rural Polish town."

In a matter of days, young Koch, looking more like a burly young peddler of kitchen utensils than a provincial medical bureaucrat, arrived and set up his demonstration in Cohn's laboratories. He carried with him his own animals, microscope, and bacteriological equipment, much of it of his own improvisation. His demonstration of the life cycle of the anthrax rods lasted three days. It required much less time than this to make Cohn and his colleagues realize what had happened. "Within the very first hour," Cohn wrote, "I recognized that he was the unsurpassed master of scientific research."[4]

Cohn requested that the entire staff of the Pathology Institute attend the second day of Koch's demonstration. Julius Cohnheim, the director of the Institute, shared Cohn's enthusiasm for the visitor's contributions. He went back to his laboratory and told his associate, Otto Weigert (1845–1904), the pathologist who developed the staining methods Koch had used (and a cousin of Paul Ehrlich, whose stains would be equally helpful to Koch), to "drop everything and go to see Koch. This man has made a great discovery, all the more amazing is that he has developed simple, precise, and definitive methods entirely on his own. There is nothing to add. I consider this the greatest discovery in the field of bacteriology and believe that Koch will continue to surprise us and shame us with further discoveries."[5]

On the third day of Koch's demonstration, the unknown district doctor from a rural Polish town was no longer a neophyte seeking learned criticism; now the novice had become the professor, imparting major new knowledge and demonstrating successful new laboratory techniques in a laboratory crowded to the rafters with professors of medicine, biology, chemistry, pathology, and histology. "Davaine has demonstrated decisively that anthrax could be transmitted with fresh or dried blood from infected animals only when the blood contained characteristic rods, and that these rods were bacteria," read the opening line of Koch's written report. Now, in three days of convincing demonstration, Koch showed exactly how these bacteria cause and transmit anthrax.

Cohn and Cohnheim set out to get Koch an appointment at Breslau or, failing that, at some other university where he could devote himself to teaching or research. These efforts did not succeed, in no small measure because, for all their international stature, both Cohn and Cohnheim were Jewish in a university system in which this was a great drawback. In 1880 they were successful, however, in obtaining a major appointment for Koch in the Imperial Health Office in Berlin. This gave him his own laboratories as well as a salary that freed him from the need to supplement his income by private practice.

In the four years that he continued to do research on a part-time basis at his family's expense in Wollstein after his three-day visit to Breslau, Koch was far from nonproductive. He continued to develop new techniques of working with bacteria, employing the aniline dyes first used by Weigert and Ehrlich to stain bacteria to prepare them for microscopy, and experimenting with the new illuminating system based on the Abbé condenser in the Zeiss microscopes and with different methods of connecting cameras to microscopes to photograph bacteria. In 1878 Koch published his small (eighty-page) book *Investigations into the Etiology of Traumatic Infective Diseases,* in which he showed that—at least in experimental animals—specific infectious diseases were caused by specific microbial agents.

To be sure, all the findings in this book were based on animal and not human experiments. However, many of the animal diseases that he studied, such as anthrax, were also crippling and often fatal infections of people. Anthrax, also known as woolsorters' disease and often contracted from infected sheep and other farm animals, caused sudden chills, high fevers, great pain, shortness of breath, and extreme prostration. Cerebral anthrax caused violent delirium; the common cutaneous anthrax caused malignant pustules, or carbuncles, in people. Tuberculosis, as Villemin had shown, could be transmitted from beast to man, and from people to animals. Koch did not have to go beyond animal models to show the pathogenic potential of bacteria in our species.

In his book Koch first made the statement that proof of the disease-inducing nature of specific organisms had to be established by meeting certain defined criteria. Proof could be demonstrated by "finding the parasitic micro-organisms in all cases of the disease in question, when we can further demonstrate their presence in such numbers and distribution that all symptoms of the disease may thus find their explanation, and finally when we have established, for every individual traumatic disease, the existence of a micro-organism with well defined morphological characters." The brilliant work of his old student was, at last, turning Henle's philosophical postulates into a firm biological law.

Another passage in Koch's book spoke for both his powers of careful observation—and for the need truly to understand the meaning of what one sees under the microscope. Of the bacilli found in the blood of septicemic mice, Koch reported that, "Their relation to the white blood cells is peculiar. They penetrate into these and multiply. *Hardly one is without bacilli* [emphasis added]. Many contain only isolated bacilli, others have thick masses of bacilli with a recognizable nucleus, in others the nucleus can no longer be distinguished, and finally some cells may appear as a cluster of bacilli about to fragment."

Koch had seen exactly what other scientists had seen under their microscopes, but only two had suspected that they were looking at one of the major inborn defenses against microbial parasites. In 1874 the Danish pathologist and physiologist Peter Ludwig Panum (1820–1885) speculated that the white blood cells—the leukocytes—might actually be destroyers of invasive bacteria. In 1881 Élie (Ilya) Metchnikoff (1845–1916), another of the many young people advised by Ferdinand Cohn, was working with starfish larvae and water fleas at Messina, Italy, and made the first of many observations of intracellular digestion that would lead quickly to proof of Panum's hunch, and to a new word for white blood cells, phagocytes (from the Greek and Latin words for eaters of cells).

In a sense, Koch was so absorbed in developing an entirely new methodology of bacteriology that he could be forgiven for failing to grasp instantly the significance of some of the new information this improved methodology made available. Koch's exhibit of his techniques were the sensation of the International Medical Congress in London in 1881. Among the many people who flocked to Koch's demonstration, held in Joseph Lister's laboratory at King's College, was Louis Pasteur, who warmly congratulated Koch on his great advances. However, as Lechevalier and Solotorovsky were later to observe, "Pasteur's remark [*"C'est un grand progrès, monsieur"*] was not the beginning of a beautiful friendship; contact between the two great men remained infrequent, and on some occasions they disparaged each other's work."[6]

That same year, working with tissue taken from an ape that had died of tuberculosis, which was then inoculated into guinea pigs, Koch began to search for the elusive subtle principle in tuberculous sputum and body materials that had eluded Villemin. This time he not only produced tuberculosis in the guinea pigs, but also isolated the germs found in the newly infected rodents, grew the bacteria in pure culture, and then inoculated healthy animals with these bacteria. The healthy animals developed tuberculosis, and bacteria that appeared in their bodies with the disease transmitted tuberculosis to other healthy animals.

Koch's discovery of the tubercle bacillus, announced at a small meeting of the Berlin Physiological Society in May 1882, created a scientific sensation around the world. Paul Ehrlich, one of the seventy people present, remarked many years later that "that evening has remained my greatest experience in science." It was also the high point of Koch's scientific career, for of all the killing and crippling infectious diseases rendered endemic by the new environments of industrialization and urbanization in the nineteenth century, only pneumonia ranked with tuberculosis as a widespread killer of people. What made the isolation of the tubercle bacillus so much more dramatic was the fact that one year earlier, in 1881, Pasteur had demonstrated that vaccines made of weakened strains of bacteria could protect animals from developing anthrax and fowl cholera after being inoculated with the active germs of these widespread farm diseases.

Although not a physician, Pasteur was elected in 1873 an associate member of the Academy of Medicine, largely because of his discoveries on the nature of fermentation and silkworm diseases. He was by then actively studying infectious diseases of animals and people. Many of his young assistants, like Émile Roux and Charles Chamberland, were qualified physicians. They took him to various hospitals to observe patients, and to sit in on postmortem examinations. During most of these visits, samples of blood and sputum and organ tissues were taken from patients and cadavers for microscopic examination at Pasteur's laboratories at the Sorbonne.

At times Pasteur's lack of early training in medicine, and conditioning in its psychic shocks, was painfully apparent. "It was to the Hospital Cochin or to the Maternité that we went most frequently, taking our culture tubes and sterilized pipets into the wards of operating theaters," Roux wrote. "No one knows what feelings of repulsion Pasteur had to overcome before visiting patients and witnessing post-mortem examinations. His sensibility was extreme, and he suffered morally and physically from the pains of others; the cut of the bistoury [a long, narrow-bladed surgical knife] opening an abscess made him wince as if he himself had received it. The sight of corpses, the sad business of necropsies, caused him real [anguish]; we have often seen him go home ill from these operating theaters. But his love of science, his desire for truth were stronger; he returned the next day."[7] Nor did his queasiness in the presence of acute disorders and death ever interfere with Pasteur's systematic collection of pathological materials.

When Dr. Émile Ducleaux in his Sorbonne laboratory developed a series of furuncles, boils originating in a hair follicle, Pasteur had the bacteria he isolated from these boils cultured and characterized. Later when pus taken from the inside and outside of a bone of a little girl operated on for osteomyelitis at the Trousseau Hospital was shown to contain the same kind of bacteria, Pasteur saw it as evidence that "osteomyelitis is the furuncle of bones." Osteomyelitis is caused by more than one kind of bacterium, with most infections caused by streptococci and staphylococci. In these two instances, the staphylococci had caused the infection.

Like many family men, Pasteur was particularly concerned with childbirth fever, the great maker of orphans and widowers. From what he could observe in the maternity wards, Roux wrote, "Pasteur does not hesitate to declare that microscopic organism is the most frequent cause of infection in recently delivered women. One day, in a discussion on puerperal fever at the Academy, one of his most weighty colleagues was eloquently enlarging upon the causes of epidemics in lying-in hospitals. Pasteur interrupted him from his place. 'None of those things cause the epidemic; it is the nursing and medical staff who carry the microbe from an infected woman to a healthy one.' As the orator replied that he feared the microbe would never be found, Pasteur went to the blackboard and drew a diagram of the chain-like organism, saying: 'There, that is what it is like!' "[8]

Like osteomyelitis, puerperal fever can be caused by many pathogenic bacteria, but the usual culprit is the chainlike *Streptococcus pyogenes*. Pasteur not only knew the cause of childbed fever; he also had some very effective techniques of preventing its causal organisms from inducing infections.

On April 30, 1878, Pasteur addressed the Academy of Medicine on germ theory and other researches he had carried on with the physicist Jules Joubert and the physician Charles Chamberland. Pasteur declared that "if I had the honor of being a surgeon, convinced as I am of the dangers caused by the germs of microbes scattered on the surface of every object, particularly in the hospitals, not only would I use absolutely clean instruments but, after cleansing my hands with the greatest care and putting them quickly through a flame, I would only use bandages, cloths and sponges that would have been exposed to air heated at 130 to 150 °C. I would only employ water which had been heated to a temperature of 110 °C to 120 °C. All that is easy in practice, and, in that way, I should still have to fear the germs suspended in the atmosphere surrounding the bed of the patient; but observation shows us every day that the number of those germs is insignificant compared to that of those which lie scattered on the surface of objects, or in the clearest ordinary water."[9]

To Pasteur the techniques of preventing bacterial infections were as important as the creation of the germ theory of infectious diseases. "There are not two kinds of science—practical and applied," he told the students of Lille. "There is only Science and the applications of Science, and one is dependent on the other, as the fruit is to the tree." Curiously, Pasteur never gave much thought to cures per se for bacterial infections; from the beginning of his researches, he saw the prevention of infection as the best of cures.

There was a very powerful reason for Pasteur's bias toward immunization: Jenner's vaccine against smallpox. Although nobody had yet isolated the agents of either smallpox or cowpox (which were not bacteria but true submicroscopic viruses), it seemed reasonable to assume that the cowpox was a milder form of smallpox, which was capable of inducing immunity to both pox diseases in people infected with cowpox. In all his experiments with the bacteria of anthrax, chicken cholera, and other diseases, it is quite probable that Pasteur consciously kept an eye open for agents of milder versions of major infectious diseases. Even when the task at hand was primarily to prove that specific bacteria were responsible for specific infections, Pasteur was very likely also looking for analogs of cowpox.

Around 1878, when Pasteur's attention was devoted mainly to two infections, anthrax and chicken cholera, his first problem was to prove that specific bacteria cause the diseases. In each instance the agents had been isolated and categorized by others. Davaine and Koch had shown that anthrax was probably caused by the anthrax bacillus originally isolated by Davaine. The bacterium of chicken cholera, now called *Pasteurella multocida,* had been isolated by Dr. H. Toussaint, who had tried with little success to culture the organism in neutral urine.

Toussaint sent the head of a chicken that had died of chicken cholera to Pasteur, who also isolated the causal bacteria. Culturing the organism, however, was more of a problem. It did not thrive in neutralized urine, which was a fine nutrient for *B. anthracis.* In other culture media, such as yeast water, the bacteria of chicken cholera simply vanished after forty-eight hours of incubation. Finally, Pasteur learned that heavy growths of the chicken cholera bacteria could be obtained very quickly by growing them in "a broth of chicken muscle neutralized by potassium hydroxide and sterilized by heating at 110 °C–115 °C."

In his first report on chicken cholera, published in 1880, Pasteur described how a few drops of a culture of this microbe, "deposited on bread or on meat fed to the chicken, are enough to cause the disease by intestinal invasion. The small microscopic organisms multiply abundantly in the intestine so that the excrements of the diseased animals are deadly. One can thus understand the manner of natural dissemination. Evidently the disease could be arrested by isolating the affected animals for a few days."

Pasteur had also made an even more important finding, but in this report he stopped just short of describing it. "Certain modifications in the method of culture of the infectious microbe can decrease its virulence." He described these modifications in only one word, "attenuation," but begged the indulgence of the Academy for not describing it any further.

A few months later, however, he informed the Academy of Sciences that attenuated cultures of highly virulent chicken cholera germs grew less virulent with age. If the interval of time between transfers of the culture from one bottle of broth to another were a day or even a week, he reported, the bacteria remained deadly to fowl. However, Pasteur now revealed, "If we wait three, four, five or eight months or more before we study the virulence of the cultures, then the whole picture has changed." Where the original cultures killed ten chickens out of ten inoculated, the greater the age, the lesser the infectivity of the cultures of these age-attenuated bacteria.

With increasing attenuation by aging in the same batch of nutrient medium, when chickens are inoculated, he reported, "only nine, eight, seven, six, five, four, three, and then only one chicken in ten dies. Sometimes mortality might be nil and all the inoculated chickens may be sick, but they all recover. In other terms, by a simple change in the mode of cultivation of the parasite, by a mere increase in the length of time elapsing between the successful transfers of the virus [i.e., the chicken cholera bacterium], we can obtain a true vaccinal virus, which does not kill, but gives a benign form of the disease and protects from the fatal disease."

The discovery of the detoxifying effects of attenuation on pathogenic bacteria had come about by chance. During the summer of 1879, cultures of virulent chicken cholera microbes had been stored in the laboratory refrigerator while Pasteur and his assistants went on vacation. After the vacation season, these accidentally attenuated cultures failed to produce fowl cholera when inoculated into healthy chickens.

Chance now began to favor prepared minds. Pasteur kept these chickens until a natural outbreak of chicken cholera provided his laboratory with fresh cultures of virulent fowl cholera germs. The fresh bacteria were then inoculated into the birds that had resisted the attenuated organisms, and into a batch of new chickens obtained from the market for this experiment.

The new chickens all came down with chicken cholera. Nearly all the chickens that had previously been inoculated with the attenuated cultures remained healthy and free of cholera. Pasteur, who used to insist that "we must immunize against the infectious diseases of which we can cultivate the causative microorganisms," now had what he had long sought: an analog of Jenner's cowpox.

This immunizing agent, attenuated chicken cholera bacteria, was as much a product of deliberate laboratory manipulation of the natural processes of bacterial infection and immunity as it was of nature. Although, unlike Jenner's vaccinia, it did not come from cows, Pasteur, in honor of the revered M. Jenner, named his immunizing agent against chicken cholera a vaccine. Within the next few years, he called his immunizing agents against both anthrax and rabies vaccines, and the term vaccination became a synonym for inoculations of any source that protected people and animals against specific infectious diseases.

Chicken cholera is not related to human cholera, and does not affect people. Anthrax, on the other hand, is a deadly disease that affects people as well as cattle, sheep, and horses. In 1880 Pasteur used heat high enough to alter but not high enough to kill anthrax bacilli in order to attenuate them. Like the age-attenuated chicken cholera organisms, the heat-weakened anthrax bacilli made excellent and safe vaccines.

While developing his anthrax vaccine, Pasteur also discovered that when animals who died of anthrax were buried, earthworms carried the infectious spores of the anthrax bacilli from the dead animals to the grass growing on the surfaces above, and thereby infected healthy grazing animals with anthrax. Fencing off such burial plots, therefore, provided one way of protecting animals from infection. The vaccine Pasteur and his colleagues developed by attenuating cultures of B. anthracis provided an even more effective way to prevent anthrax.

The dramatic public trials of the anthrax vaccine in 1881 were conducted only on sheep, horses, and cattle, but the implications for people were immediately apparent. The trials were barely over when Pasteur was delegated to represent his government at the International Medical Congress in London. By then, as Pasteur reported in a lecture on the attenuation of bacteria, vaccination had become the answer to the menace of anthrax. Within two weeks of the conclusion of the trials, "in the Departments surrounding Paris, we vaccinated nearly 20,000 sheep, and a great many oxen, cows, and horses."

Pasteur concluded his report at the Congress with a graceful tribute to Edward Jenner. In making the Congress aware of vaccination against a disease "more terrible perhaps for domestic animals than is smallpox for man," Pasteur said he had also "given to the word vaccination an extension which I hope Science will consecrate as a homage to the merit and immense services rendered by your Jenner, one of England's greatest men."

Nearing sixty, Pasteur returned to France to resume work on still a third disease, rabies, for which nobody had yet succeeded in isolating a causal microbe.

* * *

Three things were very well known about rabies at that time. The first was that it produced a raging condition, hydrophobia, for which medicine had never been able to provide a cure. Victims of hydrophobia or rabies suffered a constellation of acute symptoms that combined to cause death after a few days of terrible suffering. These symptoms included painful spasms of the throat muscles, which made trying to swallow even a sip of water an agony, while concurrent fevers, delirium, and paralysis added to the other burdens.

The second thing known about rabies was that it was definitely a transmissible infectious disease. In 1794 the British surgeon John Hunter had suggested that rabies could be caused in rabbits by inoculating them with saliva from a rabid dog. This transmission was achieved in Germany by Georg Gottfried Zinke ten years later. In 1810 the Parisian neurophysiologist François Magendie began a decade of experiments during which, among other things, he demonstrated that saliva from people with rabies could transmit the fatal disease to healthy dogs. Magendie also showed the affinity of the unknown rabies agent for the neurological systems of animals.

V. Galtier, a professor at the Lyons Veterinary School, whose work was known to Pasteur, in 1879 published accounts of how he had transmitted rabies from dogs to rabbits, and then from rabbits to rabbits. Galtier observed that because rabbits developed the paralytic and convulsive symptoms of rabies but not the "furious rages" of hydrophobia suffered by animals and people, they were probably ideal laboratory models in which to study rabies. Galtier reported that he had also tried but consistently failed to immunize rabbits against rabies with the tissues of rabid animals.

A third important fact about rabies—which Pasteur was soon to exploit—was its fairly long incubation period. People bitten by rabid dogs, cats, and other animals did not develop rabies or hydrophobia overnight. Fracastorius, writing on rabies in 1546, observed that after the infectious process was initiated by the bite of a rabid animal, "Its incubation is so stealthy, slow and gradual that the infection is very rarely manifest before the 20th day, and in most cases after the 30th, and in many cases not until after four or six months have elapsed. There are cases recorded in which it became manifest a year after the bite."

Rabies was not, like smallpox or anthrax, a very common disease. It was nevertheless a disorder that struck terror into the hearts of all who witnessed its effects on man and beast. When Pasteur was a boy of nine, a rabid wolf had created a wave of horror in Arbois, his native town, biting people and animals, and leaving eight people with hydrophobia in the immediate neighborhood of the Pasteur family. Our person bitten by a rabid animal during this outbreak escaped the fatal consequences. He was a man named Nicolle, and young Pasteur had stood by and watched with growing horror as the fresh animal-bite wound was cauterized with a red-hot poker by the local blacksmith. The cauterization, of course, terminated the rabies infection at the very onset of its long incubation period. Nicolle survived both the animal bite and the cure, which left him terribly scarred, and he lived on as a walking reminder of the horrors of rabies.

In the absence of such visualizing tools as the electron microscopes which, after World War II, made viruses visible, let alone the knowledge that infectious and nonbacterial virus particles infinitely smaller than bacteria even existed, all Pasteur's efforts to isolate the infectious agent of rabies ended in frustration. This did not deter him. By 1884, four years after he started his search, Pasteur's meticulous observations of brain and other tissues from healthy and rabid animals had enabled him to distinguish between rabid and nonrabid materials. If he could not isolate and describe the rabies virus (which Pasteur mistakenly envisioned as a submicroscopically small species of bacteria), he could at least separate tissues bearing the rabies virus from healthy tissues. In rabbits with rabies, the tissues that bore the heaviest concentrations of the virus were their spinal cords.

Since he could not attenuate living cultures of the "germ" of rabies, Pasteur settled for attenuating the active rabies agents he presumed to be in the spinal cords of rabid animals. Rabbits with rabies were killed, and their spinal cords hung from inside the stoppers of glass bottles to which caustic soda, used as a desiccating or drying agent, had been previously added. After two weeks, the viruses in the rabid spinal cords suspended in these bottles became completely inactivated.

Each day, for fourteen days, broth suspensions of medulla oblongata, the marrowlike extensions of the spinal cord in the brain, were made from one or more of these suspended spinal cords. These were carefully graded as to age and virulence. A fourteen-day-old suspension had no rabies virulence or infectivity at all; a seven-day-old suspension was half as active as a fresh virus suspension; a day-old suspension was still very infective.

Pasteur took fifty dogs and inoculated each of them with a completely inactivated fourteen-day-old suspension of medulla from the spinal cords of rabbits with rabies. On each successive day, he inoculated the same dogs with suspensions of slightly greater virulence, starting with thirteen-day-old preparations. Each succeeding suspension was one day younger, and correspondingly that much more infective. Finally, after the fourteenth inoculation of increasingly virulent medulla suspensions, the dogs were rendered completely immune to an inoculum of fully virulent saliva from rabid animals. The graded inocula from the spinal cords of rabbits with rabies had done for this group of dogs what the red-hot poker had done for M. Nicolle in 1831 in Arbois—they had inactivated the rabies viruses before they could incubate hydrophobia.

The increasingly attenuated rabies virus preparations—which Pasteur again named vaccines—were patently preferable to cauterization with a hot poker or a caustic chemical for two reasons. The least was that the two-week series of graded-for-virulence vaccinations, while not free of pain, was infinitely less traumatic. More important, cauterization was effective only if done before the rabies viruses started incubating, replicating, and spreading from the wounds to the cells of other tissues and then to the bloodstream, which disseminated them throughout the body. This meant that unless a rabid animal-bite wound was cauterized within a few hours after the bite it would not terminate the rabies virus infection. Given too late, cauterization only added great pain to the natural agonies of hydrophobia.

Pasteur's vaccine treatment—which could be begun even a few days after the animal bite (or a laboratory syringe) had inoculated a healthy individual with saliva bearing the rabies virus—delivered daily doses of antirabies virus antibodies to the body of an animal or a person exposed to rabies virus for at least two weeks. The vaccine—at least in animals—was far more efficient against disseminated rabies viruses than cauterization alone.

Pasteur tested his rabies vaccine in two sets of experiments in a total of 125 dogs. In the first series of experiments, the graduated vaccine treatments succeeded in making the dogs immune to rabies virus. In the second series of experiments, the immunized dogs were either bitten by rabid animals or inoculated with saliva from rabid dogs. None of the vaccine-immunized dogs so exposed to the rabies virus developed rabies.

It was a triumph for Pasteur's earlier discovery, the immunizing powers of attenuated microbes. He was, however, far from fully satisfied with his work. He had now demonstrated in three infectious and fatal diseases that the attenuation by aging and/or by controlled heat of both visible and invisible agents of fatal transmissible diseases could produce safe and efficient vaccines. The first two vaccines, which prevented fowl cholera and anthrax, were purely prophylactic. The latest vaccine, against rabies, was in a real sense as much a cure as a preventive, since it had to be used shortly after one was bitten by a rabid animal but before the rabies virus had time to finish incubating.

What was missing was obvious to the aging chemist: The theoretical reasons and the mechanisms that would explain *why* the attenuation of disease agents, or tissues believed to contain them, would lead to immunity against their pathological effects. After Pasteur's death, a revealing memorandum written to himself was found among his papers. Dated January 29, 1885, and written during a session of the Académie Française, it read:

"I do not know how to hide my ideas from those who work with me; still, I wish I could have kept those I am going to express a little longer to myself. The experiments have already begun which will decide them.

"It concerns rabies, but the results might be general.

"I am inclined to think that the virus which is considered rabic may be accompanied by a substance which, by impregnating the nervous system, would make it unsuitable for the culture of the microbe. Thence vaccinal immunity. If that is so, the theory might be a general one: it would be a stupendous discovery."[10]

This unknown immunizing substance was, in Pasteur's mind, quite obviously of a chemical nature. Prior to this, he had noted that in the spinal cords of rabid animals used to make his vaccine, "the heated cord which had become non-infectious was still effective as a chemical vaccine." In 1888, in the first issue of the *Annals of the Pasteur Institute,* Pasteur predicted, "It will not be long before the chemical vaccine . . . of rabies is known and utilized."

Freed of other pressures, Pasteur might possibly, during the years of work left to him, have devoted more attention to investigating some of his chemical concepts of infection and immunity. He had long suspected that the immune reaction in people protected by vaccines was not necessarily related to the whole attenuated or unaltered microbial agents used in his and Jenner's vaccines. It was quite probable, Pasteur thought, that the infective or immune actions might involve only some of the components of the bacteria (or viruses) or even only their chemical products (none of which had yet been isolated).

Unfortunately, Pasteur would never have time to test these working hypotheses, or to see if they could be developed into "stupendous" universal theories or abandoned as attractive but wrong. He was an old sixty-two, and had been paralyzed on the left side by a stroke for eighteen years, when he succeeded in immunizing dogs against rabies. History had its own inevitable demands to make of the inventor of this vaccine. As surely as day followed night, Pasteur would be forced to test this vaccine in human beings bitten by rabid animals. From all over the world, people from all walks of life began to beg Pasteur to use his antirabies vaccine on humans. Many of the letter writers were related to victims of hydrophobia, a goodly number were doctors, and their ranks even included at least one emperor, Dom Pedro II of Brazil.

In a letter to the emperor dated September 22, 1884, Pasteur replied that his studies of hydrophobia "are making good and uninterrupted progress," but that he believed it "will take me nearly two years more to bring them to a happy issue." He wrote that "until now I have not dared to attempt anything on men, in spite of my own confidence in the result and the numerous opportunities afforded to me since my last reading at the Academy of Sciences." He added that "even when I shall have multiplied examples of the prophylaxis of rabies in dogs, I think my hand will tremble when I go on to Mankind."

Ever the practical correspondent, Pasteur ended with a frank plea for subjects on whom to test his antirabies vaccine. "It is here that the high and powerful initiative of the head of a State might intervene for the good of humanity. If I were a King, or an Emperor, or even the President of a Republic, this is how I should exercise my right of pardoning criminals condemned to death. I should invite the counsel of a condemned man, on the eve of the day fixed for this execution, to choose between certain death and an experiment which would consist in several preventive inoculations of rabies virus, in order to make the subject's constitution refractory to rabies. If he survived this experiment—and I am convinced that he would—his life would be saved and his punishment commuted to a lifelong surveillance, as a guarantee towards that society which had condemned him. All the condemned men would accept these conditions, death being their only terror."

Pasteur was not to have his two years of added animal experiments, nor the terrified convict volunteers on whom to test his rabies vaccine. On July 4, 1885, a nine-year-old schoolboy named Joseph Meister was bitten by a mad dog on his way to school at Meissengott, in Alsace. The local doctor who treated the boy cauterized the bite wounds with carbolic acid that same night, but he also advised the boy's mother to take the boy to Paris, "where she could relate the facts to one who was not a physician, but who would be the best judge of what could be done in such a serious case." Two days later, the boy was brought to Pasteur, who called in two doctors, Grancher and Vulpain, to assist him in examing young Meister. On their advice, he began to treat the boy with his vaccine. In their minds and in Pasteur's, the clinically untested vaccine represented the boy's only hope of ending the incubation of the rabies viruses in the bite wounds.

The treatment worked, and on July 27 young Meister went home, having suffered no hydrophobic or other fatal symptoms of rabies. It was the last moment of peace Pasteur would ever have. Patients and reporters poured in from all over the world. Public subscriptions and government funds set up the new Pasteur Institute and its foreign branches to manufacture vaccines and provide laboratories for full-time medical and biological research. Despite himself, the fragile old investigator spent his last years as a more or less full-time celebrity.

By the time Pasteur died in 1895, few people in medicine or biology doubted that by, or at least shortly after, the turn of the century the world's scientists would have developed, and made universally available, vast arrays of efficient vaccines against the leading causes of death in the Western or industrialized world. Chief among these major killers were such transmissible infectious diseases as pneumonia, tuberculosis, cholera, dysentery and other diarrheal disorders, diphtheria, scarlet fever, typhoid fever, and septicemia (then considered a specific infection rather than disseminated blood poisoning caused by any of a score of infectious agents).

The most advanced physicians of the Western world lived by what could be termed a central dogma of infectious diseases. Few authors expressed this dogma more succinctly than the great medical generalist, Sir William Osler (1849–1919), Bart., M.D., F.R.S., former professor of medicine at Johns Hopkins, later Regius Professor of Medicine at Oxford, and author of

Principles and Practice of Medicine, one of the world's most utilized textbooks of medicine. In 1900, when Pasteur's son-in-law, Dr. René Vallery-Radot, wrote his authorized biography of Pasteur, Sir William was chosen to write the introduction to the English translation.

In this introduction Osler summarized and wholeheartedly seconded the gist of the report the French scientist Paul Bert prepared for the French Chamber of Deputies when they met to consider how to reward Pasteur for inventing the vaccine against the plague of anthrax, which, prior to the vaccine, had annually killed "20 million francs worth of horses, sheep, cattle and oxen a year" in France alone.

Osler wrote, "Pasteur's work constitutes three great discoveries, which may thus be formulated.

"1. Each fermentation is produced by the development of a special microbe.

"2. Each infectious disease is produced by the development within the organism of a special microbe.

"3. The microbe of an infectious disease culture, under certain detrimental condition, is attenuated in its pathogenic [disease-causing] activity; from a virus it has become a vaccine."

It was a dogma of hope. Good vaccines made of attenuated microbes were, however, not to be achieved against any of the major infectious diseases of humankind by the end of the nineteenth century, nor indeed by 1919, when Osler himself died.

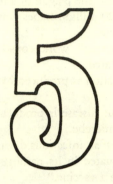

TRANSFORMATION OF THE INSTANT VACCINE DOGMA

Without theory, practice is only routine governed by the force of habit. Only theory can breed and develop the spirit of invention.

—LOUIS PASTEUR, 1854

Once Pasteur showed that the attenuation of the bacteria of fowl cholera and anthrax, and the presumably submicroscopic virus of rabies, converted some pathogens into vaccines, there was, predictably, a worldwide rush to isolate and convert to vaccines the microbial agents of the leading causes of death in the Western or industrialized world: tuberculosis, pneumonia, cholera, dysentery, diphtheria, meningitis, influenza, typhoid, puerperal (childbed) fever, and venereal diseases in particular.

Two years after the public trials of Pasteur's anthrax vaccine in 1881, the discoverer of the cholera vibrio, Filippo Pacini, died in Florence at the age of seventy-one, his isolation of the agent of cholera still unrecognized by his peers. In 1882 Koch isolated and demonstrated the pathogenicity of the tubercle bacillus. In 1884, a year after Pacini died, Koch isolated the cholera vibrio in Egypt; this time the comma-shaped bacterium was indeed recognized for what it was, and Koch was celebrated as its discoverer. There were however some detractors.

Not everyone accepted the idea yet that cholera was a bacterial infection. The July 12, 1884 edition of the *Journal of the American Medical Association* in an editorial on Koch's vibrios, concluded that "the popular germ theories and associate doctrines of contagiousness, greatly exaggerated by the newspaper press, are adding to the terror of all classes of people, and will correspondingly increase the destructive effects of the epidemic wherever it makes its appearance. For of all the predisposing causes of cholera, fear, dread, and mental trepidation are among the most efficient."[1]

The isolation and description of the specific germs of infectious diseases were facilitated by the development of the pure culture techniques of Koch in 1881. It was not by accident that most of the major isolations of specific disease microbes made between then and the end of the century were accomplished by German and Austrian workers of the Koch school. In 1884 Drs. George Gaffky and Friedrich Loeffler isolated the typhoid and diphtheria bacilli, while Berlin physician Julius Rosenbach grew pure cultures of the ubiquitous streptococci and staphylococci. In 1885, while searching for the germ of dysentery, the Viennese pediatrician Theodor Escherich isolated *Es-*

cherichia coli, the gut bacterium that after World War II was to help various biologists make basic discoveries in virology (and win many Nobel Prizes) and, after 1950, would emerge suddenly as a major cause of hospital-acquired infections. That same year, the Berlin gynecologist Ernst von Bumm grew pure cultures of the gonococcus that Dr. Albert Neisser, of Breslau, had isolated from the purulent urethral discharge of a gonorrhea patient in 1879, and used them to cause gonorrhea in a brash volunteer. In 1887 Anton Weichselbaum isolated the related meningococcus of bacterial meningitis.

The world impact of the work of Pasteur and Koch soon made itself evident. In 1885 the veterinary pathologist Daniel E. Salmon, of the U.S. Department of Agriculture laboratories in Washington, D.C., isolated what he believed to be the cause of hog cholera, which he named *Salmonella cholera-esuis,* and which was soon to figure in a major advance in the principles of bacterial vaccination.

Salmon was assisted by Theobald Smith, a twenty-six-year-old graduate of the Albany (New York) Medical College, which had not yet started to teach bacteriology before Smith graduated in 1883. Like other American medical school graduates too poor to pursue postgraduate studies in bacteriology under Koch and his associates in Berlin, or under Pasteur and his coworkers in Paris, Theobald Smith had had to teach himself what bacteriology he knew by working from articles by Pasteur, Koch, and their schools, and by developing his own laboratory skills and techniques. Smith was quite fluent in German; he was the son of a tailor named Philip Schmidt, who emigrated from Germany after the failure of the Revolution of 1848, changed his name to Smith, and opened a one-man tailoring shop in Albany in 1850. The tailor's son, born in 1859, was to become America's greatest bacteriologist.[2]

Shibasaburo Kitasato, who started his postgraduate studies in Berlin under Koch in 1885, learned quickly. He isolated the tetanus bacillus in 1889 and then, after collaborating with Emil Behring in the discovery of tetanus antitoxin, returned to Tokyo where he founded a bacteriological institute. His pupil and later assistant, Kiyoshi Shiga, discovered the dysentery bacillus in his Tokyo laboratory in 1898.

During this rash of bacterial isolations, Alexandre Yersin of the Pasteur Institute discovered the bubonic plague bacillus in 1894 in Hong Kong. Prior to joining the Pasteur Institute, Yersin had trained under Koch in Berlin in 1887. The bacillus of leprosy was first described in 1874 by the Norwegian physician G. Armauer Hansen.

The excitement of the hunt made the first round of results all the more anticlimactic: None of the newly discovered disease germs could, by attenuation, be converted to vaccines as safe and as effective as Pasteur's aging-attenuated and temperature-attenuated vaccines against chicken cholera and anthrax.

* * *

If the initial dream of a vaccine against every disease germ was not to be realized so quickly, this did not spell failure for the germ theory of infectious diseases. As early as 1886, when Theobald Smith and Daniel Salmon showed that injections of heat-killed cultures of their hog "cholera" bacillus—*Salmonella*—protected pigeons against multiple doses of living *Salmonella* as great as those that proved fatal in unvaccinated pigeons, it was shown, at least in animals, that attenuation of infectious bacteria was not the only route to the development of good vaccines. Killed bacteria might also make good vaccines in people.

As we saw earlier, in the absence of germ theory to explain just what it actually was in urban filth that caused both foul smells and contagious diseases, the early sanitary reformers were at times betrayed into taking well-intentioned actions that created rather than prevented outbreaks of cholera and other water-borne environmental infectious diseases.

Even the most medically engaged of the sanitary reformers, Dr. John Simon, Victorian England's important and productive governmental health officer, did not accept the realities and the health implications of germ theory until 1890, when he was seventy-four and near the end of his brilliant career in public health. Florence Nightingale, the nineteenth century's most influential sanitarian, went to her grave secure in the conviction that smallpox was not a specific disease caused by a specific virus, but, rather, a later and usually terminal stage of a condition she termed fever.

The fervent faith of Chadwick and the other sanitary reformers in soap and water, fresh air, sunshine, clean linen, and clean drinking water led to hygienic improvements that, before germ theory was ever envisioned, improved the human environment by reducing the population densities of bacteria, viruses, and other microbial disease agents. Filth and foul air were considered unhealthy, but no allowance was made for specific principles or agents of disease that might be present.

One of the first contributions of germ theory to environmental hygiene was the new, firm knowledge that bacteria and other microbial parasites can neither survive nor proliferate without food. For example, pure water was not necessarily found in a running brook—whose motion would collect organic wastes and plants and other nutrients and deliver them to water-borne bacteria—but it should be stored in clean tanks or reservoirs free of organic wastes and other sources of nourishment for at least thirty days, or long enough for the microbial disease organisms to starve to death. Knowledge of the chemistry of bacteria and viruses led to techniques of treating water with chlorine and other chemicals in dilutions strong enough to kill microbes but not toxic enough to harm people.

Knowledge of the actual natures and weaknesses of microbial disease agents led to improved strategies of cleanliness designed to destroy microbial pathogens. The knowledge that heat kills bacteria and inactivates viruses began to be used in many ways. High heats were used to kill pathogens in packaged foods, in laundry waters, and in the sterilization of cooking and eating utensils. Lower heats for definite time intervals were used, as originally prescribed by Pasteur in 1867 to protect wines from bacterial contaminants, to make milk and other foods free of harmful bacteria by "pasteurization." New bactericidal and virucidal drugs were developed for use in dilutions of cleaning water, or they were added to soaps and other cleansers used in households and public buildings. New antimicrobial techniques of ventilation and sewage disposal became common in all industrial nations.

Germ theory, in short, did not supplant sanitary reform but made it far more rational and effective.

In the field of antisepsis, particularly in hospital and public health medicine, sanitary reformers and physicians had been involved in efforts to reduce the prevalences of what they correctly perceived to be contagious diseases for at least a century before germ theory. Earlier, we saw how at the same time that Jenner tried to convince his medical peers that smallpox was a contagion that could be prevented by vaccination, some of his equally far-sighted professional contemporaries had learned the tragic way that, as Dr. Gordon of Aberdeen declared in 1795, not only was "the cause of puerperal fever a specific contagion, or infection," but also that "I myself was the means of carrying the infection to a great number of women."

Over the next half-century, various other doctors in Europe and America made very similar confessions. In 1843 Dr. Oliver Wendell Holmes, Sr., then professor of anatomy and physiology at Harvard Medical School, quoted many in his classic essay "The Contagiousness of Puerperal Fever," published in the *New England Quarterly Journal of Medicine and Surgery*. Like his clinical precursors, Holmes also urged physicians to wear clean clothing and to keep their hands clean when attending women in labor. Holmes quoted, with obvious approval, an 1843 letter from a Boston physician which related, "While I attended these women in their fevers I changed my clothes, and washed my hands in a solution of chloride of lime after each visit. I attended seven women in labor during this period [1830], all of whom recovered without sickness."

Holmes shared one other characteristic—speaking bluntly—with the many doctors who since 1795 had written about puerperal fever as a disease in which he quoted a Dr. Blundell as saying, "The infection is principally conveyed [by] gossipy friends, wet-nurses, monthly nurses, [and] the practitioner himself." This bluntness of expression showed itself in the eight rules for the prevention of puerperal fever with which Holmes ended his 1843 essay.

Rule 2 stated that if a physician is even present at the autopsy of a woman who died of puerperal fever, "he should use thorough ablution, change every article of dress, and allow 24 hours or more to elapse before attending to any case of midwifery." Rule 7 held that the "occurrence of three or more closely connected cases [of puerperal fever] in the practice of an individual . . . is prima facie evidence that he is the vehicle of contagion." The eighth and final rule was a masterpiece of nondiplomacy: "Whatever indulgence may be granted to those who have heretofore been the ignorant causes of so much misery, the time has come when the existence of a *private pestilence* in the sphere of a single physician should be looked upon, not as a misfortune, but a crime; and in the knowledge of such occurrences the duties of the practitioner to his profession should give way to his paramount obligations to society."

Three years after Dr. Holmes printed these rules in a Yankee medical journal, Ignaz Philipp Semmelweis (1818–1865), a young Hungarian physician trained in Budapest and Vienna, took a job as assistant at the first obstetrical clinic of the Vienna General Hospital. Semmelweis would far surpass Holmes and all others concerned about puerperal fever in two major respects: (1) in the massive thoroughness of his studies of both its environmental causes and its prevention; and (2) in the contempt he exhibited for physicians whose "teaching . . . is based upon the dead bodies of lying-in women slaughtered through ignorance," and who therefore had to be denounced (by Semmelweis) "before God and the world" as murderers.

During the nineteenth century at least, life dealt more kindly with doctors who denounced their peers as murderers in Boston than in Vienna. Doctor Holmes died at the age of eighty-five in Boston on October 7, 1894, in his own bed, laden with honors and widely mourned. Doctor Semmelweis died at the age of forty-seven on August 13, 1865, in a madhouse near Vienna, unhonored and little mourned. During his much shorter lifetime, however, Semmelweis managed to make more numerous, and professionally more important, enemies than did Holmes. He also succeeded in saving the lives of more pregnant women than did Holmes and all his like-minded predecessors combined in the British, Scottish, and American medical crusades for cleanliness at childbirth.

Shortly after the twenty-eight-year-old Semmelweis started to work at the Vienna General Hospital, the newly qualified physician experienced two shocks. The first was the death of his close friend Dr. Kolletschka, whose finger had been pricked with a dissecting knife during a postmortem examination, and who had then developed and died of septicemia, or systemic blood poisoning. The second shock was Semmelweis's discovery that the childbed fever death rate was much higher in the first lying-in ward, which was used to train obstetricians and medical students, than in the ward reserved for training nurses and midwives.

Semmelweis was quick to note "the close resemblance of the malady from which Kolletschka had died to that from which I had seen countless numbers of women perish after childbirth." Hindsight shows this to be a very acute observation, since as any modern intern knows, the symptoms of beta-hemolytic *Streptococcus pyogenes* septicemia following surgical wound infections, and those of puerperal fever, are indeed identical.

Semmelweis's observation of the daily routines followed in both of the hospital's obstetrical wards soon revealed what was probably at least a major contributing reason for the higher puerperal fever rates in the first ward. Doctors and medical students frequently came to the bedsides of pregnant women in this ward directly from the pathology laboratory, where they participated in postmortem examinations. Like poor Kolletschka, the pregnant women were being given fatal infections of puerperal fever by what Semmelweis deduced were toxic but invisible traces of putrefied matter carried from the cadavers to the ward on the hands of doctors and students.

Semmelweis ordered every doctor and student on his service to wash their hands well in a solution of chlorine and water before entering any obstetrics ward. As did Holmes and other doctors who wrote on the subject, Semmelweis also observed that "it is owing to the doctors that there is so high a mortality in childbed." Again in the tradition started by Dr. Gordon of Aberdeen in 1795, Semmelweis felt driven to confess that "as a logical outcome of my conviction I have to acknowledge that God only knows how many women I have prematurely brought down into the grave."

Many of his peers and hierarchical superiors took umbrage at both the content and the tone of these observations. On the other hand, the already measurable continental effects of the British sanitary movement had created a clinical climate of opinion that was far from antagonistic to the sanitary procedures Semmelweis ordered for the prevention of childbed fever. While Holmes's essay on the role of sickroom filth in puerperal fever was scarcely known on the Continent, the British sanitary reformers had already started to disseminate their data and to influence medical thinking in Europe and America. Chadwick's 1842 parliamentary *Report on the Sanitary Conditions of the Labouring Population,* as well as the 1843–1844 study on the Health of Towns, conducted for Parliament by Drs. Southwood Smith, Joseph Toynbee, and Neil Arnott, were known to many doctors and medical professors in Vienna. The Health of Towns Association, founded in 1844, was actively disseminating its reports and suggestions to physicians and sanitarians on both sides of the Atlantic. Sanitary reform, of which Semmelweis's antisepsis was a natural component, had by 1846 gained many European adherents within and outside of medical circles.

The results of Semmelweis's own sanitary reforms in the obstetrical department of the Vienna General Hospital were not long in attracting attention. In short order, the high puerperal fever death rates of the first lying-in ward, where all doctors and students now scrubbed with soap and rinsed with chlorinated water before approaching the bed of a pregnant woman, quickly fell to the low levels of the second ward, where nurses and midwives in training never participated in postmortems. Despite the counterattacks of Establishment doctors on Semmelweis himself, the practice of ordering doctors to disinfect their hands before examining or treating pregnant women had started to take hold as the benefits of this sanitary practice became evident.

In 1847, when an admiring friend published an account of Semmelweis's work and included its results in an article, the effects on the treatment of pregnant women were immediate and widespread. The impact of this article, as well as the series of open letters Semmelweis now took to issuing to various well-known doctors, on the medical profession were equally stunning. In these open letters, Semmelweis attacked doctors who questioned his puerperal fever findings and antiseptic procedures as "assassins," and "murderers," and "medical Neros," as well as disseminators of what he mistakenly perceived as the heresy of maintaining that "puerperal fever is an ordinary epidemic disease."

The more the battle raged, the harder it became for Semmelweis's medical friends and academic supporters to protect him from the enemies he made every time he put pen to paper. Although his fine work on the wards led to a faculty appointment by 1851, in that year—in effect backing his way to the exit with guns blazing in each hand—Semmelweis quit Vienna and retreated to his native Budapest. There he published a book on the etiology of puerperal fever, in which he quite correctly described it as a wound infection. After birth, he wrote, the uterus is like a large open wound in which putrefying organic materials that often contaminate wounds can cause fatal blood poisoning. However, since chlorine and other chemicals could neutralize the poisons caused by putrefaction, puerperal fevers, Semmelweis insisted, could always be prevented by chemical antisepsis.

This, of course, was just what Holmes and other doctors had also recommended. That Semmelweis did not isolate or even look for the active agents or toxic principles of wound infections speaks only for his intellectual limitations as a biological scientist; it does not in any way detract, however, from his success in teaching doctors how effectively to use antisepsis to prevent deaths from childbed fever.

The rest of the Semmelweis story is not a joyous one. His experiences in Vienna left residues of psychological traumas that eventually started to affect his behavior. In 1865, when Semmelweis was only forty-seven, his friends arranged to have him admitted to a mental hospital outside of Vienna. Unknown to any of them, a few days before Semmelweis left Budapest he had pierced his finger with a surgical instrument while performing an operation. As in his friend Kolletschka's case, this wound became infected. By the time Semmelweis was in residence in the madhouse, septicemia set in and it killed him.

He deserved better during his lifetime, and better since his death. It has become the custom, among hucksters of fake (and costly) cures for cancer, arthritis, and other feared chronic and/or fatal conditions—as well as among well-meaning ignoramuses with equally useless cure-alls who zealously believe in their remedies—to wrap themselves in the mantle of Ignaz Philipp

Semmelweis whenever they are arrested and tried for fraud or manslaughter. Whatever his sins, Semmelweis never deserved such disciples. All he did was to save lives; the only life ever shortened by his work was his own.

History always being more ironic than any fiction, it was inevitable that in the very year that Semmelweis died as a martyr to the cause of hospital antisepsis, an English surgeon named Joseph Lister would find, in the early work of Louis Pasteur, the theoretical biological foundations of modern antisepsis and sepsis.

Hospital-acquired infections had for centuries plagued not only pregnant women but all other patients. Few doctors were more sensitive to hospital infections than surgeons, particularly in the eras before anesthesia when they saw great pain, as well as the fevers of infections, doom most surgical patients to agonized exits from life. The great Ambroise Paré (1510–1590), surgeon-in-ordinary to three of France's sixteenth-century kings, hated to operate in the Hôtel Dieu because ambient infections in that hospital always killed too many of his patients. Two centuries later, the Scottish surgeon and anatomist John Bell (1763–1820), lamenting the pestilence of gangrene in all of Europe's great hospitals in 1801, observed that "such were its ravages at the Hôtel Dieu of Paris, that great storehouse of corruption and disease, that the surgeons did not dare call it by its true name [Hospital Gangrene]."

When hospital gangrene appeared, Bell wrote, "no operation dare be performed! every cure stands still! every wound becomes a sore, and every sore is apt to run into gangrene." The main victims of this hospital infection were those with open wounds, but few hospital patients were immune to its toxins. "What then is the surgeon to do?" Bell asked. No dressings, no quantities of wine or bark had ever checked the hospital infection. Let the surgeon "bear in mind that this is a hospital disease; that without the circle of the infected walls the men are safe; let him, therefore, hurry them out of this house of death ... let him lay them in a schoolroom, a church, on a dunghill or in a stable ... let him carry them anywhere but to their graves."

Bell was not the only surgeon to deplore hospital infections before Semmelweis was born; he was simply a better writer than most other concerned doctors. English sanitary reformers, from doctors like Southwood Smith to nurses led by Florence Nightingale, had all tried, with varying degrees of success, to make hospitals somewhat less apt to generate preventable infections in the sick and the sound. It was not until the English surgeon Joseph Lister, then professor of surgery at the University of Glasgow, encountered the "philosophic researches of M. Pasteur" concerning the function of "the germs of various low forms of life, long since revealed by the microscope" to be the "essential cause" of putrescence and the decomposition of organic substances, that the moral imperatives of the sanitary movement and the scientific potentials of germ theory were joined.

In a sense, Lister represented—in himself, his antecedents, and his work—three influential aspects of European life. To begin with, he was born an outsider; his father, the London wine merchant and amateur mathematician and optical physicist Joseph Jackson Lister, was a Quaker. The son, born in 1827, could not as a Dissenter attend either Oxford or Cambridge. Joseph Lister was educated at London's University College, and grew up under the influence of his family.

When Lister was two years old, his father worked out the method of joining with Canada balsam the doublets of the achromatic lenses developed by Euler and Selligue between 1776 and 1823. The new Lister microscope increased the effective light of the device by nearly 100 percent. "With the advent of achromatic lenses microscopy became an important science," wrote R. M. Allen. "The medical profession sensed the microscope's value; scientists and amateurs alike took it up enthusiastically, quickly creating sufficient demand to justify manufacturing it on a commercial scale."[3]

Not until the physicist Ernst Abbé produced his two-lens condenser and started to work with the Zeiss Company on new lens and lighting systems was the light microscope to receive improvements of equal value. It was on the basic Lister microscope that Pasteur made his original and most of his subsequent discoveries about the roles of bacteria and other microbes in the processes of life and death.

Young Lister grew up with the advanced light microscope as part of his learning and recreational experiences; this youthful exposure to the world of microscopy gave him an early awareness of scientific work involving the major instrument of bacteriology and germ theory. In 1854, shortly after he qualified in medicine in London, Lister became house surgeon at the Edinburgh Hospital in Scotland. Seven years later, Joseph Lister was made professor of surgery at the University of Glasgow.

By then, Lister had seen far more deaths by wound-infection septicemias than Semmelweis ever had, particularly in such common injuries as compound fractures of arms and legs, contused wounds, and industrial injuries, and in ordinary operations. The techniques of anesthesia, introduced by Horace Wells and William Morton in the United States and by James Simpson in England between 1846 and 1848 on the eve of Lister's medical education, had made surgery less agonizing for patients and surgeons alike. The elimination of surgical pain had not, however, eradicated the risk of hospital infections. In the best of hospitals, the endemic presence of gangrene, septicemia, and other treatment-associated infections meant that more than half of all surgical patients died following surgery regardless of the results of their operations.

Sanitary conditions in British and Scottish hospitals had, thanks to the sanitary reformers in general and to Florence Nightingale in particular, improved greatly since John Bell, in 1801, pleaded with his fellow surgeons to take their patients outside of the "infected walls" of the average hospital. In 1854, the same year that Lister graduated from medical school in London, Florence Nightingale and her company of intrepid military nurses introduced the life-enhancing mix of soap, water, and nourishing food to the Barracks Hospital at Scutari. The vigorous application of sound sanitary and nutritional techniques quickly reduced the patient death rate at this Crimean War pesthole of a military hospital from forty-two to twenty-two per thousand hospitalized soldiers. During the three years between 1859 and 1861, the same array of Nightingale-inspired sanitary and nutritional reforms reduced the total peacetime military death rates by half, so that they attained parity with the civilian death rates of the era. However, infectious and deficiency diseases remained the chief causes of civilian and peacetime military deaths. Hospitals were cleaner, hospital infections fewer than in 1850, but they were still endemic.

As a surgeon, Lister was acutely aware of the deaths associated with surgical and nonsurgical wounds in every hospital in which he worked. Early in his career in Glasgow, Lister's studies of inflammation led him to conclude that "the essential cause of suppuration [formation of pus] in wounds is decomposition, brought about by the influence of the atmosphere upon blood or serum retained within them, and, in the case of contused wounds, upon portions of tissue destroyed by the violence of the injury." At first, he thought it was impossible to prevent suppuration, "since it seemed hopeless to attempt to exclude the oxygen which was universally regarded as the agent by which putrefaction was effected. Then, however, Lister turned to the current scientific literature and learned otherwise.

He described what followed in a series of articles on antiseptic principles in the practice of surgery in *Lancet* and in the *British Medical Journal* in 1867.

"When it had been shown by the researches of Pasteur that the septic properties of the atmosphere depended not on the oxygen, or any gaseous constituent, but on minute organisms [bacteria] suspended in it, which owed their energy to their vitality, it occurred to me that decomposition in the injured part might be avoided without excluding the air, by applying as a dressing some material capable of destroying the life of the floating particles."[4]

Lister had been quite taken by Pasteur's demonstration that bacteria could resolve "complex organic compounds into substances of simpler chemical constitution, just as the yeast plant converts sugar into alcohol and carbonic acid." At the same time, as one who had come to maturity during the rise of the great sanitary movement, which preached that the foul odors of organic decomposition and putrescence were actually the causes of infectious diseases, Lister was culturally conditioned to associate stench with contagion.

"In the course of the year 1864," he wrote, "I was much struck with an account of the remarkable effects produced by carbolic acid upon the sewage of the town of Carlisle, the admixture of a very small proportion not only preventing all odour from the lands irrigated with the refuse material, but, as it was stated, destroying the entozoa [gut parasites, including Salmonella and other enteric bacteria] which usually infest cattle fed upon such pastures."

By then Lister had learned from Pasteur that it was from bacteria in the atmosphere that "all the mischief arises" in decomposition. He had already concluded that the prevention of surgical wound infection would be a simple matter of dressing "the wound with some material capable of killing these septic germs, provided that any substance can be found reliable for this purpose, yet not too potent as a caustic."

Carbolic acid, which prevented foul odors in human waste sewage, struck Lister as possibly just such an antiseptic material. His first experiments with carbolic acid, in the case of a patient with a compound leg fracture in Glasgow in 1865, failed. Subsequent changes in his carbolic acid preparations, and his techniques of applying them full strength and in oil dilutions to wounds and injured tissues, proved that killing the bacteria that cause infections can protect surgical patients from postoperative blood poisoning and disease.

Lister started to apply carbolic acid to wounds and contused tissues in his surgical practice. Soon he adopted the practice, introduced in 1865 by the Italian surgeon Enrico Bottini, of spraying the operating room with phenol (carbolic acid), a custom he followed for close to twenty years before he could admit it was not really necessary. But his introduction of chemical sterilization of wounds and, in due time, of surgical instruments started to save patients' lives by killing postoperative wound-infection bacteria.

During the Franco-Prussian War of 1870, surgeons on both sides resorted to what they termed "Listerism" to reduce combat-wound-infection deaths. The excellent results they obtained turned Lister into the only real hero of that war. Because of these war experiences, it was in postwar Germany and France that his methods of antisepsis were first appreciated. Long before they became routine infection-control procedures in British hospitals, Lister's antisepsis methods were employed widely to reduce the risks of fatal infections acquired in the operating rooms and the wards of most French and German hospitals.

Not until 1877, when Lister was appointed professor of surgery at King's College, London, did his domestic reputation start to match that which he had gained in Europe for his contributions to safer medical care. Few practitioners of the period matched Lister's knowledge of and inventive skills in bacteriology. In 1878, three years before Koch published his techniques for isolating and growing pure cultures of bacteria, Lister had some special equipment made and used it to isolate from milk and grow in pure culture a new microbe, which he named *Bacterium lactis*. In due time, he accepted other suggestions of Pasteur's, including the use of high heat to sterilize medical instruments and equipment.[5]

Celebrity did not turn Lister's head. As honors and titles flowed his way—he was raised to the peerage as Baron Lister in 1897 and awarded the Order of Merit in 1902—he continued to credit Pasteur and others for their contributions to his work. When Pasteur became embroiled in his battles with Pouchet over spontaneous generation, Lister was one of the first foreigners to rally to his support. Toward the end of his long life (he died in 1912 at eighty-five) Lister paid a fervent if sentimental tribute to Semmelweis, saying (according to a Hungarian doctor writing in 1965), "Without Semmelweis my work would have been nothing; to this great son of Hungary owes surgery most."[6]

This gracious man, Lister, saved millions of lives during his own years on earth, most of them those of people in cities and countries he never saw. The antiseptic uses of bactericidal chemicals soon spread not only to the operating rooms of other countries, but also to other areas of the hospitals themselves. Carbolic acid was shortly joined by other bactericidal chemicals, which were used alone or added to the soap and water used to clean hospital floors, rooms, beds, and equipment. Some of these sterilizing chemicals, such as ethyl alcohol and the everyday laundry bleach sodium hypochlorite (known commercially as Clorox), not only killed bacteria but also inactivated disease-causing viruses, like the causal agents of smallpox and rabies which were soon to be discovered and distinguished from bacteria.

Chemical sterilization of hospital microbes—started by Lister in 1865, the year Semmelweis died of a very common operating room streptococcal infection—turned germ theory into a serious clinical reality for physicians in many countries. More than a decade before Pasteur made his first attenuated bacterial vaccines against chicken cholera and anthrax, Lister wrote that the scientific work of Pasteur had "long since made me a convert to the germ theory, and it was on the basis of that theory that I founded the antiseptic treatment of wounds in surgery."

Lister accomplished more than antisepsis through his work. In basing his rationale for preventing hospital infections on killing the "atmospheric septic germs" Pasteur had already shown were the cause of putrefaction and decomposition, Lister helped convince growing numbers of doctors and laymen that bacteria were the causal agents of most infectious diseases.

During Lister's lifetime, the antiseptic uses of carbolic acid in wounds and spraying the air in operating rooms with phenol were gradually replaced by the techniques of asepsis—the absence of bacteria and other microbial disease agents—based on disinfecting hospital air and equipment, from operating instruments to bed linens, by combinations of sterilizing chemicals, heat, and such physical germ killers as ultraviolet light. The bactericidal (and virucidal) objectives of antisepsis and asepsis were identical; the two sterilizing methods differed only in the strategies they used to kill or inactivate bacteria and viruses. Both asepsis and antisepsis derived their guiding principle from germ theory, and both approaches to the sanitary reform of hospitals helped validate its implications for human health.

The search for the specific microbial agents of infectious diseases, triggered by the success of Pasteur's vaccines against fowl cholera, anthrax, and rabies, soon led to bacterial findings that put the validity of germ theory itself in doubt. Many investigators, including Pasteur himself, began to find the germs of dread diseases—such as the pneumococci of pneumonia—alive and proliferating in the sputum and bodies of perfectly healthy people suffering from no symptoms or signs of the diseases the same agents caused in experimental animals.

Some biologists speculated that healthy people who carried live colonies of known disease-causing bacteria in their systems had been immunized, like people with naturally acquired immunity to smallpox and cowpox, by earlier mild and forgotten infections. It soon became clear that pneumonia and most other diseases caused by the bacteria found in healthy people were not among the infections that, like cowpox, mumps, and measles, conferred immunity to reinfections on their survivors.

It soon became apparent that in possibly a majority of the people found to be carrying bacteria known to cause specific infections in laboratory animals no signs of the same diseases were evident. To some opponents of germ theory, such findings were added proof that bacteria did not cause infections. A few even took to public engorgements of pathogenic bacteria to prove their beliefs. Among them were people of genuine scientific talent, such as the professor of hygiene at the University of Munich, Dr. Max von Pettenkofer, the man who brought the teachings of the English sanitary reformers to Germany.

Pettenkofer knew that the pneumococci and other bacteria isolated from healthy human carriers could induce pneumonia (and other specific diseases) in laboratory animals, and that descendants of these germs isolated from these infected animals would cause pneumonia (and other specific infections) in other healthy animals. He was certain, however, that the comma vibrios isolated by Pacini and later by Koch were not the cause of cholera; Pettenkofer was, in fact, the one scientist who kept the international community of sanitary officers from taking Pacini's cholera vibrios seriously for nearly thirty years. On October 7, 1892, the seventy-four-year-old Pettenkofer tested his hypothesis on himself in public. First, he issued a statement calculated to rank with the final orations of Socrates and Giordano Bruno if the experiment should prove him wrong about what he called "Koch's comma bacillus."

"Even if I be mistaken, and this experiment that I am making imperils my life, I shall look death quietly in the face," the statement began, "for what I am doing is no frivolous or cowardly act of suicide, but I shall die in the service of science as a soldier perishes on the field of honor." Having followed these words with equally operatic pronouncements about the nature of man and beast and the need to be "ready to sacrifice even life and health on behalf of higher and more ideal goods," Pettenkofer proceeded to swallow publicly a broth culture of cholera vibrios.

Two days later, writes Howard-Jones, "Pettenkofer experienced borborygmi, some diarrhea, and some colic." He would not be free of these symptoms of enteric infection until he had a normal stool on the morning of October 15, six days after ingesting the cholera germs. On October 17 Rudolf Emmerich, Pettenkofer's assistant, swallowed an equal amount of cholera vibrios. The results were a bit more drastic: For the next forty-three hours, Dr. Emmerich had a nearly nonstop case of diarrhea, passing a stool nearly once each hour.

Although the results of both of these experiments convinced Pettenkofer that "the living comma bacillus in the intestine does not produce the specific poison that results in cholera," he conceded that Koch and the other "contagionists" could also, with good reason, describe the outcomes of the two experiments as mild attacks of cholera.[7]

Opponents of germ theory were not the only scientists to be intrigued by Pettenkofer's public demonstration of the nonfatal effects of deliberately swallowing cholera germs. One of the most thoughtful believers in germ theory who was tempted to repeat the Pettenkofer experiment was the Russian-born embryologist and zoologist Élie Metchnikoff (1845–1916), who in 1888 joined Pasteur at the Pasteur Institute, where he was to remain for the rest of his life.

Metchnikoff had been one of the first scientists to concern himself with the mechanisms of natural resistance against "harmful intruders," such as the parasites that cause diseases in water fleas. By 1882, based on observations in starfish larvae and water fleas, Metchnikoff had worked out the concept that the body contains motile cells that swarm around and digest invasive yeasts, fungi, bacteria, and other disease-causing parasites. He named these host defense cells phagocytes—from the Greek word for eaters of cells—and within a year published a paper on his phagocytic theory of inborn or natural immunity. (Phagocytes are nowadays divided into two classes. There are the macrophages, such as the histiocytes and the monocytes, discovered and named by Metchnikoff. These are large white blood cells, or leukocytes, which engulf and destroy or phagocytize degenerated cells and foreign materials. There are also the smaller microphages, such as the polymorphonuclear leukocytes, which engulf and destroy invasive bacteria.) Metchnikoff found that in animals immunized against anthrax by Pasteur's temperature-attenuated vaccine, the process of phagocytosis was always more lively than it was in nonimmunized animals.

In 1884, in a paper titled "Struggle of Phagocytes Against Pathogens," Metchnikoff had put forward the belief that "the bacilli are destroyed by the phagocytes, although the influence of other factors that may hinder their development is not eliminated." This willingness to believe that there were factors other than the white blood cells in our inborn defenses against bacteria and other disease agents led Metchnikoff to wonder if some of these factors might have been responsible for Pettenkofer's apparent immunity to infection by the cholera germs.

Metchnikoff had long entertained "the idea of producing a vaccine against [cholera] with attenuated microbes, or if not, to prevent its inception by preventive microbes."[8] What he meant by a "preventive microbe" was an organism that, like Jenner's cowpox virus, immunized people against infection by a more virulent close relative of the benign preventive [immunogenic] agent. This not only derived from Jenner; it was also a conscious application, by Metchnikoff, of Darwin's law of natural selection. He wondered if by the laws of natural selection, nature itself would select out aberrant strains of cholera vibrio that would be only weakly infective—i.e., infective enough only to produce transient diarrhea, as caused by the germs Pettenkofer swallowed—but, at the same time, act like the cowpox virus in conferring immunity against fully infective strains that cause fulminating cholera infections.

Metchnikoff's belief that such an organism might exist in the cholera vibrio family was reinforced when one of his pupils, a Dr. Sanarelli, discovered a strain in a river in Versailles, a community strikingly immune to cholera during the great nineteenth-century epidemics of the disease. After the negative results of the Pettenkofer vibrio-swallowing experiment, Metchnikoff speculated that the cholera vibrio Sanarelli had isolated in Versailles, "or some similar choleriform bacillus ... probably served as a natural vaccine against cholera in those localities which were spared by the epidemic though the cholera vibrio was brought there." This was a question, he felt, "that could only be solved by experiment."

In 1892 Metchnikoff repeated, first on himself and then on three of his volunteer assistants, the Pettenkofer experiment of swallowing live cholera vibrio cultures. The specific strains of the cholera germs used in these experiments were descendants of the vibrios Metchnikoff believed could have been the "natural vaccines" that had immunized the populace of Versailles against cholera.

Like Pettenkofer in Munich earlier the same year, Metchnikoff did not develop cholera after ingesting the live cholera vibrio cultures. Neither did his assistant, M. Lapatie. Following this, according to his wife's authorized account, Metchnikoff "did not hesitate to accept the offer of a second volunteer, M. Jupille. The preceding results having led him to suppose that the cholera vibrio became attenuated *in vitro* [i.e., outside a living host's body] and might perhaps serve as a vaccine against cholera, he gave a culture of long standing to the young volunteer."

155

The effect of this time-attenuated cholera vibrio culture on young M. Jupille soon took form as a severe and near-fatal case of classic cholera. It was months before Metchnikoff dared to repeat this experiment on himself and other volunteers, again with attenuated cultures of cholera bacilli taken from a river near Versailles that was still "free from cholera." This time another volunteer showed some symptoms of cholera, recovered, and only a short time later died "from a cause which remained obscure." Metchnikoff, shocked by the outcome, "finally resolved to perform no other experiments on human beings," not even convict "volunteers."

In reply to Pettenkofer and other peers who persisted in attacking the germ theory of the "contagionists," Metchnikoff wrote that "it is no longer Koch's theory that should adapt itself to the facts of epidemiology, but the facts should be reconciled with the fundamental truth that the comma bacillus [vibrio] is the specific agent of Asian cholera." There was yet another fundamental truth this episode in germ-swallowing helped establish: The processes of infection were as dependent on the state of a host's natural defenses against their agents as they were on the nature and the number of the microbial pathogens themselves.

Metchnikoff's seminal demonstration that white blood cells are a major component of our hereditary defenses against invasive parasites was, if not the birth of the biological science of immunology (which really begins with Jenner), the first of the major discoveries of the continuum of interacting biological and chemical mechanisms of immunity. It had all started in Italy, in 1882. After a rising wave of political and social reaction in Russia led to Metchnikoff's resignation as professor of zoology at the University of Odessa, he fled to Messina with his young wife, Olga, and five of her brothers and sisters. He had been studying intracellular digestion in microscopic animals, and continued these studies in Italy.

"One day, when the whole family had gone to a circus to see some extraordinary performing apes, I remained alone with my microscope," he wrote, "observing life in the motile cells of a transparent star-fish larva, when a new thought suddenly flashed across my brain. It struck me that similar cells might serve in the defense of the organism against intruders."

Metchnikoff wondered if "a splinter introduced into the body of a star-fish larva, devoid of blood-vessels or of a nervous system, should soon be surrounded by motile cells as is to be observed in a man who runs a splinter into his finger. This was no sooner said than done." He fetched a few rose thorns "and introduced them at once under the skin of some beautiful star-fish larvae as transparent as water.

"I was too excited to sleep that night in the expectation of the result of my experiment, and very early the next morning I ascertained that it had fully succeeded.

"That experiment formed the basis of the phagocyte theory, to the development of which I devoted the next twenty-five years of my life."

Metchnikoff had discovered, in "the motile cells of the transparent star-fish larva," the mechanisms of one of the primary inborn host of immune defense systems in all animals against an array of intruders that range from rosebush thorns to disease-causing microbes, larger parasites, and even foreign proteins.

During the same quarter of a century Metchnikoff devoted to the development of the phagocyte or cellular theory of natural immunity, various additional and interacting mechanisms of natural immunity were discovered in different countries.

In 1888 a young expatriate American doctor, George Nuttall, showed that "independently of leukocytosis [an increase in the number of white blood cells, or leukocytes, in the blood], blood and other tissue fluids may produce morphological degeneration of bacilli." Nuttall was one of a number of observers who had noted that blood and other body fluids, such as lymph, inhibited putrefaction and microbial infections. Some had attributed this to qualities in the oxygen carried by the red blood cells.

Nuttall, working in Carl Flügge's Institute of Hygiene in Göttingen, Germany, showed that independently of the leukocytes, defibrinated blood— blood free of the clotting factors that might trap bacteria—destroyed colonies of anthrax bacilli in rabbits, dogs, sheep, pigeons, and mice. His observations led to a very interesting finding: "Indeed," Nuttall wrote, "we have been led to the assumption that the bacilli that were phagocytized were not completely normal and had been subjected to the damaging effect of extra-cellular fluids." By extra-cellular fluids Nuttall meant the blood and lymph circulating outside of the white blood cells, the humoral (from *humor,* the Latin word for fluid) system of the body.[9]

The infinite capacity for foolish controversy that distinguishes the human race from all other species was quick to convert the early evidence of humoral immunity into the catalyst of a long and time-wasting controversy over whether all the mechanisms of inborn immunity were cellular or humoral.

The Belgian physician Jules Bordet, from 1894 to 1901 assistant to Metchnikoff at the Pasteur Institute, discovered that the blood serum of healthy people contained a substance that he named alexin (from the Greek word for to ward off) that has "a destructive influence on diverse cellules [cells] and on certain microbes." Bordet also found that the body tissues of animals vaccinated against bacteria started to give off a sensitizing substance that combined with serum alexin to destroy specific bacteria. Bordet named this second humoral agent, "substance sensibilisatrice."

In Frankfurt, Paul Ehrlich (1854–1915), director of two research institutes, founder of hematology, and soon-to-be discoverer of the first systemic chemical cure for syphilis, and founder of chemotherapy, was quick to appreciate the great significance of Bordet's findings. Ehrlich renamed alexin, and it is still known by the name he gave it—complement. Ehrlich also renamed the sensitizing agent associated with complement to amboceptor.

Although he deserved and could with justice have been awarded Nobel Prizes for at least four major discoveries, Ehrlich won only one, the award he shared with Metchnikoff in 1908 for his work in immunology. Ehrlich's side-chain theory of immunity, which figured in this award, caused him to be dubbed "Doctor Fantasy" by prominent opponents of this concept.

As Ehrlich explained the theory to a colleague, "the cells have the ability to attract foreign chemical substances which have a specific chemical relationship to the substances of the cell itself. Whenever such substances come in contact with a cell, a chemical binding takes place. This [bond] is as close . . . as a key is to its lock."[10]

The lock-and-key analogy to the chemicals and the receptors on the cells in the host body made the side-chain theory easy for laymen as well as biologists to comprehend. Once, in a conversation with a Silesian landowner and member of the Reichstag he had met on the train during a journey from Frankfurt to Berlin, Ehrlich launched into an impromptu exposition of his side-chain theory.

"Now if there is an infection in the organism, producing a toxin by which the living cells of the organism are attacked," Ehrlich began, "the organism creates a corresponding antitoxin,[11] to defend itself, by a process in which the 'arms' or 'receptors,' with a specific affinity for the toxin, are produced in the cells, to replace those with which the toxin first combined."

An inveterate cigar smoker, Ehrlich always traveled with a box of cigars under his arm, and a collection of varicolored pencils and pads in his briefcase. Now, half-hidden by clouds of tobacco smoke, Ehrlich began, as was also his habit, to draw whole series of diagrams to better help his fellow traveler grasp his side-chain theory of immunity. "You see, you understand, I have chosen this diagrammatic explanation of the manner in which immunization takes place in the living organism, to show how the antitoxins are formed in the living body, by a process analogous to the excessive replacement with which the body tissues repair any kind of injury."

During another trip on the same train, this time from Berlin to Frankfurt in the company of two English professors, William Bulloch and Almroth Wright, Ehrlich used the lock-and-key specificity of the antibodies and their targets (antigens) on the cells of microbial parasites as a model for possible antimicrobial chemicals. "In my study of immunity," he said to his friends, "it has occurred to me that by systematic and extensive chemical and biological experiments it should be possible to find artificial substances which are really and specifically curative for certain disease. . . . Such curative substances must directly destroy the microbes provoking the disease," and not harm the cells of the body itself.

When his friends agreed, they pointed out that he had now found his "real life-work: chemistry in medicine."

Ehrlich warmed to the idea. The man-made chemicals would, he cautioned, have to be synthesized to match the characteristics of the bacterial chemicals produced in the body by human host defense systems. "The marvelous effect of an antibody in a serum," he told his colleagues on that night train, "is due to the fact that in no case has it any affinity for the body substances, but it flies straight onward, without deviation, upon the parasites. The antibodies, therefore, are Magic Bullets, which find their target by themselves."

The side-chain theory, considered too complex to understand when Ehrlich introduced it, in time proved to be too simple to explain the growing complexes of interacting and interdependent biological and chemical processes involved in our immune systems. As late as 1949, however, Sir Henry Dale, himself a Nobel laureate in medicine, described it as "a startling theory of the nature of the reaction by which the body of the patient makes itself immune from a further similar infection." Dale observed, with justice, that "this side-chain theory of Ehrlich rapidly permeated and gave shape and direction to the researches in this field of workers in all countries; it has continued to be a principal factor in the rapid expansion of knowledge of the phenomena of immunity, allergy and related conditions."

In 1903 Ehrlich's friend Almroth Wright, together with his assistant at St. Mary's Hospital in London, Stewart Douglas, published the results of a study that did much to end the needless flap over phagocytic versus humoral theories of immunity. Their report, "An Experimental Investigation of the Role of the Blood Fluids in Connection with Phagocytosis," offered "conclusive proof that the blood fluids modify the bacteria in a manner which makes them a ready prey to the phagocytes."

They understood the implications of this finding very well. "We may," they wrote, "speak of this as an 'opsonic' effect (*opsono*—I cater for; I prepare victuals for), and we may employ the term 'opsonins' to designate the elements in the blood fluids which produce this effect." The terms opsonic and opsonizing antibodies are still among the more useful concepts in modern therapeutics.

The work of many investigators, much of which we shall review in later pages, added to the roster of major and measurable factors involved in inborn natural immunity to agents of infection—and of equally life-threatening foreign bodies.

Cancer, for example, is a disorder in which an individual's own cells become so transformed by the carcinogenic chemical or radiological or biological insult that triggers the disease that they become—as far as the host immune systems are concerned—cells foreign to the body of their origin. Just as invasive bacteria and viruses bear, generally on their outer surfaces, specific antigens—substances that elicit immune responses, such as antibodies that combine with microbial antigens and neutralize the infectious agents—cancer cells may develop specific tumor or cancer antigens that cause the body's own defense system to attack the transformed cells as if they were hostile foreign invaders. The cancers that become medical problems are possibly only those that overwhelm the host immune systems.

If the rise of immunology altered many areas of medical cure, the first century of the immunological sciences also produced some logical scientific explanations of conditions that acute doctors were reporting in some detail for at least a century before Élie Metchnikoff stuck a rose thorn or two under the skin of "some beautiful star-fish larvae." During the eighteenth and early nineteenth centuries, Drs. William Buchan of Scotland and Charles Hall of London had written about how much more likely the poor were than the affluent to contract diarrheal and contagious diseases, and of how much more frequently the families of the rich survived such diseases than the families of the poor. Of course, these early observers had never heard of such bacteria as *Salmonella* and *Shigella* which cause typhoid and dysentery, let alone the tubercle bacillus or the array of cold viruses or the ubiquitous streptococci and staphylococci. What they did observe was that such bacterial and viral diseases were most likely to infect and kill people in families that lacked such "necessaries of life" as adequate nutrition, uncrowded and well-ventilated and heated housing, and adequate health care. Just as germ theory told doctors about the specific agents of the infectious diseases of industrial civilization, immunology revealed the roles of the various inborn and interacting systems of cellular and humoral immunity that give every human being, in theory, the competence to fight off such infections.

The more immunologists study our natural inborn immune defense systems, the more confirmation they receive of the essential role of the "necessaries of life" in maintaining these mechanisms at maximum efficiency. This is one medical observation that has not changed but merely become more documented and more precise since 1789, when Dr. Buchan published *Domestic Medicine* and warned that the basic necessities of life, starting with adequate nutrition, were as important as medical care in fighting diseases.

As I write, I have on my desk the manuscript of a textbook now in press.[12] The book deals with infectious diseases in surgical patients; Chapter 20, written by Professors Wesley Alexander and Dwight Stinnett, of the University of Cincinnati, is called "Immunotherapeutic Approaches to the Treatment of Infection in the Surgical Patient."

Under the heading "Modes and Rationale of Nutritional Repletion," these three sentences appear: "Perhaps of greatest importance is the observation that correction of nutritional deficiencies can result in restoration of immunological competence. Several means are available to correct malnutrition. The best is the presentation of an adequate normal meal."

Germ theory, by identifying the specific disease agents that proliferate in filth, provided a needed scientific rationale for civic and personal hygiene. Immunology, the scientific product of germ theory, provided our species with the biological and chemical reasons why adequate nutrition, housing, and, above all else, family income are—along with a sanitary environment—the essential prerequisites of normal health.

Immunology was far from the only addition to the literature of the human condition since 1789. There was also, among many other pearls, the Fourth Axiom of Mae West: "I've been poor and I've been rich. Rich is better."

This, however, was a semantic rather than a substantive contribution to human understanding, since it was in essence merely a bright new way of stating a proven old truth. The studies of infection and immunity, on the other hand, contributed important new truths to the human treasury.

Germ theory illuminated the specific causes and mechanisms of infection, and made the search for microbial disease agents and vaccines against them the proper study of the biomedical sciences. Immunology introduced life scientists to the complexes of inborn human biological and chemical defense systems against microscopic disease agents which could be mobilized and enhanced by effective vaccines. This new study of the mechanisms of natural and induced immunity to infectious diseases would ultimately turn immunology into one of the core sciences of twentieth-century medicine.

In the end, immunology, and such of its branches as immunochemistry and immunogenetics, provided much of the basic knowledge that is essential in the development of better new vaccines.

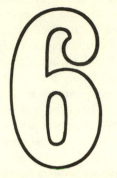

DIPHTHERIA YIELDS
TO PASTEUR'S DREAM OF A
"CHEMICAL VACCINE"

Wherever the densely crowded tenements were located, there the [diphtheria cases] were very numerous, while in the districts occupied by private residences very few cases were indicated as having occurred.... With stricter isolation of patients and intelligent and systematic supervision of schools and tenements, we can certainly reduce the number of cases of diphtheria in the city, but the total extermination of the disease under the existing conditions of life here does not seem probable unless we can acquire new means to combat the disease.

—WILLIAM H. PARK, M.D., Bacteriological Diagnostician and Inspector of Diphtheria, New York City Board of Health, in his first annual report, May 5, 1894

T he first of the two types of chemical vaccines—that is, those made from chemicals produced by bacterial cells, and those created from chemicals found in the cell walls and other cell structures—that Pasteur postulated in the memorandum written to himself in 1885 was not long in appearing.

This could have been predicted. What could not as easily have been predicted by Pasteur and his European peers and contemporaries was that much of the work that led to the development of this chemical vaccine was going to be done in America by three very young doctors, Theobald Smith (1859–1934), William Hallock Park (1863–1939), and Henry Sewall (1855–1936). Sewall and Park had had some postdoctoral training in Europe, but in physiology and laryngology, not in bacteriology. Smith graduated from the medical college at Albany before bacteriology was taught in America, and, using the journal articles of Pasteur, Koch, and their coworkers as his texts, was completely self-trained in bacteriology.

During their lifetimes, all three young Americans were very well known to European bacteriologists. The London professor of bacteriology William Bulloch, author of the classic work *The History of Bacteriology* (1938) and a fine scientist himself, spoke for all leading European biologists in his obituary essay on Theobald Smith in the *British Journal of Pathology* (1935): "It is certain that America in days to come will look on him [Smith] with that veneration with which France cherishes the name of Pasteur and Germany that of Koch."

Smith was not the only one of the three to be compared to Pasteur. In 1922, when the American Public Health Association awarded the Sedgwick Medal to Park, their citation described him as "the American Pasteur."

Kudos from such impressive sources, and the doctors' own towering achievements in biology and medicine, are logical prerequisites for lasting if not undying fame. Fate mocks logic, however. Few major American scientists are less well known and venerated by most living Americans than are Theobald Smith, who was among other things the first to show that blood-sucking insects transmit parasites of killing infectious diseases to mammals, and William H. Park, who as both bacteriological investigator and public health physician probably did more than any other individual to eradicate diphtheria from the United States and other industrial nations during the first half of the twentieth century. Dr. Henry Sewall happens to be one of the few giants in American scientific and medical history who is today even less known in America than either Smith or Park.

Born in 1855 in Winchester, Virginia, where his father was minister of a Methodist church, and removed to Baltimore, Maryland, with his family before he was a year old, Henry Sewall liked to refer to himself as "a Virginian by mistake." He also liked to talk about at least one of his Colonial ancestors, Judge Samuel Sewall, one of the hanging judges in the Salem witch trials of 1692. Unlike the other judges of Salem, four years later Samuel Sewall saw the error of his ways, and issued a public recantation of the part he had played in the extermination of twenty human beings for the false charges of being supernatural witches.

Henry Sewall's grandfather, Thomas Sewall (1786–1845), was a prominent physician and medical scientist who for the last three decades of his life was professor of anatomy and physiology at the Columbian College (later George Washington University) in Washington, D.C. His book, *An Examination of Phrenology, Errors of Phrenology Exposed* (1837), appeared at a time when many American medical scientists, college presidents, statesmen, physicians, anatomists, and psychologists had accepted with great enthusiasm the patently absurd tenets of this pseudoscience that "analyzed" human character by the shape of and bumps in one's head.[1] Sewall was the leading academic opponent of this farce, and his rational dissection of its claims survives as a classic essay in scientific method. Like his wife and daughter, Mary, Thomas Sewall died of tuberculosis.

His son, the Reverend Thomas Sewall (1818–1870), Henry Sewall's father, also died of tuberculosis. Because of his father's death, and his uncle's innocent but costly mismanagement of Professor Sewall's legacy, Henry Sewall was unable to go to Harvard as he had always dreamed of doing. Instead, primarily because the sons of Methodist clergymen paid much lower fees than other boys, Henry Sewall entered Wesleyan University in Connecticut in 1871, when he was sixteen. He stayed on for an extra year of work in chemistry and other sciences before taking Wesleyan's first science degree when he emerged as an honors graduate in 1876.

It was the year that the then experimental Johns Hopkins University opened in Baltimore, where Sewall's family still resided. Because the family lacked enough money to send him to Harvard, or for that matter to any other school away from home, the twenty-one-year-old honors graduate entered the new Johns Hopkins University in 1876 as a graduate student and staff assistant in biology. The Johns Hopkins Hospital, also endowed by the Baltimore merchant whose name it bore, was not opened until 1889, and the Johns Hopkins University College of Medicine opened in 1893.

Young Sewall was given a job as assistant in the laboratory of the university's first professor of biology, H. Newell Martin, a physiologist who had studied abroad under Thomas Huxley and other mentors. Not until a month after the first semester began did Sewall learn that his salary of $250 per term was paid out of Martin's personal funds; the first budget of the well-endowed new institution included no provision for laboratory assistants.

After taking his doctorate in physiology in 1879, Sewall went to Leipzig, Germany, where he worked under the physiologist Carl F. W. Ludwig. Three years earlier, Ludwig had given postdoctoral training to the American physician William H. Welch, who in 1884 would become the first professor of pathology at Johns Hopkins and when its medical school opened nine years later, its first dean. Sewall returned to Baltimore for another year of work under Martin, and in 1881 went to the medical school of the University of Michigan at Ann Arbor as professor of physiology. It was the start of a long personal association with Dr. Victor C. Vaughan (1851–1929), then dean at Michigan and one of the most formidable figures in nineteenth- and twentieth-century medicine and public health in America.

In 1933, toward the end of his years, Sewall penned his own memoir of one of the great adventures in ideas—the genesis and details of the work he did at Ann Arbor in 1887 that was to change bacteriology and lead to the advent of serotherapy and the creation of the first chemical vaccine. "My early training with Martin, a pupil and colleague of Huxley's and Foster's, found its lure in the mechanism of life in general, unhampered by shibboleths," Sewall wrote.[2]

"About 1880 Louis Pasteur was at his peak. I was fascinated with his feats of vaccinating animals by the inoculation of attenuated pathogens. But obviously that procedure had inherent dangers. It seemed to me that if one could get the metabolized excreta of germs, which could not reproduce, an animal inoculated with such products might be protected from the living deadly organism."

At about that time, Sewall also read the "classic essay by Weir Mitchell and [Edward T.] Reichert on Snake Venom" and was struck by their technique of extracting venom from the poison glands of live snakes. "Then as now," Sewall recalled, "fancy found its stimulus in the field of analogy. I thought: Why should not one assume that the malignant microbe found its animal counterpart in the salivary cell of the snake's poison gland? Why should not the snake's poison, properly diluted, be inoculated into an animal in increasing doses with the prospect of protecting it against an otherwise deadly dose?"

The idea, he wrote, "lay dormant for a long time. Meanwhile the tubercle bacillus had picked me for his game and I felt unequal to the strain of ordinary physiological research—but research there must be!" Eventually, subsequently recurring bouts of tuberculosis were to end Sewall's career in laboratory research, but in the fall of 1887, as he prepared to go to the North Carolina mountain resort town of Asheville for mid-winter because of his lung infection, Sewall decided to "start something in the line of the snake idea, which might work itself out while I was away."

The idea was tested on some cooperating live rattlesnakes provided by a faculty colleague, and on some nonconsenting pigeons, in the Old Medical Building at Ann Arbor in 1887. Sewall started his experiment by first determining the smallest amount of snake venom—the minimum lethal dose—that would kill a pigeon. After this, he set out to find out what nonlethal but continually increased doses of venom would do to pigeons. He learned that these gradually larger doses of venom, inoculated over a period of time, protected (i.e., immunized) pigeons against the toxic effects of inoculations containing ten times the minimal lethal doses of the same venom. In terms of the new vocabulary of serotherapy and immunology that was about to be born, he had by the use of immunologic techniques caused the pigeons to synthesize the first reported antitoxin.

The young and ailing Sewall knew exactly what he had accomplished. His work, he wrote in his paper "Experiments on the Preventive Inoculation of Snake Venom," published in the *Journal of Physiology* in 1887, "was undertaken with the hope that it might form a worthy contribution to the theory of Prophylaxis." He hoped that his results would "induce investigators more fortunately situated for the performance of such experiments to take up the same line of observation. I have assumed an analogy between the venom of the poisonous serpent and the ptomaines [toxic substances or poisons] produced under the influence of bacterial organisms.

"If immunity from the fatal effects of snake-bite can," Sewall continued, "be secured in an animal by means of repeated inoculation with doses of poison too small to produce ill effects, we may suspect that some sort of resistance against germ disease might follow the inoculation of the appropriate ptomaine [poison or toxin] . . ."

It was a brilliant hunch, and had the young physiologist been able to test this concept by searching for and isolating the toxins of bacteria, and then testing them in animals as he had tested the immunizing powers of graded doses of snake venom in pigeons, the history of science would undoubtedly have gained a sparkling chapter or two. He was, however, a member of the third generation of Sewalls to pay the price of being exposed to infective doses of the tubercle bacillus before Pasteur, Lister, and Koch helped create germ theory. Since nobody, from professors of medicine and clergymen to drovers and drapers, knew what actually caused tuberculosis until Henry Sewall was nearly thirty years old, once the dread infection appeared in any family—rich or poor—it was handed down from parents to children and from their children to their grandchildren like a legacy "in the blood."

It was only when people learned how to keep the tubercle bacilli acquired by one member of the family from being transmitted from his or her lungs to the rest of the family that intelligent doctors finally understood that there was no such thing as biologically hereditary tuberculosis. Familial active or dormant tuberculosis infections are transmitted by acquired germs, not inherited genes.

By the time Henry Sewall was ready to cut his self-earned swath in history, the probably childhood-acquired, dormant tuberculosis infection that was part of his social legacy became active. He had to leave his job at Michigan in search of health. After stops at the Trudeau Sanitarium in the Adirondack Mountains and other way stations, Sewall and his wife wound up in Denver, Colorado, where the climate was then salubrious for people with tuberculosis and other lung conditions. There he qualified as a physician, went into private practice, became a specialist in tuberculosis and public health, held chairs as professor of physiology and medicine at the University of Colorado School of Medicine—and saved his life. His father had died at fifty-two, his grandfather at fifty-nine. Henry Sewall died at the age of eighty-three, in 1936.

Sewall was always aware of the importance of the work he had done with snake venom as an antitoxin, but he was never able to continue it himself. He was also a very modest man. In a memoir written in 1933, Sewall wrote that "it is interesting to note that my close friend, V. C. Vaughan, in Ann Arbor, and W. H. Welch in Baltimore, alone saw anything in the paper."

In this, Sewall was completely mistaken. Many leading investigators, such as the clinician Ludolf Krehl in Strasbourg and Albert Calmette, the noted deputy director of the Pasteur Institute—personally selected by Pasteur himself to establish the Pasteur Institutes of Indochina and of Lille, France—wrote of the importance of Sewall's discovery long before World War I. In 1908, the year he wrote about Sewall's "important paper on rattlesnake-venom," Dr. Calmette led a group of French scientists on a visit to Ann Arbor. Of this visit, Victor Vaughan recalled that "twenty or more years after Sewall had been compelled by ill-health to give up his work with us, I received a call from a delegation of learned Frenchmen who introduced themselves by saying that they had journeyed to Ann Arbor to see the place where Henry Sewall had demonstrated that pigeons could be immunized to the venom of the rattlesnake, because they said that work had pointed out the way to the discovery of diphtheria anti-toxin."

Calmette's colleagues at the Pasteur Institute of Paris, Drs. Émile Roux and Alexandre Yersin, accepted Sewall's invitation to perform experiments with pathogenic bacteria that would "take up the same line of observation" Sewall had made with the snake toxins. They chose to work with the bacilli recently (1884) proven by Dr. Friedrich Loeffler, an assistant of Robert Koch's, to be the microbial pathogens involved in diphtheria. There was a very good reason why Roux and Yersin, inspired by Sewall's work with snake venom as an antitoxin, elected to seek similar chemical systems in the diphtheria bacillus (since renamed *Corynebacterium diphtheriae*). Of all the urban scourges of the century, diphtheria was one of the most devastating in terms of deaths of people of all ages, but most tragic because the majority of the deaths occurred (and still occur) in children under three years old.

Following the dramatic successes of the vaccines against rabies and anthrax, Pasteur and his associates were deluged with letters from doctors and laymen alike, each with a particularly devastating candidate for eradication by vaccination. Many of them begged Pasteur to work on a vaccine against diphtheria. One, signed by a woman who identified herself simply as "A Mother," was circulated to all the investigators at the new Pasteur Institute. It read: "You have done all the good a man could do on earth. If you will, you can surely find a remedy for the horrible disease called diphtheria. Our children, to whom we teach your name as that of a great benefactor, will owe their lives to you."[3]

Diphtheria is not new to the human experience. However, it was not nearly as widespread before as after the Industrial Revolution brought in its sooty wake the overcrowded warrens of the working poor in the old cities, such as London and Paris, and in many new mining and factory towns—and even cities like Manchester—where overcrowded new tenements and converted hovels were the only housing the mine and factory workers ever knew from cradle to grave. In such living conditions, particularly when crowding is exacerbated by the adverse effects of hunger, stress, and secondary infections, formerly infrequent killing and crippling infectious diseases like diphtheria (and pneumonia, scarlet fever, tuberculosis, cholera, typhoid fever, measles, rubella, otitis media) become ubiquitous or endemic.

The disease, called by many names, was known to Hebrew healers before the birth of Christ, and was described in the oral lore of the Babylonian Talmud for centuries before it was compiled in writing in the sixth century A.D. Ancient medical literature abounds in descriptions of the disease under its different names, many of which vividly describe one or more aspects of diphtheria. Arateus the Cappadocian, a Greek physician who practiced in Rome between approximately 120 and 200 A.D., called diphtheria the Egyptian or Syrian ulcers of the tonsils. He wrote of these tonsillar ulcers that from the tonsils, they spread "outwardly to the mouth," and if they "extend to the tongue, the gums, and the alveoli [and] the inflammation seizes the neck" then death follows "within a few days from the inflammation, fever, fetid smell, and want of food. But, if it spread to the thorax by the windpipe, it occasions death by suffocation." He observed, quite accurately, that "the manner of death is most piteous; pain sharp and hot as from a carbuncle; respiration bad, for their breath smells strongly of putrefaction, as they constantly inhale the same again into their chest; . . . fever acute, thirst as if from fire, and yet they do not desire drink for fear of the pain it would occasion . . ."[4]

Whether called malignant ulcerous sore throat, or croup, or angina maligna, or angina interna, diphtheria was almost always marked by the final formation of a tough, leathery membrane in the throat and its components. This blue-white membrane, composed of the debris of bacteria, white and red blood cells, killed cells from the tissues of the throat, and fibrin (the essential portion of blood clots), can cause death by respiratory obstruction. As of 1900, diphtheria was the tenth leading cause of all United States deaths.

Until late in the nineteenth century, death claimed 90 percent of people with diphtheritic membranes on the larynx, and 35 percent of all diphtheria cases. Not until the mid-twentieth century was it known that many diphtheria deaths are also caused by the actions of the bacterial cell's chemical products on the heart, the nervous system, the kidneys, and other vital organs. We also know now, as a modern specialist in infectious diseases wrote in a standard textbook, "Myocarditis [inflammation of the muscular walls of the heart] develops in about two-thirds of patients with diphtheria, but is clinically evident in about 10 percent." This and other effects of diphtheria can and do cause chronic heart conditions and death.

Diphtheria is often accompanied by secondary infections at the site of its primary lesion, frequently by the opportunistic agents of pneumococcal pneumonia as well as the beta-hemolytic streptococci that cause mastoiditis, erysipelas (St. Anthony's fire), scarlet fever, and the recurrent strep throat infections that can lead to rheumatic fever and nephritis (inflammation of the kidneys). Pneumococci, streptococci, and other potentially lethal microbial pathogens are normally found, in small and therefore safe proportions, in the flora of all people. When these other microbial organisms find masses of nutrients, like the debris coating the leathery membranes of diphtheria, they often colonize these sites and start to proliferate to levels pathogenic to their human hosts.

At the time of the 1578 diphtheria outbreak in Paris, the physician Guillaume de Baillou speculated on the wisdom, "after all else has failed," of making an opening from the outside of the neck to the larynx to keep a patient with an obstructive diphtheritic membrane from choking to death. Baillou wrote of a young man who was afflicted with a diphtheritic membrane "which threatened to suffocate him. He opened his throat with the aid of a sword: he lost much blood but he recovered. In an urgent case [of diphtherial asphyxiation] would it not be possible to attempt a similar operation?"

Other doctors, most notably the early seventeenth-century Italian Marco Aurelio Severino, did perform such surgery, but on the trachea (or windpipe) rather than on the larynx—and albeit with a surgical scalpel instead of a sword—to keep diphtheria victims from choking to death. In 1821 the French physician Pierre Bretonneau discovered that croup, malignant gangrene of the gums, and scorbutic gangrene of the gums were not three separate disorders, but a single contagious disease for which he proposed the name diphtheria, from the Greek word for leather. Bretonneau is possibly most remembered, however, for something he did four years later.

In 1825 a friend, who had previously lost three children to diphtheria, sent for Bretonneau. The friend's fourth child had come down with diphtheria, and the leathery membrane caused by the infection was slowly killing this child, too. Bretonneau cut an air passage through the child's windpipe, or trachea. The child survived, and lived to the age of seventy-one—or long enough to see Bretonneau's tracheotomy joined, in 1885, by intubation, another procedure that enables diphtheria victims to breathe. Intubation, invented by the New York physician Joseph P. O'Dwyer in 1885, calls for the nonsurgical insertion of a flexible tube between the vocal cords in the larynx into the trachea to relieve blockage of the windpipe by the diphtheritic membrane. (Intubation has since been widely used, for the passage of oxygen and anesthetic gases during anesthesia and for other needs.) Both techniques kept thousands of diphtheria patients from choking to death. Many of them, however, were infected by deadly microbes that colonized the intubation sites. To this day, for all our antibiotics, patients intubated for diphtheria and other causes are much more prone to hospital-acquired infections than are nonintubated patients.

In 1883, shortly after Pasteur had created the first of his vaccines against specific bacterial diseases, the Swiss pathologist Edwin Klebs isolated from patients with diphtheria the bacilli he felt were the agents of the disease, and described their appearance. Many investigators looked for and found bacteria that matched Klebs's description in the throats and sputa of diphtheria patients. Friedrich Loeffler grew these bacteria in pure culture and then used cultures of the Klebs bacilli to induce a diphtheria-like disease in guinea pigs and pigeons. What quickly became known as the Klebs-Loeffler bacillus was, indeed, the causal agent of diphtheria.

The medical world was so excited by this proof that most physicians failed to grasp the potential significance of one of the other observations in Loeffler's eighty-page paper in the Reports of the Imperial Health Office. Loeffler had written that in his laboratory animals, "death resulted not from a generalized dissemination of bacilli, but from an effect induced by the bacilli at the site of the injection [of diphtheria germ cultures]." Loeffler then postulated that "the hemorrhagic edema [swellings], the pleural exudate, the brownish-red areas of consolidation in the lungs, where bacilli could not be demonstrated, were conclusive indications that a toxin generated at the site of the injection and transmitted through the blood stream, induced severe damage to [blood] vessel walls. The toxin generated by the bacilli in the guinea pig is undoubtedly similar to the toxin of human diphtheria."

A "conclusive indication" is a very far cry from a working and replicable proof. Nevertheless, here was a first-rate investigator in one of the world's leading laboratories of bacteriology writing about a toxin presumably produced by the bacteria of diphtheria—and nobody, except for Loeffler himself, followed this up by searching for the toxin he so logically postulated to exist. Over the next four years, Loeffler's attempts to isolate and purify this toxin were far from fruitful.

One of the reasons that no investigators at that time—1884 was a year of great expectations in bacteriology—were ready to drop everything and start hunting for the "toxin generated by the bacilli" of diphtheria was the prevailing conviction that once the germs of any disease were isolated, one could then attenuate these germs and turn them into vaccines to prevent the disease. This was just what medical people started trying to do after Loeffler's report was published.

Since people are extremely loath to advertise their failures, very few of the many early attempts to make a diphtheria vaccine starting in 1884 were ever described and published in the medical journals of the day. Experimental diphtheria vaccines, made of live attenuated bacillus cultures, were undoubtedly produced by many over the next decade or more. Some of them might even have worked to a limited extent, but only occasionally and never consistently, for reasons that any junior bacteriologist understands today.

By 1888 when, inspired by the work of Henry Sewall in 1887 at Ann Arbor, Michigan, Roux and Yersin started to search for the diphtheria toxin that Loeffler had postulated four years earlier, the world's medical armamentarium still lacked a safe and effective diphtheria vaccine. The only way to prevent the disease was to isolate children from their classmates by keeping them home from school, and to isolate parents from their own workplaces. With the identification of the causal microbe, good evidence accumulated to show that diphtheria is spread by droplet infection; that is, the diphtheria germs are spread by microscopic moist droplets in the breath of people with active cases or who are healthy carriers of the infective organisms.

What was needed now was a way of keeping these germs from colonizing the noses and throats of potential victims or carriers. Because of the role of snake toxin in immunizing pigeons, as described by Sewall, Roux and Yersin were more than curious about the potential role of the still-sought diphtheria toxin in prophylaxis, that is, protection against the disease.

In 1888 Loeffler was still actively searching for the diphtheria toxin. At that time there were only two hospitals in Paris, the Hospital for Sick Children and the Trousseau Hospital, where children with highly contagious cases of diphtheria were admitted. It was to these hospitals that Roux and Yersin turned for cultures of bacteria swabbed from the throats of infected children in 1888, the year the new Pasteur Institute was opened.

After a month of heavy growth in nutrient broth, flourishing colonies of diphtheria bacilli were passed through a graded series of filters fine enough to separate out all the living bacteria and bacterial debris from the liquid filtrate. The bacteria-free filtrate was injected into healthy guinea pigs. It caused a diphtheria-like disease that inside of a week killed the little animals. Further tests of similar diphtheria-broth-culture filtrates killed rabbits, sheep, dogs, and birds, although mice and rats proved to be as naturally resistant to the toxin-bearing filtered broth as they were to diphtheria in nature.

Roux and Yersin now used calcium chloride to separate, by precipitation, the fraction of the filtered diphtheria-broth culture that contained the toxin. This precipitate was so toxic that only four tenths of a milligram was able to kill eight guinea pigs. It was the partially purified toxin itself.

Sewall's postulated bacterial analogy of the snake venom toxin was, at least in diphtheria, no longer a challenging hypothesis but a confirmed chemical fact. As Roux explained in a lecture to the Royal Society in London the following year, the work he and Yersin did demonstrated that after three or four weeks of active growth, the cultures of the diphtheria bacilli become "so full of toxin that, without microbes, and in infinitesmal doses, they cause the death of the animals with all the signs observed after inoculation with the [diphtheria] microbe itself. The picture of the disease is complete, even presenting the ensuing paralysis if the injected dose is too weak to bring about a rapid death. Death in infectious diseases," Roux concluded, "is therefore caused by intoxication [poisoning]."

The toxin of bacteria now being isolated and purified, the new task that faced bacteriologists was to use this purified bacterial toxin in the same way Sewall had used the snake venom toxin in 1887—to see whether inoculations of tiny amounts of the toxin, in gradually increasing doses, might ultimately protect (the word immunize was yet to be coined) a healthy person against inoculations of lethal doses of the same toxin. This put Roux and Yersin into a friendly competition with known and unknown investigators worldwide.

In 1890 this race was won by a Japanese postdoctoral graduate, Shibasaburo Kitasato (1852–1931), who after completing his studies at the Imperial University of Tokyo went to Berlin to work under Koch in 1885, and under Dr. Emil Behring, a German army doctor assigned to work as an assistant to Koch in 1889. In the same year, Kitasato isolated the tetanus bacillus and showed it was the cause of lockjaw, or, as it is now called, tetanus.

Tetanus was known to Hippocrates, who, more than four centuries before the birth of Christ, described it as a common killer of women in childbirth, wounded soldiers, and infants. In the nineteenth century, when horses were used in urban and battlefield transportation, horse manure—in which the tetanus bacillus proliferates—made cuts, abrasions, and battle wounds highly subject to infection. Nearly a century after Kitasato isolated the bacterium that causes it, tetanus remains a muscle-paralyzing disease for which there is still no specific medical treatment. Even today, when people get tetanus the chance that it will kill them ranges from 30 percent to 50 percent in all cases. Tetanus is common among drug addicts, who use contaminated needles for injections of hard drugs.[5]

Shortly after Kitasato isolated the tetanus bacillus, the young Danish physician and medical scientist Knud Faber (1862–1956) showed that the bacillus itself was harmless and only its toxin caused lockjaw. Behring and Kitasato together started to work with the toxins of both tetanus and diphtheria bacilli. Once these toxins were extracted and purified, it then became only a matter of time before some investigator or team of workers using the toxins would repeat procedures analagous to the method Sewall had used to immunize pigeons against rattlesnake venom.

On December 3, 1890, another Koch assistant, Dr. Carl Fraenkel, published in the *Berliner klinische Wochenschrift* a detailed report on how he had taken three-week-old broth cultures of virulent diphtheria bacilli, subjected them to one hour of germ-killing heat, and then—after the broth cooled—injected measured doses of it into healthy guinea pigs. A few weeks later, these inoculated guinea pigs were injected with cultures of live, virulent diphtheria germs of the same strain. The animals previously inoculated with cultures of heat-killed diphtheria proved to be immune to infection by the subsequent inoculations of live microbes. The live bacterial inoculations neither grew nor produced diphtheria toxin in the now apparently immunized guinea pigs.

For a time it seemed to Fraenkel and other doctors that at long last there was a safe and effective vaccine against human diphtheria. It is highly probable (although without published documentary evidence) that after Fraenkel's article was published, many batches of killed-organism diphtheria vaccines were produced in various laboratories and injected into a large number of experimental patients. Fortunately, since the organisms had been heat-killed, whatever toxin might have been present in the bacteria was also denatured, and so the vaccines poisoned nobody. It probably did not take very long, however, for the optimistic doctors who tested their variations of Fraenkel killed-organism vaccine to learn that they did not protect people against either diphtheria or the diphtheria toxin.

The actual reason for the failure of the Fraenkel heat-killed bacteria vaccine to immunize people would not be known for another sixty years. Meanwhile, the bacteriophages, or viruses that parasitize bacteria, had to be found in 1915; and the existence of a special type of mutant strains of bacteria called the lysogenic strains had to be discovered and studied between 1925 and 1950.

Unlike most normal bacteria, which are invaded and quickly destroyed by viruses whose nucleic acids (genes) take over the chemical machinery of the bacterial cells to produce new viruses, the lysogenic organisms are not immediately destroyed by invasive viral genes. Instead, the lysogenic bacteria simply combine viral genes with their own, and for many subsequent bacterial generations, the virus-genetic materials remain inactive or dormant. After the virus infection, the lysogenic bacteria continue about their business, replicating themselves and perpetuating their species. When they replicate, however, they pass their dormant virus genes on to their daughter bacterial cells, and this generation and its descendants pass the dormant virus genes down through many generations of lysogenic bacteria. Eventually, stimulated by radiations or certain chemicals (which are also mutagens and carcinogens in people), the dormant genes in the genetic legacy of the lysogenic bacteria suddenly become activated, and quickly take over the metabolic or chemical machinery of the bacteria, transforming them into producers of new virus particles, which multiply and soon shatter and kill their bacterial hosts.

Most strains of *C. diphtheriae* are normal, not lysogenic. The normal *C. diphtheriae* bacilli found in patients and healthy carriers are harmless. It is only the lysogenic strains which, under very special circumstances, become toxic. In the absence of viruses specific to the lysogenic strains of particular species of bacteria, the lysogenic bacteria are harmless. However, when a lysogenic bacterium takes the nucleic acids of its virus into its own collection of genes, it undergoes a process known as lysogenic conversion. The converted cell begins to produce, along with its normal quota of chemicals, a new metabolite that it never synthesized before. These new metabolites constitute the toxins of bacteria produced by lysogenic *Corynebacteria;* and the toxins of scarlet fever manufactured by lysogenic *Streptococci pyogenes.* This makes such diseases as diphtheria and scarlet fever actually virus infections produced by the toxic metabolites of sick bacteria.[6]

None of these reasons for the failure of killed-organism vaccines against diphtheria could even be suspected in 1891, the year of early euphoria and blessedly quick awakening concerning their clinical worth. But the dream of immunization against diphtheria was soon revived by a series of new developments. On the day after Fraenkel's paper on his heat-killed vaccine appeared, Behring and Kitasato published an even more earthshaking article in the *Deutsche Medizinische Wochenschrift.* It described how, in an elegant series of experiments, they had discovered that "the immunity of rabbits and mice, immunized [by Sewall's technique of graduated doses of toxin] against tetanus, consists in the power of the cell-free blood fluid to render innocuous [or neutralize] the toxic substance which the tetanus bacilli produce."

One week later Behring published the results of an identical set of experiments he had performed, alone, with the diphtheria bacillus. His results with the diphtheria toxin were identical to those of the concurrent tetanus experiments.

Behring and Kitasato coined a new word—antitoxic—to describe the toxin-destroying nature of blood serum taken from animals immunized by a series of progressively larger doses of bacterial toxin. It was clear that the blood of animals immunized by the toxins of such bacteria as the tetanus and diphtheria species soon acquired the ability to neutralize or destroy the bacterial toxins.

This was quickly recognized as a historic advance, for the antitoxin proved to be the first known antibody—that is, an antitoxin or antibacterial or antiviral or other host-protective chemical produced in the body in response to stimulation by a specific antigen. In this pioneer instance, the antigen was the toxin itself. Antigens are any substances that activate the antibody-forming cells of the body against specific microbial agents and other foreign invaders; thousands of different kinds of antigens are found in the structures of bacteria and viruses, on blood and tumor-cell membranes, and even on the pollens and other parts of plants. The various types of antibodies include, in addition to the antitoxins, the bacteriolysins (which lyse or shatter bacteria), the opsonins (which make invasive bacteria subject to phagocytosis, or engulfment and destruction, by our white blood cells), and the agglutinins (which combine with specific antigens, such as those of bacteria and viruses, and cause them to agglutinate, or clump.)

In 1890, when Kitasato and Behring demonstrated the protective nature of bacterial antitoxins (antibodies) in animals, they wondered if these antitoxins could be used to prevent or even to cure diphtheria, tetanus, and other diseases caused in people by bacterial toxins. Like the idea of using the newly discovered antitoxins to prevent infectious diseases, the concept of using the antibodies to microbial disease agents to cure infectious diseases also derived from the nearly hundred years of clinical experiences with Jenner's 1796 vaccine against smallpox.

Had the initial attempts to attenuate the newly isolated germs of diphtheria and tetanus and use them to make vaccines not failed, it is quite possible that in 1890 or thereabouts, serotherapy—that is, using antitoxins and other antibodies found in the blood serum to cure rather than to prevent infectious diseases—might never have been developed. Failure to make effective and safe vaccines against diphtheria and tetanus caused serious researchers in Germany, France, and other countries to reexamine the clinical lessons of smallpox vaccinations.

During the years when doctors were growing painfully aware of the temporary nature of primary smallpox vaccination immunity, it was also discovered that when previously vaccinated people—usually adults unless their primary vaccine had been useless—did get smallpox, it was invariably a milder and rarely lethal form. Clearly, to the principal investigators in Koch's and Pasteur's institutes, this had to mean that even after the levels of antismallpox activity originally induced by vaccination became too low to prevent smallpox, they could still moderate the course and outcome of an infection. The problem then became to learn whether the knowledge Sewall had gained with snake venom could be used to moderate and possibly even cure tetanus, diphtheria, and other medically untreatable and often fatal diseases caused by bacterial toxins.

In 1890 many investigators began to consider the glycerinated calf lymph that was used to vaccinate people against smallpox as a model for immunizing people against diphtheria, tetanus, and infections caused by other yet unidentified toxin-producing bacteria. Vaccines made of live or killed whole diphtheria bacilli having failed to protect people against that disease, it made sense to speculate about preventing diphtheria and tetanus in the same way people were then being immunized against smallpox—by inoculating them with one of the body fluids of an animal immunized with the virus or toxin of the disease itself. Instead of lymph, the idea was to use inoculations of "the cell-free blood fluid [serum]" Kitasato and Behring had found "to render harmless the toxic substance which the tetanus" and diphtheria bacilli produce in the blood of animals, and to shoot it into healthy human beings to protect them against these diseases.

In our own times, nearly a century later, federal laws demand elaborate tests of any new vaccine or drug in three or more distinct species of animals before laboratories can run even preliminary human trials of only the safety of new vaccines or drugs. At the close of the nineteenth century, the mixture of curiosity and enthusiasm that caused Jenner to scrape pus and other materials from the pustules on the arm of a dairymaid and inoculate it into the arm of a minor child was as legally unregulated as it had been in 1796. The only question was whether people in the general vicinity of Berlin circa 1890 were "vaccinated" against diphtheria and tetanus with the immune sera of rabbits and goats before it was discovered in laboratory animals that the immunity induced by the antibodies in those sera lasted only as long as the antibodies themselves lasted—at the most, for a few weeks. Unlike the cowpox virus vaccines, which caused people themselves to start to produce antibodies that neutralized both cowpox and smallpox viruses for many years, the experimental shots of immune sera rich in antitoxins (antibodies) offered effective but short-lived passive immunity with their borrowed antibodies.

The new candidate vaccines made of immune sera had a very short life indeed. However, Behring was surrounded with more scientific talent than most. For example, there was a thirty-six-year-old unpaid worker in Koch's laboratories, Dr. Paul Ehrlich, born into a clan of affluent Jewish innkeepers in Silesia, who had survived an active siege of tuberculosis and other handicaps to get through medical school, marry, and settle down to a life dedicated to research. As an undergraduate he had become a pioneer in the applications of new dyes to stain tissues, bacteria, and other biological materials. In 1878, after qualifying as a doctor, Ehrlich spent some time as a senior house physician at the Charité Hospital in Berlin, where he developed some laboratory techniques of making clinical diagnoses. When Koch isolated the tubercle bacillus in 1882, Ehrlich threw himself into the self-imposed task of developing chemical stains that would help in the diagnosis and study of the germs of tuberculosis. His intensive studies of the tubercle bacillus is believed to have played some part in the active pulmonary tuberculosis Ehrlich developed.

Fortunately, he had some independent means. In 1887 Ehrlich and his wife went to Egypt during his recuperation from tuberculosis. By 1889 he was back in Berlin. He knew how difficult it was for a Jew to get an academic appointment in medicine, and he felt that, given the ability of tuberculosis to recur, if he returned to clinical practice he would endanger both his patients and himself. Rather than tempt the academic slings and bureaucratic arrows of endemic anti-Semitism that sought out the tenderest spots in his cousin Carl Weigert's anatomy,[7] Ehrlich opened a small private laboratory in which to conduct his own researches in Berlin. Koch invited Ehrlich to work as an unpaid research associate in his own government institute, a post Ehrlich gladly accepted. Koch and his associates were stimulating people, and the facilities Ehrlich needed for his own research were all there.

Ehrlich, above all others, soon determined by measurement, analysis, observation, and experiment exactly what had to be done to put the life-enhancing potentials of immune sera to two major clinical uses. Theoretically, sera drawn from people or animals immunized by graded doses of diphtheria and/or tetanus bacteria toxins should have been able to modify and cure those diseases, particularly if given early enough in the course of an infection. There was also a sound theoretical basis for expecting that if the families, friends, schoolmates, teachers, doctors, and other contacts of people with diphtheria or tetanus were also inoculated with antitoxic immune sera, the passive immunity the "borrowed antibodies" produced in their bodies would last long enough to protect them during the time they were at greatest risk of acquiring diphtheria and tetanus.

In short order Ehrlich worked out quantitative methods of standardizing the lethal and immunizing doses of the toxins as well as the potency of the antitoxins in each batch of immune serum. In medical practice this was esssential because it gave doctors the information required to order precise doses of antitoxins based on the patient's age, weight, and condition.

Without Ehrlich's very basic techniques for transforming Behring's important immunologic findings from laboratory curiosities to safe and effective medical modalities, it might have been years before they could be used to cure and temporarily prevent diphtheria and tetanus. As things worked out, as early as Christmas night, 1891, enough animal trials had been run to permit the first use of immune sera in the clinical treatment of diphtheria. A young girl at von Bergmann's clinic in Berlin became the first patient to be so treated. In this instance the noted physician Ernst Geissler injected her with a few doses of serum from a sheep that had previously been hyperimmunized with graded inoculations of diphtheria toxin.

The little girl recovered. During the next three years, an estimated twenty thousand patients, most of them children, were treated with antitoxic sera derived from sheep, goats, rabbits, and other small animals. Not all the children recovered, but the rates of cure in those treated with immune sera were considerably higher than among the children not given the same therapy.

At that time such therapeutic agents could be patented. Behring had a friend at the German chemical house of Fabwerke Hoechst, in Halle-on-Salle. Behring also had friends in high places in the German government. Hoechst showed great interest in controlling the patents on the antitoxins against tetanus and diphtheria. The profit potentials were staggering, and they offered a generous royalty arrangement.

Behring promised Ehrlich that he would use his considerable influence to obtain for him the directorship of the Prussian State Institute for Research. Ehrlich had no reason to doubt his colleague's word. In 1893, during a meeting with one of the Hoechst directors at the company's headquarters, Behring told Ehrlich that if he accepted commercial royalties for the antitoxins, Ehrlich would not be able to run a government research institution. It might create too nasty a public scandal.

Ehrlich opted for the directorship of the research institute. The Hoechst director quickly produced a quitclaim, and Ehrlich signed away all his financial rights to royalties on the commercial sale of the diphtheria and tetanus antitoxins. His share, he later estimated, would have come to 500,000 marks, a tidy fortune by any standards.

Ehrlich was bilked, and he knew it, if only belatedly when Behring was unable to deliver on his promise to obtain the directorship for him. However, he was not destroyed by this swindle. If it rankled when in 1901 Behring became the first winner of the Nobel Prize for Medicine, this frustration was erased seven years later when Ehrlich shared the 1908 Nobel Prize for Medicine with Élie Metchnikoff for their respective contributions to immunology. In 1896, without Behring's help, Ehrlich became director of the government Institute for the Investigation and Control of Sera (analogous to the U.S. Bureau of Biologics). In 1899, after the serum institute was moved to Frankfurt, the Speyer family endowed the new Royal Institute for Experimental Therapy, which was built next door to the government institute and dedicated solely to work on the new field of chemotherapy created by Ehrlich. For the next sixteen years until his death in 1915, Ehrlich directed both institutes.

Behring was raised to the nobility and became von Behring. Some time later when Ehrlich's fame became worldwide, he was raised to the rank of privy councillor with the title of Excellenz in 1911. Behring and Ehrlich never met or spoke to one another again after the Hoechst affair. In 1915, after the second of two strokes finally killed Ehrlich, von Behring—rich in money and honors but with an unbroken string of failed attempts to create vaccines to prevent, and antitoxins to cure, tuberculosis to show as the fruits of his subsequent scientific researches—appeared as Ehrlich's body was being lowered into a grave at the Jewish cemetery of Frankfurt. He stood at the graveside and said, "If we have hurt you forgive us!"[8]

Ehrlich had long since recovered from the hurt von Behring would never forget inflicting. He had been much too busy studying the many aspects of biology and chemistry, health and disease. Along the way he had discovered that antibodies are associated with the blood globulins and that, as Dr. Béla Schick observed on the centennial of Ehrlich's birth, "Ehrlich realized the limitations of antitoxic serotherapy and developed his own original ideas of chemotherapy."

As early as 1908, Ehrlich spelled out the goals and guiding principles of the new chemotherapy. He was, he wrote, after "a cure which I have called *Therapia Sterilans Magna.* That is to say, a complete sterilization of a highly infected organism with one dose." These single doses would consist of what Ehrlich termed his Magic Bullets, chemicals formulated to seek out and destroy germs and other microbial agents of infection while at the same time causing no harm to the tissue and organs of the people treated with these Magic Bullets.

One chemical, found in Ehrlich's laboratory in 1910, was the famous substance number 606, known as arsphenamine or Salvarsan. It provided a long-needed effective treatment for syphilis. Two years later, Ehrlich's laboratory also introduced Neosalvarsan, a water-soluble form of this arsenical drug.

Meanwhile in 1894, Drs. Émile Roux and Louis Martin, at the Pasteur Institute in Paris, had inoculated a horse with gradually increased doses of diphtheria toxin. Some weeks later, by this variation of Sewall's method, the animal was immunized against diphtheria. The Parisian doctors then drew blood from the hyperimmunized horse's jugular vein. They allowed it to coagulate in a sterile container, and then harvested the serum or liquid portion of this blood. In February of that year, they used this equine immune serum to treat all the diphtheria patients at the Hospital for Sick Children. All the children recovered and went home. At the Trousseau Hospital, the only other one in Paris that admitted children with diphtheria, the new antitoxin was not used, and the hospital's diphtheria mortality rates remained unchanged.

At the Hospital for Sick Children, during the years 1890–1893, there had been an average of fifty-one deaths in every one hundred cases of diphtheria (2,029 deaths in a total of 3,971 pediatric diphtheria cases). Inside of four months, the use of antitoxic sera cut the toll down to twenty-four deaths per hundred diphtheria cases. At the Trousseau Hospital, where the immune sera was not administered, the diphtheria deaths were sixty in one hundred cases. Prevention was still superior to cure, but the cure by antitoxin nevertheless cut the diphtheria deaths in half.

If doctors still lacked a vaccine to induce long-term active immunity against diphtheria (and tetanus), they now had antitoxins that performed two functions new to the human experience: the cure of at least half of the diphtheria victims on whom they were used, and the transfer of passive immunity against the disease to the parents and other contacts of the victims during the times when they critically needed this protection.

The importance of these antitoxins in the 1890s was not lost on any parent, teacher, or, for that matter, newspaper editor. In Paris the newspaper *Figaro* started a public subscription to a fund to provide free antitoxins for everyone who needed them. Within a few days readers contributed nearly a million francs. These funds were turned over to the Pasteur Institute, which used them to build new stables, immunize many horses under sanitary conditions, and inside of a few months produce fifty thousand doses of diphtheria antitoxin to be given away free.

A full course of life-saving antitoxin treatment used up only twenty to forty cubic centimeters (ccs). The world not only had immune sera to cope with diphtheria and tetanus, but when these antitoxins were made in horses enormous quantities could be produced daily.

Now that the newly isolated bacterial toxins could be used to cure diphtheria and tetanus, investigators redoubled their efforts to determine if they could be altered or otherwise manipulated to provide more than short-lived passive immunizations.

At that time, American doctors still looked solely to France and Germany for scientific guidance in the management of diphtheria and tetanus. As early as 1884, Dr. Joseph J. Kinyoun, of the fledgling U.S. Public Health Service in Washington, made the first of many visits to the Pasteur Institute, where he studied under Roux and purchased for American use large batches of antitoxic or immune sera against diphtheria and tetanus. In 1885, Dr. T. Mitchell Prudden of the Columbia University College of Physicians and Surgeons (P and S) and Dr. William H. Welch of Johns Hopkins University became the first Americans to study under Koch in Berlin.

That same year Prudden gave the first course (a short one) in bacteriology to be offered at P and S. One of the students in this two-week laboratory class was a very serious twenty-two-year-old graduate of New York's City College, William Hallock Park. The son of a prosperous wholesale grocer and chandler, young Park had two goals in life. The first was to become a specialist in rhinolaryngology—disorders of the nose and throat. The second ambition was to become a medical missionary in Persia, ministering to both body and soul. His affluent but practical father, Rufus Park, was very supportive of his son's first ambition. Perhaps because too many of young Will's ancestors lay buried in lonely Christian missionary graves in Ceylon and other heathen lands, the successful merchant took a very dim view of the future of medical-missionary work as a career for his son.

In 1886, when young Park graduated from P and S and prepared to enter Roosevelt Hospital as an intern, his father read him a little speech. "Will," he said, "if you give up your damned fool idea of becoming a medical missionary, I will stake you to a year's postgraduate study in Austria, after you have finished your internship." When his three-year internship was nearing its end, young Park asked if it would be all right if after his postinternship studies in Vienna, he continued on to Peking for a few months' trial of field missionary work. The merchant put his answer in writing, and said that after Vienna it was straight home to New York "or no Europe at all, my boy. And remember, from Europe to America, one travels west, and not east."[9]

Young Park did just this after his year in Vienna, a tour of Europe, and a one-month postgraduate course in obstetrics and gynecology at Dublin's Coombe Hospital. His four years of postgraduate training behind him, Park looked forward to setting up a lucrative private practice as a nose-and-throat specialist in the largest and wealthiest city in the United States. His earlier experiences with diphtheria while an intern, and an error made concerning the causal agents of this disease by his mentor T. Mitchell Prudden, gave his career an entirely unexpected complexion. Instead of becoming a medical missionary, Park was to spend his life in an equally unselfish and economically just as unrewarding calling, that of public health or, as it was called in those times, state medicine. Whether Park ever saved a single soul is a question for theologians, but there can be no question that his work in the control and prevention of infectious diseases would save millions of lives, many of them during the remaining years of his own life.

In 1887, while Park was still an intern, Prudden had become a consulting bacteriologist at the New York City Board of Health. In this position, as well as in his medical school laboratories, Prudden had cultured the throat swabbings of many cases diagnosed as diphtheria by doctors in the city's better hospitals. Although he was aware that most European experts agreed that the Klebs-Loeffler bacillus was the agent of diphtheria, Prudden found so many streptococci in the throats of children with a diphtheria diagnosis, and in which he never found Klebs-Loeffler bacilli, that he published papers asserting that the streptococci were the actual disease agents.

Park returned to New York in 1890. He set up a private practice, took extra jobs as attending physician at Bellevue and three other hospitals, and started to make daily rounds in the diphtheria wards of the city's main contagion hospital, the since-closed Willard Parker Hospital for Contagious Diseases.

Nearly fifty years later, Park wrote a private memoir of his reunion with Prudden. He recalled that "the question of the relationship of the diphtheria bacilli to diphtheria came up." Prudden noted that he had been unable to culture any Klebs-Loeffler bacilli from the many diphtheria cases in which he had found thousands of streptococci. Park thought he knew why this had happened. "You know, Dr. Prudden," he said, "in children streptococcus laryngitis may frequently seem to us like laryngeal diphtheria, and I am sure," he said of Prudden's cases, "this was an epidemic attacking little children in a ward, and spread by contagion; it seemed like diphtheria but it was really a strep infection."

Under normal circumstances, this was not the most tactful statement for a young beginning physician to make to his medical school professor. It was one thing to disagree about the possible roles of newly discovered bacteria; it was quite another to tell a distinguished professor that what he had diagnosed as diphtheria was an ordinary strep throat. However, Prudden was no ordinary man. Far from resenting Park's statement, he said simply, "Don't you want to stay and work with me on this question?"

Park was flabbergasted. He reminded the professor that "the only instruction in bacteriology that I have ever had is the two weeks' course which you gave me when I was a medical student." He was also just as quick to tell Prudden that "I will be delighted if you will let me, and only require me to work after four o'clock," since he had daily clinics at four different hospitals.

The upshot was that Park was given a five-hundred-dollar-a-year scholarship to work under Prudden on the etiology of diphtheria. Two years of work in Prudden's laboratory yielded all the evidence needed to convince the older man that the Klebs-Loeffler bacillus, not the streptococcus, was the actual agent of diphtheria. This experience was also enough to convince Park that controlling diphtheria and other communicable diseases was what he most wanted to do with his life.

Park's two-year study involved close to two hundred cases of hospital patients diagnosed as having diphtheria. When the patients and the bacteria in their throats were examined by Parks, however, only fifty-four proved really to have diphtheria. Often, he noted, the same patients who had true diphtheria also had a secondary "pseudodiphtheria" caused by streptococci and other common bacterial pathogens. His recommendations included bacteriological examinations of all cases of suspicious throat infections. Since the tools and techniques of medical bacteriology were still unfamiliar to most physicians, and "as the early detection of diphtheria is important for the general health, and as this disease occurs most frequently and is most dangerous among the crowded poor, who are unable to pay for special examination, it would seem particularly the business of the Boards of Health to undertake it." Historically, state or preventive medicine was and still is responsible for keeping the preventable contagions of the poor from spreading to the families of the well-to-do.

Shortly after Park's diphtheria study was awarded the annual prize of the P and S Alumni Association and published in two issues of the *Medical Record* in 1892, Park was made assistant director of the New York City Board of Health Research Laboratory, a new unit born of the typhus epidemic that saw 241 reported cases and forty-five typhus deaths in the first weeks of the same year. On May 4, 1893, the Board of Health gave Park an additional appointment as its first official diphtheria diagnostician and inspector of diphtheria. The diagnostic laboratories were to be set up in two rooms in a. Bowery tenement; the job paid $1,200 a year; and as Park remembered, "it offered an opportunity for full-time research." In time these two rooms were to grow into the largest municipal health laboratories in the world, with Park as their director. Long before that, however, the modest-sized laboratory, devoted solely to the bacteriological diagnosis of clinical cases and to research on the natural history, cure, and prevention of diphtheria, would become a model for the world.

From the start Park's municipal diphtheria unit concentrated on both the bacteriological diagnosis of suspected cases, and the production and improvement of the antitoxins or immune sera. By May 1894 about forty depots were established, most of them in neighborhood drugstores, where physicians could obtain instructions for taking throat-swab cultures from patients and their families and contacts, as well as free kits containing sterile swabs, culture kits, and case-history forms. Dr. Anna Williams, a graduate and recent instructor in pathology at the Women's Medical College of New York and now a member of Park's staff, was sent to the Pasteur Institute for training under Roux.

In short order Park and his colleagues produced horse-serum antitoxins much more potent than any made in France or Germany. Requests for batches of the Park antitoxin poured in from health departments all over the United States and Europe. When the New York Herald started a public subscription for a fund to provide free diphtheria antitoxin to the poor, it won the support of Émile Roux, who in December 1894 sent the newspaper a letter of support for "the good cause in America." In France Roux wrote, "The mortality from diphtheria in the hospitals of Paris is no more than fourteen percent instead of fifty percent, which was the figure during the preceding years [before serotherapy]. This will suffice to show you what a benefit we owe to M. Behring, who introduced into science the anti-diphtheritic serum."

Before Park's laboratory started to turn out vast amounts of immune horse sera, a one-dose phial of diphtheria antitoxin imported from Europe retailed at twelve dollars—when it was available—as of December 1894. On January 1, 1895, the municipal laboratory started to produce superior antitoxin. By October of that year, the city was producing enough low-cost antitoxin to be able to offer free doses to the physicians of patients too poor to pay. The doses were available at the neighborhood depots, and the physicians were obligated merely to report on the outcome of each case in which they were used.

Even before Park's laboratory started to produce antitoxins, immune sera imported from Berlin by Dr. Herman Biggs, the head of the municipal

Board of Health, was used by Park to end a serious outbreak of diphtheria in a Mt. Vernon, New York, children's institution. Orphan asylums and children's hospitals were traditionally particularly subject to such devastating outbreaks. Park persuaded his chief "to let us use half of his supply in stamping out diphtheria" in the Mt. Vernon institution. The next morning they gave "a small injection of antitoxin to each of the children and the disease stopped. Twelve days later a very mild case developed. We again immunized all the children in the building, and from that time no more diphtheria developed. This taught us two important things—the diphtheria antitoxin prevents diphtheria but also that the prevention is only for a short time."

The clinical and research accomplishments of Park's laboratories became world-famous. Many American city health departments sent doctors to Park to be trained in his bacteriological and clinical techniques. Noted scientific workers, including Ehrlich and Koch, visited them to observe and to compare notes with the young director and staff. Koch recommended to the German government that it appropriate money to apply to the German people the knowledge of the diagnosis and treatment of diphtheria developed by the New York City Board of Health. His request was denied.

Park's efforts were not free of opposition. Some of it was based on the traditional fear of innovation, some on more interesting grounds. For example, there was Dr. Joseph E. Winters, professor of pediatrics at Cornell and senior medical physician at the Willard Parker Hospital. Far from being a reactionary, Dr. Winters had been one of the first physicians in the United States to accept, at face value, Koch's 1890 claims that injections of his tuberculin—a protein derived from the tubercle bacillus—could cure human tuberculosis. It was only after he injected tuberculin into some of his New York patients that Winters became one of the first to learn that, far from curing tuberculosis, tuberculin injections exacerbated the disease and often killed people who might otherwise have lived. After that, Winters was understandably opposed to injecting any other "miracle" cures into living people.

The chief critics of all that the Park laboratories did to conquer diphtheria were Park himself and his closest coworkers. The first annual report of his unit, presented in 1894 when Park was thirty, noted that diphtheria was most prevalent "wherever the densely crowded tenements were located . . . while in the districts occupied by private residences very few cases" were found. There was little physicians could do about ending the poverty that caused overcrowding in those tenements. "With stricter isolation of patients and intelligent and systematic supervision of the schools and tenements, we can certainly reduce the number of cases of diphtheria in the city," Park concluded, "but the total extermination of the disease under the existing conditions of life here does not seem probable unless we can acquire new means to combat the disease."

Park knew that diphtheria would remain unconquered until the medical armamentarium included a preparation that protected against it for at least as long as the vaccines against smallpox and anthrax protected against those deadly pestilences.

When he could find the time, Park worked, in his own mind and at the laboratory bench, on the quest for a vaccine that would produce a long-lasting immunity. As his duties for the Board of Health started to embrace all infectious diseases and the direction of all the research laboratories, Park also maintained a regular teaching schedule at the Bellevue-New York University School of Medicine, where he became instructor in contagious diseases in 1895. By 1900 he had risen to full professor of bacteriology.

During the first decades after the causal links between the Klebs-Loeffler bacillus and diphtheria were demonstrated, the attempts to produce a vaccine against the deadly infection were confined to working with either killed or attenuated (weakened) whole bacilli. Given the previous successes of the fowl cholera vaccine and the anthrax whole bacterial organism vaccine, this was logical and inevitable. However, each of these early whole diphtheria organism vaccines was a clinical failure.

Early in the quest for techniques of best using the serum antibodies (antitoxins) induced by injecting bacterial toxins into animals, Paul Ehrlich wanted to see what happened when specific amounts of antitoxin were added to specific quantities of toxin to hyperimmunize healthy animals. When these altered toxins were injected into guinea pigs, they neutralized unaltered toxins inoculated into the same animals. Ehrlich reasoned that the altered toxins became what he called "toxoids"—that is, toxins which failed to act as poisons and yet retained the ability to cause the body to start producing antibodies that neutralized active toxins.

Ehrlich did not carry his study of toxin-antitoxin mixtures much further. Five years later in 1903, Park presented a paper before the New York Pathological Society describing how when he neutralized diphtheria toxin by combining it with antitoxin, as Ehrlich had done to create his toxoids, injecting these toxin-antitoxin mixtures into animals yielded interesting results. "In an emergency," Park reported, "antitoxins [antibodies] of a good grade can be obtained from at least 50% of the horses within a period of three weeks," instead of the month or more it took to obtain immune sera with ordinary toxins.

Curiously, neither Ehrlich nor Park seems to have investigated whether the toxin-antitoxin mixtures (toxoids) increased or decreased or left unchanged the duration of toxin-induced immunity against diphtheria or tetanus. Theobald Smith, however, did determine in 1907 that the toxoids produced "an active immunity" that lasted in guinea pigs for at least two years.

In 1909, in a longer report on the active or long-lasting immunity against diphtheria produced in guinea pigs with balanced toxin-antitoxin mixtures, Smith suggested that his method of making and utilizing toxoids "invites further regard to its ultimate applicability to the human body." He cautioned that "the proportion of toxin and antitoxin which would produce the highest desirable immunity consistent with the least discomfort would have to be carefully worked out for the human subject."[10]

Once Smith's papers were published in the *Journal of Medical Research* and the *Journal of Experimental Medicine,* the medical world possessed the principle of an immunizing preparation or vaccine that would confer on guinea pigs and horses and, one hoped, also on people a long-lasting active immunity against diphtheria and tetanus, and, quite probably, against other contagious diseases caused by bacterial toxins. However, after the tragic Koch tuberculin fiasco, people in experimental medical bacteriology were no longer prone to shoot foreign substances into other people's bodies without first subjecting all candidate vaccines to carefully organized and lengthy safety and effectiveness tests in animals and human volunteers (the doctors themselves, medical students, nurses, and convict "volunteers").

Theobald Smith's articles were read by Behring and Ehrlich, Roux and the Pasteur Institute group, and Park and the dedicated men and women who collaborated in all his studies at the New York Board of Health Research Laboratory. After Smith published his findings, there was no longer any serious doubt that active immunization against diphtheria would eventually be induced by injecting people with toxin-antitoxin mixtures. The question now was how soon this extended immunization could be accomplished safely and most effectively.

The major consideration of safety was resolved in 1912 when Behring gave subcutaneous injections of toxin-antitoxin mixtures to two small groups of people in Berlin. The first group had trace amounts of diphtheria antitoxins in their systems, the second group was free of antitoxins. Behring's methods, as Park described them later, were very complicated. According to Park, Behring "found that in those who had had a trace of antitoxin before the immunization the antitoxin had increased greatly; but that in the others tested there was no increase [in antitoxin]." This only partial effectiveness was not nearly as significant to Park and his coworkers as Behring's basic "demonstration in a few human beings of the safety of the [toxin-antitoxin] injections."[11]

Now that the safety of the toxoids—or altered toxins—had been demonstrated in people, it was only a matter of carefully planned manipulations of the proportions of antitoxin used to neutralize the diphtheria toxins before safe and effective mixtures would be developed. Park's group soon produced just such mixtures.

Park wrote with some pride, after World War I, that starting in 1913, "the practical value of toxin-antitoxin injections were subjected to continuous investigation by workers in the Bureau of Laboratories of the Department of Health of the City of New York." In the fall of 1913, he reported,

"We began the practical use of toxin-antitoxin injections for the immunizing of children against diphtheria, and established the facts that the procedure was harmless and after three injections about 80 per cent of those individuals possessing no antitoxin or insufficient antitoxin to protect from diphtheria, developed immunity. . . . We soon realized that the most important problem was the duration of the antitoxin immunity in those that had developed antitoxin. A satisfactory answer to this question required that immunizations be carried out in institutions where the children would be under observation for a number of years."[12]

The clinical and social necessity for extended active immunization were plain to all physicians and parents. Thanks to serotherapy, the death rate for diphtheria had been cut in New York City from 129 deaths per 100,000 in 1905 to 85.6 in 1915. In absolute numbers, this meant a drop from 1,544 deaths in 1905 to 1,278 in 1915. The number of all diphtheria cases, fatal and nonfatal, reported by doctors to the Board of Health rose from 12,913 in 1900 to 15,279 in 1915. This was a remarkably small increase in view of the fact that until 1914 poor immigrants from Europe arrived in New York in record numbers, and added mightily to the density of the already overcrowded tenements.

In 1913 when Park and his collaborators started to test the toxin-antitoxin vaccine on children in New York City schools and orphan asylums, twenty-three states outside of New York, representing 60 percent of the national population of ninety-seven million people, reported a combined rate of 18.1 diphtheria deaths for every 100,000 people. While in rough numbers this represented a drop of from 30,666 deaths in 1900 to a total of around 17,600 in 1913, the human and social costs of diphtheria now were considered to be intolerably high. The only partial successes of serotherapy had inspired what was seen as the very feasible goal of wiping out diphtheria by induced active immunization as thoroughly as Jenner's vaccine had nearly eradicated smallpox in some countries.

Unlike smallpox and syphilis and certain other infectious diseases, which generally conferred extended active immunity on their survivors, diphtheria did not always protect people who lived through it. Although they usually emerged immune to further attacks, only too often those with their hearts and other organs permanently compromised by one siege of diphtheria suffered a second case. However good the new cures, prevention was still to be preferred.

In the New York Board of Health Research Laboratory, day-to-day work involving all infectious diseases continued to claim the highest priority. Salaries in the municipal laboratory were low, and most of the physicians and bacteriologists who worked with Park also had part-time teaching and clinical jobs, as did their chief himself. None of them could devote their full time to work on toxin-antitoxin preparations against diphtheria, but for a half dozen years Park and his staff gave this project their own seal of urgency. Their other responsibilities were not the only reasons for the six-year lag between Smith's first publication in 1907 and the first clinical trials of the Research Laboratory's toxin-antitoxin mixtures.

In 1913 Park and Drs. Abraham Zingher and H. M. Serota tested the accuracy of Dr. Béla Schick's test for susceptibility to diphtheria on patients at the Willard Parker Hospital for Contagious Diseases. In this newly developed test, the injection of a tiny drop of diphtheria toxin (one fiftieth the amount needed to cause diphtheria in a guinea pig) caused no effects in people naturally immune to diphtheria. In those susceptible to diphtheria, the same amount of toxin caused a reddish-brown swelling at the site of the injection.

Of the seven hundred patients in the hospital's scarlet fever pavilion who were given the Schick test, four hundred gave negative reactions, and none developed diphtheria during their stays in the hospital. In contrast, forty-two of the three hundred patients shown by the Schick test to be susceptible to diphtheria did, indeed, come down with it. What made this trial more interesting was the fact that an attempt was made to immunize each patient with toxin-antitoxin preparations—and not one attempt succeeded.

Different mixtures, these slightly more toxic, then were tested in 115 children, aged from four to sixteen, whom the Schick test showed were susceptible to diphtheria. Each child was inoculated two or three times at weekly intervals with these mixtures. Nearly three quarters of them were actively immunized inside of forty days, and thereafter were shown by their Schick tests to have been converted from susceptible to immune by the toxin-antitoxin preparations.

Park and Zingher made their toxoid more efficient, and by 1914, at the annual meetings of the American Medical Association, recommended, "For the general prophylaxis against diphtheria in schools and communities, excluding immediate contacts, a mixture of toxin-antitoxin alone (85 percent to 90 percent of the L+ dose of antitoxin to each unit of antitoxin) or toxin-antitoxin plus vaccine of killed diphtheria bacilli."

In due time the killed-bacteria vaccine proved ineffective and was dropped, but the toxoid—the toxin-antitoxin mixture—was ready now for mass use.

Unfortunately, the total extirpation of diphtheria—at least in the United States and other affluent countries—had to be postponed until the termination of a plague even worse than diphtheria and smallpox combined. It was called World War I, and between 1914 and 1918 it would kill at least one million people and wound another twenty million. One of the first scientific casualties of this war was the end of all German, English, French, and other European research on diphtheria and its prevention. Behring, who died in 1917, and Ehrlich, who died two years earlier, never worked on diphtheria again.

In the United States, which was not drawn into the carnage until

April 1917, Park and his close collaborators were able to make significant advances in the prevention of diphtheria by artificially induced immunizations until the new priorities of total war demanded that they devote all their laboratory resources to meet military orders for diphtheria and tetanus antitoxins and toxoids. During 1916, the great poliomyelitis epidemic—the worst in America's history—demanded most of the laboratories' attention and services. Then, as always, diphtheria was only one of many diseases on which they worked.

The years 1913 and 1914 had been devoted primarily to making the toxin-antitoxin toxoid (TAT) as effective in prophylaxis as the smallpox and anthrax vaccines. This was accomplished, and by 1915 the assistant directors of the New York Board of Health laboratories, Drs. Abraham Zingher and May Schroeder, took charge of the next phase of the orderly planned conquest of diphtheria. This called for determining how long the TAT-induced active immunity lasted.

"Even if we could make every child immune," wrote Dr. Schroeder, "this would be of little practical value unless the condition remained permanent. We decided that the most favorable means of determining the truth as to this point was to seek institutions where the children were held for a number of years. Dr. Zingher and I picked out a number of institutions and we have followed the children from year to year. . . . We have also tested 4000 inmates of the State Institution for the Insane."

Zingher obtained the cooperation of schools and parochial institutions in the boroughs of Manhattan and the Bronx, Schroeder did the same in the borough of Brooklyn. Until Zingher was called up for military duty in 1917, they shared these tasks for two years. Afterward, Schroeder carried on alone, injecting, testing, and retesting children and mental patients periodically for the duration.

In 1915 Alfred Hess, who divided his time between the municipal laboratories and the Home for Hebrew Infants in Manhattan, where he served as medical director, succeeded in getting that orphan asylum to agree to Schick test all children admitted to the home, and to immunize them with TAT if they proved susceptible. Of the 1,076 children (whose ages ranged from one month to six years) who were Schick tested here, 406 or 37.7 percent proved to be Schick positive, susceptible to diphtheria. During the year 1915, "Diphtheria had been endemic at this institution, and there were six deaths due to the disease. . . . In not a single instance did a child with a negative Schick test contract the disease."[13]

The municipal laboratories supplied the toxins for the Schick tests, the TAT for the immunizations, and they even sent along Dr. Julius Blum of the health department to run the diphtheria tests while Dr. Hess attended to his regular medical tasks in this fragile population. The Home for Hebrew Infants that year became the first institution in the world to make routine the eradication of diphtheria in its child population by Schick testing and TAT immunizations. Subsequently, within a few months two larger institutions outside of New York City, the St. Agnes and St. Dominic orphan asylums in the town of Sparkhill, New York, established routine Schick testing in their populations of 1,200 children each.

These orphan-asylum efforts represented an impressive start on the eradication of diphtheria, but just as they were proving their worth, all additional mass immunization projects were dumped into limbo for the duration of World War I.

In 1917 in the city of New York alone, there were 12,624 reported cases of diphtheria, and 1,158 diphtheria deaths. In 1918, although the municipal death-certificate data showed 1,245 diphtheria deaths, the city's doctors reported 11,455 cases of diphtheria—clearly a bit of underreporting due to the war-caused shortage of physicians. Most of the individuals who suffered and died of the disease in the nation's greatest city were under six years of age.

Nationally, the combined rate for 1917–1918 was 14.8 diphtheria deaths per 100,000 population—in rough numbers, over 30,000 diphtheria deaths. Most of these occurred in very young children. They, too, had been condemned to die for the mistake of catching diphtheria while the world war raged.

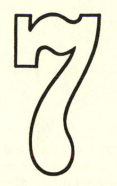

WORLD WAR I AND THE MORE DEVASTATING INFLUENZA PANDEMIC

The only time I ever saw Dr. [William Henry] Welch really worried and disturbed was in the autumn of 1918, at Camp Devens, near Boston. . . . When the blue swollen lungs were removed and opened, Dr. Welch turned and said, "This must be some new kind of infection or plague," and he was obviously quite excited and obviously very nervous.

—Dr. Rufus Cole, in a letter to Dr. Simon Flexner, May 26, 1936[1]

The total deaths [in the influenza pandemic of 1918–1919] throughout the world were estimated at 15–25 million—the greatest visitation ever experienced by the human race.

—W.I.B. Beveridge, 1977[2]

The diphtheria vaccine was far from the only medical advance to be disrupted or postponed by the ravages of World War I. What made this particular disruption more tragic was the fact that most of the human beings infected and killed by diphtheria were children under six years old. Children, however, are far from the only victims of the cruel national priorities of any modern military conflict.

Armed fighting men—many of them barely out of their own childhoods—are as entitled to life as are infants, toddlers, and mothers. It is not soldiers who make war but statesmen, and it is the statesmen who make the wars—not the soldiers who kill and are killed in wars—who collect Nobel Prizes for peace between the conflicts born of their statesmanship. Wars, however, create their own scales of national values. Because of these value systems, research, development, and the introduction and wide pediatric applications of medical innovations like safe, effective vaccines against common and deadly infectious diseases all come to a grinding halt in any military emergency as sweeping as World War I.

During the four years of that war, and the two or three years of acute disruption and reconstruction which followed it, military and military-linked priorities alone determined who would benefit the greatest, or even at all, from the most effective of the vaccines and antitoxins developed between 1880 and 1914. There were many on the market whose sellers made many claims for their worth: Putative vaccines were available for gonorrhea, scarlet fever, cholera, pneumonia, meningitis, syphilis, streptococcal infections other than scarlet fever, tuberculosis, and nearly every other major infectious disease. Doctors were urged to shoot all sorts of preparations into human bodies. In terms of safety and effectiveness, however, there were very few real vaccines and antitoxins of proven value, and of these not all were of equal clinical worth. Some, like the cholera vaccines of Kolle and Haffkine, were weakly effective; some, like the killed-organism typhoid fever vaccine of Almroth Wright, were of mixed value; still others, like the BCG (*Bacillus Calmette-Guérin*), attenuated, live tubercle bacillus vaccine that Calmette and Guérin of the Pasteur Institute had developed in 1906, but which was not made available for general use until 1921, are as controversial today as they were then.

Not only were many of the available vaccines of little value, some were capable of causing great harm. The only safe and fully effective human vaccines available as of 1914 were the glycerinated calf-lymph vaccine against smallpox, the Pasteur vaccines against rabies and anthrax, and Bordet's vaccine against pertussis (whooping cough). The antitoxin preparations against diphtheria and tetanus were 100 percent effective if used during the first twenty-four hours of the infections, and of rapidly decreasing effectiveness thereafter. In practical terms, on the battlefield this meant that if a soldier was treated with tetanus antitoxin immediately after being wounded, his chances of getting lockjaw were virtually nil; if less than three days elapsed before he received the antitoxin, his chances of surviving a tetanus infection were fair to poor; if more than three days passed, the odds were better than even that he would wind up with lockjaw, an incurable and usually fatal disease.

It is a matter of military history that thanks to antitoxin or serotherapy, in some World War I armies soldiers infected by the tetanus bacilli or exposed to the diphtheria bacilli were spared the fatal and crippling consequences of fulminating tetanus and diphtheria infections, and were able to return to no-less-lethal combat. Since the first function of war is to kill enemy soldiers, the anthrax and smallpox vaccines, and the tetanus and diphtheria antitoxins, performed handsomely in the military interests of the warring nations.

Wright's typhoid vaccine did not establish that clear-cut a record. Prior to the war, there was a universal laboratory belief that this killed-organism vaccine—whose side effects of fevers, chills, and general malaise were and remain formidable—would have prevented the ghastly toll of fatal typhoid cases among the British troops in the Boer War (1899–1902). Many bacteriologists believed that had the hidebound medical corps of the British Army made the use of Wright's typhoid vaccine compulsory for all troops, there would have been no typhoid deaths. Wright was permitted to solicit military volunteers, but the active interference of many army officials—and the even more devastating word-of-mouth reports of the adverse side effects of this vaccine that spread from vaccinated volunteers through the ranks—kept the numbers of vaccinated soldiers down to a minimal total.

Wright's friend Lord Haldane, who was then Minister of War, had Wright knighted in 1906 to give his typhoid vaccine more political clout. Although this vaccine was still not compulsory in the British Army in World War I, it was used very extensively. So, too, were more rigorous efforts made by the army's sanitary corps to keep the water the British soldiers drank and washed with free of the enteric organisms that caused typhoid, cholera, and other diarrheal infections. After the war, some studies showed statistically that the Wright vaccine had been a great success against typhoid fever. However, when these studies were examined by skilled epidemiologists, they indicated that sanitary measures played a much greater role in the reduction of typhoid and other enteric fevers. In fact, in some areas the soldiers inoculated with the Wright vaccine developed more cases of typhoid than did the uninoculated soldiers.[3]

Failure of another available vaccine, the one against streptococci, led to another historic triumph of the earlier modality of sanitary reform in protecting the health of soldiers. This time two diseases were involved, meningococcal meningitis (then called cerebrospinal fever) and rheumatic fever. The first is caused by different strains of *Neisseria meningitidis,* the second by throat infections due to hemolytic streptococci (strep throats, in today's vernacular). Penicillin and other antibiotics act very effectively against both families of bacteria, but in World War I the antibacterial drugs had not yet been discovered. Alexander Fleming, the future discoverer of penicillin and Wright's assistant since 1906, was working under Wright in the military laboratory set up in the old Casino of Boulogne primarily to produce typhoid fever vaccine for the allied troops. During World War I, there were no antibacterial drugs or effective antitoxins against either meningococci or streptococci. However, generations of public health experience before and after Florence Nightingale helped confirm what observant physicians had known before her day—filth and overcrowding generate contagious diseases.

In October 1916 a dual epidemic of rheumatic fever and cerebrospinal meningitis broke out among four thousand recruits undergoing three months of intensive training while housed in the overcrowded and poorly ventilated barracks and tents of the Guards Depot at Caterham, England. During this epidemic, which peaked in February 1917, there were twenty cases of meningitis and twenty-one of rheumatic fever. In the absence of effective drugs and antitoxins, the army camp's doctors ordered an improvement in ventilation and a minimum spacing of two and a half feet between each cot in the barracks or tents.

After the spacing eliminated the overcrowding, a small outbreak of both diseases occurred in October 1917, but it did not spread and the camp remained free of epidemic meningitis and rheumatic fever. During the great military callup of April 1918, the camp again suffered overcrowding, and a new epidemic of rheumatic fever and meningitis broke out and was not contained until after the overcrowding was relieved at the end of May.[4]

There was a less productive episode involving military overcrowding and another fatal infectious disease for which no remedies or antitoxins or vaccines existed in 1917 and 1918. This one took place in the United States, and in its inception had to do essentially with overcrowding and not with any specific disease.

In January 1918, nine months after the United States entered the war, the Surgeon General of the U.S. Army, Dr. William Crawford Gorgas, testified before the Senate Military Affairs Committee. He told the senators that overcrowding was the rule rather than the exception in most stateside military training and staging camps. This testimony was based on a personal inspection tour Gorgas had made a few months earlier as reports of increasing cases and deaths from infectious diseases, particularly from pneumonia, meningitis, and measles, came to his office in Washington from military bases around the country.

Gorgas, who had vanquished yellow fever, malaria, and (a fact not nearly as well remembered) pneumonia in Havana and the Canal Zone, had sound medical reasons for urging the government to delay the general mobilization for "two or three months" until at least clinically adequate hospitals and other health facilities had been installed, and the medical and paramedical personnel found to run them. Without adequate medical facilities, Gorgas reported to the Secretary of War, the palpable overcrowding in all United States military camps would make disastrous contagious diseases inevitable.

Gorgas's fame, as the intrepid military doctor who had conquered yellow fever and malaria and had thereby made the Panama Canal possible, meant that his report to the Secretary of War and his subsequent public testimony would be treated as a major event in the daily press. What this American folk hero had to say was more than just major news to the parents and wives of the nearly five million drafted civilians then serving in army bases. A plainspoken man who brooked no compromises with what he saw as his military, medical, and moral responsibilities to the nation, the Surgeon General pulled no punches. Here, for example, is what he had to report about conditions he found in Camp Sevier, South Carolina:

"Sanitary conditions here are serious. Sixty men have died of pneumonia in the last month. The camp has been exposed to a general epidemic of measles, about 2,000 cases having occurred within the last month. During the same period they have had 175 cases of pneumonia and fifteen cases of meningitis. The new conscripts of this command are men who are non-immune to measles. They come from the neighboring Southern states, where population is sparse, and therefore have not had measles in childhood. Always with measles a certain number of cases of pneumonia occur. The mortality of pneumonia from any cause is always high.

"The basic sanitary condition, however, in my opinion, is overcrowding. In the past, in this camp, the division commander has had to put eleven or twelve men in a tent, due to shortage of tentage. At present, he has to put nine men in a tent, which gives about twenty-eight square feet to the man. I urge that the division commander be directed to furnish at least fifty square feet of floor space to the man, which would give about five men to the tent."[5]

Gorgas's military superiors, as well as the civilian Secretary of War, a noted civic reformer and lawyer, Newton D. Baker, disregarded his pleas for more living space and adequate medical care. The newspapers had a field day with Gorgas's testimony.

The War Secretary and his equally liberal President, the erstwhile historian and college president Woodrow Wilson, were well aware of the health, political, and military implications of Gorgas's testimony. There were only two things they could do in response. They could take his medical advice and make the military bases safer for the millions drafted to serve in the armed forces, or they could get rid of Gorgas.

They continued to ignore Gorgas's urgent medical recommendations. On October 3, 1918, Gorgas was due to reach the mandatory retirement age of sixty-four. He wanted to stay on the job. Many medical associations and civic and public health leaders petitioned the President to permit him to remain in his position. Most of the nation's newspapers wrote editorials endorsing these petitions. An editorial in *The New York Times,* for example, wrote that "At 64 a surgeon or scientist—General Gorgas is both—may be at the meridian of his usefulness. Some of the most eminent medical men in this city are well past that age, and they still practice their profession. In France and England there would be no question of retiring an army officer of the attainments of General Gorgas while the war lasted. It would be considered fatuous, without the shadow of reason. The President has authority to keep the present Surgeon General in active service, notwithstanding the statutory requirement, and it would seem that it was not necessary to memorialize the President to hold fast to our most distinguished army doctor."

On October 28, 1918, Newton Baker wrote to Gorgas to tell him that his official term as Surgeon General had expired and that he was being dropped with thanks. Gorgas finally had been fired.

The great influenza pandemic of 1918–1919 had already started in many parts of the world. It would hit the overcrowded United States military bases first and hardest, and become one of the worst plagues in recorded human history. While it raged, nobody knew what caused it. Most doctors, including the Surgeon General of the U.S. Public Health Service, Rupert Blue, mistakenly believed it was caused by "the bacillus influenza of Pfeiffer" (now known as *Haemophilus influenzae*), for which there was a vaccine which, Dr. Blue said, worked with "only partial success." (It had no effect on the influenza virus, but possibly at times—very few times—it did block secondary pneumonias due to Pfeiffer's bacillus.) The only medical advice that made sense was to avoid contact of any sort with carriers of the agent of this infection—that is, to avoid overcrowding. There was no known cure for influenza, nor for the secondary infections of bacterial pneumonia that killed so many influenza victims.

At a conservative estimate, more than twenty million people around the world were to die in this influenza pandemic. Over a half million of these deaths from the disease and its complications would occur in the United States, most of them in the space of a few months starting in the fall of 1918. More American servicemen died of influenza and its secondary bacterial pneumonias than from enemy fire during what President Wilson proudly hailed as the war to end all wars.

There was nothing very new in this. All wars produce epidemics and pandemics of infectious diseases. Civilians and combatants alike have traditionally suffered the lethal consequences of war-born plagues. More than one great war has been won or lost not by military genius or ineptitude, but simply because the pestilences of war—from smallpox and typhoid to cholera, syphilis, diphtheria, and other scourges—reached the losers before they infected the winners.[6] World War I had more than its share of the classic contagions of battle: typhus, typhoid, tuberculosis, rheumatic fever, spinal meningitis, cholera, poliomyelitis, and influenza. Of them all, none killed as swiftly, as widely, and with as many military and political consequences as influenza, whose secondary infections included the far more deadly pneumococcal and other bacterial pneumonias.

Since the viral cause of influenza was not, as of 1918, even suspected, it would not be accurate to suggest that because of the war, work on a vaccine against influenza was impeded. What was seriously impeded, however, was the development of the fledgling but significant new field of virology. This critically important area of medical microbiology went into involuntary hibernation for the duration.

The agents of pneumococcal pneumonias, which caused very many of the deaths associated with the influenza pandemic, had been known since 1884. Work on vaccines against these bacteria had been going on since 1886, spurred by repeated failures to produce a safe and effective vaccine against pneumococci.

The success of serum antitoxins against diphtheria after 1892 caused many research workers to try to make similar antisera against the pneumococci. These efforts had no practical results until after 1910 when it was found that more than one strain or type of pneumococci caused pneumonia, and that antisera against one strain would not act against pneumonia organisms of any other types. By 1914 when it was determined that nearly half of all medically diagnosed cases of pneumococcal pneumonia in New York were caused by organisms of the strain designated as Type I, and that serum from horses immunized by the method of Sewall with this strain of pneumococci helped cure Type I pneumonias, the Rockefeller Institute for Medical Research began to prepare and distribute immune sera against this specific strain. In patients with Type I pneumococcal pneumonia, the specific antisera (rich in immunoglobulins or antibodies against Type I pneumococcus) conferred enough passive immunity to keep the infections from growing worse and kept people from dying of pneumonia. The passive immunity was very short-lived, however, and did not protect against subsequent infections by Type I and other pneumococcal strains for which effective antisera were later developed and marketed.

These specific antisera were frequently and incorrectly called vaccines by doctors and laymen alike. Under any name they were in too short supply and did not protect against each of the dozen or so specific types of pneumococci most frequently responsible for pneumococcal pneumonia. They did not cause even a minor dent in the avalanche of bacterial pneumonia deaths secondary to viral influenza in 1918–1919.

Once the influenza pandemic took charge of the world, in the absence of drugs and enough types and doses of antisera to cure and vaccines to prevent viral influenza and its secondary bacterial pneumonias, there was only one way to cope with the pestilence. This involved using the well-tested, universally proven strategies developed by the sanitary reformers, the civilian and military public health officers, and the social reformers of the nineteenth century—that is, to see first of all that people who lived in overcrowded hovels and tenements, inadequately heated, ventilated, and lit, were moved to less crowded housing. To preserve health and avoid common contagions, it was also medically well established that human beings had to be well nourished. They should be protected from such environmental contaminants and pollutants as filth, stress, and noise; should work in factories, farms, offices, and shops safer for human life than trenches and military barracks; and should sleep every night free from the stresses and disruptions of shellings, bombings, rifle and machine-gun firings, and nightmares about wars. The only sensible way to have brought about such means of protection against the pestilences of Armageddon would, of course, have been to end the war.

In all wars, however, the leaders and the patriotic citizens take leave of their civic senses for the duration. In the absence of any real demand for more sensible alternatives to war and mass killings—and the pandemics of filth, hunger, and stress diseases that always come with the bombs and the bugles—the war ground on for four years of the most frightful slaughter we have ever been able to inflict upon ourselves in the names of patriotism, righteousness, and divine will.

It is a matter of historical record, rarely examined in most official military accounts of World War I, that the carnage came to a halt only when the pneumonia/influenza pandemic managed in a few short months to kill more combatants and civilians than the shells and bullets of both sides in all the military battles since the guns of August 1914 started to mass-produce hunger, hovels, contagions, widows, and orphans. As the deaths from what was called the Spanish flu or the swine flu or the American military training camp flu swelled, at long last peace began to seem infinitely more rational to the western world's political heads, and to even a few atypical military leaders, than did the continuation of the war.

The millions of deaths were the least of the peacemaking effects of the great 1918–1919 pandemic. For every flu victim killed by influenza and/or its secondary bacterial pneumonias, there were a dozen or more survivors so debilitated by their infections that they were many weeks in recovering full control over their bodies. This postinfluenzal debility or chronic weakness was disruptive enough among civilian populations. In the trenches, where the armies of all the warring powers had been engaged in the most physically taxing forms of warfare since 1914, the impact of the influenza pandemic on combat soldiers was a military catastrophe. Imperial Germany's supreme military leader, Field Marshal Erich von Ludendorff, later wrote in his memoirs, "It was a grievous business having to listen every morning to the Chiefs of Staffs' recital of the number of influenza cases, and their complaints about the weakness of their troops."[7] Ludendorff wrote that in 1918 influenza, which his foot soldiers cursed as the *Blitzkatarrh,* sapped both his troops' physical strength and their will to fight, and contributed to the failure of the last desperate offensive of the German armies in July 1918.

In view of the role of the influenza pandemic in speeding the end of World War I, the failure to develop effective vaccines against viral influenza and/or pneumococcal and other bacterial pneumonias by August 1914 might even be considered a somewhat mitigated disaster. Unchecked by the great pandemic's morbidities and mortalities, government leaders on both sides of the conflict might have continued to find enough teenage and middle-aged live bodies to prolong the war until well into the 1920s.

When the war ended, work on vaccines to eradicate diphtheria from the human legacy resumed.

France and Germany were in shambles. England had been bled dry in meeting the price of her victory. Inflation, hunger, and chaos reigned in Vienna and the old Hapsburg empire. Russia was torn by revolution, civil war, armed intervention, hunger, typhus, tuberculosis, cholera, and most of the other classic pestilences of war. In all of Europe there were neither the laboratories nor the investigators nor the funds to resume work on the development, clinical trials, and mass uses of a vaccine against diphtheria.

Thanks to a much shorter period of military participation in the war, and to the lack of German bombing planes capable of nonstop round-trip flights across the Atlantic Ocean, the United States emerged more or less intact. (Minus, of course, the 500,000 Americans killed by the influenza pandemic; the 53,000 servicemen killed in battle, and the lost work potentials of many of the 204,000 who had suffered nonmortal wounds.) None of our cities had been shelled, bombed from the air, or turned into battlegrounds; none of our farms had been ravished and torn by trenches; and none of our research institutions had been laid waste by battles, bombs, and homeless squatters.

The most important of the centers of research on the prevention of diphtheria, the Research Laboratory of the New York City Board of Health, its director, William Hallock Park, and his associates, were ready to resume work on the vaccine as soon as demobilization was started. The most important of the European diphtheria researchers to survive the carnage, Dr. Béla Schick, the Hungarian rabbi's son who had trained under the great pediatrician Theodor Escherich in Vienna and invented the Schick test for immunity to diphtheria, was now on staff at New York's Mt. Sinai Hospital and was available to collaborate with Park.

Thanks to the Schick test, Park and his associates starting in 1913, had been able to determine in weeks if their early experimental diphtheria toxin-antitoxin (TAT) vaccines were or were not producing immunity. When the killing ended, Park, Schroeder, and Zingher used the Schick test to make the happy discovery that school and orphan asylum children and adult mental hospital patients injected with their diphtheria TAT preparations as early as 1914, were in 1919 and 1920 still immune to diphtheria toxin.

By 1921 field and laboratory work had told Park and his close associates a number of significant things about diphtheria. The first was that thanks to remembered and never-noticed subclinical diphtheria infections, about half of the children and adults given Schick tests proved to have acquired lifetime natural immunity to diphtheria. This was important for many reasons, not the least of them the fact that this knowledge enabled physicians and public health workers to single out those individuals who did not need to be immunized by the diphtheria TAT vaccine.

The work of the Research Laboratory doctors also showed that in 50 percent of the diphtheria cases the disease was transmitted to them by healthy carriers. Theoretically, this meant that once half the total population of children in any nation or continent was immunized, diphtheria would be eradicated very quickly. By 1940 this was to be proven in New York City.

By the end of 1919, Park, Schroeder, Zingher, and Schick sought and obtained permission from parents to Schick test and if necessary immunize thousands of New York City public schoolchildren against diphtheria. In 1920–1921 Dr. Schroeder personally supervised the immunization of 50,000 Brooklyn schoolchildren, while Dr. Zingher did the same in the treatment of 52,000 public schoolchildren in Manhattan and the Bronx.

They understood, perhaps as well as parents of young children, how urgent this work was. As Dr. Schroeder told her peers at the New York Academy of Medicine in 1921, "Over 28,000 cases of diphtheria occurred in New York City during the years 1919–1920, and of the 2,284 persons who died, over 90 per cent were children, and that at least 90 per cent of these cases of sickness and death could probably have been prevented by means of the Schick test and immunization with diphtheria toxin-antitoxin (TAT). When we realize all this should it not spur us on to work toward that day when diphtheria shall become like smallpox—one of the rare diseases?"[8]

Since all the children to be tested and immunized were gathered in such central locations, Dr. Zingher noted, "We were able to apply the Schick test and the control test to as many as 500 or 600 children per hour. In one school we tested, on one day, during school hours, 2400 children; in another double school, over 2700 children."[9]

The logistics of conducting these tests did not interfere with Zingher's capacity to discover and record some findings of major significance in the future control of diphtheria. He found that "children from the homes of the more well-to-do have a much higher percentage of positive Schick reactions [i.e., no naturally or otherwise acquired immunity to diphtheria] than those from the homes of the poorer classes of the population, who live in closely crowded neighborhoods . . . in some schools as many as 67% of the children were found to give a positive reaction. The percentage diminishes . . . until we reach the schools located in the densely congested sections of the East Side, where not more than 16 to 20 percent give positive [susceptible] reactions."

Zingher did not neglect to spell out the reason for the greater susceptibility of well-to-do children to diphtheria. "Contact immunity seems to be an important element in the establishment of the so-called 'natural immunity,'" he reported in 1921. "Repeated exposure to diphtheria bacillus in the congested districts causes not only actual clinical cases of diphtheria to develop but also produces mild infections of the mucous membranes which are not recognized as diphtheria, but which may well lead to the gradual development of an antitoxic immunity." He cited the 79 percent and 75 percent positive Schick reactions of boys tested in exclusive prep schools as indications that "segregation of the children, either among the well to do or in rural and sparsely settled sections, plays an important factor in retarding the development of natural immunity to diphtheria."[10]

Municipal, state, and foreign health officers from around the nation and the world flocked to New York to observe what was happening in the city's free schools under the supervision of the Research Laboratory doctors. Soon, similar diphtheria control programs were launched in other cities and states.

In 1925 Gaston Ramon at the Pasteur Institute in Paris developed a superior diphtheria toxoid. Instead of mixing toxin with antitoxin, he allowed the toxin to stand with a 0.5 percent solution of formaldehyde for a month. Five years later it was learned that the addition of 0.2 percent of alum added to the immunogenicity of the chemically treated toxoid. Both advances in toxoids were quickly adopted by the Research Laboratory and, indeed, by most American pediatricians.

By 1928 "fully 500,000 school children had received injections," Park would write later. "It was then decided that the time had come to make a determined drive to treat the preschool children, especially those under 1 year of age. . . . Between 300,000 and 400,000 children have been immunized by the medical inspectors of the Health Department or by private physicians." That was in 1931. Since Park had started to work on the antitoxic treatment and immunologic prevention of diphtheria in 1893, New York City diphtheria deaths had diminished from 150 per 100,000 population to 2.8 per 100,000 population.

Nationally, and in countries such as England and France, diphtheria cases and deaths fell in line with the New York City figures. By 1940 the disease was for all practical purposes eradicated in New York City. Elsewhere in the nation, it took a little longer. In 1933, when for the first time all of the then forty-eight states reported their vital statistics to the U.S. Public Health Service, there were 50,462 cases of diphtheria cited and a total of 4,937 diphtheria deaths. The 1933 diphtheria death rate was 3.9 per 100,000 population. By 1950 the United States death rate had fallen to 0.3 per 100,000 population, and 5,796 cases, 410 of them fatal, were reported.

By then, most children born into families that could afford comprehensive pediatric or even family medical care were routinely immunized against diphtheria, tetanus, and pertussis (whooping cough) in one trivalent vaccine starting at the age of two months. Booster doses of the DTP vaccine are now given at the ages of four, six, and eighteen months. When the children are between four and six years old, they are given combined booster shots against diphtheria and tetanus. Ten years later they are given a final booster immunization of diphtheria toxoid alone. Many less affluent children receive the same immunizations at low-cost or free well-baby clinics and hospitals, but only two thirds of all infants and young children at risk in the United States are now immunized against diphtheria, tetanus, and whooping cough.

Since more than half of all children at risk were immunized against diphtheria by the mid-1950s in this country, by 1957 the United States death rate for this disease fell to below .05, and has remained there since. In 1980, for example, there were only three cases reported. In 1978, the last year for which diphtheria death data are available, there were only four deaths. Diphtheria had become what Dr. Schroeder and her peers strove to make it back in 1921—one of the diseases as rare as smallpox—but only in the United States and other affluent nations.

In the rest of the world, diphtheria remains one of the major killers and maimers of children. Few conditions suffer more from underreporting than do the endemic diseases of poor countries; this is not because their rulers are corrupt—which they often are—but because the costs of setting up and operating an effective health statistics service are far beyond the resources of those countries. In 1977, for example, India reported an annual figure of 15,127 cases of diphtheria and failed to report any deaths, although in 1973 India had reported 648 diphtheria deaths. However, in 1961, the late Professor W. Barry Wood, Jr., of Johns Hopkins observed that "at the 1960 Asian Pediatric Conference, a single Indian physician reported more than 2000 cases of diphtheria [in his own practice]. In the same year, only half this number was reported in the entire United States." Diphtheria, as the World Health Organization now recognizes, is a major world health problem.

Park lived long enough—he died at the age of seventy-six in 1939—to know that he had led most of the major efforts to create a vaccine against diphtheria, and to use it in the eradication of the disease from the United States and other industrialized nations. Like Pasteur, Park was never in any doubt about where the scientific future of most vaccine work would materialize. His friend, colleague, and official biographer, Dr. Wade Oliver, wrote in a very revealing passage:

"Even as early as 1897 Park visioned the future role of chemistry in bacteriology and immunology. And as the years passed he became more firmly convinced, from the innumerable discoveries made, that in the chemical approach lay the ultimate conquest of disease. When asked a few months before his death, "Where does the future of bacteriology lie?" he unhesitatingly answered with conviction in his voice, "In the chemistry laboratory!"[11]

Not the least of the reasons for this belief was the long and often maddening quest for a pneumonia vaccine that Park had followed, and for a time joined, since 1890.

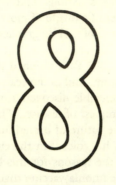

INDUSTRIAL CIVILIZATIONS' "CAPTAIN OF THE MEN OF DEATH": PNEUMONIA

That poverty was the greatest single cause of bad sanitary conditions was very early impressed upon me. If I should again go into a community such as Cuba or Panama, and were allowed to select only one sanitary measure, but were at the same time given power to select from all sanitary measures, I would select that of doubling wages.

—WILLIAM C. GORGAS, Surgeon General, 1914[1]

At the opening of this century, the three leading causes of all United States deaths were (1) pneumonia and influenza (with nearly all these deaths caused by pneumonias, not influenza), which were responsible for 11.8 percent of all reported deaths; (2) tuberculosis, the cause of 11.3 percent of all reported deaths; and (3) diarrhea and enteritis, the cause of 8.3 percent of all American deaths. The tenth leading cause, diphtheria—which killed 40 in every 100,000 Americans and was the cause of 2.3 percent of all reported mortalities—was, like the first three diseases, a primary cause of infant and child mortality. These four common bacterial diseases combined were responsible for over one third of all reported United States deaths in 1900, killing at the rate of 579 per 100,000 population per year.

Of all the killing infectious diseases of 1900, pneumonia—inflammation of the lungs—characterized by Sir William Osler as the "captain of the men of death," was, in his words, "The most common as well as the most serious acute infection of this country, with a mortality exceeding that of all other acute fevers put together, measles, scarlet fever, diphtheria, whooping-cough, typhoid fever and dysentery."

It was not unusual for pneumonia to develop in and kill affluent people in the prime of healthy life. However, observant physicians had long known that pneumonia was far more likely to strike bedridden hospital patients than healthy people going about their lives outside of hospitals. They also knew that pneumonia, like other infectious diseases, was more prone to develop in underfed families in unheated, overcrowded tenements and farmhouses, or in children warehoused in county orphanages, than in well-to-do families and children.

Even as far back as the turn of the century, astute physicians were aware that many other diseases, from common colds to cancers, could develop into precursors of severe and often fatal cases of pneumonia. Then and now bacterial pneumonia was a leading hospital-acquired disease. All of these and analogous pneumonia-associated factors led doctors to recognize that the physical condition of the human hosts of the pneumococci had as much to do with their catching and either surviving or dying of pneumonia as did the pneumonia germs themselves. These physicians, incidentally, understood the importance of host health factors in pneumonia long before it was established that encapsulated (i.e., virulent) pneumococci are found in the mouths of a majority of all perfectly healthy people.

What no doctor could foresee in 1904 was that nearly a half-century before we had antibacterial drugs to cure bacterial and mycoplasmal pneumonias, and more than a half-century before we had good vaccines against the major pneumococcal pneumonias, the successful completion of the Panama Canal would be dependent upon first conquering pneumonia in a tropical isthmus known for many years as "the White Man's Grave."

As we near the end of this century the building of the Panama Canal (begun by Ferdinand de Lesseps in 1880) still ranks as one of the greatest single accomplishments of this or any previous century of recorded human history. "The French occupants found the Isthmus a death trap and during the nine years of occupancy they lost 22,818 laborers from yellow fever," wrote an American general. "When the United States took charge of the Canal in 1904, the death rate was as high as ever and a yellow fever epidemic was actually going on."[2] Four years later, in his presidential address to the American Medical Association, Dr. William Crawford Gorgas (1854–1920) stated that by 1908 in the Panama Canal Zone, "Yellow fever was nonexistent, and the annual malaria mortality down from more than five deaths per 1000 workers [or 500 deaths per 100,000] to a rate of one death per 1000 [or 100 per 100,000]. The overall death rate for Americans residing in Panama—once considered a pestilential swamp—was now lower than in most parts of the United States."[3]

Gorgas's well-documented successes in Cuba and Panama against malaria and yellow fever easily merited all the praises and honors they won for him. Curiously, in all the kudos that came his way for the control of these two tropical diseases, little attention is paid today by doctors and laymen to Gorgas's equally historic and on the whole equally successful efforts to protect the Canal workers against what was then the leading cause of death on both the mainland and the Canal Zone: pneumococcal pneumonia.

We were taught that the dauntless army surgeon Gorgas cleaned up the swamps where the mosquitoes that carried the agents of malaria and yellow fever proliferated. Once this environmental cleanup was accomplished, said our history books, then the equally dauntless army engineer Goethals led brigades of well-sanitized healthy Americans, who climbed into the cabs of huge steam shovels, pulled the levers that started huge cement mixers, and built a record canal in record time. There is no doubt that all this actually did happen. What the books left out, however, also had a major bearing on the proud saga: the very existence of the majority of the workers whose muscles, sweat, and blood ultimately built the Canal.

It was impossible to get low-paid white workers from the mainland to fill these jobs. Some showed up, in response to offers of free fares to the

Zone. Of these pioneers, Army Lieutenant Robert E. Wood, detailed to the Isthmian Canal Commission, wrote, "The beginnings of the force recruited in 1904 . . . were largely Americans who had left the United States for this country's good—railroad men who were blacklisted on the American railroads, drunks, and what we called tropical tramps, American drifters in Latin America."[4]

They did not last very long at their Canal jobs. Like the French before them, the American Canal authorities tried to import foreign workers, but the reputation and the realities of the Zone defeated these recruiting efforts. American union leaders attacked the idea of sending large numbers of their workers to "that deathtrap," particularly, writes the fine modern historian of the Canal David McCullough, "after an inspection team from Japan, representatives of large contractors of Japanese labor, reported the Isthmus too unsafe to risk the lives of their men."[5]

What was needed were large numbers of men conditioned by evolution and experience to put in a day's work in the brutal climate of the Zone and survive to work many other days. In the perceived wisdom of the directors of the project, this meant black men. There was no shortage of blacks in the southern states of the mainland, but the importation of black workers "met with strenuous opposition from southern congressmen who foresaw their home states suddenly drained of their natural supply of cheap labor."[6]

Cheap labor, that essential ingredient of the Industrial Revolution and of the pyramids the Pharaohs had built for their tombs in earlier millenia, was also considered by the Commission's chiefs to be the essential key to the construction of the Panama Canal. Since it had to be black labor, and could not be composed of North Americans, it had to be recruited in the West Indies, where cheap labor was not only black but also English-speaking. The imported Jamaican and other West Indian blacks learned many of the construction skills. Lieutenant Wood, in his final official report to the Canal Commission, declared that "the bulk of the building work on the Canal has been done by West Indian carpenters, masons, and painters . . . and toward the end of the construction period the West Indian remained on the job as steadily as the Spaniard or even the American."[7]

Because they were black, the West Indians who did the bulk of the work on the canal were not allowed to move into the model American homes, or attend the model American schools, or eat in the hygienic model American mess halls, or become patients in the fine American hospitals when injured on the job or felled by major sickness, such as pneumonia.

During the first years of American operations in the Canal Zone, the West Indian blacks were housed "in barracks containing about 84 men each, and of such dimensions as to give them about 30 feet of floor space." William C. Gorgas, the former president of the American Medical Association (AMA) and then Surgeon General of the U.S. Army, observed, "This is ordinarily considered very crowded," since "it is a well-recognized fact in military hygiene that overcrowding of a barrack is coincident with inflammation of the upper respiratory passages, which at times becomes epidemic." Such inflammation, "in many cases due to the pneumococcus, resulted in lobar pneumonia in some persons [and] in others a certain amount of immunity. . . . If we have 85 men in a crowded barrack, and the pneumococcus gets in, the probabilities of its spreading to the other men are considerable."[8]

At the time (1906) Gorgas personally observed these conditions, most of the imported black Canal workers lived in these Jim Crow barracks. A minority of them quit the barracks and built squatters' shanties for themselves in the bush from scraps of wood, canvas, and other waste materials. The effects of these formal and informal living arrangements were only too predictable. "It is not generally known but it is true that pneumonia was far more fatal to Canal workers, especially Negroes, that either yellow fever or malaria, or even the two of them combined. In 1906, for instance, when malaria killed only 224 employees of the Canal Commission and the Panama Railroad Company, and yellow fever was not even included in the mortality tables, there were 413 deaths from pneumonia, or more than half as many as from all other causes combined, including accidents."[9]

The Canal's imported black workers, whether they lived in the steamy barracks or the squalid shantytowns, suffered most of the Zone's pneumonia morbidities and deaths. Of course, this was a half century before antibiotics, and when vaccines against pneumonia, diphtheria, and other contagions of crowding were still unrealized research goals. With one exception, none of the members of the highest echelons of the great Canal project—for whom the personal health risks of the Zone vanished with the elimination of malaria and urban yellow fever—were unduly concerned with the fact that pneumonia killed so many of their black Canal workers. Curiously, the one high authority who concerned himself with the health and welfare of the black people and their families was a man who by birth and tradition happened to be the last ranking official in the Canal Zone who could be expected to concern himself with their fate. Although born to a U.S. Army ordnance officer, William Crawford Gorgas was a child of eight when his father, a Pennsylvanian, chose to side with his southern fellow officers against his country during the Civil War.

Young Gorgas not only became a loyal son of the Confederacy, but as he grew into youth and man's estate, he never foreswore this allegiance. While fighting yellow fever in Havana, he wrote to his mother for his dead father's Confederate Cross, which he promised to wear "on the outside of my full dress coat. Because I wear the blue now does not make me any less an ardent Confederate." In the same letter he said the southern people would have been better off had the rebellion succeeded, and that "we would have been one of the world powers and would gradually have abolished slavery. . . .

As it is, the intelligence of the country has been impoverished and everything that our people can save is taxed away for the benefit of the Northern states."[10]

Despite the victory of the Blue over the Gray during the Civil War, Gorgas had grown up with the dream of attending West Point, like his father Josiah, and becoming a professional U.S. Army officer. President Ulysses S. Grant, however, declined to approve an appointment to West Point for the son of a fellow officer who had deserted to the enemy. The only way William Gorgas could get into the army was as a doctor. Accordingly, in 1876 he entered New York City's Bellevue Hospital Medical College, from which his future army colleague Walter Reed had graduated six years earlier. At Bellevue, where Gorgas took the cram course offered by Professor William H. Welch, he was known best for his Christian faith and his amiability. After completing his medical studies and a year of internship at Bellevue Hospital, Gorgas was accepted by the army, and in June 1880 he entered the U.S. Army's Medical Department as a $133-a-month lieutenant.

For the incurably romantic young doctor, who saw military service as a selfless means of doing good in this world, army service during the closing decades of the nineteenth century—except for meeting, falling in love with, catching yellow fever from, and in 1884 marrying his colonel's sister-in-law, Marie Doughty—was a far cry from his youthful dreams of chivalry. The years 1880–1900 were decades in which the chief task of the U.S. Army was to complete the job begun by the Spanish conquistadors in the opening years of the sixteenth century—to drive the Native Americans off the face of this land and to kill as many as possible in the process. From time to time this essentially genocidal task of killing Indians was varied by the equally unchivalrous task of breaking railroad and other major labor strikes.

The Surgeon General of the army, George Miller Sternberg (1838–1915), who like Gorgas was a man with an acquired immunity to yellow fever, was quite intrigued to have under him an immune army doctor whose wife was also immune to the mosquito-borne plague. Wherever there was an outbreak of yellow fever, there Lieutenant Gorgas was assigned. Through all these experiences and notwithstanding the fact that he had been ushered into this world by Dr. Josiah Nott, an early proponent of mosquito-vectored yellow fever and malaria, Gorgas remained unconvinced that mosquitoes transmitted these diseases.[11] Like Florence Nightingale and the English sanitary reformers, Gorgas held it was not mosquitoes but filth that carried yellow fever, and he remained steadfast in this belief in 1898, when he was placed in charge of the army's yellow fever camp at Siboney, outside of Havana, during the Spanish-American War.

One of Gorgas's patients at Siboney was Major Victor C. Vaughan, a doctor who in 1881, as dean of the medical school of the University of Michigan, had brought Dr. Henry Sewall to Ann Arbor as professor of physiology.

"It was largely through Dr. Gorgas' skill in the management of yellow fever that the death rate in our army was so low," Vaughan was to write later. "His kindly words to his patients served as a better tonic than any name in the pharmacopoeia."

Vaughan did not describe what subsequently happened at Siboney, but one of Gorgas's biographers, John M. Gibson, writes of how, at Gorgas's urging, the commanding officer decided to do what the people of Philadelphia, Memphis, Tennessee, and hundreds of other American sites of yellow fever outbreaks had done: "Fight yellow fever with the lighted torch. The little military community ... made a lively bonfire. After it had burned itself out, it was hopefully believed that the flames had destroyed the germs of yellow fever as effectively as they had consumed the blankets, wooden beds, clothing, and other hospital paraphernalia which had burned so briskly that day. Gorgas was soon to learn that they had not."

What ensued, after Gorgas was appointed sanitary officer of Havana in 1898, is now common knowledge. In the spirit of Florence Nightingale, but with the resources of the U.S. Army of Occupation and the limitless manpower of its sanitary corps, Gorgas quickly turned the war-ravished city of Havana into one of the cleanest cities on earth. Dead animals in the streets, garbage piles, backyard accumulations of trash, swamps, any containers bearing stagnant waters, food stores, public markets, private businesses, and even private homes were cleaned up by Gorgas's men or ordered cleaned up by his medical officers. All contagious diseases were affected by this hurricane of sanitation—from smallpox, which was still endemic in North and South America, to pneumonia, typhoid, dysenteric disorders, streptococcal infections, and other major causes of death. In one year, thanks largely to the cleanup of the filth in which contagions proliferate, the Havana death rate fell from 9,130 to 3,667 per 100,000 population. The same cleanup was also the linchpin of the Reed-Gorgas war on mosquitoes which wiped out malaria and urban yellow fever in Havana and in most of Cuba.

In 1906 when Gorgas became aware of the ravages of pneumonia in the Canal Zone, he completely accepted the role of the pneumococci in the causation of the disease. In the absence of a drug to control and kill these pneumonia germs, or a good vaccine to immunize the Canal workers against them, Gorgas was also in no doubt about what had to be done to control pneumonia. One of the first things was to find out why black people suffered the most cases of pneumonia; during the first eight months of 1906, for example, all but fifteen of the 390 Canal workers who died of pneumonia were black.

Havana had given Gorgas an obvious clue to this condition. The single group in the Canal Zone least free of the types of filth Gorgas had eradicated in Havana were the blacks who made up the bulk of the Canal's work force. Even President Theodore Roosevelt, who had visited the Zone earlier in the year, was shocked by what he had seen, and in a letter to one of his aides, the President observed that of all the things he found there, "the least satisfactory feature ... was the arrangement for feeding the negroes. Those cooking sheds with their muddy floors and with the unclean pot which each man had in which he cooked everything, are not certainly what they should be." Roosevelt was particularly bothered by "the very large sick rates among the negroes, compared to the whites," as well as by the housing in which he had seen the crowded and unsanitary environment in which the blacks had to live.

Gorgas saw all this, and more. As a doctor, he not only saw that crowding hardworking men into steaming and ill-ventilated barracks guaranteed rapid and multiple transmissions of the pneumonia organisms and impaired inborn immune or host defenses against the pneumococci, but he also saw quite clearly the only clinically intelligent alternative. "If," he wrote, "the pneumococcus establishes itself in a man living in a hut alone, or with his family, it is not apt to spread to the men with whom he works, and with whom the contact is not intimate."

As a southerner who had experienced at first hand the tax burdens and poverty that the victors of all wars impose on the losers, let alone as a former Bellevue intern, Gorgas understood better than most doctors the causal relationships of family income to family health. He knew that the wages paid to most of the black workers were much too low to allow them to afford decent food, clean linens, and—if houses in the Canal Zone towns were available to nonwhites—anything resembling adequate housing. The wages were too low even to enable the blacks to afford more than the clothes they wore on their backs, so that they had no dry clothing to change into at the end of a day of working rain or shine in the tropical heat.

There was little Gorgas could do about either the climate or about raising the wages paid the black workers. He did, however, have the power to convince the Canal authorities to set aside cultivable plots in the unused government land in the hills, where the workers could build clean cabins, raise garden vegetables and fruits, and to which they could bring their families from their native Caribbean islands. The blacks were also given the right to rent or even buy houses in the new government-built towns, which had potable piped water and sanitary sewage disposal systems.

At about the time the blacks started to move out of the barracks, the Canal Commission, Gorgas later noted, "found that in order to attract labor, and keep it on the Zone, they had to increase and, within a very few months, double the wages of the manual laborer ... It does not take more than a moment of thought to show you how such a measure acts and reacts. Results take place in many directions, but particularly with regard to increasing the ability of the people to live well and get better food and clothing."[12]

To physicians, as well as to laymen concerned with the prevention of infectious diseases, the results of Gorgas's planned efforts to control pneumonia—and of the equally meaningful efforts of the Canal Commission to hang on to its black workers by more than doubling their wages—were most impressive. How great a change this double boon of decent housing and doubled family incomes proved to be was summarized by Gorgas in the *Journal of the American Medical Association* of June 13, 1914. "In 1906, our work force was an average of 21,000 negroes and 12,500 white men. Among these negroes, we had 396 deaths from pneumonia, a rate of 18.74 per 1,000 [or 187.40 per 100,000] per annum." During the same year, on the United States mainland the total pneumonia death rate for people of all races stood at 14.1 per 1,000 or 146.10 per 100,000 resident population.

In 1907, one year after housing, wages, and family life started to improve for the black Canal workers, Gorgas wrote that "we had an average of 28,600 negroes and 10,700 white men. Among these negroes we had 304 deaths from pneumonia," a rate of 10.61 per 1,000, or 106.1 deaths per 100,000—while on the mainland, pneumonia was killing at the significantly higher rate of 129.70 per 100,000 Americans of all races.

By August 1913 the total Panama Canal Zone work force consisted of 46,000 blacks and 12,500 whites. At that time, mainland deaths from pneumonia were reported at 130.7 per 100,000 population. However, increased wages and healthier living conditions had helped lower the black pneumonia death rate on the Zone to a low 0.42 per 1,000, or 4.2 per 100,000 population. This was still higher than the white pneumonia death rate on the Zone, but it did represent a reduction of 97.76 percent in only seven years "in the face of an increase of more than 100% in the number of prospective [black] pneumonia victims."

In short, Gorgas's efforts—social and clinical—had resulted in an 18.82 percent decrease in the pneumonia death rate of black Canal workers between 1906 and 1907—while during the same period on the mainland, the total pneumonia death rate for all Americans fell from 146.10 per 100,000 population to 129.70, a decline of 11.23 percent. Between 1906 and 1913 the decline in the pneumonia death rate of black workers in the Canal Zone was far greater than that of the total pneumonia death rate on the mainland. In the Zone during these seven years, the pneumonia death rate among the black Canal workers was slashed by 97.76 percent: from 187.40 per 100,000 in 1906 to 4.2 per 100,000, or 0.42 per 1,000, in 1913. The United States mainland death rate for pneumonia in people of all races fell from 146.10 per 100,000 population in 1906 to 130.70, or 13.07 per 1,000, in 1913, a drop of 10.54 percent. It was a historic lesson in the comparative public health values of improved individual and family living conditions—that is, of making human life fit for human beings—that Dr. William C. Gorgas was never to forget, or dishonor.

* * *

If Gorgas's victory over pneumonia never made the headlines the daily press gave his successes against yellow fever and malaria, the Canal Zone statistics were not lost upon certain people who had the most to lose to the ravages of pneumonia. While the makers of public health policies on the mainland seemed uninterested in Gorgas's expert advice on how to control this largely urban and industrial infection, people like Samuel Evans, chairman of the Crown Mines Company in Johannesburg, South Africa, paid very close heed.

This company mined gold. In the South African gold and diamond fields, as in the mines and mills of Europe and America during the first century of the Industrial Revolution, the most coveted of all resources was an abundant supply of cheap labor. In the South African gold mines, as in the Panama Canal Zone, both geography and demography demanded that the vitally needed cheap labor be black men.

The South African gold mining industry and the Panama Canal Zone had one other thing in common: endemic pneumonia, which decimated low-paid, barrack-housed blacks. In 1904, the year that Gorgas arrived in the Zone to make it a safe place to work, a South African doctor, F. W. Waldron, wrote that "pneumonia in endemic form with epidemic outbreaks is certainly one of the scourges of the mining compounds in this country. . . . The mortality of the disease is so high that humanitarian reasons on behalf of the native, and economic reasons on behalf of the employer of labour call for active measures."[13]

In 1910 Evans read an article by William Osler in which the Oxford professor of medicine described in some detail how Gorgas was making great inroads against pneumonia in black Canal workers.[14] This caused Evans to seek out Gorgas's own reports on Panama and to note their pneumonia statistics carefully. As a businessman, Evans understood health problems in terms of net productivity: A black miner sick and/or dead of pneumonia digs up very little gold, or worse—none at all.

Samuel Evans was not the only South African gold-mine owner to grasp the causal relationships between miners' health and profits, miners' diseases and losses. Between 1893 and 1899, the number of native Africans recruited from villages in the bush to work in the gold mines and live in the mine compound barracks increased from 25,049 to 111,697.[15] J. P. Cartwright, in a book published in South Africa in 1973, notes that "the system by which these men were brought to the mines was a somewhat rough-and-ready one, and it is perhaps best not to inquire too closely into the methods employed by the recruiters who delivered the first 'kaffirs' at so much per head."

In a recent paper on the history of pneumococcal vaccines in South Africa, Robert Austrian notes that many newly "recruited" blacks arrived suffering from malnutrition, and if they survived "the arduous journey from their kraals to the mine compounds, they worked for periods of six to nine months before returning to their homes." This resulted in a constant turnover of the mining force and the continuous introduction of new individuals susceptible to pneumonia into the mine compounds.

These conditions were roundly and frequently denounced, and "from press, platform, and pulpit had come ringing denunciations of this form of human exploitation and demands, in humanity's name, that it end," wrote Gibson. "A strike of Rand gold miners, who emphasized the prevailing health conditions among their grievances and insisted that something be done to reduce the appalling death and morbidity rates, threw the pneumonia situation into dramatic focus and fanned the flames of popular resentment."

The South African mineowners went on recruiting cheap native backcountry labor as before, but as "mounting deaths from pneumonia sent the general death rate [of gold miners] up to 350 per 1000—more than one out of three—the British government took official cognizance of the situation by announcing that the recruiting of these laborers would have to end unless they could be assured better health protection. The Bureau of Native Affairs went even further. It actually prohibited the employment in the mines of workers from tropical Africa, who had proved particularly easy prey to the disease [pneumonia]."[16]

All these developments made the owners of gold and diamond mines in South Africa very interested in the control and eradication of pneumonia in their workers. In February 1911 the chairman of the Central Mining and Investment Corporation of London, Sir Julius Wernher, sought out the pathologist and medical bacteriologist Almroth Wright, the codiscoverer of opsonic antibodies and developer of the partially effective typhoid vaccine. At the moment Wright was studying the problems of curing and preventing pneumonia. He wanted to test a new drug, optochin, recently developed by Professor Julius Morgenroth in Berlin. This drug killed pneumococci in mice, and Wright was anxious to test it in people with pneumonia. He also was anxious to test killed-bacteria vaccines in both the treatment and prevention of pneumonia.

Wright agreed, for a stipend of two thousand rands a month paid by the Witwatersrand Native Labour Association, to go to South Africa for six months with a small group of collaborators. Shortly after he got there and started testing optochin in native Africans, Morgenroth informed him that the drug was as toxic to human optic nerves as it was to pneumococci in mice, and had caused amblyopia—partial loss of vision—in a number of European volunteers. This put an end to the Wright field study of the "pharmaco-therapy of pneumococcus infections."[17]

The tests of the heat-killed pneumococcal vaccine in the cure and prevention of pneumonia were not quite total failures, but they came very close and certainly offered no immediate solution to the mineowners' public relations problems with endemic pneumonia in the mine compounds. As of now, there are eighty-three known types of pneumococci that cause pneumonia in man. As of September 1911, when Almroth Wright made up his vaccine from pneumococci isolated from black miners with pneumonia, only three types of virulent pneumococci had been identified. What was known about them was that they comprised two general groups, one with a slimy capsule surrounding its smooth outer walls, the other was an unencapsulated type with rough walls. Only the encapsulated strains or types caused pneumonia, while the rough types were harmless.

In making his vaccine, Wright made no distinction between the different capsular types he found; if the bacteria he isolated in patients had capsules, they went into the cultures from which he made his vaccine. The vaccine, which contained one or more capsular types, failed as a cure, and on October 14, 1911, Wright began a series of trials of the vaccine as a preventive agent against pneumonia in 50,000 people. The trials were completed in 1912, and Wright, in a two-part report in *Lancet*, pronounced them to be a resounding success in the reduction of pneumonia attacks and deaths. He recommended that the vaccine be "applied as a routine measure to every native on recruitment."[18] (In the first part of his report on his studies in South Africa, Wright also declared that the then available "staphylococcus and streptococcus vaccines are effective in acute localised staphylococcic and streptococcic infections," a verdict that, like these two vaccines, did not survive the test of time.)[19]

Prior to Wright's report, Dr. G. D. Maynard, statistician of the South African Institute of Medical Research, analyzed the outcomes of the vaccine trials and, Austrian tells us, "concluded that the attack rate of pneumonia was lessened in the first four months following inoculation but that vaccination had no significant effect on the case fatality rate. The conclusions are not surprising when one considers that the number of pneumococcal types in the vaccine was unknown and may have been quite limited and that the doses of vaccine employed were, in the light of later knowledge, marginal at best."[20]

Even before the Maynard analysis was published, Samuel Evans visited the Panama Canal Zone to seek Gorgas's advice and, if possible, to talk him into making his own investigation on the Rand. Weary of his years of fighting the good fight for sanitary reform with the Zone's top military and civilian brass, and tempted by the chance of repeating in darkest Africa his Caribbean triumphs, Gorgas accepted the invitation of the South African Chamber of Mines. On December 3, 1913, Colonel Gorgas and his staff arrived in Johannesburg "to make investigations into the cause of the high death-rate from pneumonia among the native laborers working in the mines of the Rand."

En route to South Africa, Gorgas had stopped off in London to consult with Almroth Wright and to review the clinical outcomes of the vaccine trials. What he found in the way of housing and sanitation in the mine compounds was pretty much the same he had found earlier in the Canal Zone. In his report to the mineowners, Gorgas spent almost as much space describing how improvements in housing and the resumption of family life had reduced the incidence of pneumonia in the Zone as he did in his analyses of the conditions he found on the Rand and his recommendations that they repeat his Canal Zone reforms. He also suggested that some of the barracks then used to house the miners under crowded conditions be converted into regional hospitals once the miners were moved into individual huts.

Gorgas's opinion of the pneumonia vaccine was not as negative as Maynard's, nor was his reading of the clinical results as discouraging. "I recommend that the question of immunization for pneumonia as recommended by Sir Almroth Wright be more carefully looked into," he wrote. "So far the evidence on the subject is more or less contradictory. As tried on the Rand the inoculated do not show any greater protection than the controls, but as used at the Premier Mine in 1913, the results seem very striking. In 1912, the 17,000 inoculated had a death-rate from pneumonia of 6.89 per thousand, and the 6,700 [uninoculated] controls a death-rate of 17.72 per thousand. . . . I can see no reasonable explanation for the marked difference between the pneumonia death-rate of the inoculated and that of the controls, except that the inoculation gave a large degree of protection to the inoculated."[21]

Gorgas's associate, Dr. Samuel T. Darling, probably hit on the reason for the success of the vaccine at the Premier Mine: "The vaccine used at the Premier may be from the [pneumococcal] organisms of a different strain from those used on the Rand."

Before he could pursue his studies of the Wright vaccine any further, Gorgas learned from the local press that in February 1914, President Wilson had appointed him to succeed the recently deceased Surgeon General of the U.S. Army. The daily newspapers and the medical publications of the United States applauded this appointment. The *Journal of the American Medical Association* spoke for everyone when it declared that "probably not since the days of the Civil War has it been possible to make an appointment that will cause so much general satisfaction." Gorgas sailed for Washington and a hero's welcome from an admiring nation.

On September 28, 1914, Surgeon General Gorgas and Harvard civil engineer Professor Lewis J. Johnson delivered addresses on public sanitation and taxes at a dinner at the Business Men's Club in Cincinnati, Ohio. During his years in the Canal Zone, Gorgas had, as a born victim of unfair and discriminatory tax policies, become attracted to the single-tax movement. This movement promised to solve, by more equitable taxes based solely on the real value of land, the problems of poverty for the poor, of trade union pressures for employers, and of public sanitation and well-being for the entire population.

In his talk, "Economic Causes of Disease," Gorgas declared that "sanitation is most needed by the class of people who would be most benefitted by the single tax." Then he quickly moved from theory to experience, his own experience. "That poverty was the greatest single cause of bad sanitary conditions was very early impressed upon me. If I should again go into a community such as Cuba or Panama, and were allowed to select only one sanitary measure, but were at the same time given power to choose from all sanitary measures, I would select that of doubling wages. This in my case is not altogether theory."[22] And he proceeded to spell out how doubling wages in the Canal Zone brought public health benefits.

Had anyone in the same high position, but of lesser national and world esteem, made the same statement at the same dinner, he would not have lasted out the week in his job. Gorgas was much too popular to fire, but from that moment on President Wilson counted the days before he could safely rid his administration of this courtly prophet of dangerous truths.

Although the synergistic combination of Gorgas's efforts to end overcrowding and unsanitary living conditions in the Zone, plus the Canal Commission's doubling of black Canal workers' wages, had in only seven years reduced by 97.76 percent their pneumonia death rate, when it was all over and he had to write his recommendations to the mineowners of the Rand gold fields, Gorgas urged the continuation and expansion of all research that might result in a practical vaccine against pneumococcal pneumonia. He knew that it would never be as easy to end overcrowded living conditions for the working poor of urban centers like New York, Philadelphia, and Chicago as in the subtropical Canal Zone. He had lived through four New York winters as a medical student and Bellevue Hospital intern, and he knew by firsthand clinical observation how easy it was for inadequately dressed people living in overcrowded and unheated tenements to catch and die of pneumonia once winter came. Like William Park, who knew that more social and sanitary reforms—much as they helped reduce diphtheria cases and deaths—would in the end not be enough to eradicate diphtheria, Gorgas looked to vaccines to ultimately eradicate the major infectious diseases.

When the Rockefeller Institute for Medical Research was established in New York City in 1901, there were still no cures or vaccines for pneumococcal or any other form of pneumonia. Many species of microbial pathogens can, like the viruses and the pneumococci, cause pneumonia. They include such common bacteria as beta-hemolytic streptococci, staphylococci, *Haemophilus influenzae* (which also causes meningitis in infants but does not cause influenza), *Escherichia coli, Legionella, Klebsiella,* anthrax, *Pseudomonas aeruginosa,* and *Pasteurella pestis,* better known as the agent of the bubonic, pneumonic, and septicemic plagues. Pneumonia is also caused by *Mycoplasma,* bacteria-like organisms without the rigid cell walls that surround bacteria, which are close evolutionary relatives of the much larger bacteria; by fungi;

and even by nonbiological chemicals, anesthetics, and heavy oils that get into the lungs and cause inflammations.

While most cases of pneumonia diagnosed and treated by doctors are caused by bacteria, Robert Austrian reminds us that "more than three-quarters of all human pneumonias are caused by viruses. Most viral pneumonias are never seen by doctors, or even get to a hospital. It is only when routine X-rays of all people with respiratory infections are done in hospitals and clinics that you find out that most of the pneumonias revealed by the X-rays were caused by viruses. Only about one-quarter of all pneumonias seen by hospital doctors are bacterial pneumonias, with most of them acquired outside of the hospitals. Nor are all bacterial pneumonias predominantly pneumococcal."

However, 80 percent to 90 percent of all medically diagnosed cases of bacterial pneumonia are caused by the lancet-shaped pneumococci originally found and described in 1881 by Pasteur in France and by George Sternberg in the United States. Pasteur found the organism in the saliva of a child who had died of rabies, but lost interest in the pneumococcus when it failed to cause rabies in animals. Sternberg found it after inoculating his own saliva into a rabbit and growing it in a broth made of rabbit flesh, but he was unable to cause any diseases in rabbits with this bacterium. He did, however, correctly classify it as a streptococcus.

Three years later in Berlin Dr. Albert Fraenkel isolated an encapsulated type of the same bacteria from the lung of a thirty-year-old man who had died of pneumonia. Fraenkel injected these encapsulated organisms into a healthy rabbit, which promptly sickened and died of a pneumonia-like disease. Subsequent laboratory and clinical work, notably by Professor Anton Weichselbaum of Vienna (who would in 1886 discover the meningococcus), soon established the encapsulated lancet-shaped bacteria as the agents of many of the pneumonias that killed vast numbers of people.

Weichselbaum proposed the name *Diplococcus pneumoniae* for this entire species, and the name survived in the United States until very recently, when it was changed to *Streptococcus pneumoniae,* as it had been known in England for generations. This put the pneumococci, at least taxonomically, into the same bacterial family as the hemolytic streptococci that cause streptococcal strep throat infections, and tonsillitis, erysipelas, and meningitis of the newborn; and whose late consequences include poststreptococcal nephritis, rheumatic fever and rheumatic heart disease, and Sydenham's chorea (St. Vitus' dance), a complication of rheumatic fever. Although *S. pneumoniae* is known primarily for its role in the etiology of bacterial pneumonia, present-day doctors also know it as a significant cause of nonmeningococcal bacterial meningitis, and as the causal agent of more than half of the middle-ear infections (otitis media) that strike between 76 percent and 95 percent of all children in the United States at least once before they are six years old.

After the work of Fraenkel and Weichselbaum, most doctors believed that protective vaccines made of either attenuated or killed whole pneumococci would be developed imminently, and that these whole-organism vaccines would swiftly make pneumonia as rare as Jenner's vaccine had made smallpox in late nineteenth-century Western Europe and America. Many such vaccines, including the killed-organism variety Wright had tested in over 50,000 black African gold miners on the Rand, were indeed developed and tried, with results that were at best equivocal—as on the Rand—and at worst, utter failures.

By the end of the nineteenth century, when work done by Sewall in America, Behring and Kitasato in Berlin, and Park in New York made possible the immunizing of animals against diphtheria, and the extensive use of antitoxins from the sera of these animals in both the cure of many diphtheria cases and the temporary passive immunization of the families and other close contacts of diphtheria patients, many serious research workers started to try to make analogs of the diphtheria antisera against other deadly bacteria. At a time when bacterial infections, beginning with the major killer pneumonia and including tuberculosis, diarrhea and infectious enteritis, poststreptococcal nephritis, and diphtheria, constituted five of the ten leading causes of death in America, it was quite logical that vast efforts would be made to develop antisera against the pneumococci, the tubercle bacilli, the meningococci, the gonococci, enteric bacteria, including *Salmonella, Shigella,* and *E. coli,* and other disease germs.

The antisera that were developed during the first few years of these efforts were, despite many premature success stories in the scientific journals and the lay press, almost total failures. At times, some of these experimental antisera seemed to work very well, only to fail utterly the next time they were used in other patients. In 1909 Franz Neufeld and Ludwig Handel, at the Robert Koch Institute for Infectious Diseases in Berlin, discovered one of the major reasons for the occasionally successful but always unpredictable results of some of the experimental immune sera against pneumococci.

Neufeld found that the morphologically identical (and encapsulated) strains of pneumococci consisted of at least two, and most probably more than three, antigenically or chemically specific strains or types. They showed that antisera against one type of pneumococcus could not protect mice against infections caused by pneumococci of either of the other two specific types.[23]

This suggested that—particularly as the isolations of other antigenically distinct types of pneumococci multiplied—the concept of effective serotherapy against the polytypic species of pneumococci would prove to be illusory. At the new Rockefeller Institute, where in 1909 Drs. Alphonse R. Dochez and L. J. Gillespie started to work on the serological or antigenic typing of different strains of pneumococci isolated from patients at the Rockefeller Hospital, their findings soon provided good evidence for believing that serotherapy would undoubtedly be very effective in the cure of many cases of human pneumonia.

Dochez and Gillespie found that roughly 80 percent of all cases of human lobar pneumonia diagnosed in New York were caused by pneumococci that corresponded, roughly, to Neufeld's Types I and II, and of the newly isolated Type III. They also found a fourth, heterogeneous group of pneumococci that comprised various subtypes with different characteristics, but which all failed to react to antisera against the first three types. They called this strain Group (or Type) IV, but some European bacteriologists termed it the American Scrap Heap.[24]

Within the three types of bacteria, antisera to which protected mice against 80 percent of all pneumococci isolated from New York patients, immune sera against Type I pneumococci protected mice against 45 percent of the isolations, while antisera against Types II and III organisms protected mice against 20 percent and 14 percent of all isolations, respectively. In short, these three "typical" strains were now practical targets for all doctors concerned with pneumonia. Further work showed that while it was now possible to use antibodies in the blood serum globulins of animals previously immunized with graduated doses of Type I pneumococci to cure people with pneumonia caused by this capsular type, various problems had to be resolved before safe and effective antisera against Types II and III could be produced.

However, since Type I pneumococci caused nearly half of all medically treated pneumonia cases, Dr. Rufus Cole, director of the Rockefeller Hospital, decided to go ahead with the development and production of antisera against this strain. There were no commercially produced antisera available, so the Rockefeller Institute, like the Pasteur Institute with the diphtheria antitoxins a generation earlier, set up clean stables, purchased horses, and prepared to produce Type I antisera in these animals. Eventually, as the technique of producing immune sera against other types were improved, and as other of the now eighty-three known types of pneumococci were identified, the Institute started to produce pneumococcal antisera in horses (and later in rabbits) against other of the most common strains of the pneumonia germs.

Years later, on the eve of the debut of the sulfa drugs and the antibiotics, Dr. Cole was able to report that in 1936–1937 immune sera were used in more than fifty patients "suffering with lobar pneumonia due to pneumococcus Types I, II, V, VI, VII, XIV, XVIII there has been but one death and this occurred in a patient five weeks convalescent from pneumonia. In untreated patients with similar [pneumococcal] type distribution, the death rate would have amounted to about 34 percent"; that is, seventeen of this group of fifty pneumonia patients would have died.

Because commercially produced antisera against the Type I pneumococcus and various other common strains of pneumococci were widely available after World War I, it became routine practice in military and civilian hospitals to culture the bacterial organisms isolated in all pneumonia patients, and to type the pneumococci that were recovered from these hospital-admission cultures. This routine typing made the serologic treatment of certain cases of pneumococcal pneumonia very practical.

The antisera were not risk-free. From time to time, pneumonia patients inoculated with immune globulins derived from the blood serum of hyperimmunized animals got serum sickness—a form of severe allergic reactions to the proteins foreign to people in the blood of the animals from which the antisera were taken. The first bout of serum sickness was generally painful but nonfatal. However, once a person had serum sickness, he or she could rarely if ever again be treated with antisera from this particular animal species, since severe and even fatal anaphylactic shock could accompany a second bout of this allergic disorder.

When the Rockefeller Institute started producing pneumococcal antisera in 1913, Oswald T. Avery, a thirty-six-year-old graduate of the Columbia University College of Physicians and Surgeons (P and S) in the class of 1904, was hired by Rufus Cole to be responsible for the inoculation of the horses with Type I pneumococci, the processing of the immune globulins in their blood serum, and the "measurement of its antipneumococcal activity. He was also made responsible for much of the diagnostic work, and developed a rapid culture method for determining the pneumococcal types recovered from the patients" at the Rockefeller Hospital.[25] His official title was Bacteriologist, and his salary was $2,000 per year, no vast sum for a physician who had graduated from P and S nine years earlier, but he was a bachelor of modest and ascetic habits who often forgot to eat and consumed very little when he did.

Oswald Avery had come by his modest life-style by being born into the genteel poverty of a Baptist preacher's manse in 1887 in Halifax, Nova Scotia, shortly after his parents, Joseph and Elizabeth Avery, had emigrated from England. When Avery was ten, his father accepted a call to a Baptist mission church, the Mariners' Temple, on Henry Street in the heart of New York's teeming Lower East Side. Born or converted Baptists were few and far between in the fetid, overcrowded tenements, where with grim impartiality tuberculosis, pneumonia, rheumatic fever, diphtheria, measles, typhoid, and other contagions of poverty decimated the families of the immigrant Irish and the Eastern European Jews.

The Reverend Avery edited a church paper, *Buds and Blossoms,* and, with the aid of modest sums from more affluent local Baptists, like John D. Rockefeller, strove to convert the neighborhood Jews, Irish, and unchurched transients to Baptism. In his spare time, the pastor, himself the son of an inventive English papermaker, found time to invent and patent a new medicine, Avery's Auraline, which he described as a remedy for "the relief and cure of deafness, earaches, and noises in the head." Nothing came of it commercially.

A German cornetist hired to provide music when the church's organ broke down taught young Oswald and his older brother, Ernest, to play the cornet. For some time, the Avery boys blew their horns on the steps of the Mariners' Temple every Sunday to attract passersby. Eventually, they won scholarships at a local music conservatory. Oswald Avery played cornet in the Colgate University band, and on at least one occasion he played in a symphony orchestra conducted by Walter Damrosch.

The Reverend Joseph Avery died in 1892 of Bright's disease, shortly after his firstborn, Ernest, died of an apparent lung disease. His widow, Elisabeth, was given a job by the Baptist City Mission Society, which kept her and her surviving son alive in their accustomed modest circumstances. Sometimes Avery spent summer vacations at "great estates" owned by some of New York's wealthiest families, but by then nothing could change Oswald's abstemious ways. He had learned not to expect or need very much of life's material wealth, which were traits sorely needed by the sons of poor men who went into medical research as a full-time career.

About three years after Avery joined a group general medical practice in New York, he recalled, "Sir Almroth Wright came to New York from England and gave a lecture at the [New York] Academy of Medicine on his newly invented opsonic technic. The New York City Health Department was interested in this and arranged to have a colleague of Sir Almroth give a short course of instruction to a small group. I was one of those to take this course. At its completion, Dr. William [H.] Park gave me a job doing opsonic indices [measurements of the rates at which opsonic antibodies are taken up by bacteria to make them subject to engulfment and destruction by phagocytes, or white blood cells] for the Board of Health at a stipend of $50 per month for part-time work. I also found part-time employment doing milk bacteriology for the Sheffield Company. Pasteurization of milk was just coming in; I made bacterial counts of milk before and after pasteurization at a stipend that was also $50 per month."

This was the beginning of the end of Avery's career as a private medical practitioner. In 1907 Dr. Benjamin White, a physiological chemist who had taken his doctorate at Yale and pursued postdoctoral studies in Germany, Austria, and England, and whom Avery knew socially, was appointed director of the Hoagland Laboratory, a privately endowed medical bacteriology institution opened in 1888, the year the Pasteur Institute was built. White, who was not a physician, "mentioned to me that he needed a young doctor to be his assistant director. I responded enthusiastically and so I was invited over to the Hoagland Laboratory," at a starting salary of $1,200. Avery was to remain with that pioneer American bacteriological research laboratory until 1913, when Rufus Cole brought him to the Rockefeller Institute to supervise the production and testing of Type I pneumococcal antisera.

The Hoagland Laboratory, situated in a Syrian neighborhood in Brooklyn, owed its inception to a diphtheria infection which in 1884 killed the grandson of Cornelius N. Hoagland, founder and head of the giant Royal Baking Powder Company. Hoagland had practiced medicine for over a dozen years until the baking powder business made him rich. Although he was sixty-six years old when diphtheria took his grandchild, Hoagland went back to the practice of medicine. Three years later, he incorporated and endowed the laboratory for "the promotion of medical science and the instruction of students in special branches thereof."

The Hoagland Laboratory opened its doors in 1888, the same year that Drs. Émile Roux and Alexandre Yersin at the Pasteur Institute isolated the toxin of the diphtheria bacillus and, using Sewall's method, inoculated it into healthy animals to hyperimmunize them against diphtheria. The main speaker at the dedication of the Hoagland Laboratory was the Johns Hopkins professor of physiology H. Newell Martin, under whom Sewall had taken his doctorate eight years earlier. Cornelius Hoagland was among those who hailed the birth of antitoxin therapy in 1892–1893, which cured at least half of all diphtheria cases. He died in 1898 at the age of eighty, only fifteen years before William H. Park developed and started mass trials of the first of the safe and effective toxoid vaccines that would eradicate diphtheria in the United States by mid-twentieth century.

Because of the profound interest the Hoagland family had in diphtheria antitoxins, Avery spent his summer vacation in 1911 at the bacteriological laboratories of a large manufacturer of antisera and vaccines, the H. K. Mulford Company. He was there primarily to train the staff in the latest bacteriological techniques, but he also learned a great deal about the problems of large-scale commercial production of antisera. This knowledge was to stand Avery in good stead when he went to the Rockefeller Institute three years later.

Very early it became clear that there were smooth-walled and rough-walled subtypes of pneumococci, with the smooth pneumococci being surrounded by a slimy capsule. By 1915 when Victor C. Vaughan wrote his book *Infection and Immunity*, published by the American Medical Association as a contribution to the Panama Pacific Exposition, the consensus of advanced medical opinion was that while the capsule probably had something to do with virulence, little was known about either the composition or the precise pathological function of the pneumococcal capsule. "The formation of the capsule is dependent on conditions. Highly virulent organisms taken from the animal are capsulated. On the other hand, subcultures grown on artificial media through many generations have no capsules or show imperfect ones. Growth in blood serum seems to favor capsular development. It seems most probable," Vaughan concluded, "that the formation of the capsules is a protective function."

He was absolutely right; more than a half-century later, it became apparent that the capsule protected the pneumococci against leukocytes, the white blood cells that take up and consume, or phagocytize, bacteria and other microbial pathogens. In 1915, however, it was not even known what the capsules were made of, let alone what they contributed to pneumococcal infection.

Earlier, in 1897, A. G. Auld, a pathologist working in the joint laboratories of the Royal Colleges of Physicians and Surgeons in London, had made an interesting but unexplained discovery in germ-free filtrates of pneumococci cultures isolated from patients with pneumonia. When inoculated into healthy rabbits these nutrient broths, from which all living and dead pneumococcal and other bacteria had been filtered, these filtrates caused various disturbances, Auld reported, including a rise in temperature to 106.2°F, pleurisy, shortness of breath, and a pneumonia-like symptom in which "the entire lower lobe of the right lung was completely consolidated."[26] The rabbits survived, and other researchers started to examine germ-free filtrates of broth cultures of pneumococci and other bacteria.

In 1917 Dochez and Avery, working with hospital-isolated pneumococci, found what was probably the same substance Auld had isolated twenty years earlier. They determined that this soluble, germ-free material, which they named the specific soluble substance (SSS), was an integral chemical of live pneumococci. They also showed that when the cultures of pneumococci isolated from patients had high levels of this SSS, the prognosis for a patient's recovery was poor—while low levels of SSS indicated that the patient would probably recover. The relationship between virulence and these pneumococcal chemicals and infection was now fairly evident.[27]

The problem then became to determine the nature of these chemicals, and a few months later Avery and Dochez completed some studies that convinced them that the SSS "is of a protein nature or is associated with protein."[28] Before they could verify or disprove this conclusion—it happened to be incorrect—the First World War, and the associated Spanish influenza pandemic, made more pressing demands on their time. It would be a half dozen years before Avery could get back to his investigation of the chemical nature of the SSS of encapsulated pneumococci.

To do this right, Avery knew that he needed a chemist with more skills in chemical determinations than either he or Dochez possessed between them. There was just such a bright young chemist already at the Rockefeller Hospital, the thirty-four-year-old organic chemist Michael Heidelberger, then working under the biochemist Donald Van Slyke. From time to time, Avery would seek him out in Van Slyke's laboratory, wave a small vial of a brownish powder in front of his eyes, and say, "When can you work on this, Michael? The whole secret of bacterial specificity is in this vial." The brownish powder was SSS.

In 1923 Heidelberger was transferred from Van Slyke's section "to the pneumonia group, although 'Van' generously let me continue to use the same laboratory. Thus began my career," he wrote more than fifty years later, "as a microbiologist."[29] Thus also began something Heidelberger at ninety was still too modest to mention: the birth of immunochemistry, the core science of all the vaccine work that was to follow the world over.

Like Avery, Heidelberger also played a wind instrument—in his case it was the clarinet—and had also grown up in New York City. However, Avery was the son of a Baptist missionary who had come to the great city to convert the Jews—while Heidelberger had been born "on East 127th Street in New York City," the grandchild of "Jewish Germans who emigrated between 1840 and 1850, apparently because of the greater opportunities in the United States." Avery had not decided to study medicine until he was almost ready to graduate from Colgate University. Heidelberger recalled that "because I was known as an obstinate child, and, having made up my mind at the age of eight that I wanted to be a chemist, though without knowing why, I stuck to it and became one." Avery earned his doctorate in medicine at Columbia in 1904; Heidelberger got his doctorate in organic chemistry at Columbia in 1911. The organic chemist was destined to revolutionize the immunological sciences; Avery, at the age of sixty-seven, would make the twentieth century's single most important discovery in all the biological sciences, including immunology.

Heidelberger, in two autobiographical essays written when he was ninety and still at work daily in his laboratory at the New York University School of Medicine, painted a portrait of a New York quite different from the metropolis Avery recalled of his childhood, and of second- and third-generation Jewish people who lived far differently than had the immigrant generation the Reverend Avery hoped to convert. "I know little of my father's parents, except that his father, Michael, died in Silver City, Idaho. David, my father, was born in Philadelphia and left school early to earn a living. He became a partner in a firm that made carriage robes, but with the advent of automobiles he went 'on the road' almost six months of the year selling lace curtains for another manufacturer."[30] He remained a traveling salesman selling, Heidelberger remembered, "anything you could think of," and on his earnings raised a family that included a Norfolk-born wife, Fanny, who had been sent to live with relatives in Nuremberg for a year after she graduated from finishing school, and three children. "As a consequence of her year abroad," Michael and his younger brother, Charles "were required to speak German at the table and were accompanied to Central Park two afternoons a week by a governess who would tolerate nothing but French. We hated both burdens, and it was only years later, when these languages became essential, that I realized what a head start I had had."

Like many other children of the same cultural background, "Charles and I wandered in safety all over Central Park . . . we also gravitated often to the Metropolitan Museum of Art and the Museum of Natural History. All of these excursions were possible because my mother taught us all the primary school subjects in an hour or two each day, leaving the remainder for reading (I read *David Copperfield* and was taken to opera and concerts when I was eight years old), wanderings such as those above, and playing in the street with other children just out of school."

Like many New York families of all backgrounds, the Averys and the Heidelbergers paid the penalties of having children before there were antibiotics to cure (and some vaccines to prevent) fatal infectious diseases. Oswald's older brother, Ernest, with whom he played the cornet on the steps of the Mariners' Temple on Sundays, died in 1892 of what appears to have been tuberculosis. In 1913 Heidelberger's younger brother, Charles, developed postrheumatic heart disease bacterial endocarditis—inflammation of the lining membrane of the heart. Early in his illness, Dr. Park's research laboratory at the municipal health department had "immunized a horse with the strain of *Streptococcus viridans* isolated from Charles' blood," and antisera from this hyperimmunized horse had been inoculated into the sick brother. "This first contact with immunology was not encouraging, for large injections of the horse's serum failed to help," and Charles died of this common end result of rheumatic heart disease.

When after taking his doctorate in organic chemistry young Heidelberger wanted to do a year of postgraduate work in Europe, his parents were willing to "stake me to this, and I was selfish enough to accept what I knew was a sacrifice. But first they wished me to seek advice from old Dr. Samuel Meltzer, who had listened with his massive head against my chest as our family physician throughout my boyhood and had then become the distinguished head of Physiology at the Rockefeller Institute for Medical Research. He tried, wisely, I think, to discourage me, saying a scientific career was nothing for a poor man's son, but he gave it up and turned me over to the [Rockefeller Institute] chemists, who would know the best person under whose direction to work. Thus I had the luck to meet P. A. Levene, Walter A. Jacobs, and D. D. Van Slyke at tea that same afternoon."

Heidelberger's postdoctoral year under Richard Willstatter in Zurich was a period of intensive work and learning, but it was not entirely without its diversions. He played clarinet in the student orchestra, and the leading daily newspaper duly reviewed his performance in the Mozart Quintet for Clarinet and Strings. In the fall of 1912, Heidelberger became a Fellow of the Rockefeller Institute at a salary of $1,200 a year. "The position was to assist Dr. W. A. Jacobs in synthesizing drugs for the cure of poliomyelitis, as part of the study of the disease by Dr. [Simon] Flexner," the director of the Institute.

The quest to find or synthesize an antipolio drug failed, and, with Flexner's encouragement, both Jacobs and Heidelberger "turned to African sleeping sickness, or trypanosomiasis, which was making whole regions of that continent uninhabitable." The trypanosomes of African sleeping sickness are protozoa, parasites transmitted from animals to other animals, including people, by bloodsucking tsetse flies. Paul Ehrlich's quest for an anti-African sleeping-sickness drug had in the end yielded a drug that killed the protozoa but was far too toxic for people. (However, the same study also found Ehrlich's drug number 606, Salvarsan, to be the first effective albeit very toxic drug against syphilis.) Guided by Ehrlich's mistakes, Jacobs and Heidelberger developed a far less poisonous arsenical drug, which Flexner named tryparsamide, which was field-tested in the Belgian Congo after World War I and was to be the mainstay of sleeping-sickness treatment for decades. Jacobs and Heidelberger won Belgian decorations and monetary awards for its development.

After the First World War, "Dr. Flexner, an ardent believer in chemotherapy, insisted that we tackle bacterial infections, notably pneumococcal and streptococcal diseases," wrote Heidelberger in 1977. "Lloyd D. Felton joined us for testing in animals, and we started to synthesize active bactericides.... However, the combination of 'drug and bug' usually killed the test mice more quickly than the drug alone. One of the intermediates that we converted into such useless substances was para-aminophenyl sulphonamide, or sulfanilamide, which the Tréfouels, Nitti and Bovet found to be the [medically] active portion of the purple dye for which Domagk received the Nobel Prize in 1939. That so simple a substance could cure bacterial infections by a mechanism other than the drug killing of the microorganisms never occurred to us. If it had, we might have saved hundreds of thousands of lives in the 20 years before Domagk, the Tréfouels, Nitti and Bovet made their discoveries. I always told this story in lecturing on chemotherapy in the course on biochemistry at the College of Physicians and Surgeons of Columbia University and begged the students never to allow themselves to become slaves of an idea."[31]

Unlike the antibiotics, which are bactericidal drugs that act to kill or cause the destruction of bacterial organisms, the sulfas are bacteriostatic drugs that cure bacterial infectious diseases by inhibiting the growth and proliferation of living pathogenic bacteria. The sulfonamides act by preventing bacteria from synthesizing folic acid, one of the vitamins (and metabolites) essential to bacterial metabolism. For this reason, the sulfa drugs are classified as antimetabolites. The sulfas do not kill the disease-causing bacteria present in a person's body at the time the drugs are administered, but they do slow the growth and reproduction of such bacteria to levels that render them harmless to the laboratory animals in which new drugs are first tested, and in people.

When Heidelberger approached the new task of determining the chemistry of the SSS of the pneumococci, he did not allow himself to become a slave to Avery's idea that the specific soluble substances of these pneumonia-causing bacteria were proteins. He showed that they were, rather, carbohydrates, in the form of the polysaccharides that make up the capsules of pathogenic pneumococci and other bacteria. Although only proteins were believed to be antigens, Heidelberger suspected that these capsular polysaccharides might have some antigenic capacities. However, as he and Avery reported in 1923, their "attempts to stimulate antibody production by the immunization of animals with the purified substance yielded negative results."[32] Nevertheless, they continued to work on the further purification of the SSS, using larger amounts of starting material, in the hope of learning more about the capsular polysaccharides.

Their distinguished Rockefeller Institute colleague, Dr. Karl Landsteiner, suggested that the SSS was what he termed a hapten, which he defined as an incomplete antigenic molecule incapable of causing antibody production except when coupled with a completely antigenic protein. Heidelberger, however, continued to work on the further purification of the polysaccharide molecule.

He was by then a married man with a three-year-old son, Charles. Flexner had been urging him to improve his economic condition by seeking a job in a better-paying institution, but Heidelberger had found his life's work, and he knew it. For the next six decades he would concentrate on studying the relationships between chemical structure and immunological specificity, mainly with bacterial polysaccharides. Avery and other colleagues made experimental artificial antigens by coupling the bacterial polysaccharides to specific proteins, but Avery by that time had also become fascinated by the work of the British bacteriologist Fred F. Griffith. Griffith had succeeded in transforming noninfective and nonencapsulated pneumococci into capsulated and fully virulent or infective organisms.

In 1927 Heidelberger left the Institute to accept a better-paying job as chemist of the Mt. Sinai Hospital in New York. Avery was by that time devoting more and more attention to the work in which "Griffith found that mice injected subcutaneously with a small amount of a living R [Rough] culture derived from Pneumococcus Type II together with a large inoculum of heat-killed Type III (S or Smooth) cells frequently succumbed to infection, and that the heart's blood of these animals yielded Type III pneumococci in pure culture." To Avery this was a biological mystery that demanded solution, because "the fact that the R strain was avirulent and incapable by itself of causing fatal bacteremia and the additional fact that the heated suspension of Type III cells contained no viable organisms brought convincing evidence that the R forms growing under these conditions had newly acquired the capsular structure and biological specificity of Type III pneumococci."

Eventually, when Avery did solve the riddle of what caused what became known as the Griffith transformation effect in pneumonia bacteria, this would be the least of the questions his discovery would answer in bacteriology, genetics, immunology, transplantation surgery, drug sensitivity and resistance, virology, evolution, mutation, and the chemical nature of the individual variations that simultaneously make each member of the human race unique and different from any other person and yet brother or sister to all people.

In 1923 when Heidelberger and Avery published their first report on the SSS of the pneumococci, one of the many people who read it was a twenty-two-year-old, third-year medical student in Berlin, Wolfgang Casper, the son of a Berlin dermatologist and the grandson and great-grandson of other German physicians. Young Casper, like young Heidelberger, enjoyed the benefits of ambient music, art, and literature from the time he started to speak. He had a passion for taking apart complicated things like toy trains, clocks, old microscopes, and music boxes and then reassembling them. "They didn't all have the same number of parts in them when I was finished," he remembered years later when he was living and practicing medicine in Staten Island, New York. "But by God they still ran."

Like Heidelberger who knew at the age of eight what he wanted to be, when he was a child Casper knew he wanted to be a doctor, even though as a physician he never lost his zeal for experimentation. "But first of all I was a clinician who treated patients."

In 1926, during his first year out of medical school, Casper went to work as an intern in the dermatology and venereology department of the three-thousand-bed Rudolf Virchow Hospital in Berlin. His chief was one of the world's most noted dermatologists, Dr. Abraham Buschke, who had studied under Albert Neisser at Breslau from 1895 to 1897, "where he developed his interest in bacteriological research in infectious diseases.[33] Neisser, who discovered the agent of gonorrhea, the gonococcus (now called *Neisseria gonorrhoeae*), was a dermatologist in an era when, as for many succeeding generations, venereal diseases were treated by dermatologists. When the Rudolf Virchow Hospital, then the largest hospital in the world, was opened in 1906, Buschke was made director of the dermatology department with the title of Professor.

With Buschke's permission, Casper also went to work as an after-hours unpaid volunteer assistant to the microbiologist in the Robert Koch Institute for Infectious Diseases, Oscar Schiemann. Schiemann was working with the SSS, repeating the work Heidelberger and Avery had published, and trying further to purify the materials. At that time, because as Heidelberger put it, "all immunologically active substances were supposed to be proteins," and because of Karl Landsteiner's huge and well-earned prestige, it seemed most prudent to conceive of the pneumococcal SSS, the carbohydrates of which the capsules of pneumococci are made, as haptens that had to be coupled to proteins to produce antibodies in mammals, birds, and other creatures.

As part of his investigation, Schiemann was working up tables of the minimum lethal doses of specific pneumococci in mice—that is, the smallest amount of a specific strain of a specific type of encapsulated pneumococci that will kill an average-sized mouse. At the same time, Schiemann, who was a very methodical and thorough investigator, conducted parallel studies of the possible toxicity or lack of toxicity of the pneumococcal capsular polysaccharides. This he did by injecting measured and gradually increasing doses of purified pneumococcal capsular polysaccharides into the bodies of healthy mice.

In the summer of 1927, Schiemann decided to go on vacation. He asked Casper to inoculate a last test batch of healthy mice with specific different doses of a very powerful strain, and to time and record the results, "and then finish up. Put gas in the glasses, kill the control mice, and close up the lab until I get back." With that, he was off to the train. What followed during that Berlin summer was still fresh in Casper's mind half a century later.

"I took a very virulent culture of pneumococci, with which I knew from experience that I could kill any mice in from 30 minutes to an hour. But just before I inoculated the experimental mice, I had an idea. Instead of the mice Schiemann had selected, I injected the pneumonia germs into mice we had previously injected in toxicity tests with our purified capsular carbohydrates, taken from the same strain of pneumococci.

"And then I waited for them to get pneumonia and die. And waited. And waited. I began to think that possibly I'd made a mistake, used the wrong culture. No. It was the right culture. Only the results were wrong. The germs were not bothering the SSS-inoculated mice.

"The mice were in a cage on the lab table. I pulled up a chair and sat there and watched them for signs and symptoms of anything. Nothing was going on. They did not die in one hour. Or two hours. Or four hours. I fell asleep with my head on that table. Remember, I had 600 beds in my service, and whatever I did at the Koch institute was moonlighting.

"I woke up the next morning with my head still on the table. I had a stiff neck. I looked up and the mice were still alive—and hungry. Then I got angry. But before I threw the whole batch of culture out as a mistake I dug up the tiny amount of purified pneumococcal polysaccharides we had left. I made up a much greater dilution than I'd used the day before. I now divided another batch of mice into two groups. In the first group I injected the pneumococcal polysaccharide dilution. In the other, my control population, I injected plain saline water. After an hour went by, I inoculated both batches of mice with the virulent pneumonia bacteria. The same results. Inside of a few hours, the control mice previously injected only with the saline were all dead of pneumonia. But the mice protected by the capsular polysaccharides of the pneumococci were still alive.

"I was tired. I fed all the mice and went home to get a few hours sleep. I think I slept around the clock.

"When I went back to the Koch, the mice inoculated first with the pneumococcal carbohydrates and then later with the virulent pneumococci were still alive. I sat down and sent off a four-word telegram to Schiemann. It read: 'The mice didn't die.' Schiemann understood immediately what had happened. He knew me better that I thought he did. He cut short his vacation and rushed back to Berlin. Together, we re-did the experiment, again and again and again, with three different types of pneumococci. Each time, and with each type of pneumococcus, the mice previously injected with dilutions of the pneumococcal polysaccharides lived after inoculations of each type of pneumococcus that killed the unprotected control mice."

In 1927 Casper and Schiemann published their account of this work under the title of "Are the Specific Soluble Substances of the Three Types of Pneumococci Haptens?" in the German *Journal of Hygiene Infectious Diseases*. Their answer was—no, the polysaccharides of the pneumococci are complete antigens in themselves.

So perished the dogma that only proteins could be antigens—and so began the era of vaccines made from purified capsular polysaccharides of bacteria.

From Avery at the Rockefeller Institute in New York came an invitation for Casper to join the Rockefeller Hospital's pneumonia group, which was looking for a reliable pneumonia vaccine. Casper wanted to accept the offer to go to New York. Buschke was horrified. *"Dumkopf!"* he said, not in anger but in horror at Casper's naïve unworldliness. "Don't you read the newspapers? Don't you know what's going on in America? Al Capone! Gangsters in the streets! They'll shoot you down the first time you try to take a walk in New York."

Buschke believed every word of this, and he got Casper's father, an old friend, to help him talk his son out of needlessly risking his life. Young Casper listened to reason. He had always loved Berlin, and now that he had pointed the way to a pneumonia vaccine, he would be able to concentrate on another prophylactic problem that the Puritan conscience of America might inhibit if he did move to New York. He went to work on a gonorrhea vaccine made along the same principles.

The further development of pneumococcal capsular polysaccharide vaccines—from the vaccine with which Casper protected mice against single strains of pneumococci to capsular polysaccharide vaccines which in one shot protected people against over a dozen disparate types of pneumococci—now followed in slavish accordance with Mirsky's law.

As defined by the late Rockefeller University biochemist Professor Alfred E. Mirsky, this law holds that while we would never have had the music of Beethoven, the paintings of Rembrandt, and the plays of Shakespeare had these three men never lived, we would still have had, and at roughly the same times, cell theory, germ theory, the theory of natural selection and evolution, and immunology if Schleiden and Schwann, Pasteur and Koch, Darwin and Wallace, and Metchnikoff and Ehrlich had never been born. Art is unique and individual, the personal work and legacy of its creators. Science is a cumulative and, in the end, an impersonal process. Scientific developments follow new scientific discoveries, and each discovery raises questions and leads to inquiries that, in turn, lead to new scientific developments which result in new scientific discoveries.

Thus, the 1923 discussion by Avery and Heidelberger in New York of the probable immunological significance that "the capsular material of many microorganisms consists, at least in part, of carbohydrates" led inevitably to young Casper's impulsive use of these bacterial capsular sugars as pneumococcal antigens in mice in Berlin in 1927. Once he and Schiemann published their results, it was inevitable that regardless of what they did at the Koch Institute themselves, various other researchers in different countries would try to duplicate their work in humans.

At the Rockefeller Institute in 1929 and 1930, Drs. Thomas Francis, Jr., and William S. Tillet demonstrated that purified pneumococcal capsular polysaccharides when injected into human volunteers could produce in their blood antibodies against the specific capsular type of pneumococcus from which the polysaccharides were derived.

Even earlier than this, at Harvard, Dr. Lloyd D. Felton repeated Casper's work from the beginning. After he duplicated this mouse-protective pneumococcal capsular polysaccharide vaccine, he then made one up of a much larger dose. This he tried on himself, and then on volunteers in his laboratory. The first doses were four times as high as they had to be, and left Felton and his colleagues with painfully swollen arms. In properly small doses, these dilutions caused human volunteers to produce antibodies, and their blood sera had enough of the antibodies to protect mice inoculated with these sera against pneumococci of the same capsular types.

In 1929 Felton started to inject nontoxic dilutions of polysaccharides from the same strains of pneumococci that caused a small group of patients to have repeated bouts of pneumonia. None of the patients got pneumonia again for over a decade. When the Great Depression started in the fall of 1929, it terminated the dollar support of many promising lines of clinical research. As unemployment soared to record-breaking levels, jobless veterans of World War I, older Americans who lost their own businesses and shops, youths who came into their teens after the crash of 1929 and never had a job, farm families forced to abandon their farms, and other people now suddenly without income built squatter settlements along the waterfronts of New York and other great cities (called Hoovervilles after the Depression-era President) or slept in abandoned factories and barns. In 1933 one of the first emergency measures of the new Roosevelt administration was to take over unused military camps and tents and set up the Civilian Conservation Corps (CCC) under the direction of the U.S. Army. The CCC proposed to provide food, shelter, and much needed medical care to two groups of Depression victims: the homeless and unemployed veterans of World War I, who were men in their early thirties to late forties, and unemployed young people of seventeen or over. The CCC camps were set up in unused army bases all over the nation, and the CCC men went to work at much needed outdoor jobs related to such conservation measures as planting trees to combat or prevent soil erosion, clearing swamps, and reforestation.

Felton went to the army personnel in charge of the CCC with a simple idea: Because during the First World War bacterial pneumonia had killed over 20,000 American soldiers, he proposed that the army help him run mass trials of a polyvalent pneumococcal polysaccharide which, if it worked, would protect the CCC men against Type I or Type II pneumonia, and would do no harm if it failed, since the capsular polysaccharides, which were not whole bacterial organisms, were unable to cause any disease.

The army accepted the offer, and the laboratories of the National Institute of Health, then headed by Felton, turned out the new vaccines. Between 1933 and 1937, it was tested in five trials in the CCC camps. Over 32,000 men were inoculated in CCC camps in New England and in California. The New England CCC camps' case-incidence rate for Types I and II pneumonia was 4.34 per 1,000 years of life in the inoculated group, as against 7.28 for the uninoculated control group. The West Coast rates were 1.73 for the inoculated CCC men, as against 15.69 cases per 1,000 years of life for the control population. By 1940 a total of 120,000 CCC men received this capsular polysaccharide vaccine.[34]

The results seemed promising. So much so that by the time the trials were concluded, E. R. Squibb and Sons, Inc., started to go into the capsular polysaccharide vaccine business. By then Michael Heidelberger had been at the Columbia University College of Physicians and Surgeons (P and S) as a professor of biological chemistry for five years. These were important years, during which he proved that antibodies were globular proteins (immunoglobulins), and clarified the differences between various types of blood complement, and continued his lifelong studies on the chemical composition of the surface structures of encapsulated microbial pathogens. During the same years, he was also chemist for the medical service at Presbyterian Hospital.

When World War II began, Heidelberger and his old colleague Avery were both made consultants in infectious diseases to the Secretary of War. "Because of a continuing large series of pneumococcal pneumonias during several years at a training camp for aviators at Sioux Falls, South Dakota, it became advisable," Heidelberger wrote later, "to find out whether or not human subjects could be protected by immunization with purified capsular polysaccharides of the causative types. Felton had attempted this during the Great Depression by immunizing many thousands in camps of the Civilian Conservation Corps. His massive experiment was ill-fated, however, because healthful, outdoor living conditions led to almost no pneumonia in any of the camps, unimmunized or immunized," and there was really no way of measuring the actual immunological results of the massive trials of Felton's bivalent vaccines. Heidelberger presumed that the results had been good, but this was not scientific proof of a vaccine's efficacy.

He asked for volunteers from the entering 1942 and 1943 classes at Columbia P and S to be injected with the capsular polysaccharides of pneumococcal Types I, II, and V. In these inoculated students, the antibodies to these pneumococci appeared quickly and continued to be produced at effective levels for years. Further tests led Heidelberger to recommend to the Surgeon General that the personnel at the CCC training camp in Sioux Falls be vaccinated against pneumococcal pneumonia. It was decided to make a vaccine from polysaccharides of pneumococcal Types I, II, V, and VII, as the resident microbiologist at the military installation "had found these types in about 60% of the pneumonias."

The actual production of the polyvalent vaccines was never a problem, since by then Squibb had built a plant to turn out such vaccines for civilian use once the war ended, and they agreed to supply the vaccines needed. In 1944 "the camp's population was randomly marshalled into two lines of 8,500 each. Those in one line were injected with 1 cc of saline as control subjects. Those in the other line were given 1 cc containing 50–70 micrograms each of the polysaccharides. . . . Within two weeks there were no more pneumonias caused by the four types among those vaccinated. Even the nonvaccinated were partially protected because, as the microbiologists found, the vaccinated personnel no longer carried these pneumococci in their noses and throats. Pneumonias due to pneumococcal types not in the vaccine remained equal in both groups, which showed the strict specificity of the protection. The entire study, so beautifully organized and monitored in the field under [Dr.] Colin MacLeod's direction, showed that epidemics of pneumococcal pneumonia in closed populations could be terminated within two weeks after vaccination with the polysaccharides of the causative types."[35]

It was a brilliant climax to what Heidelberger and Avery had started in Avery's laboratory in 1923. Avery himself was not in on this particular development because, with the collaboration of Colin MacLeod and Maclyn McCarty, Avery had finally identified and defined the chemical nature of the substance that induced transformation of pneumococcal types first described by Fred F. Griffith in England. In 1944 they revealed the name of the transforming chemical—it was "a nucleic acid of the desoxyribose (DNA) type," which they described as the fundamental unit of the transforming principle.[36] In a private letter sent a year earlier to his younger brother, Roy, Avery had suggested that this DNA might be capable of inducing predictable and hereditary changes in cells, and that these changes would be permanent. "Sounds like a virus—may be a gene," Oswald Avery told his brother.

Some scientists understood at once the significance of this transforming function of DNA. Publication of the Avery, MacLeod, and McCarty paper was, the Columbia P and S biochemist Erwin Chargaff wrote, the "really decisive influence, as far as I was concerned, to devote our laboratory almost completely to the chemistry of the nucleic acids."

It took a little longer for other scientists to realize, with the help of workers like MacLeod, Chargaff, and others, that the nucleic acids were the critical constituents of the genes. By the time Avery died quietly of cancer at the age of seventy-eight in 1955, not enough of his peers understood this to assure him of a Nobel Prize for medicine or physiology or chemistry. The full recognition of what he had accomplished was yet to come.

The triumph of the pneumococcal polysaccharide vaccine that his earlier work on pneumonia bacteria had helped make possible was aborted by the postwar flood of sulfas and antibiotic drugs. This was not entirely unexpected. After 1938 when the first of the sulfa drugs were introduced, they helped reduce the death rates from all types of pneumococcal pneumonias. When sulfapyridine, for example, was used, it cut the normal death rate for pneumococcal pneumonias from 25 percent of all cases to around 12 percent, a far better record than the more expensive antisera, and the adverse side effects of the new sulfa drugs were not as severe as those from serum sickness.

Between 1900, when pneumonias were the leading cause of all deaths and killed 175 out of every 100,000 Americans yearly, and 1929, when the Great Crash turned life into a shambles for the nation, pneumonia deaths had been reduced to 91 per 100,000 population. In 1937 American pneumonia deaths stood at 85 per 100,000. In 1938, the first year in which the sulfas were available, pneumonia deaths were already reduced to 68 per 100,000. In 1945, the first year in which penicillin was available to civilians, pneumonia deaths were reduced to 44 per 100,000. By 1950 they were down to 27 per 100,000 and by 1960 they stood at 32.9.

Suddenly America's doctors had something they had never had before—two groups of drugs that actually cured people of bacterial and mycoplasmal pneumonia. In the immediate postwar years, Squibb could not even give away the adult and pediatric six-antigen polysaccharide vaccines against pneumococcal pneumonias. Doctors require only two qualities of any vaccine: It has to be safe, and it has to be effective. Pharmaceutical companies look for the same qualities and one additional one in a vaccine or any other medical product: It has to be marketable at a profit.

The two perfectly good vaccines were taken off the market as soon as it was clear to Squibb that no market could be made for them. Henry James Parish, M.D., F.R.C.P.E., D.P.H., former clinical research director of the Wellcome Research Laboratories in England, spoke for the vast majority of his pharmaceutical industry and his medical peers in 1965 when he wrote in his authoritative *A History of Immunization,* "Controlled clinical trials with any [pneumococcal] vaccines are now unnecessary: drugs have proved much more effective in medical practice and have replaced vaccines entirely."

By then, the death knell had already sounded for pneumococcal and all other bacterial vaccine research.

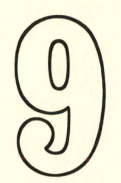

"... VIRUS, A CREATURE OF REASON"

The quantity of filtered sap necessary to inoculate a tobacco plant is extremely small ... The sap expressed from a diseased portion or portions permits one to inoculate an undetermined number of healthy plants and to transmit the disease to them. This shows that the virus, even though liquid, propagates itself in the living host.

—MARTINUS WILLEM BEIJERINCK, 1898

The smallest known bacterium is Pfeiffer's influenza bacillus which is 0.5 to 1.0 microns long. Were the hypothetical agent of foot-and-mouth disease 1/10 or even 1/5 this size, it would be beyond the resolving power of our microscopes, even with the best immersion systems. This simple consideration would explain our failure to demonstrate the agent in the lymph under the microscope.

—FRIEDRICH LOEFFLER and PAUL FROSCH, 1898

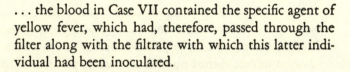

... the blood in Case VII contained the specific agent of yellow fever, which had, therefore, passed through the filter along with the filtrate with which this latter individual had been inoculated.

—WALTER REED and JAMES CARROLL, 1901

Five hens were inoculated with the clear filtrate. Two hens developed leukemia. These experiments indicate that cell-free filtrates can produce leukemia. The transplantation of cells is not involved. It is likely that the disease is caused by an organized virus.

—WILHELM ELLERMAN and OLUF BANG, 1908[1]

The successes of antibiotics against bacterial pneumonias in the immediate postwar years were matched and even exceeded when new and aptly named "wonder drugs" significantly reduced the killing and maiming results of a wide array of other hitherto untreatable and incurable bacterial infections.

Consider, for example, some of the ravages and deaths caused by only one family of bacteria, the streptococci of many pathogenic types, before and after common antibacterial drugs were developed.

During the preantibacterial drug era, every county and municipal hospital had its erysipelas wards, whose patients were in the main, aging derelicts dying in agony of what could well have been a biblical plague. A then common streptococcal skin disease, erysipelas, tortured as it killed. It was marked by raging fevers, spreading inflammations, and complications including post-streptococcal nephritis and pneumococcal pneumonia. Erysipelas, thanks to penicillin, is rarely seen today in this country.

Post-streptococcal nephritis, a once common product of streptococcal throat and skin infections, has been nearly eradicated since the bacteria that cause the infections which often result in this kidney inflammation proved to be so exquisitely sensitive to penicillin, the first and least expensive of the antibiotic drugs.

Tonsillitis, an inflammation of a tonsil subsequent to infection, usually caused by streptococci, was and is for all of the twentieth century the major stated cause of tonsillectomies. The tonsils removed by these operations are part of the inborn host defense (i.e., immune) system against all bacterial, viral, and other microbial disease agents in all people. Medical prudence has long dictated that tonsils should be left intact unless they become so irreversibly swollen (by repeated infections) that they threaten life.

For many years, starting before World War I, internists, laryngologists, immunologists, and pediatricians warned parents against insisting upon needless tonsillectomies. When medically required, a tonsillectomy can be a life-extending, even a life-saving operation. But by the 1920s so many parents ignored medical advice and demanded that the operation be performed on toddlers with perfectly healthy tonsils in order to prevent such end effects of strep throats as chronic nephritis, rheumatic valvular heart disease, bacterial endocarditis, rheumatic fever, and such side effects as Sydenham's chorea (St. Vitus' dance), that for many decades tonsillectomies became the most performed major operation in the United States. Not even a massive and well-publicized study between World Wars I and II, conducted over a period of more than twenty years by a highly regarded professor of pediatrics, Albert D. Kaiser, in nearly 5,000 children in Rochester, New York, and which showed that in only about 20 percent of these children were there ever any medical grounds for tonsillectomies, had any effect on family demands for the routine removal of preschool children's tonsils.[2]

Then, in 1960 Dr. Charles H. Rammelkamp, Jr., published the results of the six-year study he and a team of civilian and military doctors had conducted in close to 7,000 airmen at a training base in Wyoming. The Rammelkamp group showed that "tonsillectomy did not reduce the rate of infection by Group A streptococci" in tonsillectomized airmen; that rheumatic fever was more likely to hit tonsillectomized people than it did individuals with intact tonsils; and, most important of all, that "therapy with one of the antibiotics eliminated the suppurative [pus-forming] complications [of streptococcal infections] in the presence or absence of tonsils."[3]

Now physicians began to take the matter more seriously, and to explain firmly the facts of life to parents who demanded tonsillectomies for which there were no medical indications. It took a little time to sink in, and in 1965, tonsillectomy and/or adenoidectomy still ranked first in the six most common major surgical operations performed annually in the United States. A staggering total of 1,215,000 T and As were performed in 1965—but in 1977, a dozen years later, T and A no longer ranked first but third, down nearly 50 percent to a still considerable total of 617,000.

By then, the value of antibiotics had been well established, huge numbers of children had been spared preventable mastoid and needless tonsillar surgery, and millions of people who might otherwise have been killed by streptococcal, staphylococcal, enterobacterial, clostridial, and other bacterial lung, gut, organ, and septicemic infections were alive and functioning because of the growing arrays of antibacterial drugs. The postwar vital statistics made this amply clear. Nevertheless, when a national Centers for Disease Control (CDC) study headed by Dr. John V. Bennett took a look in 1976 at what was written on the year's death certificates, they learned that "infections and their sequelae accounted for 123,000 deaths annually in the United States, and were the fourth commonest cause of death."[4]

For various reasons, starting with postmortem studies that suggest that upward of one third of death-certificate diagnoses would be contradicted by autopsies performed by qualified pathologists, these vital statistics can seldom be taken at face value. Additionally, doctors at the CDC and other health agencies have long known that the numbers of notifiable infectious diseases actually reported by doctors to local health departments, as required by law in most states, represent only 10 percent to 20 percent of the actual totals.

There was still no doubt that the antibiotics could cure just about every known bacterial disease, nor that 86 percent of the infections that caused 311,000 deaths annually were caused by bacteria susceptible to antibacterial drugs. This meant only two things. The first, not enough antibiotics were used on enough bacterial infections, most of which could be cured by proper dosages of the right antibacterial drugs early enough in the infection. The second—and for a long while ignored—clinical lesson was that while the sulfas and the antibiotics could generally cure, they could rarely prevent primary bacterial infections.

Of the remaining 14 percent of all fatal infections suffered by Americans, most were caused by viruses. Since viruses are not living organisms, and have no metabolism, they could not be inhibited by sulfa drugs that prevented them from synthesizing the folic acid vitamin, the metabolite so essential to all metabolisms, or killed by antibiotics that stopped them from developing cell walls or fatally disrupted their metabolisms. There were no drugs that worked against the common cold, viral pneumonia, poliomyelitis, measles, mumps, and hepatitis; nor did they protect against such serious causes of acquired, albeit congenital, mental retardation and much more devastating birth defects as the fetal rubella virus and cytomegalovirus. For these *in utero* viral diseases, as for smallpox, rabies, and yellow fever, the best way to cure them was to prevent them from ever happening, as Jenner in 1798, and Pasteur in 1885, and Max Theiler in 1936 had demonstrated could be done by vaccines.

As a logical result, after the treatment values of the antibacterial drugs brought all research on bacterial vaccines to a long halt, whatever work was done on infectious-disease vaccines between 1946 and about 1960, was done almost exclusively with viruses.

In 1796 when Edward Jenner developed the first safe and effective vaccine against a virus disease, neither the germ theory nor its lexicon existed to explain its ability to protect (immunize) people against smallpox. All that was understood of the virus—which in Jenner's day meant simply what it meant in Latin, a poison—of smallpox was that it was in some inexplicable way neutralized, or rendered harmless, by something in Jenner's cowpox vaccine.

For generations after the death of Jenner in 1823, little was known about what he and his medical peers termed the virus of smallpox. Nobody knew whether it was a liquid like other poisons, a solid, one of Leeuwenhoek's microscopic "animalcules," or a toxic vapor. Doctors did not have to see the virus of cowpox in order to use it to neutralize the virus of smallpox, nor did they have to know whether it was animal, mineral, or the essence of nut-brown ale. The nature of viruses themselves were not, for the first half of the nineteenth century, considered a fruitful or even a proper study of medicine.

On the eve of germ theory, the father of experimental medicine, Claude Bernard (1813–1878), in an essay on the quite visible skin mite, *Acarus*, discussed the still vague microscopic disease-germ hypothesis and postulated on the existence of "... a virus, a creature of reason." When his contemporary Casimir Joseph Davaine, at about the same time isolated the anthrax bacilli, he initially called them viruses. Later he named them bacteria, from the Greek word for short rods, *bacter*, and ultimately settled for the name bacteridia.

As the term bacteria was gradually accepted by Cohn, Pasteur, Koch, and the other founders of germ theory and bacteriology—although Pasteur later was most partial to the term microorganisms—the first bacteriologists (or microbiologists) started to develop filters with pores fine enough to hold back the germs or bacteria of disease and fermentation in blood, urine, lymph, and other fluids from milk to drinking water. The diameters of the different filter pores enabled them to make fairly reasonable measurements of the actual sizes of microbes visible only under the microscope.

When germ theory slowly became a fact of scientific life, most if not all of the early microbiologists were certain that the "virus" of smallpox was merely a very tiny bacterium that in due time people would learn to culture in proper nutrient media and to isolate under the light microscope. Some early researchers believed that the viruses of variola (smallpox) and vaccinia (cowpox) were actually one and the same thing, a belief still held by a few today.

In 1872 Ferdinand Cohn found and described two species of micrococci that he was certain were the viruses of variola and vaccinia. One year later, Robert Koch isolated from vaccine lymph several strains of the same micrococci in the form of tetrads, and gave them the name of tetracoccus vaccine. Koch remained steadfast in his certainty that these micrococci, and only these bacteria, were the causal agents of smallpox. Several years later, when the director of a smallpox vaccination clinic in Berlin isolated some different species of bacteria from vaccine lymph and termed them the true germs of smallpox, Koch casually injected the newly found "smallpox germs" into himself to prove otherwise. Koch, however, was also bacteriologist enough to endorse Muller's earlier (1868) suggestion that glycerin be added to all vaccine lymph to inhibit bacterial growth.

Dr. John Brown Buist of Edinburgh isolated three varieties of micrococci from vaccine lymph in 1886 and characterized each as vaccinia. Buist also isolated from other lymph different bacteria he described as the agents of true smallpox, or variola, and published drawings of both "variola" and "vaccinia" germs in his book *Vaccinia and variola: a study of their life history.*

Buist's British contemporary, the pathologist S. Monckton Copeman, now best remembered as the head of the English official commission that made glycerinated lymph the standard vaccine in England, found some very suspicious "minute bacilli" in vaccine lymph. He had great difficulty in growing or culturing them until he hit upon the idea of seeding hens' eggs with these bacilli through a platinum needle, sealing the needle openings in the eggshells, and then incubating the inoculated eggs at 37° C (98.6° F) for a month. The pure culture of the bacillus found in these inoculated eggs, Copeman told the Royal Society in 1898, was then injected subcutaneously into a calf. According to Copeman, this yielded a strain of lymph that "after being passed through a series of calves, was successfully employed for the [smallpox] vaccination of children."[5]

This achievement was remarkable in that Copeman was unaware of course that smallpox was not a bacterial but a viral infection (a fact known to Drs. Ernest Goodpasture and Alice M. Woodruff who in 1931 quite independently reinvented Copeman's technique of using egg cultures to grow fowl pox virus at Vanderbilt University). In his quest for the elusive and filtrable bacterium of smallpox, Copeman had quite possibly become the first medical microbiologist to grow viable animal viruses in chickens' eggs. Copeman lived long enough (he died in 1947 at the age of eighty-five) to witness the birth of modern virology.

In 1892 a Russian graduate student, Dmitri Iosofovich Ivanovski, was sent to investigate the tobacco mosaic disease in Bessarabia and the Ukraine. He found that even after sap from the infected tobacco plants was passed through the Chamberland bacterial filters, it remained toxic enough to induce the disease when brushed on the leaves of healthy plants. Ivanovski's published paper concluded that tobacco mosaic disease was caused by ultramicroscopic bacteria small enough to pass through bacterial filter candles.

The scene shifted now to the neat little Dutch town of Delft, which through the centuries had become world-famous for three very excellent reasons: the blue-and-white and brown-and-white Delft pottery it produced; the paintings of Jan Vermeer (1632–1675); and the discoveries of bacteria, protozoa, and other animalcules by the executor of Vermeer's estate, town-hall janitor, draper, amateur microscopist and scientist, and, for nearly a half century, corresponding member of the British Royal Society, Anton van Leeuwenhoek (1632–1723).

Starting in 1897, the bacteriologist of the Delft yeast works, Martinus Willem Beijerinck (1851–1931), used the new bacteriology laboratory and heated glass house of his alma mater, the Delft Polytechnical School, to resume his study of tobacco mosaic disease. A year later he was appointed professor of general bacteriology at the Polytechnical School, from which he had graduated before going on to the University of Leyden, where his roommate was Jacobus H. van't Hoff, who became his lifelong friend and in 1901 won the first Nobel Prize in chemistry.

Earlier, in 1886, Beijerinck had worked under Adolf Mayer at the

Wageningen Agricultural Experimental Station on the economically costly tobacco mosaic disease. He had been unable to find "either bacteria or parasites of other types in diseased leaves," and abandoned work on the problem. Ivanovski's paper inspired Beijerinck to resume his search for the now proven filtrable agent of tobacco mosaic disease. During the intervening years, Beijerinck realized that in 1885 his "bacteriological knowledge was very incomplete," and that his dozen years of continuous bacteriological investigations after he left Mayer's laboratory now enabled him to "perform a faultless series of experimental inoculations" of the infected sap filtrates into healthy plants.[6]

In 1900 Beijerinck published the results of these experiments in which, like Ivanovski, he had infected healthy plants with what he was certain were germ-free filtrates of sap from diseased plants. As in the Russian's experiments, these filtrates were infective in themselves. Unlike Ivanovski, however, Beijerinck concluded that "(1) The infection is not caused by microbes, but by a living liquid virus. (2) Only growing plant organs where cellular division takes place are susceptible to infection. There only does the virus multiply."[7]

Beijerinck named the agent of tobacco mosaic disease a *Contagium vivum fluidum*. Since it passed through bacterial filters that held back bacteria, the virus was not "corpuscular" (cellular) but, Beijerinck insisted, "molecular," closer in form to a chemical molecule than to a living organism. He described the virus as a molecule that like living organisms could replicate itself, although not independently like bacteria or people, but solely when it was "incorporated into the living protoplasms of the cell, into whose reproduction it is, in a manner of speaking, passively drawn."

Beijerinck's description, published on the eve of the twentieth century, was very close to the modern concept of a virus as an ultramicroscopic obligate parasite that can reproduce itself only in the living cells of unicellular organisms like bacteria, and in the cells of multicellular organisms like potatoes, pigs, and people. This concept was quite difficult for most biologists to accept then and later, since the bacteriophages, the viruses that attack only bacteria, had yet to be found—and the electron microscope, which enabled people to visualize the viruses of smallpox, cowpox, influenza, yellow fever, and other diseases, was more than four decades in the future.

During the same year in which, inspired by Ivanovski's work, Beijerinck resumed his study of tobacco mosaic disease in Delft, the imperial German government ordered the Koch Institute for Infectious Diseases to look into the nature and cure or prevention of foot-and-mouth disease of cattle and sheep, whose periodic outbreaks cost Germany dearly in food and money. The job was given to Dr. Friedrich Loeffler, the army physician who had suggested that the Klebs-Loeffler bacilli of diphtheria produced toxins, and Dr. Paul Frosch, a veterinary bacteriologist. In the interim between Loeffler's work on bacteria and that on foot-and-mouth disease Roux and Yersin, inspired by the antitoxin work of Sewall, isolated the diphtheria toxin that had eluded Loeffler, and Behring and Ehrlich used it to inaugurate the era of serum antitoxins—serotherapy—against bacterial diseases.

Loeffler and Frosch took lymph from vesicles in the mouths and on the udders of cattle with foot-and-mouth disease. They diluted these filtrates in sterile water, and passed the dilutions through fine infusorial-earth-filter candles. They hoped that all that would remain in these sterile, germ-free filtrates would be the natural antitoxin of foot-and-mouth disease analogous to the smallpox antitoxin they presumed was the active immunizing principle in germ-free glycerinated cowpox vaccine lymph. What followed after these cell-free filtrates were injected into healthy animals quickly wrecked Loeffler's and Frosch's initial hopes of producing a vaccine against foot-and-mouth disease.

"The results were always the same: animals injected with filtrates succumb as often as those injected with unfiltered lymph." Loeffler and Frosch were very careful workers, and took great pains to ensure that after filtration the lymph from diseased animals "was found sterile by bacteriological examination." Despite this, these filtrates "still produced typical foot-and-mouth disease three days after injection into the mucous surfaces of the upper and lower lips of calves and heifers. The fact that the disease had been transmitted to stall-mates by animals that had been injected with filtered lymph indicated that the disease was not due to a toxin."[8]

The investigators were, happily, quite prepared to admit that their working hypothesis that the disease was caused by a bacterial toxin was now untenable. But the disease-causing effects of their toxin-free filtrates were replicated in experiment after experiment. "How was this striking fact to be explained?" they asked. "There were two possible explanations: Either (1) an unusually effective toxin was dissolved in the lymph or (2) the filtrate contained a previously undiscovered agent of disease, so small as to pass through the pores of a filter capable of retaining the smallest known bacteria."

They could only conclude that the agent of foot-and-mouth disease was a non-toxin-producing bacterium too small to be seen under the microscope, and tiny enough to pass through filters that screened out all other known bacteria. Even after Beijerinck published his findings on the filtrable agent of tobacco mosaic disease, Loeffler and Frosch never made a connection between the filtrable agents of the plant and the cattle diseases. Roux and his colleagues at the Pasteur Institute also dismissed Beijerinck's conclusions as "interesting but unproven."

In 1900 when Walter Reed was put in charge of the U.S. Army's Yellow Fever Commission to investigate and control yellow fever in Cuba in the wake of the Spanish-American War of 1898, "Dr. William H. Welch kindly called our attention to the important observations which have been carried out in late years by Loeffler and Frosch relative to the etiology and prevention of foot-and-mouth disease in cattle," Reed and James Carroll wrote in 1901. "It was for the purpose of ascertaining whether observations conducted along these same lines ... might throw additional light upon the etiology of yellow fever that the following experiments were undertaken."[9]

The experiments involved testing Cuban doctor Carlos Finlay's 1880 suggestion, oft restated to unlistening medical ears, that the causal agents of yellow fever were transmitted to people by the bites of bloodsucking mosquitoes of the genus *Stegomyia* (now *Aedes aegypti*). Some doctors insisted that the germ of yellow fever was the *Bacillus icteroides,* one of various bacteria that would be put forward as the agent of yellow fever over the next thirty years. Yellow fever itself was not native to the Western Hemisphere, having been brought over on slave ships from Africa to Barbados in 1647.

On December 8, 1900, a soldier volunteer bitten by a mosquito obtained from a yellow-fever ward three days earlier came down with yellow fever. The next day the jubilant Reed wrote to his wife that "just 18 days from the time we began our experimental work we have succeeded in demonstrating this mode of propagation of the disease, so that the most doubtful and skeptical must yield. Rejoice with me, sweetheart, as, aside from the antitoxin of diphtheria and Koch's discovery of the tubercle bacillus, it will be regarded as the most ablest piece of work, scientifically, during the 19th [sic] century.... It was Finlay's theory and he deserves great credit for suggesting it, but as he did nothing to prove it, it was rejected by all, including [Surgeon] General Sternberg ... Major Kean says that the discovery is worth more than the cost of the Spanish War, including lives lost and money expended."

Reed and Carroll did not sit back and rest on these laurels. In the same series of elegant experiments, they diluted and filtered the blood sera of people with yellow fever, made certain that they were sterile, and then injected these clinical filtrates into the bodies of healthy (and very brave) soldier volunteers. The filtrates caused yellow fever in some of the soldiers. The world now knew that yellow fever was a filtrable virus disease, and that the *Stegomyia* mosquito was its vector.

Like most of his competent peers, Walter Reed continued to think of the virus of smallpox as an ultramicroscopic bacterium. He died in 1902, the year after he and Carroll reported on their work before the Society of American Bacteriologists in Chicago. His death, at the age of fifty-one, was caused by peritonitis following appendectomy, an inflammatory condition responsible for many postsurgical deaths before antibiotic drugs were available.

Most of the world's clinical bacteriologists would go on perceiving the virus as a tiny bacterium until close to midcentury, but one by one, as different viruses were shown by careful laboratory studies to be the probable agents of many specific diseases, laboratory chiefs quit trying to find the visible "germs" of these diseases. In 1905, for example, when the Italian microbiologist Adelchi Negri showed that vaccinia (cowpox virus) and variola (smallpox virus) were two separate filtrable viruses, biologists stopped using their microscopes in search of the smallpox germ—and doctors stopped making what they firmly believed to be curative immune sera against smallpox by hyperimmunizing goats and horses with the bacteria they had isolated from vaccine lymphs. Many patients with smallpox had been inoculated with sera from these hyperimmunized animals. Since, like all uninoculated people with smallpox, at least half of them did not die of it, these survivors were often trotted out as living testimonials to the efficacy of the smallpox-germ antisera used to cure them.

The many species of bacteria that contaminated calf-lymph smallpox vaccines played an interesting role in the 1915 discovery of the bacterial viruses by Dr. Frederick W. Twort, a pathologist and bacteriologist. Twort was, at the time, superintendent of London University's Brown Institution, a hospital endowed by a Mr. Thomas Brown of London and Dublin in 1871 "for care and treatment of Quadrupeds or Birds useful to Man." Twort, whose previous studies of microbial nutrition had found what he named the "Essential Substance" in bacterial nutrition, a nutrient now known as vitamin K, was continuing his investigation of the growth patterns of microbial entities. One of them was vaccinia, which Negri had shown in 1905 was a virus.

"It was well known," Twort wrote nearly thirty-five years later, "that the [vaccine] lymph at that time nearly always contained not only the virus of vaccinia but a certain number of bacteria, and micrococci such as are capable of producing pustules." Twort also considered "the possibility of a direct infection of the living micrococci by the living virus of vaccinia."[10]

Twort discovered that a filtrable material found in his cultures of micrococci originally isolated from vaccine lymph lysed, or dissolved, growing cultures of the same bacteria. He termed this material the bacteriolytic agent, and suggested it could be either a virus that entered bacterial cells or an enzyme produced by bacterial cells. When Twort dipped a sterile glass rod into a micrococcal culture lysed by this invisible agent, and then touched a healthy growing culture of micrococci with the same rod, they too were dissolved inside of a few hours.

In his first report on this phenomenon, published in *Lancet* in 1915 and entitled "An Investigation on the Nature of Ultra-Microscopic Viruses," Twort observed that it seemed probable "that the material [the bacteriolytic agent] was produced by the micrococcus."

Twort added a comment that bears repeating. "Incidentally," he wrote in that 1915 *Lancet* article, "this apparent spontaneous production of a self-destroying material which when started increases in quantity might be of interest in connection with cancers."

While still not certain that his bacteriolytic agent was a virus, Twort added that "in any case, whatever explanation is accepted, the possibility of its being an ultra-microscopic virus has not been *definitely* disproved."

At about the same time, and ignorant of what Twort had found in vaccine lymph in London, Felix d'Herrelle (1873–1949), born in Montreal, taken to France at six by his newly widowed mother, educated in France and at the medical school of the University of Leiden in Holland, and a staff member of the Pasteur Institute since 1908, was making similar findings in cultures of locust dysentery bacilli in North Africa. In 1910 while working on the Yucatan Peninsula in Mexico, d'Herrelle had found a species of locust coccobacilli that caused diarrhea in insects. He soon found, he wrote, that "I could start epidemics in columns of healthy insects by dusting cultures of the coccobacillus on plants in front of the advancing [locust] columns: the insects infected themselves as they devoured the soiled plants."[11]

During the five years that followed, d'Herrelle traveled from the Argentine to North Africa for various governments to fight locust invasions, making and drying his bacterial cultures, dusting them on growing food and fruit crops, and carefully noting the results in his journal. "At various times," he observed, "I noticed an anomaly shown by some cultures of the coccobacillus which intrigued me greatly . . ." When the bacilli were grown on agar plates in small flat dishes, "the anomaly consisted of *clear spots* (plaques), quite circular, speckling the cultures grown on agar. I scratched the surface of the agar in these transparent patches, and made slides for the microscope; there was nothing to be seen. I concluded from this and other experiments that the *something* which caused the formation of the clear spots must be so small as to be filtrable, that is to say able to pass through a filter of the Chamberland type which will hold back all bacteria."

In March 1915, during the second year of World War I, d'Herrelle, then a French Army doctor, was sent to Tunisia to start an epidemic of dysentery among locusts threatening the North African wheat crop. He dusted the wheat and adjacent leaves with his powdered coccobacilli and not only caused the planned locust dysentery epidemic but also, "As the result of the infection there was a considerable [locust] mortality, and, even more interesting, when the following year all the rest of North Africa was again invaded [by locusts], Tunisia remained free [of locusts]; the illness had continued to rage among these swarms of locusts which had survived long enough to move South at the end of the season, and had brought about their destruction during the winter."

In the course of this campaign, d'Herrelle noticed the clear spots in some of his plate cultures of the coccobacilli, and stayed on to "investigate their significance" at the Pasteur Institute of Tunis. The director of this outpost, Charles Nicolle (1866–1936), the son of a physician in Rouen, was as fine a poet, novelist, and philosopher as he was a physician, epidemiologist, and microbiologist. Hans Zinsser's classic *Rats, Lice and History* was affectionately dedicated to Nicolle. In 1928 Nicolle won another honor—the Nobel Prize in medicine for his work on the transmission by body lice of typhus fever *Rickettsia* from sick rats to healthy people. While still in medical school,

Nicolle took the new course in medical microbiology given by the Pasteur Institute in 1892. After qualifying in medicine, he taught and practiced in Paris and Rouen until 1903, when his approaching deafness made it difficult for him to treat patients. In that year Nicolle moved to Tunis as head of the local Pasteur Institute, and remained there for the rest of his life.

When Nicolle saw the clear spots (or plaques) in d'Herrelle's bacterial cultures and studied the records he had carefully compiled, he was as impressed by the dysentery that continued to plague the swarms of locusts who flew south after the season as he was by the plaques. The clear spots, he told d'Herrelle, "may be a sign of a filtrable virus carried by your coccobacilli, a filtrable virus which is the true pathogenic agent, while the coccobacilli is only a contaminant." This was a shrewd guess, but when d'Herrelle filtered coccobacilli-culture emulsions showing the clear spots and then tried to infect healthy locusts with the filtrates, nothing happened.

Nicolle's guess was not completely wrong. The coccobacilli did carry viruses that killed other coccobacilli, but these viruses had absolutely no effects upon locusts or anything else but other coccobacilli. All viruses are kingdom-specific: Bacterial viruses attack only bacteria; plant viruses attack only plants; animal viruses attack only animals. Some animal viruses, such as the smallpox virus, are also species-specific, so that they attack people but not other animals. Bacterial viruses are the most selective of all, being not only kingdom- and species-specific, but also strain-specific. If the lytic agent in d'Herrelle's coccobacilli cultures did not attack locusts, it was at least a virus.

In August 1915 when d'Herrelle returned to Paris, Roux asked him to investigate an epidemic of human dysentery then raging in a cavalry squadron at Maisons-Lafitte. "I thought that the hypothesis put forward for explaining the locusts' illness might be helpful in understanding human dysentery. I therefore filtered emulsions of the feces of the sick man, let the filtrates act on cultures of dysentery bacilli, and spread them [the filtrate-treated bacterial cultures] after incubation on nutritive agar in petri dishes. On various occasions I again found my clear spots, but the feeding of these cultures to guinea pigs and rabbits produced no disease."

D'Herrelle went on adding filtrates from the feces of a gravely ill dysentery patient daily to cultures of *Shiga* dysentery bacilli taken from his own bloody stools. For the first three days nothing happened, and the sick cavalryman's condition remained unchanged. On the fourth day d'Herrelle repeated this procedure, and then placed the tube of *Shiga* bacilli broth cultures as well as the agar plate seeded with filtrates and bacilli from this culture in the incubator kept at human body temperature, 37°C or 98.6°F.

"The next morning," d'Herrelle recalled, "on opening the incubator I experienced one of those rare moments of intense emotion which reward the research worker for all his pains: at first glance I saw that the broth culture, which the night before had been very turbid, was perfectly clear: all the bacteria had vanished, they had dissolved away like sugar in water. As for the agar spread, it was devoid of all growth and what caused my emotion was that in a flash I had understood: what caused my clear spots was in fact an invisible microbe, a filtrable virus, but a virus parasitic on bacteria.

"Another thought came to me also: 'If this is true, the same thing has probably occurred during the night in the sick man, who yesterday was in a serious condition. In his intestine, as in my test tube, the dysentery bacilli will have dissolved away under the action of their parasite. He should now be cured.'

"I dashed to the hospital. In fact, during the night, his general condition had greatly improved and convalescence was beginning."

D'Herrelle also dashed off a short communication, entitled "On an invisible microbe, an antagonist of the dysentery bacillus," which was presented by Roux to the French Academy of Sciences on September 15, 1917. Here d'Herrelle used the word bacteriophage for the first time, the suffix taken from the Greek word *phagein*, "to eat." Eaters of bacteria—bacteriophages—is an excellent word for what scientists perceived the bacterial viruses to be prior to the electron microscope, since all they could see of the bacteriophages under their light microscopes was what they did to bacteria. The word bacteriophage is usually shortened to the less cumbersome diminutive, phage.

For the next three decades, d'Herrelle devoted his life to proving at one and the same time that the ultramicroscopic phages that shattered and seemed to devour bacteria were really viruses and not enzymes or other chemicals produced by the bacteria themselves; attempting to prove that the phages could both cure and immunize people against bacterial diseases; and arguing that the phenomenon found by Twort in bacterial contaminants of cowpox vaccine lymph differed from the bacteriophagic effect d'Herrelle discovered in insect and human dysentery bacilli cultures. During these years, he went from Paris to Leiden, where he held a chair, to Egypt, where he headed the International Sanitary Commission, and in 1928 he became professor of protobiology at the Yale University medical school, where he remained for some years before returning to France.

Before he died in 1949, d'Herrelle was, with the aid of the new electron microscope which made his phages visible, vindicated on one score: the phages were undoubtedly bacterial viruses. However, it was equally clear that Twort had discovered them first, even if in 1915 he was not quite as sure as d'Herrelle and Nicolle were that the lytic agents of bacteria were viruses.

In the nearly total absence of knowledge of viruses in general—the first textbook on virology, Salvador E. Luria's *General Virology,* would not appear until 1953—and of bacterial viruses (phages) in particular, physicians and educated laymen could hardly be blamed for confidently expecting that the viruses that attacked and destroyed bacteria had major roles to play in human health. Many a promising medical career was wrecked as a result of trying to use phages as cures for bacterial infections between, roughly, 1920 and 1950. Many man years of scientific work that might have been devoted to more productive studies in prophylaxis were squandered in efforts to devise immunological strategies of using phages to prevent bacterial diseases.

D'Herrelle was neither a charlatan nor a madman, nor were the physicians who tried to use phages to cure bacterial dysentery diseases blithering idiots. Phages filtered from the stools of dysentery patients really did lyse and destroy *Shiga* bacilli from the same patient at the same time. But if these identical phages were used against patients with dysentery caused by *Shiga* bacilli of the same type but of a different strain or subtype, nothing happened. Bacterial viruses found in cultures of cholera vibrios contaminating a water well worked brilliantly when billions of them were dumped back into the same well—but only for a week or so. Then new cultures of cholera vibrios, but of strains not sensitive to the phages that destroyed the first strain, might appear in the same wells, and treatment with huge doses of bacteriophages originally isolated from the first population of cholera germs would have no effect of any sort on the succeeding strains.

The reasons for these failures were the same: There have never existed anything resembling purebred bacteria (or, for that matter, people) of the same species, type, and strain in nature. The bacterial viruses are species-, type-, and strain-specific. A phage that works only against the *Escherichia coli* species of enteric bacteria, will not work against any strains of streptococci, or pneumococci, or any other bacteria save the *E. coli* species—and, at that, the *E. coli* parasitized by specific coliphages have to be of precisely the single strain susceptible to its matched phage. Each *E. coli* cell is so specific to only specific bacteriophages that well-typed phages are used to help identify or type *E. coli* (and other bacteria) by this sensitivity or resistance, and phage typing of clinical isolates of many species of bacteria is now a standard procedure in medical microbiology.

This combination of wide type variations in nonlaboratory bacterial populations, and the highly specific type and strain limitations of bacteriophages, guaranteed that any clinical cures or immunities resulting from the uses of phages would be very temporary at best. Theoretically, by making up phages against every single type and strain of disease-causing bacteria isolated from the bodies, stools, and blood and urine of patients with fulminating bacterial diseases, and applying these phages in massive doses, this therapy would cure any bacterial disease by lysing all its agents. In practice, unfortunately, by the time all these bacterial strains and their specific phages were isolated, and literally scores of cultures seeded with phage filtrates to grow the batches of new phages required for medical treatment, in the absence of sulfas and antibiotic drugs most of the seriously ill patients would be dead, and the patients with less critical infections would have taken turns for the worse.

This did not mean that the bacteriophages had no place in medicine. When modern virology did come of age after World War II, it turned out that for all of their vast differences, a cell was a cell and a virus was a virus—and a bacterial virus, in its interactions with a bacterial cell, is able to answer many complex questions about the biology, chemistry, and physics of life at the cellular and subcellular or molecular levels where life begins, proliferates, and ends. I recall hearing Gilbert Dalldorf, the discoverer of the Coxsackie viruses, during a conference early in the phage era, saying that while we cannot crawl into a living cell to find out what goes on inside when foreign genetic material is introduced, we could send viruses inside to find out for us.

In 1931, even before we had the technology to visualize the viruses inside living cells, the Goodpasture-Woodruff technique of growing them in developing chick embryos in fertile hens' eggs enabled the study of the effects on live animals by the viruses that could be raised, and titrated (or counted), but not seen.

After World War II, with the development of the ultracentrifuge and electrophoresis to isolate viruses, and electron microscopes to make them visible, phages became the experimental model of choice in virus studies. Literally overnight, the ubiquitous bacteriophages—particularly those isolated from raw sewage rich in human fecal matter—became the "guinea pigs" of modern virology. By 1959, barely a decade into the new era, Dr. Wolfhard Weidel, director of the Max Planck Institute for Biology in Tübingen, Germany, could truthfully write that "the work with phage has led to more important discoveries than all other virus work together." Between 1958 and 1980, over a dozen scientific workers have won Nobel Prizes for genetics, medicine, physiology, and biochemistry done largely with *E. coli* and their very specific bacteriophages (a statistic that would have warmed the heart of the pediatrician Theodor Escherich, who in 1885 isolated the coliform enteric bacteria named after him during an unsuccessful search for the human dysentery bacterium).

Weidel gave one of the basic reasons for the postwar reliance on the many strains of *E. coli* and their phages: "Growing phage is no problem at all: a simple nutrient broth is infected with suitable bacteria. In a few hours the previously clear fluid will look turbid because it now contains millions of bacterial cells. A few drops of phage solution are added, and after an interval the solution again clears. If all has gone well, each cubic centimeter [there are a little under 30 ccs, or cubic centimeters, in one fluid ounce] should now contain up to a billion phage particles but practically no more whole, live bacteria. This is a large yield with a small amount of effort. A single hard-working experimenter using the egg method may have to spend up to $2000 a year [1959 dollars] for eggs, whereas one using phage can do with less than a tenth of that amount for the same purpose," since the *E. coli* and other bacteria in which bacterial viruses are grown are cheaper and far more plentiful than the fertile hens' eggs in which animal viruses are grown in laboratories.[12]

* * *

Three major developments had to occur before experimental and medical virology could each come into being.

The first development was cumulative: the half-century and more of bacteriological, biochemical, and immunological research on infectious diseases that intellectually eliminated the possibility that bacteria, protozoa, and other living microorganisms could be responsible for causing smallpox and other common infectious diseases. Starting with Reed's and Carroll's 1901 report on the experimental induction of yellow fever, decades of solid clinical studies began to point to filtrable—and, for nearly another fifty years, unseen—agents that were finally given the name of virus.

During the century after Claude Bernard spoke of this unseen agent as an artifact of human deduction, "a creature of reason," the virus was reasonably perceived to be, in turn, a submicroscopic bacterium, a fluid contagium, an infectious molecule, and, in our times, an ultramicroscopic particle consisting of a thin coat of proteins (sometimes mixed with a few traces of lipids [fats] or enzymes) surrounding a cargo of one or another but never both of the two nucleic acids—DNA and RNA. DNA (deoxyribonucleic acid) is the basic chemical of heredity, RNA (ribonucleic acid) is produced in living cells by DNA to deliver its metabolic and other chemical and hereditary instructions to the organism's single or multiple cells.

The second development that helped create modern virology came toward the end of World War II, and would have a much more lasting effect on biology, genetics, medicine, philosophy, and the human condition than even that most terrible of world wars. It was the investigation by Oswald Avery, Colin MacLeod and Maclyn McCarty of the transforming principle—which proved to be DNA—of the 1928 Griffith transformation effect of pneumococci.

Nucleic acid itself was not unknown prior to 1944; in 1869 it was first isolated from the nuclei of white blood cells in pus taken from surgical patients of the University of Tübingen hospital by a twenty-five-year-old postdoctoral student, Friedrich Miescher (1844–1895). He named it nuclein, and for the next seventy years or so, in addition to being renamed nucleic acid by the biochemist Richard Altman in 1889, it was studied by Miescher and many scientists who wondered if it might play a specific role in heredity. The great American cell biologist Edmund B. Wilson noted in 1895 that "chromatin [a major component of the chromosomes] is known to be widely similar to, if not identical, with a substance known as nuclein. . . . And thus we reach the remarkable conclusion that inheritance may, perhaps, be effected by the physical transmission of a particular chemical compound from parent to offspring."[13] Later, Wilson veered away from the concept that the chromatins carried genetic information. (Today we know that the chromatins are genetically active complexes of both DNA and RNA combined with proteins.)

The classic work of Avery, MacLeod, and McCarty carried these studies to their logical conclusion. One of the major secondary effects of their 1944 paper on the Griffith transformation effect was to help finally elucidate the roles that smallpox virus and other animal viruses play in the cause and transmission of transient, crippling, degenerative, and fatal diseases in our species. Thanks to Avery and his coworkers, we know that the disease viruses are rogue genes that invade and transform healthy living cells so that instead of producing only new normal cells, they now begin to synthesize replicas of their virus parasites, damaging or killing themselves in the process of carrying out two genetic programs, their own and those mediated by the nucleic acid of their virus guests.

The third development that helped create modern virology was technological: the continuum of new hardware—from the ultracentrifuge and the electrophoresis instruments, which made possible the isolation and separation of viruses; to the electron and scanning electron microscopes, which made viruses and their invasion of bacterial and animal cells visible; to the scores of other new laboratory devices, like inexpensive paper chromatography and awesomely costly nucleic-acid analyzers—that all combined to make it possible to grow, harvest, and study the viruses in action. There were also the high-speed electronic computers required to store and process the mountains of solid data about viruses all this new hardware produces.

These ubiquitous and inordinately expensive tools (a decent electron microscope now costs from $100,000 to $150,000 to buy and another $50,000 a year in salaries and expendable equipment to operate), which are so commonplace today in virus laboratories everywhere, were each beyond the imagination of the generations of science fantasy writers and more pretentious futurologists who wrote on the sciences during the first half of the century.

These and many related scientific developments clarified the similarities and the differences between viruses and bacteria, which both share one devastating trait: Each group of microbial or submicrobial pathogens is capable of causing debilitating, crippling, chronic-degenerative, and fatal infectious diseases in fish, fowl, insects, other bacteria, plants, and all animals including each of the races of humankind.

Both types of pathogens are far too small to be seen with the naked eye. Bacteria, most of which can be seen under the light microscope, are measured in microns. A micron (μ), often called a micrometer, is one millionth of a meter, 1/1,000 of a millimeter, or roughly 1/25,000 of an inch. Some of the most pathogenic species of bacteria, such as the staphylococci and the streptococci, are only 0.75 to 1.25 microns in diameter. Bacillary forms of bacteria, such as *E. coli* and the *Shiga* dysentery bacillus, have diameters as small as a half a micron and are only two to three microns long. None of these and most other bacterial disease agents are able to pass through the placental membrane that protects the developing embryo against environmental pathogens, but the characteristics of *Treponema pallidum,* the spiral bacteria that cause syphilis, enable them to pass the placental barrier and infect the fetus.

Viruses are measured in millimicrons (mμ). A millimicron is one billionth of a meter, or one thousandth of a micron. Viruses range from three to three hundred millimicrons in size, or about one thousandth the size of an average bacterium.

Bacteria (including the ultramicroscopic, filtrable, and cell-wall-free subfamily of *Mycoplasma*) are living organisms. Like all other living organisms, including people, their cells always contain two kinds of nucleic acid— deoxyribonucleic acid (DNA), which is found only in the cell nucleus in less primitive or eucaryotic forms of life, and in the cytoplasm of procaryotic or nonnucleated organisms, such as bacteria, which have no defined nucleus, and ribonucleic acid (RNA). Ribonucleic acid is made in living cells on the templates of DNA, and transfers hereditary information from the DNA contained in the chromosomes of the nucleus to the rest of the cell or cells in living organisms. The bacteria have only a single, circular chromosome. The higher organisms have more chromosomes, arranged in matching linear pairs, like the forty-six chromosomes (twenty-three pairs) in the nucleus of each human cell.

Similar to higher organisms, bacteria have a metabolism, which is, by definition, "the sum of all the physical and chemical processes by which living organized tissue is formed and maintained, and also the transformation by which energy is made available for use by the organism."[14] In bacteria, as in bacteriologists, the energy required to conduct the metabolic processes is derived from the nutrients taken in and processed by the cells and their organelles (the bacterial analogs of the specialized organs in the higher organisms). Bacterial metabolism, like our own, is also dependent upon metabolites, or chemicals and minerals and other substances essential to the metabolic functions. These metabolites include vitamins and other coenzymes which microorganisms and people synthesize from their nutrients or find already formed in their foods.

As a general rule, the bacteria reproduce themselves asexually, by binary fission, a process during which each cell splits into two daughter cells containing nucleic acids identical to those of the parent cells. At times, under certain circumstances that often cause trouble, they also reproduce sexually.

Like other living organisms, including people, bacteria can be killed by starvation, traumas (including radiations, osmotic shocks, and other physical forces), natural toxins and synthetic chemical poisons, and excessive heat.

Viruses are not living organisms, nor are they even cells. They are ultramicroscopic particles whose cores or cargoes consist of either DNA or RNA *but never both nucleic acids,* and whose shells or outer coats consist largely or completely of proteins, which at times also contain traces of lipids and enzymes.

The basic unit of all living things is the cell. A bacterium is a single-celled organism, with a rigid cellulose-like outer wall or shell, outer and inner membranes between the outer walls and the cytoplasm, which is a viscous or thick fluid within the membranes containing the single chromosome bearing the bacterial genes, and the organelles that perform the myriad functions of metabolism blueprinted by the genes.

The basic unit of the virus is the virion—the core nucleic acid plus the proteinaceous coat or capsid that encloses it. A mature virus is also known as a virion.

Although the mechanisms vary by which plant, bacterial, insect and animal viruses parasitize the specific living organisms they infect, the viral function in each type of virus-cell interaction is identical: to transfer nucleic acid from inside the coat of the virus to the inside or cytoplasm of the bacterial, plant, insect, or human cells they attack. Once in the host cells, the viral nucleic acids, which contain the genes, take over and reprogram the metabolic machinery of the invaded cells. The living cells continue to take in nutrients as they did before becoming the involuntary hosts of the viral genes, but now instead of reproducing new healthy daughter cells—which is the end purpose of all metabolic processes in bacteria—the parasitized cells start to use the same food proteins, carbohydrates, fats, trace-mineral elements, and other nutrients and metabolites to replicate fully formed, chemically active new virions by the hundreds.

In bacterial populations—with the exception of mutant subpopulations of various species, which are termed lysogenic (self-destructive) bacteria—this forced replication and accumulation of virus particles causes the bacteria to swell to the breaking point and ultimately lyse or burst. Lysis releases hundreds of chemically active virions into the environment of other susceptible bacteria they can attack.

The lysogenic bacteria, on the other hand, take in the phage nucleic acid, be it DNA or RNA, and incorporate it into their own circular chromosome. There it does not immediately take over the chemical direction of the bacterial cells. Instead, the viral genetic package becomes incorporated into the bacterial chromosome, and for many bacterial generations is passed down, in its dormant state, to the daughter cells and from them to subsequent generations of other descendant cells.

This alteration of the original nucleic-acid composition of the bacterial chromosome induces certain changes, but fortunately for the bacteria, few of them are damaging to the lysogenic bacteria. People, however, are not quite so lucky when these changes occur.

Consider the *Corynebacterium diphtheriae* species. One of the reasons it was so difficult for poor Edwin Klebs to get people to take him seriously when he isolated this species and claimed it was the causal agent of diphtheria was that when other nineteenth-century investigators isolated the same bacteria, they were very often unable to get it to cause diphtheria or diphtheria-like diseases in laboratory animals. At other times the Klebs (*Corynebacterium*) bacilli they isolated from patients with diphtheria did cause severe and fatal diseases in animals. They concluded at the time that the Klebs bacillus was a harmless commensal—an organism that lives on or in living tissues without causing any harm—and that diphtheria was probably caused by other bacteria, such as the streptococci, found just as frequently on the throat membranes and nasal tissues of diphtheria patients. Even when Friedrich Loeffler, at the Koch Institute, finally proved that the bacterium isolated by Klebs was indeed the agent of diphtheria, he never understood why strains of the Klebs-Loeffler bacillus that were morphologically identical with the pathogenic strains failed to produce the diphtheria toxin.

In 1951, nearly seventy years after Loeffler proved the pathogenicity of at least some strains of otherwise identical *C. diphtheriae,* when both phages and the phenomenon of lysogeny were known, it became possible to solve the puzzle. The genetic materials in the nucleic acids, of which neither Klebs nor Loeffler were aware, are not to be tampered with without risk of serious consequences. The addition of the dormant genes of lysogenic phages to the single circular chromosomes of lysogenic *C. diphtheriae* cause the bacteria to undergo what is called lysogenic conversion. This lysogenic conversion does not cause the bacteria to be born again as do other types of conversion in higher forms of life. It does, however, cause the diphtheria bacilli to synthesize a metabolite unlike any other they ever manufactured before. This metabolite is not harmful to the bacteria themselves, but it also happens to be the diphtheria toxin which kills people, as V. J. Freeman discovered at the University of Washington in Seattle in 1951.[15]

There are lysogenic and nonlysogenic strains of other bacteria. The nonlysogenic and lysogenic strains of *Streptococcus pyogenes* are far from harmless, since they are one of the two major causes of human infections and of pus formation in wounds. However, when lysogenic strains of *S. pyogenes* undergo virus-induced lysogenic conversion, they start to produce the toxin that causes scarlet fever—an infectious disease which, until the advent of penicillin, was a major cause of deafness and death in children.[16]

In all lysogenic bacteria, whether or not they are toxin-producing, the dormant prophages—or the dormant and naked nucleic acids of lysogenic bacterial viruses incorporated into their own bacterial chromosomes—do not remain dormant forever. After a few or a few thousand passages from generation to generation of lysogenic bacteria, the long-dormant lysogenic prophages suddenly revert to virulence and start acting like normal virus genomes. They take command of the chemical and metabolic systems of the bacterial cells. Inside of a few minutes, the cells start to produce hundreds of mature phage particles, enough to tear themselves apart.

Prior to the advent of the electron microscope (which was developed in Germany on the eve of World War II but not produced commercially until after peace came in 1945), all viruses, including the bacteriophages, were invisible to human eyes. The virus-infected lysogenic bacterial cells themselves, however, could be clearly observed under the light microscope, growing normally like any other bacteria for generations (under optimum circumstances a bacterial generation can start every twenty minutes) until, for no visibly apparent reason, the cells themselves suddenly started to swell and seemingly self-destruct.

Between 1922 and 1932, the Nobel laureate Jules Bordet of the Pasteur Institute of Brussels used this demonstrable series of "spontaneous" happenings as proof that bacteriophages simply did not exist, and that such swelling and shattering of the bacterial cells were caused by enzymes produced by the doomed bacteria themselves. Needless to say, neither Bordet nor anyone else ever proved the existence of these postulated enzymes, but most bacteriologists—including the ones who wrote most of the standard textbooks on bacteriology—accepted this hypothesis as a proven theory. They did not refer to bacterial viruses but to what their texts, until well after World War II, termed either the Twort-d'Herrelle effect, or the bacteriophagic phenomenon.[17]

The Russian-born husband-and-wife team of Drs. Eugene and Elizabeth Wollman, who had gone to work in Élie Metchnikoff's laboratories in 1910, started to look into the phenomenon after World War I. By 1927 they were certain that it was caused by bacterial viruses, as d'Herrelle proclaimed to all who would listen. The Wollmans, however, felt that much more work was required to elucidate fully the mechanisms of lysogeny. They were on the verge of completing this work in December 1943 when they were rounded up by the Nazis in occupied France, transported to the Auschwitz (Oswiecim) annihilation center in occupied Poland with hundreds of thousands other European Jews, and exterminated. After World War II, André Lwoff, who had trained under the Wollmans at the Pasteur Institute and served with distinction in the anti-Nazi underground forces during the Nazi occupation of France, proved that the bacteriophages do indeed replicate in and destroy bacterial cells by lysis.[18]

Variants of lysogenic and nonlysogenic states are found in the interactions of viruses and human cells. Sometimes the viruses that infect people cause different kinds of damage at different sites in the body. The poliovirus, for example, is an enteric virus which enters the human gut through the mouth and usually causes a mild, short-lived disorder marked by a very slight rise in body temperature and little discomfort. The poliomyelitis infection passes very quickly—lasting just long enough to program the host immune system to produce antibodies protecting people for life against the infecting serotype or types of poliovirus for as long as the person lives. (As a rule, wild populations of poliovirus contain all three major serotypes of this virus.)

When on some occasions the poliovirus travels from the alimentary tract to the cells of the central nervous system, and particularly to the gray matter of the spinal cord where the motor impulses of all bodily movements originate, the results can be catastrophic. Polioviruses, unlike most infectious viruses, are necrotizing, that is, they destroy the cells they parasitize and use for virus replication as do the bacterial viruses. Many cells in the human body are self-regenerative and repair themselves after a major infection. However, "the motor nerve cells, once destroyed, do not have the property of regenerating themselves as do the cells of the skin, the liver, or other organs. This is why paralysis, once established [by poliovirus infection], is often permanent."

Bulbar poliomyelitis, which results when the viruses get into the brain, as they used to in upward of 25 percent of all polio cases in the United States epidemics of this century, was more terrifying, particularly for children who had previously had their tonsils and adenoids removed and in whom bulbar poliomyelitis was present in 85 percent of all epidemic polio cases. Death was a common outcome when the disease reached the medullary respiratory center and the infected children gradually ceased breathing. In bulbospinal polio infections, the breathing muscles became paralyzed, and paralysis of the lungs often followed. Before the Salk and Sabin poliovirus vaccines eradicated infantile paralysis from this and other industrial countries, some people with lungs permanently paralyzed by poliovirus infections were kept alive in coffin-like and electrically powered mechanical respirators, popularly known as "iron lungs," often for many years.

Usually, in most human virus infections there is an uneasy and very troubled state of coexistence between the infectious viruses, their genes, and their human hosts. The human cells penetrated and altered by the infectious viruses begin to proliferate or grow at a slower rate, because their food must now be shared between the metabolic systems that produce their own daughter cells and the chemical needs of the new systems that cause them to replicate new virus particles. Unlike the normal nonlysogenic bacterial cells, the infected human cells are not destroyed by the viruses they produce. Rather, they begin to shed or leak showers of newly replicated infective virus particles that soon infect the still healthy cells in the same human bodies. These newly infected cells are now similarly altered by the viral genes, and they too begin to shed viruses that invade their neighbor cells.

In adults, as in infants and children, while viruses of various diseases, from smallpox and yellow fever to the common cold, continue to be replicated by the chemical machinery of their own cells, the diseases grow more severe.

In nature the only defenses against these disease viruses (and other microbial pathogens, such as bacteria and Protista) are the not inconsiderable inborn host or immune defense systems which—since humankind evolved—have always acted to isolate, phagocytize, destroy, and otherwise neutralize most microbial pathogens. These inborn bodily defense systems have enabled enough of us to survive a million years or so of viral and bacterial and related infections to bring us into the eras of vaccines, sulfa, and antibiotic drugs, and other man-made accessories. These natural or inborn host defense systems are probably the major reason we still survive most infections, but they do not work with equal efficiency in all individuals, since they work best in people who are in good health at the time they acquire their infections. Historically, the human inborn immune system—the array of different and often interacting types of antibodies, complement and other blood factors, interferons, and probably many other humoral and cellular defenses against infections that have yet to be isolated, named, and hailed as universal remedies—does not function nearly as well in those who are chronically undernourished, inadequately housed, and in poor health when exposed to the same viruses or other pathogens as it does in economically more fortunate individuals.

Developing fetuses *in utero* are protected against most viral infections that affect their mothers by two inborn host defenses—the temporary placental barrier formed from embryonic and uterine tissues during pregnancy, which blocks most bacteria and larger microbes, and the maternal antibodies that protect the fetus against the infections to which the mother is immune. When mothers who are not immune to certain viruses, such as the cytomegalovirus and the rubella (German measles) virus, become infected during pregnancy, the new infective particles shed by the mothers' infected cells are too small to be stopped by the placenta.

These viruses soon attack the developing fetuses. When they transfer their own genes to the fetal cells, they do not kill them, but they slow their growth to half or less than half the normal rate. This means that fetal eyes, ears, brains, spines, limbs, organs and nervous systems infected at various stages of their own genetically programmed development start to grow at slowed rates of development.

If the developing fetuses are infected by the cytomegalovirus (CMV) or the rubella virus very early in gestation, the damage caused to their cells by the viral genes is usually severe enough to kill them. However, if the virus infections start to slow the cellular growth for the duration of the nine months of pregnancy, the shedding of new virus particles made in the slower-growing cells of the infected fetuses will cause the patterns of multiple birth defects found in such children at birth: the viruses that cause blindness in the fetus during gestation continue to be shed by the fetal cells, so that they also slow the proper development of ears, limbs, and central nervous systems. Rubella- or CMV-damaged children therefore seldom have only one major birth defect.

In infants, children, and adults, permanent damage and death from viral diseases occur when their bodies are unable to produce enough phagocytes, antibodies, interferon, complement, and other intrinsic defenses against the viruses to destroy or neutralize them and end the infections. One viral disease, rabies, is 100 percent fatal. The smallpox virus, whose infection is equally incurable, kills upward of 50 percent of its victims and, unlike the rabies virus, attacks people and no other animal species. The common cold, a disease caused by a veritable regiment of different viruses, is rarely fatal by itself, but it often precedes fulminating and at times fatal bacterial infections. The one thing rabies, smallpox, and the common cold have in common with all or nearly all other virus diseases is that no drugs exist either to cure or to prevent them.

Sometimes, as in lysogenic bacteria, the genetic materials, or proviruses, of human diseases will be incorporated into the nuclei of human cells and will then fail to take over the metabolic machinery of these cells. Instead, as in lysogenic bacteria, they will become, in effect, extra but dormant chromosomes passed down through generations of healthy human cells to their descendants. Then after a few months or many years of apparently benign coexistence, something occurs that triggers the proviruses in the genetic package—the genome—of human cells to become fully virulent again.

As with the lysogenic bacteria and their guest prophages, the events that reactivate these "sleeping volcano" viral genes vary: another sickness, an exposure to radiations or mutagenic or carcinogenic chemicals, an interaction with another virus, or even the subtle and unavoidable biochemical changes that materialize with aging. Once reactivated, these no longer dormant genes cause shingles and other virus diseases, and possibly help cause some forms of cancer that seem to be associated with environmental factors or aging or both.

In at least one human disease, kuru—an agonizing, chronic degenerative condition that ends in madness and death and, so far as we know, affects only young adults in the Fore people of New Guinea—the disease is the price paid for eating the brains of vanquished soldiers of other tribes and not knowing that these tissues contained the slow-acting viruses of kuru.[19]

Since viruses have no metabolisms, they cannot be starved to death or killed by drugs like the sulfas, which act by inhibiting the bodily production of a metabolite essential to bacterial metabolism. The penicillins and other antibiotics are equally useless against viruses, since they act by disrupting bacterial metabolism.

Until the genetic function of the nucleic acids was better understood, a good deal of time and energy was wasted in the debate over whether viruses were living or dead. Viruses are not living organisms in the sense that bacteria and we are living organisms. Genetically, however, viruses are far from inert. They actually manage to reproduce themselves (a trait of living organisms), and they do this with far less effort than living organisms: All they need to do is penetrate living cells and then manipulate those cells to perform the chemically complex tasks of viral replication for them.

"Progeny virus particles resemble their parents because they contain identical chromosomes. We also see," writes the Nobel laureate and biochemist James D. Watson, "that they are no more 'alive' than isolated chromosomes; both the chromosomes of cells and those of virus can be duplicated only in the complex environment of a living cell."[20]

Whether their genetic materials are living, or nonliving, or belong to the twilight zone some say prevails at the interface where life ends and new life begins, the viruses are most significant for what they do to diminish and terminate millions of human lives yearly.

The roster of major diseases caused solely or in large measure by viruses is much greater than the list of infectious disorders now formally classified as virus diseases.

It has long been known that in addition to causing smallpox, influenza, poliomyelitis, yellow fever, measles, hepatitis, infectious mononucleosis, rubella, and chicken pox, many virus infections have a way of triggering bacterial and even noninfectious diseases. Viruses are known to cause prenatal damages that result in such immediately apparent birth defects as blindness, deafness, cerebral palsy, arms the size of fingers, and mental retardation, as well as such delayed sequelae of fetal virus infections as diabetes.[21]

There is good evidence, developed by such fine scientists as George Burch of Tulane University, New Orleans, that "viral infections occurring *in utero* produce a significant amount of heart disease." Burch has also observed, and subsequent clinical studies by other workers have further documented, that many postnatal viral infections are primarily responsible for some cases of pericarditis, myocarditis, endocarditis, and other heart diseases. Burch lists as "viruses that cause heart disease in man," many ranging from adenovirus, the herpes zoster (chicken-pox) virus, and the Coxsackie virus to, among others, those that cause influenza, measles, mumps, rubella, cytomegalovirus infections, smallpox, infectious mononucleosis, and yellow fever.[22]

Investigators in the Soviet Union and elsewhere have for some years been reporting the isolation of toxic and viral substances in the blood of patients with schizophrenia. A recent study organized by David Tyrrell and collaborators in England found a virus-like (VLA) agent in the cerebrospinal fluid of eighteen of forty-seven patients with schizophrenia, and in eight of eleven patients with serious or chronic neurological disorders, such as Huntington's chorea, multiple sclerosis, and "unexplained alterations of consciousness." This agent appears to be an RNA virus that is very difficult to grow in large quantities in egg and tissue cultures. They reported that "patients with a V.L.A. tended to have poorer outcome and to be less likely to respond to treatment" with the tranquilizers and other behavior-modifying drugs that usually work in disturbed people. "If V.L.A.[s] are found to cause illness," Tyrrell and his six collaborators concluded, "there will be a possibility of treatment or prevention by vaccination or by giving interferon or synthetic antiviral compounds."[23]

The temporal links between virus diseases and major bacterial infections were evident long before viruses were even known to be involved. Although it was not until 1931 that the British scientists Christopher Andrewes and Wilson Smith isolated the virus of influenza, the world had long since learned, during the great Spanish flu pandemic of 1918–1919, that influenza very often is followed by bacterial pneumonias which kill more people than influenza itself.[24] Between 1914 and 1917, Walther Kruse in Germany and George B. Foster in the United States proved, by inducing colds in volunteers with filtrates derived from suspensions of nasal materials taken from people with colds, that the common cold was caused by one or more as yet unisolated viruses. Few people took this proof seriously because what doctors found was that after every cold—that is, every virus infection of the upper respiratory tract accompanied by sneezing, a running nose, and general but nonfeverish malaise—noses and throats became crowded with bacteria, notably pneumococci, streptococci, staphylococci, *Haemophilus influenzae* bacilli, *Neisseria catarrhalis,* and Friedländer's bacilli. This was widely but incorrectly interpreted to mean that these bacteria were, alone or in concert, the true causes of common colds.

During the first half of the twentieth century, stock bacterial vaccines were turned out and sold in large quantities for use against nearly all pathogenic bacteria, from the gonococci of gonorrhea and the streptococci of scarlet fever to any and all germs with the possible exception of the mycobacteria of tuberculosis. As early as 1910 these stock vaccines were in common use.[25] Fortunately, they were killed-organism vaccines, so that at least they could not reinfect anyone. They were often used as "anticatarrhal" agents and as antipneumonia or other specific bacterial disease vaccines. After World War I, because of the experiences of Spencer Lister and other doctors in South Africa who had continued the work begun by Almroth Wright in 1912, some of the stock pneumococcal pneumonia vaccines prepared in this country were even type-specific, which made them quite effective against single types of pneumococcal bacteria.

These stock vaccines, used alone or followed by autogenous vaccines made of killed bacteria recovered from the patients themselves, were given orally or by injection to cure people with colds or influenza, and also to members of their family and other close contacts to protect them from the same diseases.

Dr. Anna I. Von Sholly and her boss, Dr. William H. Park, at the New York City Board of Health Research Laboratory, on the heels of the 1918–1919 pandemic seized upon the idea of creating "a vaccine made of the mixed organisms which predominate in respiratory diseases, used as a prophylactic agent in epidemic 'grippe' [i.e., influenza] and acute respiratory diseases in general."[26]

Similar combination vaccines had been made and tested before, and others would follow for the next decade in America, Europe, and Japan. In each of them, the results were quite parallel to those that Sholly and Park, after testing their mixed-organism vaccine in 1,536 volunteers of all ages in 1919 and 1920, reported in the *Journal of Immunology* in 1921.

Two vaccines were used by Sholly and Park. The first, given to 1,412 male and female volunteers, was called Vaccine L, a saline suspension of cultures of six heat-killed bacteria: *Haemophilus influenzae*, hemolytic streptococci, *Streptococcus viridans*, and Types I, II, and III pneumococci. The other 124 volunteers were given Vaccine R. This was essentially the Mayo Clinic preparation of Types I, II, III, IV, "and allied green-producing" pneumococci, plus "diplostreptococci," hemolytic streptococci, *Staphylococci aureus*, and *H. influenzae*. The vaccines were administered at four-week intervals, starting in the last week of September 1919.

After six months of close clinical observation, during which a recurrent outbreak of influenza hit New York City, Sholly and Park reported that the results were not quite as promising as those of Park's first clinical trials of his diphtheria vaccines had been earlier.

"Among the inoculated, 13.7% gave a history of no respiratory infections during this time. Among the non-inoculated, 29.77% [more than twice as many people] gave a similar history." During the influenza outbreak, there was very little difference "in their respective degrees of immunity" between those who had and those who had not had the Sholly-Park mixed-organism vaccines. "One might infer," they wrote, in an understatement, "that it were wiser not to be inoculated."

However, their multivalent vaccines did seem to make a significant difference in only one disease: pneumococcal pneumonia. There had been only one case of pneumonia among the inoculated volunteers, and eleven pneumonia cases in the control population. Sholly and Park held that "it would seem fair to make some claims for the efficacy of a typed pneumo-streptococcus vaccine as a preventive of pneumonia," and they called for more research in this area. Otherwise, they agreed, "our evidence does not make a strong case in favor of the vaccines given by us as a prophylactic agent against acute respiratory diseases—pneumonia alone excepted."

Other clinical trials of similar vaccines showed, during the next twenty years of using bacterial vaccines against viral diseases, "that ordinary *stock* anticatarrhal bacterial vaccines diminished neither the frequency nor the severity of colds," wrote H. J. Parish. These failures finally eradicated whatever support remained for them in the scientific community. "However," observed Parish, who was both a physician and the director of a pharmaceutical company research laboratory, "the popular demand for various preparations was encouraged by reports of improvement or cure in individual cases—often an opportunity for exploitation by the uncritical (or unscrupulous) doctor or commercial firm!"[27]

There was simply no bacterial vaccine against the common cold. Nevertheless, as long as doctors and laymen alike persisted in believing that bacteria caused both colds and influenza, "anticatarrhal" bacterial vaccines of stock or their own (autogenous) bacteria continued to be shot into people. If, like most, they survived their colds or grippes, they willingly wrote glowing testimonials to the efficacy of stock and autogenous vaccines.

In our times, the evidence suggesting that "ordinary" and nonfebrile upper respiratory and nasopharyngeal viral infections lead to more serious bacterial and noninfective disorders has become overwhelming. All specialists in infectious diseases now accept, for example, that otitis media is a bacterial infection of the middle ear secondary to upper respiratory viral infections usually caused by adenoviruses, rhinoviruses, and Coxsackie and other viruses, but on occasion by hemolytic streptococci. A recent longitudinal study of respiratory diseases and their complications in children aged six weeks to eleven years at the University of North Carolina School of Medicine found 348 otitis media episodes during 339 child years, with 77 percent occurring in children under three. In this youngest group there were eight otitis media epidemics, and seven of these coincided with viral respiratory disease outbreaks.

To Dr. F. W. Henderson and his collaborators at Chapel Hill these data demonstrated "that otitis media is an epidemic complication of common respiratory viral infections in children below three years of age." One of his senior collaborators in the North Carolina study, Dr. Wallace A. Clyde, Jr., concluded that while penicillin and other antibiotics can cure streptococcal and other bacterial infections which follow upper respiratory virus infections in young children, "the primary causes of otitis are the respiratory viruses, and prevention will have to begin with vaccines against the most common of the respiratory viruses."[28]

A 1980 study conducted by Dr. Victor Fainstein and others at Baylor University in Waco, Texas, in pharyngeal (throat) cells from patients with naturally acquired acute respiratory illnesses and from volunteers experimentally infected with influenza virus vaccine showed that "infections with influenza virus predispose to secondary pneumonia due to *S. aureus, H. influenzae,* and *Streptococcus pneumoniae,* and infections with other respiratory viruses may also sometimes lead to secondary bacterial complications." The Baylor group suggested that one of the reasons for the increased adherence of pathogenic bacteria to the mucosa of the throat and nose might be the alterations virus infections cause in these tissues.[29]

The Epstein-Barr virus (EBV), one of the herpes viruses, is a classic example of the role of a single virus in more than one disease of people. The EBV is the known cause of infectious mononucleosis, and there is very good evidence linking it to two types of human cancers: Burkitt's lymphoma, a disease found largely in African children, and nasopharyngeal carcinoma, a cancer found primarily in Chinese adults.

For years it was believed that the Epstein-Barr virus was transmitted by mosquitoes, since Burkitt's lymphoma seemed to be found only in regions where malaria was endemic. Later it was found that this was only half true:

the mosquitoes were, as observed, related to the onset of Burkitt's lymphoma, but only in people who had previously or recently had malaria, which causes changes in body tissues and whose protozoan parasites are indeed vectored by mosquitoes. These changes are now believed to have enhanced the possibly carcinogenic effects of EBV particles found in children with Burkitt's lymphoma.

Many tumor viruses can, under laboratory conditions in which animals are inoculated with massive viral doses, cause lymphomas, leukemia, and sarcomas in mice, rats, gerbils, guinea pigs, and cats. Similar cancers can be induced in tumor-virus-free animals of the same species by massive doses of ionizing radiations, and by exposure to chemicals known to be carcinogenic. After the radiation-induced or chemically induced cancers appear, tumor viruses that were not previously present in their mature or virion forms suddenly appear in these animals. These "radiation viruses" and "chemical viruses" can in massive doses induce the same types of cancers in the same species of animals.

Experimental vaccines made of tumor viruses offer various levels of protection against cancers in animals. If and when similar viruses are ever found to cause cancers in people, such vaccines would become obvious models for vaccines against human cancers. What seems obvious, however, frequently turns out to be only partly, if at all, true.

Research at and supported by the National Cancer Institute during the past decade suggests now that when viruses cause cancer in bird and beast, they do not do so alone. It seems likely that tumor viruses, and many others not normally considered to be related to cancers, possibly combine their nucleic acids with the proviruses or uncoated nucleic acids of other viruses already present in a host body, and that these "recombined" viruses then proceed to play a primary or secondary causal role in the induction of cancers. If this does indeed turn out to be the case, then every virus will have to be seen as a potential cancer virus—and vaccines against known tumor viruses alone might not be enough to prevent cancers.

This also suggests that in 1908 when Wilhelm Ellerman and Oluf Bang in Denmark produced leukemias in hens with filtrates from the tissues of leukemic hens, the diseases they induced in healthy chickens were not solely due to the "organized virus" in those filtrates.

Their work was developed further by Peyton Rous (1879–1970) at the Rockefeller Institute in the chicken sarcoma named after him. For many years biologists who tried to duplicate Rous's work had very mixed results, as indeed did Rous himself. Then in 1961 Dr. Harry Rubin of the University of California at Berkeley showed that "at least some strains of Rous sarcoma virus (RSV) were defective"—that is, they could transform healthy cells, but these cells were unable to "issue infectious progeny without the help of a co-infecting helper virus from the avian leukosis group."[30] Rubin isolated such a helper virus, now named the Rous associated virus (RAV), and since then, when a combined RSV-RAV inoculant is added to a culture of chick-embryo cells, it not only transforms these cells, but the transformed cells then start to shed RSV-RAV particles that can infect other cells. In 1966 when he was eighty-seven, Peyton Rous was awared the Nobel Prize in medicine for his "discovery of the tumor-inducing viruses."

In 1957 at the British government's Medical Research Institute in London, the late Alick Isaacs and his collaborator, Jean Lindenmann, found in the tissues of bodies infected with influenza an interesting protein that appeared to be one of the human body's inborn means of curing influenza. They named it interferon. It had many interesting characteristics, the most notable being that when produced by animal and human cells after attacks by any disease viruses, it seemed to act against these and all other viruses that affect people.

During the decades that followed, interferon was found to have multiple biological effects other than its well-established antiviral activity. These included the inhibition of cell multiplication, which underscored interferon's potentials in the control and possibly even cure of cancerous tumors. From the start, however, it was interferon's antiviral function that attracted the most attention.

Its discovery inspired as many instant hopes for its use in treating and preventing all virus diseases as, a generation earlier, d'Herrelle's writings on his clinical work with bacteriophages had generated for the therapeutic and prophylactic uses of the viruses that killed only bacteria. These clinical hopes survived the early expectations that interferon combined, in one molecule, the specific pathogen-killing capability of Ehrlich's Salvarsan and later chemical Magic Bullets, such as the antibiotics, with the long-term immunizing powers Jenner and his successors had provided in their Magic Shots—the vaccines against specific mass crippling and killing virus diseases from smallpox to polio.

Many ill-conceived attempts to use crude and inappropriate interferon preparations against the common cold, influenza, and other viral diseases turned the early years into a time when "much second-class research was carried out with third-class preparations slightly contaminated with interferon."[31] One of the primary reasons interferon survived the initial inferior studies, let alone the wild claims made for it in the mass media and in popular science fiction, was that from the moment it was discovered, various responsible governmental and private research institutions sponsored and funded intelligently planned investigations of its antiviral and cell-regulating activities.

Among the earliest of these more responsible studies was the one started by Dr. Ion Gresser at the French government's Institute for Scientific Research in Cancer at Villejuif, which showed that interferon acted to slow the course of leukemia in mice. Over the next two decades, other scientists in Europe, Israel, and the United States were able to repeat Gresser's work with interferon against animal cancers and ultimately even human cancers.[32]

From the beginning, in the late 1950s the United States government's investments in interferon research were channeled primarily through the National Institutes of Health (NIH). The National Institute of Allergy and Infectious Diseases (NIAID) got into interferon research first, while the National Cancer Institute (NCI) began work a few years later.

To date, the federal government has invested around $15 million in laboratory and clinical interferon investigations. In 1978 Dr. Frank J. Rauscher, Jr., discoverer of the Rauscher mouse leukemia virus, resigned as director of the National Cancer Institute and joined the American Cancer Society (ACS) as senior vice-president in charge of research. Largely at his urging, the ACS committed more than six million dollars to fund large-scale multi-university clinical studies of interferon in the treatment of cancer.

During the years since Isaacs and Lindenmann first described interferon's medical potentials, researchers in many laboratories began to make interferon-containing preparations by adding viruses to broth cultures of human leukocytes and to cultures of human fibroblast, placental, and foreskin tissues. These human cell-synthesized interferon preparations were tested against many disease viruses and also against different cancers. At Stanford University, California, for example, Dr. Thomas Merrigan used a leukocyte interferon preparation to protect children being treated with immunosuppressive chemotherapy for leukemia against chicken pox—the most frequently reported virus infection in the United States and, next to gonorrhea, the second most frequently reported notifiable disease.

Others here and abroad have reported clinical situations in which interferon seemed to act against osteosarcoma and other forms of human cancers. In 1981 a two-year controlled study led by Dr. Lawrence Jacobs in Buffalo, New York, showed that when both the diagnosis of multiple sclerosis and interferon treatment were initiated early enough, the combination prevented further nervous-system deterioration in ten patients. Like most cancers, multiple sclerosis is not presently classified as a virus disease.

A few years after it was discovered, it was found that interferon, which in nature is synthesized by all mammalian cells in response to viral invasion, can also be produced by people in response to inoculations of double-stranded RNA and other compounds. At the time it was hoped that such interferon inducers would soon enable people to produce all the extra interferon they needed whenever they were exposed to or infected by disease viruses. These early expectations were soon shattered by the toxic side effects produced by all the interferon inducers developed to date.

A more far-reaching body of discoveries—which won the 1980 Nobel Prize in chemistry for Drs. Paul Berg, Walter Gilbert, and Frederick Sanger—

led to new recombinant DNA or gene-splicing techniques that would significantly improve interferon's qualities and increase its availability, and just as markedly reduce its costs of production and purchase.

In the recombinant DNA techniques, an enzyme is used to separate from human leukocytes the specific segments of human chromosomal DNA containing the genes that direct the white blood cells to produce interferon. While this is being done, other workers remove the plasmids, or nonchromosomal gene-carrying structures, from the viscous cytoplasm within the common single-celled gut bacteria, *E. coli*. Then other enzymes are used to incorporate the human interferon genes into the bacterial plasmids. The altered plasmids then are inserted back into the bacterial cells.

As the "genetically engineered" *E. coli* cells reproduce, many (but not all) of them begin, under the influence of the human interferon genes in their plasmids, to produce interferon almost identical to that produced by human cells. These interferons produced by the "brainwashed" *E. coli* can be harvested and used in people with virus diseases and cancers.

New "genetic engineering" companies quickly came forward to develop and refine the techniques of producing recombinant DNA interferons in industrial quantities. They soon joined forces with giant American and European pharmaceutical manufacturers, who had the technical and engineering resources to undertake the mass production of recombinant interferon, and who have to date invested over $200 million in production facilities. At present, industrial interferon is being produced only in broth colonies of *E. coli*, but it will soon be commercially produced in other bacteria and even in yeast cells.

Until 1981 clinical studies in sick people were made primarily with interferons produced by adding viruses to cell cultures of human leukocytes. The resulting product, termed "leukocyte interferon," is only about 1/1,000 of 1 percent pure interferon. By contrast, recombinant interferon produced by combining the nucleic acids in bacterial plasmids with the DNA of the specific human genes that cause human leukocytes to make interferon enables the violated and altered bacterial cells to synthesize interferon that subsequently can be made 90 percent to 98 percent pure.

At present, a single genetically manipulated liter of bacterial colonies in nutrient broth can synthesize between two hundred and four hundred million units of at least 90 percent pure interferon. While the yields of recombinant production techniques are much higher than those of leukocyte interferons made in human cells, the costs are considerably lower. Instead of a course of leukocyte interferon treatments of a single cancer patient costing up to $30,000, by early 1982 it cost between $200 and $300 to treat a cancer patient with a full course of recombinant interferon—and with much purer and more potent interferon at that.

When leukocyte interferons were used, patients were given up to nine million units of 1/1,000 of 1 percent pure interferon daily. By the end of 1981 the 90 percent pure recombinant interferons were being administered in doses of two hundred million units per patient per day.

The coordinated trials of interferon in human cancers organized by the American Cancer Society were undertaken to learn two things. The first was whether interferon was as active against human cancers here as it was reported to be by reputable centers in Finland, Sweden, France, Yugoslavia, and England.

The initial ACS clinical trials were made in four forms of cancers—breast cancer, multiple myeloma, non-Hodgkins lymphomas, and melanomas. Leukocyte interferon used against the first three forms of human cancers yielded positive results, but only in about 15 percent of the melanoma patients treated. Positive results in this study were defined as reductions of 50 percent or more of tumor mass. These results obtained with leukocyte interferon were so encouraging that by October 1981, two additional forms of cancer—nasopharyngeal carcinoma and kidney carcinoma—were added to the ACS interferon study.

During the same year, Hoffman-LaRoche Inc., one of the major manufacturers of recombinant DNA interferon, started to provide five of the universities participating in this study with the newer and more potent form.

The other scientific aim of the entire project was to learn something about the pharmacokinetics of interferon in cancers. "In other words," Rauscher explains, "to learn, among other things we presently do not know: how much interferon do you give? When do you stop giving it? How long do the effects of interferon last against specific forms of cancer? Why does it work? How does it work? Might it be more effective in combination with other drugs as some doctors now suggest? How can you tell if a given cancer patient's tumor is going to respond to interferon? And, perhaps the most important question of all, how to profile the individual patient—chemically, immunologically, biologically—before putting that individual on interferon?"[33]

None of these basic questions has yet been answered. Nor, to date, have this and other clinical trials either proven or disproved the worth of interferons as anticancer substances. However, around the world most tests of interferon in cancer patients have shown that it also acts against disease viruses already present in their bodies or in their immediate environments. At the Karolinska Hospital in Stockholm, Sweden, for example, Dr. Hans Strander's studies of lymphocyte interferon in patients with osteosarcoma have shown that patients receiving interferon injections thrice weekly "have had fewer respiratory infections than other members of their families."[34] In the ACS studies of leukocyte interferon and human cancers in the United States, it was determined that interferon acted against various virus diseases present in the bodies of the same patients.

The medical and social implications of these findings are multiple. Unlike the antitoxins or immune sera used against specific bacterial and viral diseases, the interferons act against a wide array of disease viruses. In this respect, they are more like antibiotics, which act against broad spectra of bacterial organisms. Finally, like antibiotics against bacteria and immune sera against specific infections, interferon can treat and help reverse virus diseases—but it cannot induce long-term immunity against them.

Moreover, again like immune sera and rabies vaccines, interferon must be used very early in the course of a viral infection, generally during the first three or four days of the infection itself. As in the serologic treatment and prevention of symptomatic diphtheria, tetanus, pneumonia, rabies, and measles, the actual worth of interferon in the health of any nation will be determined by the structure, quality, and above all the sheer dimensions of its health-care delivery systems.

In cancers, as in virus diseases, timing is all-important, calling for early, possibly even presymptomatic diagnoses of cancers and virus diseases known to be susceptible to interferons and other therapies. This, in turn, would make it possible to start interferon therapy during the brief time when it can be most effective. The current dogma that we now have too many doctors, and that there is no longer any need to waste government funds to train more physicians, is a perilous self-delusion. It is not only untrue today, but the present cutbacks and/or termination of long-established federal programs to educate and train more physicians will deprive millions of Americans of the potential benefits of interferon in the control of most virus diseases and, possibly, of some forms of cancer.

Whether safe and effective interferons, produced and sold at low cost, prove capable of curing virus diseases and even some forms of cancer remains to be determined. What now seems certain, however, is that since most of the drugs and chemicals that can destroy viruses are equally devastating to human genetic materials, we are not about to see any great outpouring of systemic antiviral drugs analogous to the explosion of post-World War II antibiotics that made previously incurable and fatal bacterial pestilences eminently curable.

By 1976 when Dr. John V. Bennett and his colleagues at the Centers for Disease Control made their study of infectious disease deaths in the United States, viruses were responsible for only 14 percent of all such deaths. The major reasons for this low post-World War II proportion of virus disease deaths included the safe and effective vaccines developed and used on a mass scale against what had been from 1954 to 1968, widespread, noncurable, and nonpreventable crippling and killing virus infections, starting with the poliomyelitis vaccines that would rid our country and other affluent nations of infantile paralysis in less than a decade of intensive use.

As we shall see in the next chapters, some of these new, life-enhancing vaccines were made of viruses that had not even been discovered prior to 1950.

271

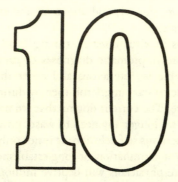

C H A P T E R

TRAGEDY AND TRIUMPH:
THE PREMATURE POLIO VACCINES
AND THE BIRTH OF
MODERN MEDICAL VIROLOGY

Dr. James P. Leake (addressing Dr. John A. Kolmer): I beg you to desist from the human use of this vaccine.

Dr. John A. Kolmer (rising to respond): Gentlemen, this is one time I wish the floor would open up and swallow me.

—Floor discussion, American Public Health
Association meeting, 1935

272

Only three safe and effective vaccines against virus diseases were created before modern medical virology emerged as a scientific discipline after World War II.

The first, Jenner's 1796 cowpox vaccine against smallpox, was the work of an acutely observant English country doctor who knew neither cell theory, germ theory, immunology, genetics, nor immunochemistry. Nor did Jenner or his medical contemporaries have the slightest inkling that his vaccine worked because the separate viruses of cowpox and smallpox were antigenically both cross-reactive and cross-protective. Jenner was not aware of even the rudiments of virology, which, like germ theory and the other basic theories of microbiology, were elaborated long after his death in 1823.

For all its early and still existing shortcomings, the Jenner vaccine ultimately eradicated smallpox. Today, thanks largely to the proper use of this vaccine by responsible governments, smallpox immunizations are neither necessary nor even medically desirable.

The second good vaccine against a virus disease was the one against rabies Pasteur developed by 1884 and used for the first time in a human being in 1885—nearly a century after Jenner first used his cowpox vaccine to immunize a human being against smallpox.

When Pasteur started to work on rabies, it was a 100 percent fatal disease. He learned how to identify and isolate rabbit spinal tissue bearing the rabies virus. He also learned how to attenuate and fix the virulence of the rabies viruses by repeated passages of virus-laden saliva from the mouths of rabid dogs through the brains of rabbits, followed by aging of the infected rabbit tissues. Graded doses of emulsions of infected rabbit spinal-cord tissues, ranging from fully attenuated to fully virulent, were then given in a series of vaccinations to people bitten by rabid animals. Pasteur's boyhood observations of the long incubation period of this disease agent enabled him to take advantage of the ten to 180 days' incubation period to neutralize the rabies virus before it caused a fatal case of hydrophobia.

Rabies (hydrophobia) is still a 100 percent fatal disease—but only if antirabies vaccines are not used in time to prevent the disease from developing after someone is bitten by a rabid animal. Thanks to Pasteur's vaccine and improved modern successors, hydrophobia is no longer a significant cause of death in industrial nations with acceptable health-care-delivery systems.

Max Theiler (1899–1972), of the Rockefeller Institute, who created the third premodern effective virus vaccine, the 17D-strain live virus vaccine against yellow fever in 1936, knew a thousand times more about viruses than Jenner and Pasteur combined. From Pasteur, Theiler took the technique of attenuating viruses from sick people by passing them through the brain tissues of other animals—in this instance, mice. The yellow fever viruses that Theiler passaged, attenuated, and fixed in their altered forms by Pasteur's cross-species technique were changed to the point where they no longer produced yellow fever but did induce the production of antibodies against wild and virulent yellow fever viruses. The electronic and optical techniques that within a decade would make viruses visible were not yet developed when Theiler created his vaccine. Originally, this vaccine was used to protect laboratory and hospital workers exposed to yellow fever viruses. Theiler himself developed yellow fever in the course of his work with laboratory cultures of its virus.

Thanks to the investigators who followed Pasteur, Theiler knew a great deal about viruses. By 1936, because of studies conducted by his Rockefeller Institute colleague Wendell Stanley, and as a result of the work done by Frederick Bawden, Norman Pirie, J. D. Bernald, and Isadore Fankuchen in England, Theiler knew that viruses could be chemically reduced to nucleoprotein crystals, and that "nucleic acid of the ribose type [RNA] could be isolated from these crystals." The work of Oswald Avery and other Rockefeller Institute colleagues on the role of nucleic acids in heredity would not be published for another eight years, but Theiler knew in 1936 that dilutions of the nucleoprotein crystals derived from tobacco mosaic viruses could, when applied to the leaves of healthy tobacco plants, cause tobacco mosaic virus disease. More than that, he was also aware that tobacco plants given tobacco mosaic virus disease by these dilutions then started to replicate fully infective mature virus particles equally capable of infecting healthy plants.

During World War II, Theiler's 17D live yellow fever vaccine was to spare the lives of thousands of American servicemen at immediate risk of yellow fever in tropical and subtropical theaters of war in Asia, Latin America, Africa, New Guinea, and elsewhere.

The 1936 yellow fever vaccine was far more sophisticated than Jenner's arm-to-arm smallpox vaccine. Theiler's viruses were not only attenuated and fixed, they were also grown in sophisticated tissue cultures.

On the eve of World War II, the Rockefeller Institute set out to conquer yellow fever in Brazil by use of the vaccine Theiler had developed in its laboratories. The Institute's vaccine-production group seeded hatching hens' eggs with fixed yellow fever viruses grown in tissue cultures. After a week of incubation, the chick embryos were removed and finely minced, and normal human blood serum was added to the mixture. This mixture of ground infected chick-embryo tissues and human blood serum was then centrifuged and the separated fluids were filtered. The resulting filtrates became the vaccines.

The Rockefeller Institute vaccine worked as well against yellow fever as Jenner's did against smallpox. However, it was not long before it was found that, like Jenner's arm-to-arm lymphs, the yellow fever vaccine also at times transmitted the agent of at least one other disease—hepatitis, or yellow jaundice. More than a million Brazilians had been vaccinated against yellow fever with the 17D vaccine before local doctors began to report outbreaks of yellow jaundice or hepatitis following vaccination. Not every batch of vaccine caused hepatitis, but there were enough cases for the Rockefeller Institute to order research on serum-free vaccines, since it seemed likely that the hepatitis agents came from the human blood serum used in the production of the vaccine.

When America's entrance into the war became imminent, the Institute undertook to supply, at no charge, all the yellow fever vaccine the armed forces would require. To save the time it would take to run massive field tests of the serum-free vaccine developed at the Institute, it was decided to make the vaccine with human sera supplied by healthy blood donors obtained through medical agencies. In Baltimore the professor of bacteriology at the Johns Hopkins School of Hygiene and Public Health, Dr. Thomas C. Turner, suggested that the medical students, interns, nurses, and laboratory workers at Hopkins would make a very healthy cohort of paid blood donors, and this suggestion was quickly accepted.

Theiler, alerted by the Brazilian hepatitis side-effect data, warned Dr. William Sawyer, who was in charge of the vaccine program at the Institute: "You are courting disaster." His prediction was not long in materializing. In March 1942 a hundred cases of hepatitis following yellow fever vaccination were reported from training camps in California. Similar reports soon began to pour in from other military installations here and abroad. During 1942 in all American military bases (30 percent of them overseas), there were nearly 50,000 cases of both infectious and what then became known as "serum hepatitis," and eighty-four were fatal. Midway through that year, the Rockefeller Institute stopped making yellow fever vaccine with human sera.

This experience showed that not only could human blood sera transmit the virus of serum hepatitis, but also that apparently healthy human carriers—such as the medical students and nurses at Hopkins whose sera was used in some batches of yellow fever vaccine—could transmit active hepatitis viruses to others via serum-based vaccines, blood transfusions, and other interchanges. It also revealed that there are at least two types of hepatitis—infectious and serum.

Smallpox, rabies, and yellow fever share a trait common to all major virus diseases: With few possible exceptions, none have ever been cured by potions, drugs, or elixirs made by people. Not that doctors have ever lacked for virus disease cures, from the tasty but medically useless fruit and vegetable extracts Thomas Sydenham (1624-1689) used for measles, to the highly toxic compounds of antimony and mercury that Hermann Boerhaave (1668-1738) prescribed for smallpox, to the debilitating and often fatal calomel (mercurous chloride) purges and massive bleedings Benjamin Rush (1745-1813) inflicted upon hundreds of victims of the great yellow fever epidemic in Philadelphia in 1793, some seventeen years after Rush put his signature on the Declaration of Independence. All these putative remedies for virus infections had their medical supporters; they each evoked glowing testimonials from laymen and physicians who took them and lived to tell the tale; none worked against any viruses, and some even caused otherwise preventable deaths.

During the Great Depression of 1929-1940, Franklin Delano Roosevelt was elected President of the United States in 1932. Roosevelt, an inheritor of vast wealth, had been paralyzed from the waist down by acute poliomyelitis since 1921. When he became President, he proved to be acutely sensitive to the human suffering of the millions of innocent victims of the gross mismanagement of the national economy that culminated in the stock market crash of 1929 and the resultant economic collapse. Roosevelt promised the victims jobs, and he created millions of them, administered by new federal public works agencies, such as the Civilian Conservation Corps, the Federal Theater Project, and the Work Projects Administration (WPA).

None of these New Deal programs really ended the economic crisis, but they and the President who created them gave millions of salvaged American families the great human gift of hope. Growing numbers of people sought some nonpolitical ways of thanking the popular President, and many were soon to find one such way in a public crusade to conquer paralytic poliomyelitis.

In 1927 during his own physical rehabilitation from polio, Roosevelt had established the Georgia Warm Springs Foundation to help individuals obtain rehabilitative treatment for paralytic polio, and to disseminate clinical information about the newest therapeutic and rehabilitative techniques to hospitals and private physicians. Two years later the New York philanthropist Jeremiah Milbank set up a fund of $250,000 for the study of the natural history of poliomyelitis. Milbank selected a small group of doctors and microbiologists, headed by Dr. William Hallock Park—who was then leading the successful effort to eradicate diphtheria—to conduct basic research on poliomyelitis.

After Roosevelt was inaugurated in 1933, some of his admirers organized a series of national Presidential Birthday Balls to raise money for his

Warm Springs Foundation. A special scientific advisory board of the President's Birthday Ball Committee (PBBC)—headed by the microbiologist and popular science writer Dr. Paul de Kruif—started to provide seed grants to different scientific investigators of polio. De Kruif, a man of many scientific enthusiasms, was convinced that only proper diet could both prevent and cure paralytic poliomyelitis.

In 1938 the Birthday Ball Committee was supplanted by the National Foundation for Infantile Paralysis (NFIP), headed by Basil O'Connor, the former law partner of Franklin Roosevelt. The Foundation soon became better known as the March of Dimes.

Throughout the darkest and bitterest years of the Great Depression, which at its peak saw twenty million unemployed Americans, people gravitated to the Stygian and anonymous comforts of their neighborhood movie theaters and the double-feature dreamworlds they opened up to all who had the price of admission. Periodically, in these Cathedrals of the Common Man, a third film, produced by either the PBBC or the NFIP, would be shown between the two feature films. This production was a ten-minute tearjerker, narrated by a reigning movie star, in which viewers were shown children paralyzed by polio being kept alive in coffin-like Drinker mechanical respirators—the iron lungs—while other paralyzed children were fitted with leg braces and trained to walk. There were scenes of polio research conducted in microbiology laboratories, and of doctors and nurses being trained in the rehabilitation of polio victims.

As the film ended, the movie star narrator would be shown in a pediatric polio ward, patting the paralyzed children and staring directly into the moist eyes of every person in the audience. Her voice, her nostrils, her entire body quivering, she would inform her viewers that the medical care, the iron lungs, the braces, and above all the scientific research on vaccines that would prevent paralytic polio were all paid for by the billions of dimes contributed by ordinary and often very poor people like the lucky men, women, and children listening to her voice. The lights would come up, and ushers would pass up and down the aisles with jingling collection cans.

The responses of simple people in movie audiences to these appeals often took on a very political character. Millions in those days were employed in the New Deal public works programs. Their jobs were funded from tax revenues, and to make such programs feasible, the Roosevelt administration had materially raised the income tax rates on high-middle-income and millionaire-income levels. These income tax increases made Roosevelt less popular among members of the nation's solvent minority than paralytic poliomyelitis itself. Many individuals in the higher tax brackets took to organizing expeditions to the newsreel and ordinary movie theaters for the express purpose of hissing "That Man!" The March of Dimes collections gave the President's supporters a heartfelt way of replying to the hissing parties.

The dimes added up to millions of dollars, as did the larger contributions made by people who could afford to give more. Many of these funds were spent by the NFIP on polio vaccine research at a time when the federal treasury was too drained to support biomedical research and experiment.

In a real sense, our current poliovirus vaccines represent a solid bridge between the old and the modern eras in medical virology.

Two very important facts about poliomyelitis were established very early in this century.

As early as 1908 in Vienna, the protean Karl Landsteiner (1868–1943) caused paralytic polio in a laboratory monkey by injecting the animal with an emulsion of the spinal cord tissues of a child who had died of polio. This proved what many had long suspected: that poliomyelitis was a transmissible infectious disease. Landsteiner then showed what was not known before: Polio is a virus disease. He did this by inducing paralytic polio in monkeys by inoculating them with germ-free filtrates of dilutions of tissues from people with active cases of the disease. Viruses pass easily through filters fine enough to block the passage of bacteria.

Landsteiner's findings were universally accepted.

The second major set of findings about the natural history of poliomyelitis were reported and abundantly documented in Sweden in 1911, during the largest polio epidemic in the history of medicine at the time. These findings dealt with the epidemiology of poliomyelitis and the routes by which its virus is normally transmitted. Unfortunately, they were not highly regarded by most of the world's polio researchers for over a generation.

By 1911 work conducted by Drs. Simon Flexner and Paul Lewis at the Rockefeller Institute in New York had repeated and amplified Landsteiner's original findings. Landsteiner had caused polio in monkeys by inoculating his germ-free polio tissue filtrates into the peritoneal cavity, the abdominal area bounded by the peritoneum, which is the tough membrane surrounding the liver, stomach, colon, and small intestine. The Rockefeller Institute investigators also used the intraperitoneal route, but they added other pathways of infection, causing polio in monkeys with tissues taken from the spinal cords of polio patients, and also by inoculating the animals with filtered nose and throat washings of polio patients.

Their results convinced Flexner and his coworkers that polioviruses entered the human body through the nose and throat, and that poliomyelitis was a serious disease confined solely to the central nervous system in the human body. They were equally certain that it would be only a matter of a short time before family doctors would have the means of preventing and curing paralytic poliomyelitis, or infantile paralysis as it was usually called then.

The Rockefeller Institute issued a press release in the spring of 1911, in which Flexner was quoted as declaring: "We have already discovered how to prevent the disease, and the achievement of a cure, I may conservatively say, is not far distant." The same press release said that this meant within six months.

Three days later on March 12, 1911, *The New York Times* ran a long interview with Flexner in which he declared, "Infantile paralysis is a germ disease that attacks the spinal marrow and the brain, and merely by injuring or by totally destroying the delicate tissues causes either a temporary or a permanent paralysis of the muscles." Flexner went on to explain, according to the *Times,* that "the germ of infantile paralysis enters the brain and spinal cord chiefly, if not exclusively, by way of the nasal passages. 'In the course of the disease,' he said, 'the germ is also thrown off from the brain through the nose and mouth.' "

The prestige of the Institute and its investigators was so great that for the next four decades, paralytic poliomyelitis, or infantile paralysis, was believed by most workers to be a disease caused by a respiratory virus that entered the human body through the nose and then headed straight for the central nervous system. This meant that it was also a neurotropic virus; that is, a virus with a tendency to be attracted to the cells of nervous tissues. Although widely accepted, this dogma was not a fact but a very tragic error.

In 1911 when the great polio outbreak erupted in Sweden, the government's State Bacteriological Institute assigned the task of helping cure and prevent infantile paralysis to a three-doctor group headed by a twenty-four-year-old recent medical school graduate, Carl Kling (1887–1967). The other two doctors, the urban sanitarian Alfred Pettersson and the pediatrician Wilhelm Wernstedt, were considerably older but no less energetic than Kling.

Together, they repeated all the work published by Flexner and Lewis. However, they also isolated enough poliovirus from the intestinal walls and contents from patients with polio and healthy members of their families (as well as from healthy people who had had no contacts with polio patients) to report that it was not exclusively a respiratory virus. On the contrary, their clinical viral isolates entered the body through the gastrointestinal system and did not usually travel from the gut to the spinal nerves.

The Swedish group's findings suggested that the poliovirus was not a respiratory but an enteric virus present in the food and water people ate and drank. Once in the human gut, the poliovirus probably caused a mild, subclinical infection—not severe enough to cause paralysis but sufficient to immunize people against further polio infections. After this, the poliovirus passed from the body in excreta.

Furthermore, according to Wernstedt, since the poliovirus seemed to paralyze primarily young children, and since older members of the family seemed immune to polio infections despite the presence of the virus in their guts and feces, this indicated that in modern industrialized environments, most children acquired immunity to the infection long before they entered school. It also meant that the immunity produced by subclinical polio infections was permanent. Far from being an infrequently epidemic neurologic disease, then, poliomyelitis was a very common or endemic and innocuous enteric disease that on rare occasions spread to the central nervous system and caused paralysis. It was only the children without naturally acquired immunity who got poliomyelitis, and in only a few of the infected children did the poliovirus travel to the brain or the spinal cord or the major nerves and cause paralysis or death.

It must be remembered that this was not a clever speculation but a working hypothesis supported by more than ample clinical findings in thousands of polio victims, their closest contacts, and their nonrelated, noninfected neighbors. Nevertheless, these findings and the conclusions made by Kling and his coinvestigators were pretty well ignored by the scientific and medical worlds.

When the Swedish group presented their work at the Fifteenth International Congress on Hygiene and Demography in Washington in 1912, "their report," John R. Paul wrote, "was somewhat overshadowed by a spectacular announcement which stole the show. The rival presentation was by two Harvard professors who had carried out experiments that were supposed to prove that poliomyelitis was an insect-born disease transmitted by the common stable fly! This news was apparently greeted at the convention with a tremendous ovation."[1]

The echoes of this ovation had barely receded into eternal silence before two Public Health Service doctors completely exonerated the common stable fly of this crime of transmission. Nevertheless, for the next thirty-eight years, or for just as long as microbiologists continued to believe that the poliovirus was neurotropic and respiratory in nature, the agent of poliomyelitis continued to be grown only in the spines, brains, and other neural tissues of expensive monkeys in most of the world's polio research laboratories. While this erroneous neurotropic dogma reigned, various major epidemics of paralytic polio broke out in, among other places, New York and the northeastern states in 1916 and again in 1931, in Philadelphia in 1932, and in Los Angeles in 1934.

In 1931 a British-born, Montreal-educated young doctor, Maurice Brodie (1903–1939), published an article on the active immunization of monkeys against poliomyelitis in the prestigious *Journal of Experimental Medicine,* a publication of the Rockefeller Institute. In the article he described experiments he had conducted at McGill University with live virus vaccines, and with combinations of these vaccines and hyperimmune sera from convalescent polio patients. This article was read by William H. Park, who quickly offered young Brodie a dual appointment on the faculty of the New York University medical school, and in the New York City Health Department Research Laboratories. Brodie left Montreal to accept both jobs, and Park was instrumental in getting him grants from the New York Foundation and the Rockefeller Foundation to expand his work on a polio vaccine. During the Great Depression, new paying academic jobs and research grants were rarer than hens' teeth—but new polio vaccines were even rarer.

Park, the honored conqueror of diphtheria and a lifelong bachelor, was one of millions of American parents, victims, family doctors, health officers and clinical investigators who bore the lifelong mental scars of the 1916 polio epidemic, the worst ever suffered in American history. He saw in Brodie's early work a chance to settle his old scores with poliomyelitis, to render it as preventable as his earlier vaccine for diphtheria had made that once major cause of death in this country.[2]

The events that followed the collaboration between Park and Brodie would be closely observed by two young members of the NYU-Bellevue Hospital community. The older of the two, Albert Sabin, was born in Russian Poland in 1906 and had lived through World War I, the postwar pogroms, and the Russian Revolution before arriving in New York as a fifteen-year-old immigrant in 1921—three years before the anti-Semitic racial quotas of the U.S. Immigration Act of 1924 would have barred him, as a racially undesirable alien, from entering the United States. He was at an impressionable age when he arrived, and one of the American institutions that was to influence him most was Paul de Kruif's *Microbe Hunters,* published when Sabin was twenty and a student at the New York University dental school. As with many young people during the 1920s, Sabin was inspired by de Kruif's overly romantic but stimulating sagas of Pasteur, Koch, Metchnikoff, Walter Reed, Paul Ehrlich, and their peers to seek a place for himself in their ranks.

Sabin transferred to the New York University medical school, from which he graduated in 1931, at which point Park hired him as a research assistant in the school's bacteriology laboratory. He held this job for the next three years, while he completed his internship and residency at adjacent Bellevue Hospital. In 1934 after a few months of postresidency training at the Lister Institute of Preventive Medicine in London, Sabin took a job at the Rockefeller Institute, where he worked under Peter Olitsky, a noted and talented polio researcher. By then Sabin was a published author of journal articles, his first one in 1931 having been on poliomyelitis.

Jonas Salk, the other member of the NYU-Bellevue community to have been touched by the Park-Brodie vaccine experiments, had been born in 1914 in the Bronx to a Russian-Jewish immigrant tailor and his immigrant wife. Salk was still in high school when Sabin earned his M.D. in 1931. It was not until Salk entered New York University as a liberal arts major that he discovered the sciences in his course work, and quickly decided to study medicine. Like Sabin, he managed to squeeze through the Jewish admissions quota and entered the New York University medical school in 1934. After taking a year's leave to study chemistry, Salk took his M.D. at the age of twenty-four in 1939.

By July 1934 Brodie had abandoned his earlier effort to make a live poliovirus vaccine and had turned out a formalin-inactivated, or killed-virus, vaccine. He and Park had tested it first on themselves, for safety, and then on a half-dozen other human volunteers at NYU-Bellevue.

Such tests, for safety alone, are required today by federal regulations during the first clinical stage of the testing of any new vaccine, but they must be run in far greater numbers of people and only after the vaccine is initially tested in more than one species of animals. When it is clear that the experimental vaccine neither harms nor kills animals or people, only then is it injected to determine if and in what quantities the safe vaccine preparation causes them to produce antibodies against the antigens of the virus or bacterium in the vaccine. If the vaccine proves to be safe and adequately immunogenic—that is, able to cause the recipients to produce antibodies against its antigens—it is then challenged with doses of bacteria, viruses, or other pathogens, first in animals and then in people. If the vaccine comes through all these tests with good marks, long-term trials are conducted in animals and people to determine the duration of antibody production and active immunity in those vaccinated.

Only after all these time-consuming preliminary trials are completed is the new vaccine approved by the Food and Drug Administration (FDA), through its Bureau of Biologics, for testing in large numbers of people of both sexes and all ages. These life-protective federal regulations did not exist in 1934 and 1935.

Brodie tested his inactivated poliovirus vaccine on twenty monkeys. After testing it on himself and his colleagues, in 1934 Park informed the newspapers that the vaccine, known as the Park-Brodie vaccine, was perfectly safe and presented no dangers.

Two days later, Dr. John A. Kolmer, director of the private Dermatological Research Laboratory in Philadelphia, called his own press conference to announce that he had developed and tested successfully, on forty-two monkeys, himself, his two children, and twenty-two other children a chemically attenuated live poliovirus vaccine. The chemical used to alter his live attenuated polioviruses was ricin, a poison found in castor oil plants. The safety of his vaccine, Kolmer said, derived not from the addition of sodium ricinoleate, but was "largely due to the fact that it is prepared from remote monkey passage virus that has apparently lost infectivity for human beings, just as the smallpox virus is changed by passage through the lower animals." (Many doctors at that time shared Kolmer's mistaken belief that the cowpox virus was merely an attenuated, fixed form of the smallpox virus.)

By the end of 1935, Brodie and his coworkers had injected his formalin-killed poliovirus vaccine into 3,000 New York City children. Before the year was over, 10,000 children in various sections of the country had been injected with the Park-Brodie formalin-inactivated polio vaccine, and 12,000 children had received the attenuated live poliovirus vaccine developed by Kolmer. In June of that year, Brodie, Park, and Kolmer presented reports on their results to date at the Eighty-sixth Annual Meeting of the American Medical Association in Atlantic City, New Jersey.

The joint Brodie-Park paper noted that "convalescent serum is inefficacious in the treatment of preparalytic poliomyelitis," since "poliomyelitis is an infection of the central nervous system exclusively," and that the serum could never reach the well-insulated cells of the nervous system. This meant that "the best means of combating the disease seems to be in the form of a vaccine."[3]

As of that meeting, they said, their formalin-inactivated poliovirus vaccine had been given, in either one or two doses, to 2,300 people, and had caused no deaths or polio infections. Kolmer reported, "Sodium ricinoleate vaccine has now been given to more than 400 children in Philadelphia during the past year with absolutely no ill effects, and enough for the immunization of 2000 individuals has been distributed."

A few weeks later, in a pair of contiguous papers in the *New York State Journal of Medicine* of August 15, 1935, Brodie and Park continued to report successes with their polio vaccine. They insisted that "there is only one strain of [polio] virus. Thus an effective vaccine should protect against any poliomyelitis infection." In the second paper, published under Park's name alone, he declared that "there is no reason to fear that the strains of virus from various cases differ from each other sufficiently to lessen the value of vaccination."[4]

Park was wrong. Brodie was wrong. Kolmer was wrong. Even before Park's article was published, doctors around the country were reporting attacks of paralytic polio in children immunized with the formalin-inactivated, and the ricin-treated and attenuated live poliovirus vaccines of 1935. An investigation headed by Dr. James P. Leake of the U.S. Public Health Service soon found that "paralytic poliomyelitis was not epidemic in any of the localities at the time of the outbreak of these cases." Leake reported that twelve people vaccinated with either the Park-Brodie or the Kolmer vaccine had developed paralytic poliomyelitis. Six of these twelve people had died. Leake minced no words: He blamed the vaccines for the deaths.[5]

Given the large numbers of children who did not develop polio after being vaccinated with either the Park-Brodie or the Kolmer vaccine, these cases could have been incubating prior to the time of vaccination—or the unharmed children, prior to being vaccinated, could have had and recovered from subclinical infections with the strain or strains of poliovirus in both vaccines and were already immune to them. However, Dr. Thomas Rivers, at the

Rockefeller Institute, showed that the Park-Brodie vaccine induced little or no protective antibodies in monkeys, and that large doses of the Kolmer live virus vaccine actually caused paralytic polio in laboratory monkeys.

There was still a third possibility, which in the absence of later precise knowledge of the existence and prevalence of specific types of polioviruses was understandably not considered in 1935. It is highly possible that both vaccines contained only ubiquitous Type I polioviruses, which caused most polio infections—and that both of the 1935 polio vaccines were quite effective against this most dominant strain or type. The two premature vaccines might actually have immunized thousands of children and adults who were still susceptible to Type I polioviruses, and the postvaccinal infections that did develop in twelve of the more than 23,000 people inoculated with the Park-Brodie and Kolmer vaccines might have been caused by the less common types of polio viruses that had not been incorporated into the vaccines.

At a meeting of the American Public Health Association in St. Louis, Missouri, at which in November 1935 Dr. Leake presented his data on the national trials of the two polio vaccines, he turned and faced Dr. Kolmer. "I beg of you," Leake said, "I beg you to desist from the human use of this vaccine."

Kolmer rose to his feet and replied: "Gentlemen, this is one time I wish the floor would open up and swallow me."

Both the Kolmer and the Park-Brodie polio vaccines were withdrawn from distribution and destroyed.

Park continued to insist to his dying day that the future of prophylaxis against paralytic polio lay with killed- (inactivated) poliovirus vaccines. Kolmer's private Dermatological Research Laboratory was taken over in 1939 by the medical school of Temple University in Philadelphia, and Kolmer became professor of medicine and also director of the laboratory.

Brodie left New York in disgrace and took a job at the Providence Hospital in Detroit. In May 1939 he died of what his death certificate described as coronary thrombosis, at the age of thirty-six—a month after Park died of a heart attack in New York at the age of seventy-six. Regardless of what the death certificate reads, the actual cause of Brodie's death was, of course, poliomyelitis, or more specifically, the somatic consequences of his failure to make a safe, effective vaccine before anyone knew enough about viruses generally and polioviruses in particular to accomplish this feat.

The essential missing knowledge was not long in coming.

For the first three decades of research on the poliovirus, it had been assumed that, as with the cowpox and rabies viruses, there was only one antigenic (or serologic) type of poliovirus. However, in 1931 two Australian doctors, Macfarlane Burnet and Jean Macnamara, working with the standard MV strain maintained in Park's New York Board of Health laboratories, and with the Victoria strain originally isolated from a patient who had died of poliomyelitis in Melbourne in 1928, showed that both viruses were antigenically different types. The MV and the Victoria viruses could both cause experimental polio in mice.

Mice given experimental polio with the Victoria poliovirus and which recovered, developed antibodies against it and were immunized or protected against further attacks by that strain. However, the mice immunized against the Victoria strain developed fatal cases of paralytic polio when injected with the MV polioviruses from New York. This indicated that if a vaccine were ever developed, it would have to contain at least two types of antigenically distinct polioviruses to be effective. [6]

At the time, this finding was ignored or dismissed by most European and American polio investigators. Macnamara, who was essentially a clinician, devoted her energies to winning public support and expansion of the then available treatments for polio victims. Burnet, a research scientist (he would share the Nobel Prize in medicine with Peter Medawar for his work in immunology in 1960), continued to investigate infection and immunity.

Fortunately, even in 1931 he was not ignored by every investigator. When the Poliomyelitis Unit was set up at the Yale University School of Medicine during that year, Drs. John R. Paul, Dorothy M. Horstman, and James D. Trask began the first of a series of careful studies in New Haven in which they repeated the Australian work and confirmed the existence of different antigenic types of poliovirus in the tissues of polio patients. Their results, published in the *Journal of Experimental Medicine* in 1933 and 1935, were most certainly read by Park and Brodie.

These early studies of type differences eventually led to the massive effort started in 1949 by the National Foundation for Infantile Paralysis (the March of Dimes) through its multiuniversity (Pittsburgh, Kansas, southern California, and Utah) typing program to classify over two hundred clinical strains of poliovirus isolated from patients all over the world. This work—considered by many to be the NFIP's major contribution to the conquest of polio—was led by Dr. David Bodian of Johns Hopkins. Prominent roles in this program were played by Drs. Albert Sabin and Jonas Salk.

The collaborative study revealed by 1951 that of the 196 different isolates of poliovirus from patients in many lands, the vast majority—161 strains, or 82.1 percent of the total—were in what was designated as Type I. Another twenty, or 10.2 percent, were Type II, and the remaining fifteen, or 7.7 percent, were Type III. There were apparently no other types of poliovirus, which meant that a safe and effective vaccine containing the antigens of each of the three serologic types was now theoretically feasible.

By 1951 the electron microscope, which finally made viruses visible to cameras and human eyes, had made it easier to visualize and identify viruses isolated from patients. However, polioviruses still had to be grown, and experimental vaccines tested but only in monkeys imported largely from India and the Philippines at great expense. Worse than the costs of buying and maintaining these animals were the temporal limits they placed on the pace of investigative progress.

While the three antigenic or serologic types of poliovirus were being established, many laboratories worked on culturing viruses outside human and animal bodies, refining and extending the then available tissue-culture techniques that would soon play major roles in growing viruses in tissue or cell cultures, along with rapid and inexpensive testing of the laboratory-grown viruses' ability to affect human and animal cells maintained in living cultures. As obligate parasites of living cells, viruses cannot be grown in anything but living cells.

In 1928 the Canadian husband-and-wife team of Drs. Hugh and Mary Maitland, working at the University of Manchester, England, succeeded in growing vaccinia (cowpox) viruses in microbially sterile flask cultures of minced kidneys, chicken serum, and mineral salts. They were soon able to culture various other viruses in this growth medium. Until the advent of the sulfa drugs, which enabled laboratory workers at least to inhibit or reduce bacterial contamination of these tissue cultures, not too many viruses could be constantly grown in the flasks. Later, penicillin and other bactericidal antibiotic drugs proved even more effective at preventing bacterial contamination of growth cultures of live human or animal cells and tissues.

The technique of growing viruses on the tissues of developing chick embryos in sealed hens' eggs, originated by Drs. Ernest Goodpasture and Alice M. Woodruff in 1931, was considerably less subject to bacterial contamination than the Maitlands' preantibiotic flask cultures.

Many kinds of human disease viruses, including those that cause influenza, yellow fever, rabies, and encephalitis, could be grown in great quantity in hatching eggs. In Australia, Macfarlane Burnet was quick to replicate this work and to use hatching-egg cultures in his own virus research. Decades later, when he reflected upon all that had happened in virology since 1931, Burnet declared, "Nearly all the later practical advances in the control of virus diseases of men and animals sprang from this single discovery." This was not an understatement, but it did not apply to any work in poliomyelitis, since the poliovirus proved to be one of the human disease viruses that could not grow in developing-chick-embryo tissues in hatching eggs.

The quest for improved techniques that would permit the growth and harvesting of human disease viruses in live tissues other than chick embryos in hatching eggs centered about improvements in the flask-culture technique of the Maitlands. On the eve of World War II, Dr. George Gey at Johns Hopkins increased the yields of viruses grown in live tissue cultures by slowly rolling the tubes or flasks containing the virus-seeded tissue cultures in liquid nutrient media over and over again in electrically turned drums. The continuous rotation facilitated the optimum oxygenation of the tissues' living cells.

At Harvard's school of medicine, John F. Enders, an associate professor of bacteriology, and two members of the class of 1940, Frederick Robbins and Thomas Weller, were each fascinated by Gey's improvement on the basic Maitland tissue-culture technique.

Prior to America's entry into World War I, Enders and Weller had both worked together with embryonic chick tissues in flask cultures, in which they grew vaccinia virus. In 1940 Weller and a classmate, Lawrence C. Kingsland, were interns in pathology and bacteriology at Children's Hospital in Boston. There they set up a small tissue-culture laboratory, in which they hoped to be able to grow viruses isolated from patients and to use these viruses in making more accurate diagnoses of infectious diseases.

A little more than a year later, however, the Japanese bombed Pearl Harbor, and the young doctors and the professor went into the services, Enders as a civilian expert.

It was not until 1948, six years after Pearl Harbor, that Weller, Robbins, and Enders were to resume work on virus cultures under the same roof. This time the roof was not at Harvard but at Children's Hospital in Boston, where after the war Enders became chief of the research division of infectious diseases. Within five years the teacher and his two former students were to share a Nobel Prize in medicine for their work with polioviruses in tissue cultures, but this would be only one of the major disease viruses their research would help render harmless to people.

They were a curiously matched trio. The younger men came by their biomedical research interests through early exposure to the biological and medical sciences by fathers they loved and admired. Weller, born in 1915 in the university town of Ann Arbor, Michigan, where his father was professor of pathology at the medical school, grew up listening to the lore of clinical laboratory investigations. Robbins was born in 1916 in Auburn, Alabama, to one of the world's leading botanists and plant geneticists, Dr. William J. Robbins, who later became head of the New York Botanical Gardens. During the war, Weller was stationed at the military microbiology laboratory in Puerto Rico, while Robbins worked in the laboratory of virus and rickettsial diseases at the Sixteenth Medical General Hospital in Italy.

Enders was born in 1897 into a family of bankers and insurance company presidents in Hartford, Connecticut. His route to a career in virus research was a curious one. He did not decide upon a life in microbiology until he was in his late twenties and a graduate student in literature at Harvard. There, like many others, Enders fell under the spell of the professor of bacteriology and immunology, Hans Zinsser. Of all the scientists who wrote and lectured about microbiology during this century, Zinsser ranked second only to the legendary Paul de Kruif as the author who attracted the most young people to biomedical research. Max Theiler, for example, although himself the son of a distinguished scientist—Sir Arnold Theiler—did not decide to become a research worker until inspired by one of Zinsser's books.[7]

287

Enders had no idea (he understood at the time that through Zinsser he had found his vocation in life) that both he and Zinsser owed their careers in research to an event that had occurred on the then new Morningside Heights campus of Columbia University during the year of Enders's birth. It is possible that Zinsser, being the raconteur he was, might have told the story to Enders before he wrote it into his autobiographical memoir, *As I Remember Him,* in 1939.

Like Enders, Zinsser, the son of an affluent chemical manufacturer, had started out as an English major and a poet. At Columbia Zinsser was one of the "young enthusiasts who were at that time sitting at the feet of [Professor] George Edward Woodberry."[8]

In his autobiography Zinsser wrote of how, "In my sophomore year, while in the Woodberrian poetic exaltation, and feeling much of the time like a young Shelley, I threw a snowball across the campus at a professor emerging from the [Schermerhorn] Natural Science Building. It was a prodigious shot, a good hundred yards, I think. I hit him in the ear, knocked his hat off, and had time to disappear around the corner. I had nothing against him. It was an impulse, and a happy one, because I became guiltily conscious of him, thereafter, and eventually I took one of his courses as a sort of apologetic gesture. He happened to be both an anthropologist of note and a philosopher, and it was he who awakened in me the realization of the philosophical implications of scientific fact. There were great teachers of science at Columbia in those days, and the junior year—largely owing to the inspiration of the man whom I had hit in the ear—found me, without cutting loose entirely from the Department of Comparative Literature, feeling as though I had suddenly entered a new world of wonders and revelations, on the top floor of Schermerhorn Hall under the reign of Edmund B. Wilson and Bashford Dean."[9]

It was not long before Zinsser switched from literature to medicine and emerged as one of the greatest resources a nation can have: a fine scientist and an inspiring teacher whose students not only included the young people who worked under him at Stanford, Columbia, and Harvard, but also the thousands of people who read and still read *Rats, Lice, and History* and other of his books.

Before going to Harvard as a graduate student in literature, Enders entered Yale College in 1914, where his undergraduate education was interrupted by two years of army service as a flight instructor during World War I, and a postwar year as a real estate salesman, before he returned to take his A.B. in 1920. Enders learned more than science from Zinsser, under whom he served as an associate professor until the older man's death from leukemia in 1940. By precept, Zinsser also taught Enders how to inspire young people.

In 1929, a year before he earned his doctorate in microbiology, Enders received an appointment as a teaching assistant under Zinsser at the Harvard medical school. At the time, Zinsser was trying to develop a vaccine against the rickettsial organisms that cause typhus fever, Rocky Mountain spotted fever, and scrub typhus. Enders helped him work on methods of cultivating the large quantities of these microbes required for vaccine production.

The rickettsia are unusual organisms. Far smaller than most bacteria but not too small to be seen under the light microscope, they, like the viruses, are obligate parasites of living cells. The rickettsia parasitize cells in the bodies of certain groups of insects, including body lice, fleas, mites, and ticks. Like the yellow fever virus, these organisms are transmitted to people by the bites of these common insects.

Today the rickettsia, which contain both DNA and RNA, are classified as bacteria and can be controlled with many antibiotic drugs. However, in the 1930s because they could not be grown in cell-free nutrient media like bacteria, but could be cultured in media enriched with minced chick-embryo tissues and horse serum—as well as in hatching hens' eggs, like the viruses—the rickettsia were generally classified as larger viruses.

In the late 1930s, Enders and William Hammon collaborated in a study of malignant panleukopenia, a fatal disease of kittens, more commonly known as cat distemper. They discovered that this disease was caused by a virus that parasitized the bone marrow. To prevent it, they made up a vaccine of viruses present in the spleen and bone marrow of kittens killed by the disease. The vaccine worked very well in protecting healthy cats against the virus infection.

When war came, Enders was made a member of the armed forces' Epidemiological Board's special expert commission on measles and mumps. Both these common childhood virus infections were so ubiquitous in American family life that by the time young men were old enough to be drafted into the armed forces, most of them had been left naturally immune to them as well as to other common infectious diseases. In the training camps, however, thousands of young recruits who had not yet acquired natural immunity to measles, mumps, polio, and other widespread viral infections were gathered together from all over the country.

The results of concentrating these cohorts of young people in crowded, stressful, and uncomfortable military training camps were, as in all wars, completely predictable. Infections "ping-ponged" from one susceptible recruit to another. Parallel epidemics of infectious diseases broke out in many camps here and abroad. Some of these infections were much more serious in men of eighteen to forty than they normally are in young children. The outbreaks interrupted training schedules, filled the sick bays, and in many instances caused permanent damage or even death as the pathogenic viruses and bacteria spread like wildfire through the ranks of the nonimmune susceptible recruits.

During the war years, special commissions set up by the military tried to make vaccines that were partially or wholly effective against major infectious diseases whose transmission was, historically, exacerbated by military drafts and crowding. Dr. Thomas Francis, Jr., under whom Jonas Salk had trained at New York University, was assisted by Salk and Fred Davenport in turning out a killed-virus vaccine that was partially effective against influenza.

In 1917–1918 mumps had been the leading cause of days lost from active service in the American Expeditionary Force. After that war Surgeon General Thomas M. Parran showed that only the venereal diseases were responsible for more disabling infections among all armed fighting men. Mumps, which attacks the salivary glands, is caused by a virus in the same family as the influenza virus. In nature the mumps virus is found only in people, although under laboratory conditions it can be grown in monkeys and other animals. Most people are familiar with the painful swelling the virus causes in the human salivary glands; less cognizant of its painful and sexually sterilizing effects in adult male testes; and rarely aware of its causal role in mumps virus encephalitis, which, until the wide use of modern vaccines in children, was a frequent cause of permanent brain damage and lifelong confinement in mental institutions.

Not until 1934, when Ernest Goodpasture and C. D. Johnson caused mumps in rhesus monkeys by injecting them with filtered and cell-free saliva from afflicted patients, was it realized that mumps was probably a virus disease. During World War II, Enders noted, "We started where Goodpasture left off." Enders and his coworkers failed to grow the mumps virus in hatching-egg or tissue cultures, but he and Joseph Stokes, Jr., did manage to grow it in monkeys.

The first result of this isolation and culturing of the mumps virus was a diagnostic skin test, similar in action to the Schick test for susceptibility or immunity to diphtheria. The Enders group made a suspension of minced parotid gland—one of the salivary glands—from a monkey that had previously been infected with and was now immune to mumps. This parotid-gland suspension was then subjected to enough heat to render it killed and noninfective but still able to react with mumps virus antibodies (immunoglobulins) circulating in the bloodstream.

Tiny doses of this killed-virus preparation were injected under the skins of soldier volunteers with a history of having had mumps. Nearly all the volunteers developed local skin rashes around the injection site, which signified the positive reactions of the circulating mumps virus antibodies to the mumps virus antigen in the skin-test suspension. This also suggested that they had acquired lifelong immunity to the virus during earlier (usually childhood) cases of mumps. Heat-treated parotid-gland suspensions from monkeys free of mumps virus caused no skin reactions. When the killed-mumps-virus-antigen suspension was injected into soldier volunteers who did not recall ever having had mumps, only half of them showed no reactions. The others—those with positive skin reactions—had indeed acquired natural immunity after unapparent or unremembered earlier bouts of the mumps.

For those soldiers shown by their antigen skin tests to be still susceptible to mumps virus infections, the Enders-Stokes team made up a vaccine preparation in which an emulsion of parotid glands from monkeys infected with mumps was chemically inactivated with formalin. It worked in both monkeys and soldier volunteers, but the war ended before it could be put into large-scale use. It was, of course, the first safe, effective vaccine against mumps, but subsequent work by Dr. Karl Habel at the National Institutes of Health, by Enders and his coworkers, by Maurice Hilleman of the Merck Institute for Therapeutic Research, and by other workers would pave the way for the more effective modern live virus mumps vaccines now in general use.

In 1946 Enders resigned his position at Harvard to accept a post as director of the laboratory of infectious diseases at Children's Hospital in Boston. He was joined by the newly demobilized Weller and Robbins. Together, they resumed the lines of tissue culture and virus research that the war had interrupted for the two younger men. Penicillin, streptomycin, and other antibiotics that killed rather than, like the sulfa drugs, retarded the growth of bacteria became available after the war to prevent bacterial contamination of cell and tissue cultures. Gey's roller-tube method of handling tissue cultures helped shorten the growing time and increased the yields of laboratory-grown virus cultures.

By March 1948 Weller succeeded in growing mumps viruses in broth cultures containing minced chick amniotic membranes. These viruses, tested in mice, proved to be infective.

Following this success in animal tissues, the Enders team decided to try to culture disease viruses in live human cells. These cells were in skin muscle tissue derived from stillborn babies or from premature babies who had died shortly after birth in Boston Lying-In Hospital.

Weller set up twelve tissue-culture flasks, each containing emulsions of these embryonic skin muscle tissues in a broth of various nutrients. Four of these cultures were seeded with throat washings from a child with chicken pox, since the varicella (chicken-pox) virus was one of Weller's particular research interests. Because the laboratory had a grant from the March of Dimes, and the NFIP had made polioviruses abundantly available, four of the twelve flasks were inoculated with the Lansing strain of Type II poliovirus.

The chicken-pox virus failed to grow in the human embryonic skin muscle cells. The polioviruses, however, did grow very well. It was a historic first: Until then, nobody had succeeded in growing polioviruses in nonnervous human tissues or cells, in part because nobody had ever really tried, in face of the dogma that poliomyelitis was exclusively a disease of the central nervous system and infected only neural tissues.[10]

For the next months, Weller, Enders, and Robbins carefully and frequently repeated the culturing of the Lansing poliovirus in human embryonic skin muscle tissues. Enders suggested that they try growing the poliovirus in other tissues. "It was in the back of my mind," he explained, "that if so much poliovirus could be found in the gastrointestinal tract [in people], then it must grow someplace besides the nervous tissue."

The Enders group seeded tissue cultures of mouse and human intestinal tracts with polioviruses. The viruses grew very well in the tissues of the abdominal viscera—from gut to stomach. This tissue-culture confirmation of the thesis put forward by Kling and his coworkers in Sweden during the great polio epidemic of 1911 was a long time in coming; in 1949 Kling, at sixty-two still very active in polio research, was one of the first to hail this work.

There was more to come from the Enders group. They grew polioviruses in penile foreskins which had been removed by circumcision from boys between four and twelve years old in Boston hospitals. They showed that anti-Lansing poliovirus antibodies in the blood serum of monkeys who had recovered from polio caused by Lansing-strain virus prevented the proliferation of Lansing poliovirus in human tissue cultures.

Enders made one other observation. He grew the human tissue cells in thin sheets on the glass walls of the culture flasks. In these flask or roller-tube cultures, he needed only an ordinary light microscope to observe what happened to the human cells when active poliovirus particles were added to the nutrient growth broths. Within a few days, the polioviruses caused the healthy growing cells to change color, shape, growth rates, and other normal characteristics. Under the microscope anyone could see how the cells in the tissue cultures fell apart as the polioviruses killed them.

Viruses remained invisible under the light microscope, but their effects on living cells could now be seen clearly under ordinary light microscopes. From the Greek word *cyto* for hollow or cell, Enders named these visible results of virus-cell interactions the cytopathogenic effects (CPE).

More than a new name was involved. Since viruses could be grown in human tissue cultures and their pathogenic effects observed and measured, monkeys were no longer necessary for the growing (culturing) and testing of the pathogenic and immunologic effects of polioviruses and their antisera. Tissue culturing had also freed investigators from dependence upon monkeys and other animals in their studies of most other infectious, necrotic, and tumor viruses.

Modern medical virology was taking shape.

Enders, Robbins, and Weller had finally liberated the minds of biomedical workers from the shackles of the dogma that the poliovirus was respiratory and neurotropic. They had also demonstrated that it could be cultured and tested in all types of human nervous and nonnervous tissues. The March of Dimes's multiuniversity typing program had shown that there were only three serologic types of polioviruses.

The way was now clear for the early development and testing of good monovalent and polyvalent vaccines against each major type of poliovirus.

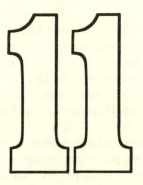

SALK AND SABIN VACCINES MAKE ERADICATION OF PARALYTIC POLIOMYELITIS FEASIBLE

The U.S. Immunization survey reveals a steady fall in the past few years in the percentage of children immunized against poliomyelitis and measles, particularly among the urban poor. The explanation for these unfortunate trends undoubtedly involves many factors, including the expiration in 1968 of the federal Vaccination Assistance Act [of 1962], which had provided funds to state and local health departments for purchases of vaccines.

—DOROTHY M. HORSTMANN, M.D., "Lagging Immunity of Our Children," *New England Journal of Medicine,* December 16, 1971

The first safe and effective virus vaccine to be developed and mass-tested after Enders, Robbins, and Weller grew polioviruses in neural and human nonnervous tissue cultures, and freed virologists from dependence upon monkeys as hosts and test animals, was the formalin-inactivated polio vaccine made by Dr. Jonas Salk at the University of Pittsburgh in 1951–1954. The Salk vaccine was a trivalent preparation containing the Types I, II, and III strains that had been grown in monkey tissue kidney cultures.

Salk's vaccine was a highly improved modification of the ill-fated, formalin-killed but untyped poliovirus vaccine of Park and Brodie. The suspicion, often voiced but never really proven, that formalin failed to kill every poliovirus in every clinical spinal emulsion Park and Brodie used in their 1934 vaccine continued to trouble many investigators and pediatricians when it became known that Salk was working on a formalin-inactivated, three-antigen poliovirus vaccine.

One of the first investigators to attempt to make a good killed-poliovirus vaccine was Paul Heinrich Römer (1876–1916), a coworker of Emil Behring's in the development of the failed and now forgotten "Bovo-Vaccine," made of human tubercle bacilli and intended for the immunization of calves against bovine tuberculosis. Römer's earlier experiences had given him good reason to be most circumspect about whatever he did and reported in vaccine work.

In 1910 Römer—one of the first investigators to suggest that polioviruses could enter human bodies via the intestinal tract as well as through the nose—made up a heat-inactivated vaccine. It failed in large part, he believed, because heat did not kill all the polioviruses in this vaccine. Some of the monkeys injected with it came down with paralytic polio. The following year Römer used formaldehyde to inactivate the polioviruses present in the spinal columns of polio patients, and used these formalin-inactivated viruses to vaccinate mice. They failed to protect the mice from getting polio. Römer abandoned all further work on a polio vaccine. During his time and later, European and American researchers tried to inactivate polioviruses with carbolic acid and other chemical germicides, used alone or in combination with blood sera from people convalescing from poliomyelitis.

Salk's decision to use formalin to inactivate the three types of polioviruses in his vaccine was based in part on his successful experiences, under the direction of his medical school mentor, Thomas Francis, Jr., with formalin-inactivated influenza virus vaccines developed for the armed forces during World War II. His faith in the capacity of formalin to inactivate or kill all poliovirus particles in any treated batch was shared by many of his peers, among them the Johns Hopkins University neuroanatomist Howard A. Howe. Like Salk, Dr. Howe had played a major role in the four-university National Foundation for Infantile Paralysis (NFIP) poliovirus typing program conducted, at a cost of $1,370,000, in 30,000 monkeys between 1949 and 1951.

In 1951–1952 Howe used formalin to inactivate viruses in a vaccine made "from large pools of the spinal cords of rhesus monkeys paralyzed by the three prototype" polioviruses. Howe's polio vaccine was tested first in ten chimpanzees, and was shown to be safe and immunogenic. The Howe vaccine then was tested in six children at the Rosewood Training School at Owings Mills, Maryland. Howe noted that each of these children "were low-grade idiots or imbeciles with congenital hydrocephalus, microcephaly, or cerebral palsy." (The prevailing and very eugenically oriented American medical ethics of the first half of this century considered mentally and physically handicapped children to be the subjects of choice for medical experimentation.) None of the mentally handicapped children bled and then injected with the Howe vaccine got polio, and he was able to report that "both children under 5 years of age and chimpanzees develop readily demonstrable neutralizing antibodies at comparable levels following the injection of small quantities of clarified monkey cord suspensions containing formalin-inactivated poliomyelitis virus."[1]

By the time Howe's report appeared in 1952, Salk at the University of Pittsburgh was already well into the development of his own formalin-inactivated vaccine. Early cell culture and animal tests suggested that the Salk vaccine was safe and effective in various species of laboratory animals. These animal trials also showed that Salk's previous formalin-inactivation procedures could be improved by some minor modifications. Hypothetically, Salk felt that the vaccine was ready for testing in people. But the differences between an attractive hypothesis and a test-confirmed theory could, as he well remembered, lead to a tragedy like the three paralytic polio deaths that had been charged to the formalin-inactivated Park-Brodie poliomyelitis vaccine in 1935.

Logic determined that the vaccine would cause minimal damage if it could be tested in people who had previously experienced and survived paralytic poliomyelitis infections. If the vaccine worked in people as it did in animals, it would cause an increase in circulating antibodies against polioviruses in their bodies. If the vaccine did not cause these people to produce antipoliovirus antibodies, there was still a good chance that the formalin had rendered the vaccine's three viruses noninfective. Because he was sure the formalin treatment did kill the polioviruses, Salk opted to test his new vaccine on children who had been previously crippled by the disease.

His field testing, amply funded by a grant of over a million dollars from the NFIP, took him to the D. T. Watson Home for Crippled Children in Leetsdale, Pennsylvania. There, with parental and school permission and cooperation, he conducted very carefully structured tests on the polio-crippled children. First, before vaccinating them, Salk and his staff bled the children for base-line measurements of the antibodies against polioviruses already present in the blood. It turned out that 87 percent—or sixty of the sixty-nine children tested—had previously acquired natural immunity to poliomyelitis and produced antibodies against Type I poliovirus. The children were given two shots of the trivalent vaccine; the second was a booster shot five weeks after the first dose. In each child, antibody production against all three types of polioviruses was either initiated or sharply increased by the Salk vaccine.

From Leetsdale, Salk and his team moved on to a different test population, mentally retarded children living at the state school in Polk, Pennsylvania. Here the levels of antibody production induced in these children by the new polio vaccine were equally encouraging. Most gratifying to Salk was the safety record: Not one child in either institution for the physically or mentally handicapped came down with anything resembling polio after receiving two shots of the Salk formalin-inactivated trivalent poliovirus vaccine. "When you inoculate children with a polio vaccine," Salk said at the time, "you don't sleep well for two or three months."

In time, it seemed that the tragedy which had haunted the aging Park and killed the young Brodie was the product of natural infections caused by wild environmental strains of poliovirus, types not included in the Park-Brodie vaccine. The formalin used to inactivate the poliovirus in the 1935 vaccine had done its job: It is simply impossible, however, to kill viruses whose antigens are not included in a vaccine.

It was small comfort now for Park and Brodie, and not quite enough to assure Salk. In the classic tradition of medical research, Salk had injected the vaccine into himself and his three sons. He had also vaccinated close to five hundred children and adults in an affluent suburb of Pittsburgh, and discovered that 60 percent of the children had no antibodies against any strain of poliovirus. In 1953, encouraged by their results to date, Salk and his colleagues, in their preliminary report on their first year of work concluded, "Although the results obtained in these studies can be regarded as encouraging, they should *not* [their emphasis] be interpreted to indicated that a practical vaccine is now at hand."[2]

Before this cautious report was published, however, the NFIP's immunization committee met on January 23, 1953. A majority of the members were far more eager to push for a mass trial than Salk and colleagues. Their number included Dr. Harry Weaver, the Foundation's research director, and

Dr. Joseph Smadel, the scientific director of the department of virus and rickettsial research at Walter Reed Army Institute of Research. "What are you waiting for?" Smadel is quoted as having said at this meeting. "Why don't you get busy and put on a proper field trial?"[3]

The matter was put to a vote, and most of the members present elected to proceed with mass trials of the Salk killed-poliovirus vaccine. The dissenters included John Enders and Albert Salk. Like Macfarlane Burnet, they believed that "sooner or later, it will become necessary to use living poliovirus vaccine given by mouth in infancy."[4]

Nobody awaited the reports of the evaluation committee more anxiously than the U.S. Public Health Service licensing committee, without whose approval the stockpile of ten million Salk vaccine doses, for which the NFIP had already paid five pharmaceutical manufactuerers $7,500,000 worth of March of Dimes offerings, could not be released to health departments and pharmacies. The five companies were sitting on orders for another nine million dollars' worth of Salk vaccines using March of Dimes money. These lucrative orders, however, were subject to the vaccine being licensed as safe and effective.

From the joint standpoint of the NFIP and the drug manufacturerers, the results of the trials as announced by Professor Francis left little to be desired. The Salk vaccine did cause children to produce circulating antibodies that neutralized all three types of polioviruses; local outbreaks of poliomyelitis during the period of the 1954 trials had produced 50 percent fewer cases in the vaccinated children than in the control children; and, most important, not one of the million children vaccinated with the formalin-inactivated Salk vaccine got poliomyelitis from that experience.

To the millions of people who, in the darkest years of the great depression, had contributed dimes, then dollars, and had given years of their lives to help the March of Dimes (and its predecessor, the President's Birthday Ball Commission) to collect hard-earned contributions from ordinary concerned people like themselves—first for the medical care of polio victims and for the iron lungs (Drinker respirators) that kept people with polio-paralyzed lungs alive, then for the basic and applied research to develop a vaccine to prevent polio—the announcement that those dimes and dollars had yielded a safe vaccine which would protect their children and grandchildren against polio was possibly the greatest moment in American life since the end of the killing in World War I. Now, as in November 1918, church bells and, in many cities, trolley bells and factory sirens hailed the development, the testing, and the licensing of the Salk vaccine as the great step forward for humankind that it was.

Chronologically, the work that had produced the Salk vaccine and the equally dedicated efforts that had gone into the Park-Brodie and the Kolmer vaccines, were only two decades apart; scientifically, the distance between both vaccines was considerably greater. Writing of the 1935 and 1955 vaccines, Yale Professor John Paul, whose career in poliovirus research spanned both eras, noted that "the situations were in no way comparable, for the Brodie-Kolmer vaccines had been launched in the face of colossal ignorance, whereas the Salk-type vaccine had been promoted under circumstances which from the start almost guaranteed success. And yet one cannot help feeling a twinge of sympathy for the two figures of 1935 who were so alone in the midst of their disgrace, in contrast to the powerful forces of the National Foundation, the U.S. Public Health Service, and innumberable advisory committees—including the (PHS) Licensing Committee—that stood back of the Salk-type vaccine."[5]

Within a few weeks of the issuance of the Francis report, the federal Bureau of Biologics released ten million stockpiled and now safety-tested doses of the new Salk vaccine. Children lined up in schools, in health department and hospital clinics, and at other stations to receive Salk shots provided gratis by the March of Dimes. Unlike most popular dreams, the Depression-born dream of a polio vaccine had come true. After April 12, 1955, over 400,000 doses of vaccine had already been shot into children before the mass euphoria was suddenly turned into numbing horror.

Reports began to come into the Public Health Service, and from them to the press, that in California and in Idaho doses of Salk vaccine manufactured by Cutter Laboratories of Berkeley, California, had induced cases of paralytic polio in children and adults. On April 27 California's health department ordered that the Cutter-made Salk vaccines be taken off the market in that state. While the gutter press and radio scandalmongers exacerbated the fears of parents whose children were already vaccinated, the U.S. Center for Communicable Diseases (now the Centers for Disease Control—CDC) investigated the tragedy and found that in seven of the total of seventeen lots of the Cutter Laboratories Salk vaccine immunization was followed in some instances by cases of acute poliomyelitis.

Their report noted that "a total of 204 vaccine-associated cases occurred. Of these, 79 were among vaccinated children, 105 among family contacts of vaccinated children, and 20 among community contacts. Approximately three-fourths of the cases were paralytic. There were 11 deaths, making a case fatality-rate of 5%." In short, the doses from these seven imperfectly inactivated lots of Cutter-made vaccine had paralyzed and killed fifteen times more children than the earlier Brodie and Kolmer vaccines combined.

No cases of poliomyelitis, however, had occurred in people given Salk vaccines from the other eleven batches made by Cutter. Nor had there been any paralytic or fatal aftereffects of vaccination with Salk vaccines from any of the lots marketed by the other four pharmaceutical manufacturers.

The government's thorough investigation of the safety of all but the seven contaminated batches of Cutter vaccine helped restore the confidence of family physicians. Two other concurrent developments also helped keep the entire polio vaccine program from collapsing in the United States. The first was the fact that in Canada, where the Salk vaccine was produced by the well-regarded Connaught Laboratories in Toronto, no cases of polio hit any of the 860,000 children vaccinated with it between April and June 1955. The Canadians were not about to abandon the use of their Toronto-made Salk vaccine merely because of laboratory errors in a California facility. Similarly, the Danes, who manufactured a Salk-type vaccine in the government's Danish Serum Institute, continued their own mass immunization program with no untoward effects on children and adults.

As the facts were clarified by responsible governmental and medical institutional agencies, confidence in the Salk vaccine was regained. Between April 12 and May 7, 1955, despite the understandable fears triggered by the Cutter incident—and the cruel exploitation of these fears by many elements of the mass media—some four million doses of the Salk vaccine had been given to American children. By November 1955 the CDC reported that "the decline in attack rates for naturally acquired paralytic cases had been from two to five times greater among vaccinated children than among the unvaccinated in the same age groups."

Albert Sabin, no admirer of Jonas Salk or his vaccine, later declared, "The development by Jonas Salk of an effective formalinized vaccine provided a tool with which the incidence of the paralytic disease could be greatly reduced and many thousands of paralytic cases had been prevented by its use in various parts of the world."[6]

This was somewhat of an understatement. By 1965, when Sabin made this statement in accepting that year's Lasker Award for clinical research, the Salk vaccine had already been licensed for ten years in the United States. During the first six of those years, the Salk vaccine was the only one licensed in this country. Between 1954 (the last of the prevaccine years) and 1961, the incidence of poliomyelitis reported to local health departments declined from 23.9 cases per 100,000 population to a mere 0.7 cases per 100,000 population in 1961. In absolute numbers this represented a decline of from 38,576 cases (15,640 of them paralytic) in 1954 to 1,312 cases (988 of them paralytic) in 1961.

It must be remembered that the Salk vaccine was not licensed until the spring of 1955, and that in 1961 the monovalent Sabin oral poliovirus vaccine was licensed. The trivalent Sabin vaccine (TOPV) was not licensed until 1963.

In the Scandinavian countries that relied exclusively on the Salk-type inactivated vaccines of their own manufacture, the trivalent inactivated poliovirus vaccine (IPV) eradicated poliomyelitis completely. In Sweden, which began manufacturing and administering the IPV in 1957, 100 percent of that nation's children and a vast majority of its adults were immunized using the Salk-type vaccine. No indigenous cases of poliomyelitis were reported in Sweden between 1962 and 1977, when an unvaccinated two-year-old girl caught a mild paralytic disease caused by Type II poliovirus. No polio cases were reported after 1977.

In Finland a recent report noted that "the inactivated poliovaccine has eliminated not only the disease but also the poliovirus itself from Finland. The last endemic cases of poliomyelitis were seen in 1961, and two were imported in 1964." The government epidemiologists conducted an intensive search to determine whether polioviruses were still circulating in Finland. It was carried out "in 1972–74 in sewage, among patients with polio-like diseases, and among healthy preschool children. Viruses, mostly Coxsackie B viruses, were isolated from sewage in 67 percent of samples, but no polioviruses were found."[7]

By 1982 the federal Centers for Disease Control reported that "the risk of poliomyelitis is generally very small in the United States today, but epidemics are likely to occur if the immunity of the population is not maintained by immunizing children beginning in the first year of life. Small outbreaks have occurred in 1970, 1972, and 1979 as a result of introduction of [polio] virus into susceptible populations in communities with low immunization levels."[8] According to the same agency's latest available immunization survey, more than 40 percent of American children between one and four years old have not been fully immunized against polio.

The United States and the Scandinavian case and mortality data since 1955 speak volumes for the safety and efficacy of the Salk-type formalinized vaccines. They do not, however, explain why perfectly competent and rational directors of health-care systems in the United States and most of the world's non-Scandinavian nations have since 1963 gradually replaced the Salk killed-virus vaccines with the Sabin live virus polio vaccines. In the United States, for example, the Salk vaccines are now available only in the state of Michigan.

Albert Sabin, in his 1965 Lasker Award lecture quoted earlier, had followed his praise of the Salk vaccine with two sentences that stated his case for live poliovirus vaccines taken orally rather than by injection. "It has been demonstrated, however," he said, "that in communities in which a large proportion of the population is protected against paralysis by the Salk vaccine, the polioviruses readily maintain a continuous cycle of transmission, and when the circulating viruses are of sufficient virulence, paralysis continues to occur among those who never acquired immunity or lost it after vaccination. This phenomenon accounted not only for the continued occurrence of many paralytic cases, but also for epidemics of various sizes in countries like the United States, Canada, Hungary, Israel, Japan, Australia, and others where the Salk vaccine had been used on a large scale."

Epidemic is possibly too strong a word to use for the rise in reported cases of acute poliomyelitis—including paralytic and fatal cases—that occurred in this country when the number reported jumped from 3.3 cases per 100,000 population in 1948 to 4.8 cases per 100,000 population in 1959. By the end of 1959, the downward trend that had begun in 1955 was accelerated, so that in 1960 the reported polio case rate fell to 1.8 per 100,000 population. Statistically, the outbreak of 1959 was merely a little blip on a steadily declining straight line. Numerically, however, the 6,389 paralytic poliomyelitis cases reported in 1959 represented a jump of 2,592 cases more than had been reported in 1958, and for those who were permanently paralyzed or killed in this very transient rise in reported paralytic polio cases—and for their families—this was no minor episode.

To doctors and microbiologists like Sabin and Enders, such postformalinized-vaccine outbreaks were predictions that had been spelled out in the Francis evaluation report of April 12, 1955. In the massive field trials of 1954, the Salk vaccine had shown itself to be only 60 percent effective against spinal paralysis, but 94 percent protective against bulbar paralytic polio. From the data at hand, the Francis report stated that the evaluation committee was not able "to select a single value giving numerical expression in a complete sense to the effectiveness of the vaccine as a total experience." Dr. Francis went on to state that "it may be suggested that the vaccine was 80 to 90% effective against paralytic poliomyelitis; that it was 60 to 70% effective against disease caused by Type I poliovirus, and 90% or more effective against that of Type II and Type III poliovirus."

These levels of effectiveness were high enough to justify the widest possible uses of the Salk formalinized poliovirus vaccine in all unprotected populations, and low enough to justify the funding of major efforts to develop and test live attenuated poliovirus vaccines whose oral mode of entry into the human body was closer to what prevailed in nature—and whose administration in one single oral dose presented fewer opportunities for infections, needle accidents, and incompleted courses of immunization inherent in the three-dose schedule of the parenteral Salk-type vaccine.

Whether or not Sabin developed his version of the live poliovirus vaccine, the time was ripe for the development and use of a poliovaccine whose immunizing antigens (immunogens) would be delivered by viruses as live as those used in the most successful vaccine in medical history: Jenner's cowpox vaccine against smallpox, a thousandfold greater scourge than poliomyelitis had ever been.

Because of the continuing successes of Jenner's live virus cowpox vaccine against smallpox, and Pasteur's attenuated live virus vaccine against rabies, and Theiler's live virus vaccine against yellow fever, the earliest efforts to develop a vaccine against paralytic poliomyelitis were based on the concept of attenuated live polioviruses as the active principle.

After Simon Flexner and Paul Lewis discovered, in 1910 at the Rockefeller Institute in New York, that the blood sera of monkeys convalescing from poliomyelitis contained antibodies against polioviruses, they swiftly proceeded to use live polioviruses to induce immunity in healthy monkeys. The Rockefeller Institute scientists employed the methods of Pasteur and Sewall to inject the polioviruses "subcutaneously in gradually increasing doses over a period of several months," until the rhesus monkeys became fully immune to polio.

These graded courses of innoculation or immunization worked equally well in monkeys who had recovered from naturally acquired poliomyelitis, and who also proved "insusceptible to re-inoculation with the virus; in other words, they had developed an artificial immunity." Flexner and Lewis held that "the successful outcome of this experiment suggested that the blood of persons who had recovered from poliomyelitis contained similar immunity principles."

This was in the spring of 1910, when millions of lives had already been saved from death by diphtheria or tetanus by the judicious uses of immune sera from the blood of horses previously immunized against either disease by series of graded doses of their bacteria. These antitoxic or immune sera conferred only passive, not active or long-lasting immunity against untreatable major infections. Nevertheless, whereas in 1900 the United States death rate for diphtheria stood at 40.3 per 100,000 population, by 1909 it had been reduced by half to 19.9 per 100,000 population. This was accomplished by using the animal immune sera first given to a little girl with diphtheria in von Bergmann's clinic in Berlin on Christmas Night, 1891. In 1894, at the Pasteur Institute in Paris, Émile Roux and Louis Martin first immunized horses with graded doses of diphtheria bacilli, and opened the way to producing large amounts of immune sera laden with antibodies against the diphtheria toxin, and producing them at very low prices. Inside of a year, the Pasteur Institute antitoxins had reduced the Paris hospital diphtheria deaths by 50 percent.

Flexner and Lewis lost little time in trying to repeat this work in horses, but with polioviruses. They had to report "the failure to produce a neutralizing serum in the horse by repeated injections of filtrate" of virus suspensions. "The horse serum, when mixed with the virulent filtrate and incubated [as in the rhesus monkeys], displayed no power whatever to inhibit the action of the virus. The monkeys injected with the mixture of horse serum and virus became paralyzed in the same average period as the controls." The Rockefeller Institute researchers were beginning to learn the hard way that polioviruses could be cultured in no other animals but monkeys and people.

More than three decades later, another Rockefeller Institute investigator, Max Theiler, who previously had succeeded in attenuating the 17D strain of yellow fever virus, was able in 1936 also to attenuate the Type II Lansing strain of poliovirus. As he had done earlier with the yellow fever virus, Theiler passaged the poliovirus continuously through the brains of living mice until, without losing its immunogenic capacities to cause mice to produce antibodies against Type II poliovirus, the attenuated virus was no longer paralytogenic. Although still immunologically active, the altered Type II poliovirus could no longer cause poliomyelitis in mice.

Theiler reported this development at an NFIP scientific meeting in 1946 in the hope that some of the others more actively involved in polio research would carry it on from there. He himself was too busy with other lines of work to explore this further. Theiler's data were carefully studied by various investigators, among them Hilary Koprowski, then at Lederle Laboratories, Joseph Melnick, then at the Yale Poliomyelitis Study Unit, and Albert Sabin, then at the University of Cincinnati (Ohio) School of Medicine. Each had been working to develop a live virus polio vaccine, and each set about applying Theiler's experiences toward this goal.

Koprowski and his Lederle coworkers passaged a strain of poliovirus through the bodies of cotton rats, and then gave twenty human volunteers this attenuated strain as a vaccine. The nonimmune volunteers promptly started to produce circulating antibodies against this strain, while the volunteers who were previously immune to polioviruses started to excrete live polioviruses. Koprowski presented these data to the NFIP immunization committee.

At about the same time, Enders, Weller, and Robbins succeeded in attenuating the Brunhilde (Type I) strain of poliovirus by cultivating it in human tissue cultures. Instead of passaging the polioviruses through live animals, virologists were now able to attenuate the viruses by passaging them through the viable cells of people and other animals which were kept alive in laboratory flask tissue cultures.

Melnick and Sabin soon produced attenuated live poliovirus vaccines they had developed independently of each other. They described these experimental vaccines at the 1953 meeting of the immunization committee. By that time the NFIP was so deeply committed to the forthcoming mass trials of the Salk vaccine that its lay leaders gave the data on the two live virus vaccines short shrift. This and similar decisions provoked a rift between the scientific members of the committee and the directors of the Foundation. For a time it seemed as if the scientists would resign in a body, not because they opposed the Salk killed-virus vaccine, but because they felt that the serious potentials of live virus vaccines against paralyzing poliomyelitis were being studiously ignored.

By December 1954 Sabin was given a decent grant by the NFIP to develop further his live poliovirus vaccine. All told, the NFIP grant programs would support Sabin's work to the tune of close to two million dollars during the next decade. Despite these grants, however, Sabin was hard put to find much support for large-scale trials of his polio vaccine.

Like Koprowski, Sabin was forced to look abroad for mass tests. Koprowski, now at the Wistar Institute of the University of Pennsylvania in Philadelphia, tested his live vaccine on a quarter of a million people in the

Congo. His former Lederle associates, led by Harold Cox, developed and tested still another live vaccine in various Latin American countries.

Over a period of three years starting in 1957, Sabin managed to have his live virus vaccine tested in a large series of international cooperative studies. "The tests proceeded step by step on increasingly larger numbers of people from hundreds to thousands, to tens of thousands and hundreds of thousands, and finally in the spring of 1959 to many millions. During this period," Sabin later recalled, "studies were carried out in the United States, Mexico, Holland, England, Sweden, Singapore, Czechoslovakia, and the Soviet Union." These trials, done on millions of people, confirmed all Sabin's claims for the safety and efficacy of the live attenuated poliovirus vaccine. It required only one dose. Shortly after the trials began, the Sabin vaccine would eradicate poliomyelitis and its viruses from all of Czechoslovakia.[9]

Despite these results, in 1959 the NFIP vaccine advisory committee, although praising the Sabin oral polio vaccine as having great potential, held that its capacity "to prevent paralytic poliomyelitis, while assumed, is at present not known." They therefore decided that "it would be unwise to embark, at this time, upon mass vaccinations with live attenuated polioviruses in the United States."[10]

When this policy statement was released by the NFIP, other nations, from the Soviet Union and Western Europe to Singapore, to Mexico, where the Sabin live virus vaccine had already replaced or was in the process of supplanting the Salk inactivated poliovirus vaccine, showed a combined population close to twice that of the United States. In August 1959 the World Health Organization (WHO) of the United Nations sent Professor Dorothy M. Horstmann, of the Yale Poliomyelitis Study Unit, to the Soviet Union to study the effects of using the Sabin live poliovirus vaccine in the entire population of the USSR. After three months of investigation, she reported that the clinical trials had gone very well and that the Sabin vaccine was both safe and effective.

It took nearly another three years of large-scale testing, but in August 1961 the pharmaceutical firm of Charles Pfizer and Company was licensed to produce and market in the United States a monovalent Sabin oral vaccine against Type I poliovirus. Three months later the Type II oral poliovaccine (OPV) was licensed, and in March 1962 the trivalent oral poliovirus vaccine (TOPV) against all three types of polioviruses was licensed and used to immunize millions of American children and adults by the end of the year.

Immunologically, the Sabin vaccine was the start of a new era, not only in the prevention and even eradication of paralytic poliomyelitis and its three types of causal viruses, but also in the development of both live virus and live bacterial vaccines against growing numbers of major infectious diseases.

*   *   *

Since the live virus vaccines were taken into the body through the mouth, as are enteric viruses in natural infections, they almost immediately caused the gastrointestinal mucosa of the upper gut to produce the mucosal, secretory IgA (alpha globulin) antibodies that are the human immune system's first line of defense against invading viral particles and bacterial organisms.

The immunoglobulins (Igs) are protein globules found in the bodies of people and other animals. All immunoglobulins are antibodies, which are proteins produced by lymphocytes or lymphoid cells in response to the presence of foreign antigens, such as those on or in viruses and bacteria. Human cells transformed by cancer at times develop new antigens (tumor antigens) that are so different from the antigens on healthy cells that they register on the immune systems as "foreign," and antibodies then are produced against the cancer-cell membrane antigens. The words immunoglobulin and antibody mean exactly the same thing and are used interchangeably in medicine.

In normal human bodies, 80 percent of all antibodies are in the immunoglobulin G (IgG) or gamma globulin class. Another 10 percent are IgA secretory immunoglobulins; 5 percent to 10 percent are IgM antibodies; 1 percent to 3 percent are IgD antibodies, whose functions are little understood; while the remaining less than 1 percent are IgE antibodies, which are active in allergic diseases and certain infections.

The IgA antibodies are found in saliva, tears, and other secretions, as well as in the moist mucosa that line the nose, throat, stomach, intestines, rectum, and other body areas. These secretory or mucosal antibodies cling to and attack microbial pathogens at their portals of entry into the body long before the IgG and IgM antibodies that circulate in the blood and lymph systems can—with the aid of other circulating immune factors, such as complement and properdin—attack and neutralize or destroy viruses, bacteria, and other infectious disease agents. The IgA antibodies also reach newborn children in the colostrum in their mothers' milk.

The IgM antibodies are the first of the circulating immunoglobulins to be produced in response to antigenic stimuli. They are very heavy globulins, five times the size of the smaller and lighter IgG antibodies that start to appear in the circulatory system a day or two later. The IgG antibodies, small enough to penetrate the placental barriers, are nature's instruments for delivering functional doses of every type of antibody present in pregnant women to the developing bodies of their unborn children. These maternal antibodies provide passive protection against virus and bacterial infections for the first six months of postnatal life; conversely, the congenital maternal antibodies in neonates often neutralize live virus and live bacterial vaccines, and cause postponement of their use until the children are a year old.

Since the IgG globulins include collections of all the disease-specific antibodies present in a human body, concentrates of IgG molecules derived from the pooled sera of thousands of blood donors are often injected into children and adults who were exposed to active cases of common infectious diseases, such as measles, polio, rubella, and influenza. The passive immunity delivered by these concentrates of pooled gamma globulins often lasts long enough to prevent infections. In some clinical risk situations, exposed individuals are injected with immune globulins—that is, antibodies from the sera of human volunteers (or paid donors) previously immunized against these and other specific diseases.

In terms of polio prevention, long before the antigens on the surface of the formalin-killed viruses in the Salk-type vaccines reached lymphocytes that produce the circulating IgG antibodies in the bloodstream, the secretory IgA antibodies would be actively binding to and neutralizing the intrusive wild polioviruses.

Vaccines cannot be injected directly into the bloodstream through the veins because of the dangerous side effects that intravenous (IV) injections of any materials can cause. Therefore, for safety's sake all parenteral vaccines, such as the Salk vaccine, are given intramuscularly (IM). From the muscles the vaccines ooze very slowly, and in minute amounts, to the vessels of the circulatory system. This often takes thirty-six to forty-eight hours. The oral vaccines, on the other hand, start to produce IgA antibodies minutes after they reach the gut or the nasopharyngeal or respiratory systems, while "inoculation of susceptible persons with parenteral killed poliovirus causes little if any production of upper gastrointestinal mucosal antibody (IgA). This finding is in contrast to the high levels of IgA observed in the gastrointestinal tract with oral live vaccine."

Despite its inability to trigger the production of IgA antibodies, the Salk-type killed-poliovirus vaccine does, after three injected doses, produce enough IgG antibodies against all three types of polioviruses to have eradicated the disease from Sweden and Finland. Nevertheless, the rapidly produced secretory IgA antibodies induced by the single needed oral dose of live trivalent oral poliovirus vaccine, which also causes the vaccines to synthesize circulating IgG antibodies, represent a great productive advantage, that most doctors and health agencies prefer their patients to acquire.

Just as Jenner's vaccine transformed smallpox from a medical disease to a societal delinquency, the Salk and Sabin vaccines converted paralytic poliomyelitis from a medical catastrophe to a societally eradicable, ordinary, vaccine-preventable infectious disease.

Once these two good American vaccines against the polioviruses became available to the entire world, any nation whose citizens—starting with its newborns, infants, and very young children—suffered paralysis and death from polio was a country in which one of three very well-defined social defects prevailed. These social deficiencies are: (1) the lack of enough government funds to mount and maintain a permanent, responsible national immunization program against polio and all other vaccine-preventable diseases; or (2) the lack of sufficient regard on the part of a government for the health and human dignity of all its people to ensure that vaccination is a heritage of birth and an irrevocable right of citizenship; or (3) a combination of the first two factors in the minds and deeds of those governmental leaders who deliberately abandon good immunization programs to extend life—while increasing funds allocated for nuclear and non-nuclear engines of death.

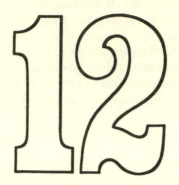

TO SAVE OUR CHILDREN: LIVE VIRUS VACCINES AGAINST MEASLES, MUMPS, AND RUBELLA

Considering how destructive [measles] is; considering how many die, even in the mildest epidemical constitution; considering how it hurts the lungs and eyes; I thought I should do no small service to mankind if I could render this disease more mild and safe, in the same way the Turks have taught us to mitigate the small-pox.

—FRANCIS HOME, M.D., FRCP, 1759

The soldiers everywhere are sick. The measles are prevalent throughout the whole army, and you know that disease leaves unpleasant results, attacks upon the lungs, typhoid, etc., especially in camp, where accommodations for the sick are poor.

—GENERAL ROBERT E. LEE, CSA, in a letter to his wife, August 4, 1861 cience, if anything, is a cumulative process. For each question about nature for which it obtains good answers, it raises a host of new questions that were never known to exist before. For each advance in the basic knowledge of the natural history of health and disease, and each resulting new strategy of curing or better yet preventing a single dread disorder, a score of new treatments and vaccines become suddenly conceivable.

The postwar findings in medical virology that resulted in the Salk and Sabin vaccines against paralytic poliomyelitis were soon applied to a number of considerably more common and costly virus diseases of children and adults. Between 1963 and 1969, this surge of basic and applied research resulted in the licensing of safe and effective vaccines against measles, rubella, and mumps—three major causes of deafness, blindness, organic birth defects, and prenatal and postnatal irreversible brain damage. Not surprisingly, John Enders and his principal coworkers played major roles in the development of all three vaccines.

Measles has always been a major disease. Even today in the poor countries, where most of the world's people live, measles is still responsible for up to half of all infant and child deaths. In the United States, as the pediatrician Louis Z. Cooper observed, "Before a measles vaccine was available, more than nine out of ten children caught measles, half of them before they were five. Measles starts with a high fever, a runny nose, a cough, and a sore throat. After five days, a blotchy red rash develops. Usually the disease runs its course in another week, but sometimes there are complications. One measles patient in every six develops pneumonia or a serious ear infection. One in every thousand gets measles encephalitis, an inflammation of the brain that can cause paralysis, mental retardation, and even death. Far from being a harmless childhood disease, measles kills more children than any other acute infectious illness."[1]

During 1946, when John Enders moved from Harvard University to Children's Hospital in Boston, there were 695,843 cases of measles reported to local health departments by physicians, most cases being in children under five—for a rate of 468.8 cases per 100,000 population. In the same year, physicians reported a total of 25,698 cases of acute poliomyelitis to their local health departments—or 18.3 cases per 100,000 population.

In terms of duly reported cases alone, this meant that measles was more than twenty-seven times more prevalent than poliomyelitis in this country in 1946. Unfortunately, the numbers by themselves are deceptive enough to be grossly misleading. Polio, like rabies and bubonic plague, is one of the "horror" diseases whose treating physicians are quick to report each and every single case they attend. Measles, on the other hand, like most other notifiable diseases doctors are legally required to report, has always been scandalously underreported. As three CDC experts observed in 1979, "Underreporting is a substantive problem; it is estimated that current reporting accounts for only 10% to 25% of the [measles] cases actually occurring."[2] This means that the actual number of measles cases suffered in 1979 came to well over 100,000, rather than the mere 13,597 actually reported.

There are many reasons for the documented failure of most physicians to obey the laws requiring them to report all notifiable diseases to their health departments. Some doctors consider the reporting of "harmless" diseases like measles to be a waste of their time and of taxpayers' money; other physicians resent all mandatory paper work; while still others are simply much too tired at the end of a busy day to take the trouble to fill out all the bureaucratic forms. Poverty, and earlier experiences with older children who recovered from measles without complications, are another reason for this underreporting. As many doctors know, poor families in which measles strikes a second child often do not spend the money required to get medical care and medication—such as aspirin for the high fever, or penicillin for the prevention and/or treatment of the bacterial bronchopneumonia that often is associated with the disease.

Measles, and the efforts to prevent it by both variolation and vaccination, have had a long and curious history. The Persian doctor Rhazes (born 860 A.D.) described measles as being merely "the safer form of smallpox." The seventeenth-century English physician Thomas Sydenham is credited with being the first doctor to differentiate between smallpox and measles, which he saw as two separate diseases. A busy practitioner who based his medical writings on often acute bedside observations, Sydenham characterized measles as a disease that usually struck children, causing fever, chills, "running from the eyes," a livid skin rash, and "other symptoms like those of peripneumony."

He prescribed various medications for the alleviation of the rashes and other symptoms, most of them compounded of different combinations of syrup of violets, oil of sweet almonds, syrup of maidenhair, black-cherry water, and syrup of poppies. Although measles was then, as now, a medically incurable (if usually self-terminating) disease, Sydenham's nostrums, apozems, and linctuses for uncomplicated cases had the then uncommon virtue of being harmless. For some of the complications of measles, Sydenham's treatments were not quite as gentle. "About the 12th day from the invasion [of bronchopneumonia] the patient may be moderately purged," while, he wrote, "the diarrhoea which follows measles is cured by bleeding."

Sydenham had no prescription for the prevention of measles. In 1757 the Scottish physician Alexander Monro (1697–1767) suggested that the technique of variolation used to prevent smallpox should be tried. However, since the skin eruptions of the measles rash were not filled with the kinds of pus present in smallpox skin pustules, Monro decided to give the matter considerably more thought.

The following year, Dr. Francis Home (1719–1813) came up with a possible solution. He decided to take blood from measles patients at the time their skin eruptions broke out, and to use it as an immunizing inoculum. Home used a fine scalpel to scarify the arms of people who had no history of having had the disease. Then after dipping cotton balls in the blood taken from measles patients, Home applied the cotton to the open cuts in the arms of the healthy individuals.

Home did this procedure in hundreds of people. In one typical cohort of twelve healthy children Home inoculated early in his experiments, ten came down with mild cases of the disease, which presumably immunized them against reexposures to it. Home believed that this was indeed the case, and he wrote of having developed a means of making measles "more mild and safe in the same way as we mitigate the smallpox." Home lived long enough (he died at ninety-four in 1813) to witness the introduction of Jenner's smallpox vaccine.

Possibly because of the by then well-known dangers of transmitting syphilis, tuberculosis, and other savage diseases by smallpox variolations, mid-eighteenth-century European physicians were in the main not at all tempted to bleed their measles patients for inocula against a much milder disease. After Jenner introduced his infinitely safer cowpox vaccine against smallpox, some doctors who rightly feared variolation quite probably looked for equally benign animal infections that would prevent measles in people. Gradually, the medical profession seemed to lose interest in vaccines against measles until Pasteur, Koch, and other germ theory pioneers revived interest in all vaccines. In 1905 Ludwig Hektoen, at the University of Chicago, injected some healthy student volunteers with blood from patients with active cases of measles. Most of the students developed the disease, particularly when the blood of the donors was taken inside of thirty hours of the time their rashes erupted.

Joseph Goldberger (1874–1929) and his Public Health Service colleague, John F. Anderson, injected a cell-free filtrate of blood from a measles patient into a monkey in 1911—with two significant results. The monkey came down with a full-blown case, which gave experimental biologists their first animal model in which to study this disease. Of far greater importance, however, was the fact that the bacteria-free nature of the inoculum showed that measles, like smallpox, was most probably caused by a filtrable virus. Subsequent work in other laboratories around the world confirmed the viral etiology of measles, although for the next decades the medical journals of the world continued to publish claims by qualified investigators in fine university centers that specific bacteria were the real cause of measles.

In 1938 Harry Plotz, an American working at the Pasteur Institute in Paris, grew the measles virus in hatching-egg chick-embryo cultures. Two years later at the Rockefeller Institute, Geoffrey Rake and M. F. Shaffer passaged cell-free filtrates of blood from measles patients in hatching eggs. Experimental vaccines made from these egg-passaged viruses were used to immunize a few people, including some children. When America was drawn into World War II, considerable work was done in armed forces laboratories on developing egg-passaged and attenuated live virus vaccines against measles, since many susceptible young recruits contracted measles during basic training. However, the vaccines caused many severe reactions after they were injected into healthy recruits. Ultimately, the adverse reactions caused the army to drop work on measles vaccines.

Until the measles virus could be isolated, visualized and photographed under the new electron microscope, and grown in pure cultures, it was not exactly easy to get a handle on what had to be known before a good vaccine could be made. After the war ended, Enders and his collaborators began to work on the problem and, much of this work was shared by Dr. Thomas Peebles. In January 1954 when measles broke out in a school near Boston, Peebles went to examine the affected children and took throat washings and a few blood samples from one of them, David Edmonston. These materials were seeded into a culture of human kidney tissues at the Enders laboratory.

The cytopathic effects (CPE) Enders and his younger coworkers had learned to recognize as signs of virus activity began to appear in each successive batch of human kidney-tissue cultures after each passage of the Edmonston virus, which now could be isolated and studied under the electron microscope. Immune serum from patients convalescing from measles neutralized it. It was no longer merely a suspect. It was the long-sought measles virus.

It took three years of painstaking laboratory work, chiefly by Milan Milanovic, a visiting Yugoslav Fellow in Enders's laboratory, to attenuate this virus by passaging it through various tissues and cells of people and birds, mice and monkeys, until it no longer caused disease in monkeys—but at the same time caused the monkeys to start producing circulating antibodies, which neutralized fully virulent measles viruses in tissue cultures. More animal and first-stage clinical tests followed, and finally by 1960 Dr. Enders's close coworker, the pediatrician Samuel I. Katz, was ready to start testing the vaccine in small and then larger groups of children.

The Edmonston live measles virus vaccine was licensed for general use in 1963. A killed-virus vaccine developed in another laboratory was also licensed at about the same time, but it was not very practical. This and subsequent live measles virus vaccines, licensed during a year in which there were 385,156 reported cases of measles, soon repaid their costs of development a thousand times over. In 1973 the CDC reported that during their first ten years of use, "Over 60 million doses of vaccine have been distributed, nearly 24 million [measles] cases have been prevented, and the economic savings total nearly 1.3 billion dollars." The CDC estimated, by projections of prevaccine-era patterns, that because of the live virus measles vaccines, 7,900 cases of mental retardation caused by measles encephalitis had been averted, 2,400 lives saved, 12,182,000 physician visits and 1,352,000 hospital days saved, and 78,000,000 school days saved.

At no point, however, during that initial decade were all children at risk immunized by their own or by public health doctors. The cases averted by vaccination made an impressive total, but during the same ten years, a total of 1,547,957 cases of measles were reported to local health departments, ranging from 458,043 cases reported in 1964 to 32,275 cases in 1972, and then as now subject to the CDC caveat that the reported numbers represented only 10 percent to at most 25 percent of all actual cases. Vaccines are valuable only when used.

Long before the measles vaccine started to prove itself, Enders's old student and postwar Fellow, Thomas Weller, had become involved in the hunt for the virus of rubella, or German measles.

For over a century, rubella (German measles) was known as a measles-like but much more common childhood disease than measles. It was often mistaken for scarlet fever, a more serious streptococcal infection. Most children had rubella before they were five and suffered no complications, other than slightly swollen lymph nodes of the head and neck. Apparently the rubella infection conferred lifelong immunity against its recurrence once a child got over it. As early as 1914, A. F. Hess had suggested that it was caused by a filtrable virus. In 1938 two Japanese doctors, Y. Hiro and S. Tasaka, succeeded in transmitting the disease by inoculating healthy nonimmune children with cell-free filtrates of nasal washings taken from children with active cases of rubella. This supported Hess's hypothesis that the agent of rubella was probably a virus, but in 1938 there was no urgent clinical rationale for launching major efforts to isolate the virus. The reason was soon provided by Norman McAlister Gregg, an Australian ophthalmologist.

In 1940–1941 a rubella epidemic broke out in most Australian communities. Within a year of an outbreak in Sydney, Gregg noticed a sharp rise in children being born with congenital cataracts. In his own practice, Gregg had a total of thirteen newborn infants with congenital cataracts. These children had two additional features in common: Most suffered from other handicapping birth defects—such as deafness, congenital heart disease, microcephaly (abnormal smallness of the head), cerebral palsy, and mental retardation—and all had been born to mothers who had had German measles during pregnancy.

Gregg prepared a query concerning children recently born with congenital cataracts and sent copies to a small number of other ophthalmologists in the country. Among the answers received, seventy-eight other cases of blindness due to cataracts were reported in newborns. Of these congenitally blind babies, forty-four had also been born with congenital heart defects. Each of the ninety-one congenitally blind babies treated by Gregg and his peers shared other common problems: They were all underweight, smaller than normal, hard to feed, and, if not born blind, suffering from strabismus (squint). As they grew older, it would be found that these birth-damaged children were also mentally retarded. The other clinical factor shared by sixty-eight of the seventy-eight congenitally blind children seen by other physicians was that their mothers recalled having had mild cases of rubella during their pregnancies. Gregg published his findings in the *Transactions of the Ophthalmological Society of Australia* in the spring of 1941, under the unambiguous title "Congenital cataract following German measles in the mother."

This seminal report was almost universally overlooked. World War II was then two years old. Japan and Australia and most of the European nations capable of conducting rubella and birth-defect studies were at war, and the United States, teetering on the brink, was soon to be bombed into that war. As in all wars, the armies on both sides had one underlying goal: the ancient and classic goal of killing as many enemy soldiers and civilians as humanly and technologically possible. Medically, the health of the soldiers trained to kill foreign enemies became the top clinical research priority, followed closely by the health of the civilians who produced the munitions and engines of war. Nothing has a lower biomedical research priority in times of war than the eyes, ears, brains, and other organs of unborn children threatened by the postulated virus of a harmless and rarely complicated transient infection.

If rubella was shunted aside for the duration, it was not forgotten by many fine scientists. Just before the bombing of Pearl Harbor, Karl Habel, at the then National Institute of Health, succeeded in transmitting rubella to monkeys using the same method used earlier in children by Hiro and Tasaka. When the war ended, laboratories in Australia and the United States, and in slowly rebuilding Europe and Japan tried without initial success to isolate the presumed virus of rubella. Gregg's continuing studies now claimed the attention of many investigators.

Largely because of Gregg's work, the congenital effects of maternal rubella made Australian doctors aware that "in Australia during the years 1939–42 there were probably 400 to 500 infants born with congenital damage of one sort or another resulting from rubella infection."[3] A retrospective study of the birth dates of those listed in Australian census records as deaf-mutes showed, as Macfarlane Burnet wrote, "that in Australia there have been several periods when many such birth dates are concentrated within a few months. In 1900, for instance, the graph of births of people subsequently registered as deaf-mutes provided a typical epidemic curve whose peak was six or seven months after that of a known rubella epidemic. The answer then is simply that congenital damage by rubella in pregnancy had been occurring for at least forty years before Gregg recognized it in 1940."[4]

Injections of gamma-globulin concentrates from pooled normal human sera did not always seem to work, after the war, in preventing rubella in children. For this reason and because German measles was so mild a disease, most pediatricians advised against subjecting healthy children to the risks and inconveniences of costly immunoglobulin injections. However, as Enders's wartime collaborator, the pediatrician Joseph Stokes, Jr., wrote in the chapter on virus diseases in the 1954 edition of Nelson's *Textbook of Pediatrics,* "It is important for girls to be exposed to German measles and to contract the disease before the age of child bearing."

In 1948 Macfarlane Burnet and his collaborators used gamma globulin from the blood of people convalescing from rubella to provide passive immunity that protected over twenty nonimmune pregnant women who had recently been exposed to the disease. Gradually, as Burnet and others extended these efforts, doctors in America and elsewhere over the next fifteen years began to use such immune sera, with demonstrably high levels of antirubella antibodies, to induce short-term passive immunity to rubella in pregnant women who had recently been exposed to individuals (often as not their own young children) known to have rubella. These immune sera were better than no protection at all, but they were still a far cry from vaccines that could confer permanent immunity to women before they became pregnant.

Enders was one of many scientific workers who tried and failed to isolate and culture the rubella virus. As Robbins and Weller left his laboratory to follow their own careers—Robbins in 1952 to Western Reserve University in Cleveland as professor of pediatrics, Weller to the Harvard School of Public Health as professor of tropical medicine—new Fellows in pediatric virology arrived to share the work load.

Although Weller was now in what seemed to be another field of work, most (but not all) tropical diseases are so named because they are endemic in the tropics long after being eradicated in the industrial nations, which, by coincidence, seem for the most part to be in the temperate climatic zones. Then as now, the major killing "tropical" diseases included such all-climate infections and infestations as malaria, measles, rubella, diphtheria, tetanus, mumps, infant diarrhea (caused by bacterial- and viral-contaminated food and water), yellow fever, hookworm, influenza, pneumonia, cholera, typhoid, and typhus, plus such all-climate deficiency diseases as rickets, pellagra, marasmus, and scurvy. Many of these infections, as well as smallpox, had been wiped out, by 1954, or reduced to insignificance in this and other industrial countries by clean water systems and other artifacts of planned environmental hygiene; vaccinations; antibiotics; and (the most basic advance in public health) wage increases that reduced family crowding and improved maternal, child, and family nutrition, and paid for measurably greater access to private and governmental medical care. This meant that in his new laboratory, Weller remained as deeply involved with the etiology and prevention of major infectious diseases as he had ever been.

In 1960 Weller's ten-year-old son developed an atypically severe case of rubella. At the same time, a major outbreak of German measles hit many new army recruits at Fort Dix, New Jersey. Both Weller and a talented team, headed by Paul Parkman, E. L. Buescher, and Malcolm S. Artenstein, at the Walter Reed Army Institute of Research (WRAIR) isolated the rubella virus, Weller from a specimen of his son's urine added to primary human amnionic-tissue cultures. The WRAIR team in February 1961 isolated the virus from cultures of African Green monkey kidney cells to which they added throat washings from seventy-nine army recruits with German measles. Weller and Parkman exchanged cultures of the viruses they had isolated and grown. Both strains of virus isolated from patients with rubella were identical in form and in cytopathic activity against cells in laboratory cultures, and were immunologically active in human volunteers. There was no longer any doubt that the rubella virus had been isolated.[5]

The newly isolated virus remained more or less a laboratory curiosity until 1963–1964, when one of the greatest rubella outbreaks in history occurred in the United States. German measles was not then a notifiable disease, and there are no records of how many people actually caught rubella during that epidemic. It is not even known how many children suffered congenital or developmental damage caused by prenatal rubella infections. The only firm figure we do have is that 20,000 children suffered prenatal brain damage caused by rubella infections during the 1963–1964 epidemic, and that (in 1969 dollars) the costs of the rehabilitation of these congenital rubella syndrome victims was put at over $2 billion five years after the epidemic ended.[6]

The human and fiscal costs of that epidemic played a large part in winning congressional approval of Title XIX—the Medicaid provisions—of the Social Security Act of 1965, as well as for the Early and Periodic Screening, Diagnosis, and Treatment (EPSDT) amendments to Title XIX that made comprehensive pediatric care, including all necessary vaccinations, the mandated birthright of every American child regardless of ability to pay for needed care. In some instances, legislators who proposed and fought for this legislation acted out of compassion for the victims of rubella; in many more cases, however, the legislation making vaccination a birthright was supported because it would always cost the federal government far less to vaccinate the entire susceptible population than to institutionalize and/or rehabilitate victims of polio and other ubiquitous infections. The EPSDT amendments, however, have been nominally administered at best and, in most states, simply ignored.

At the federal Bureau of Biologics, to which Paul Parkman moved when his military service was completed, Parkman joined forces with Drs. Harry Meyer, Jr., and Theodore C. Panos to develop an attenuated live rubella virus vaccine in 1966. Although the infection itself is generally free of postnatal complications, considerable numbers of tests had to be run in animals and small groups of children—many of them the children of doctors working on the vaccines—before mass trials were undertaken. Once the safety of the vaccine was established, the first of the large trials were conducted in children's hospitals and orphan asylums, where crowding put these children at the greatest risk of catching German measles.[7]

The Public Health Service had to be particularly cautious about issuing a license for the new attenuated live poliovirus vaccine, since it had been developed at its own Bureau of Biologics, whose functions include testing all experimental vaccines before they can be licensed. At no point since then has the rubella vaccine been administered to more than 60 percent of the children, particularly girls, for whom its use is most urgent, since it has been used primarily for the protection of children whose families can afford the continually rising costs of private medical care. Despite the underuse of the rubella vaccine, reported cases of German measles in the United States fell from 57,686 in 1969 to 11,795 in 1979 (with, of course, the probability that these reported cases represent only about 10 percent of the actual numbers during those years).

By the time the rubella vaccine was licensed, another live virus vaccine, this one against mumps, had been approved for general use. As we saw earlier, the complications of mumps are not limited to the lumpy and painful swelling it causes in the salivary glands. The complications range from orchitis, an excruciatingly painful inflammation of the testes which, in adult males, can result in sterility, to mumps encephalitis of the brain so severe that it causes brain damage and irreversible mental retardation. Mumps can also at times cause both nerve deafness and pancreatitis, or inflammation of the gland where the body produces the vitally required hormone, insulin.

The first vaccine against human infections that Enders ever developed was the killed-mumps-virus vaccine he and Joseph Stokes, Jr., made for the armed forces during World War II. When peace came Enders, who had little faith in inactivated or killed-virus vaccines, immediately went to work attenuating the mumps virus by continuously passaging it through chick-embryo cells. The vaccine worked well but not permanently, offering a term of immunity only a little longer than could be obtained from hyperimmune gamma globulin. In the Soviet Union, a similar live virus vaccine was introduced and used in millions of children. In this country, however, the short-lived active immunity offered by this early live mumps virus vaccine was enough to keep the Public Health Service from licensing it for general use.

Maurice Hilleman, who had moved from the Walter Reed Army Institute of Research to take over the virus and cell biology branches of the Merck Institute for Therapeutic Research near Philadelphia, eventually supplied a better vaccine in response to the same kind of stimulus that had sent Weller into rubella research. In 1960 his six-year-old daughter, Jeryl Lynn, caught the mumps. Hilleman took some blood and saliva from the little girl, diluted and filtered these body fluids, and passaged the filtrates through chick-embryo cultures. After only a few passages through the tissues of another species, the Jeryl Lynn strain of mumps virus was too attenuated or weakened to infect any kinds of cells in tissue cultures, let alone cause mumps in susceptible people.

Hilleman and his coworker, Eugene Buynack, developed a vaccine based on this attenuated, Jeryl Lynn strain of the mumps virus. They came up with a vaccine that worked very effectively in its preclinical trials. In the spring of 1965, the Merck group joined forces with a team headed by University of Pennsylvania pediatrics professor Robert E. Weibel to test the still experimental mumps vaccine in controlled field trials in Philadelphia and its suburbs. After children of various school districts were vaccinated, Weibel and his collaborators for the next 116 months "took blood samples from children who had either been vaccinated or developed natural mumps ... Nine and one-half years later, antibodies (against mumps virus) persisted in both groups ..." The children in the mumps program continued to be followed. "There were only three reported cases of natural mumps in 1975 and two in 1976 in a suburb of 50,000 persons,"[8] where most of the schoolchildren had been vaccinated with the Jeryl Lynn mumps vaccine in the trials of 1965.

The Hilleman mumps vaccine was licensed for general use in January 1968. One of the first to be vaccinated was Jeryl Lynn's baby sister, Kirsten Jeanne, which represented a new variation of the traditional or classic route of the transmission of mumps viruses from children with mumps to their siblings.

Prior to 1968 mumps was not a notifiable disease. In 1968, the first year of the mumps vaccine's availability, a total of 152,209 cases were reported by local physicians. By 1979 the number of cases reported around the country fell to 14,225.

As in the case of measles, the reported mumps cases probably represent 5 percent to at most 20 percent of the actual numbers since 1968, with the further caveat that upward of half of all mumps cases were and are never seen by doctors. Still, assuming that the actual numbers of mumps infections in the United States were around 1,522,090 in 1958 and 142,250 in 1979, this more than ten-fold drop represents a public health gain of considerable magnitude. Particularly, I might add, in view of the fact that at no point since 1968 have more than 60 percent of the populations at risk been vaccinated against mumps, polio, measles, rubella, or any of the other viral and bacterial vaccines now licensed for use against major infectious diseases.

In terms of viral vaccines, not all of which are medically recommended for infants and young children, the present array of licensed virus vaccines, and when and where they were developed, includes:

Smallpox (1796)	England (last documented case in U.S. in 1949, last known case in world in 1977, stockpiled but no longer used)
Rabies (1885)	France
Yellow fever (1936)	U.S., France, England
Influenza (1943)	U.S., England
Poliomyelitis (1954)	U.S.
Measles (1963)	U.S.
Mumps (1968)	U.S.
Adenovirus (1970)	U.S. (licensed in 1980 for military use only)
Hepatitis B (1980)	U.S.

The costs of purchasing and administering the measles, polio, rubella, and mumps vaccines that the American Academy of Pediatrics recommends be given routinely to all children, starting at the age of two months, can be covered with one or two ten-dollar bills. The costs of medical, hospital, and long-term posthospital care can run into tens of thousands of dollars per year for the remainder of every single human life irreversibly diminished by paralysis, blindness, deafness, brain damage, cerebral palsy, and other prenatal and postnatal damages resulting from the direct and often multiple effects of poliomyelitis, measles, mumps, maternal rubella, and other vaccine-preventable virus diseases.

Obviously, the vast amounts of federal funds invested in the development of vaccines against viral diseases since World War II have paid cash benefits far in excess of the sum total of the highly profitable tax-dollar investments in basic and applied biological and medical research.

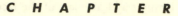
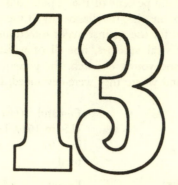

VACCINES AGAINST HUMAN CANCERS: POSSIBLY SOON, BUT NOT RIGHT NOW

There is also overwhelming evidence that the hepatitis B virus is the single most important causative factor of hepatocellular carcinoma.... Thus, mass immunization programs against HBV infection ... may ultimately reduce the morbidity and mortality from ... hepatocellular carcinoma.

—WOLF SZMUNESS, M.D., and eight co-authors, "Hepatitis B Vaccine, Demonstration of Efficacy in a Controlled Clinical Trial," *New England Journal of Medicine,* October 9, 1980

Concerning the association between the [hepatitis B] infection and liver cancer, he [Dr. Szmuness] suggested that the prevention of one may avert the other. "But that's a long way off," he stressed. "It'd be premature to call this a vaccine against cancer."

—ANON., "Efficacy of Those Hepatitis Shots Is Affirmed," *Medical World News,* October 13, 1980 ot every attempt to develop a vaccine after the agent of a major virus disease was isolated and grown in pure cultures succeeded in storybook fashion during the 1960s. For example, there was the cytomegalovirus (CMV), so named because it caused the cells it infected to swell up to giant proportions until they were at times taken for protozoa.

In 1921 these "protozoan-like" cells found in certain lesions of infant diseases were named cytomegalia (giant cells) by Ernest Goodpasture and Fritz Talbot, who described them as resembling the nuclear inclusions seen in the cells of the skin lesions of the disease called, since ancient times, herpes (from the Greek word meaning creeper or snake).

After World War II these skin eruptions were found to be caused by the cytomegalovirus (CMV), a member of the herpesvirus family. The burr-shaped DNA herpes viruses are responsible for many human disorders, including the "cold sores" or "fever blisters" caused by the herpes simplex viruses Type I. Most people carry herpes simplex Type I viruses all their lives. They were considered to be harmless until in very recent years herpes simplex Type I and the newly discovered herpes simplex Type II viruses were both found to be known agents of what is presently America's leading sexually transmitted disease, the recurrent and as yet medically incurable genital herpes infection. Between twenty and thirty million Americans are now estimated to contract this infection every year.

Other disease-causing herpes viruses include the Epstein-Barr virus (EBV) and the varicella-zoster virus. The Epstein-Barr virus is the proven cause of infectious mononucleosis, the "kissing disease," and is believed by some important investigators to be the cause of two serious forms of cancer, Burkitt's lymphoma, and nasopharyngeal carcinoma. The varicella-zoster virus is the agent of childhood chicken pox and middle-age shingles.

As early as 1936, work in various laboratories had suggested that the cytomegalia agents were filtrable viruses. For example, in 1936 at Washington University in St. Louis, Missouri, Margaret Smith showed that "the presence of greatly enlarged cells containing large intranuclear inclusions in the salivary glands of several species of rodents has been shown to be associated with a transmissible filtrable virus."[1] In 1953 Wallace Rowe, at the National Institutes of Health, found a viral agent in adenoids obtained from operations on young children, and that this transmissable agent caused cytopathogenic (CPE) effect on the tissues of people, rabbits, hamsters, and embryonic chicks.

During the next year in St. Louis, Margaret Smith recovered a similar virus from the salivary glands in mouse tissue cultures, and proposed to call it the salivary gland virus (SGV) after it caused changes in other mouse tissue cultures. However, when "Weller isolated the identical virus from a liver biopsy from an infant with a clinical diagnosis of cytomegalic inclusion disease"[2] and sent a culture to Rowe, it became apparent that Smith, Weller, and Rowe had all isolated the same virus. This soon became known as the cytomegalovirus.

Clinical studies of the teratogenic effects of maternal CMV infections on developing fetuses by Weller, the pediatrician James B. Hanshaw,[3] and others soon revealed that CMV infections were an even greater public health problem than *in utero* rubella. Like the rubella viruses, the CMV easily passes through the placenta of infected mothers and invades the cells of their developing fetuses. There, it causes mortal damage and/or permanently handicapping birth defects by infecting and reducing by half the growth rates of developing organs, limbs, nervous systems, and brains. Fortunately, only the rubella and CMV particles regularly pass the placental barrier, although from time to time other viruses also penetrate this inborn defense against fetal infection.

Today we know that "only a small proportion of people throughout the world escape infection with cytomegalovirus (CMV),"[4] and that at least 10 percent of all infants acquire CMV infections before they are born. A recent British study concludes that "one of every 1000 newborns, at least in England and the United States, will have hearing loss, psychomotor retardation, or neurological defect secondary to congenital CMV infections."[5] In a study of *in utero* infections that cause brain damage, conducted by the British scientists H. Stern and S. D. Elek in mentally retarded children living at home with their parents in London, it was shown that CMV may account for 10 percent of all these brain-damaging infections, while the rubella virus and the toxoplasma (a protozoan parasite found in uncooked meat) combined "were responsible for about 2 to 3% of all the cases of mental deficiency" in these London children.[6]

In a recent study conducted at the University of Alabama medical school and cooperating institutions pediatricians and specialists in infectious diseases and learning disorders produced data that "firmly establish clinically inapparent congenital CMV infection as a major public health problem." The authors felt that "the discovery that hearing defects may occur in as many as 17% of children born with subclinical, congenital CMV infection is perhaps the single most important finding of this study." They estimated that "approximately 4000 infants (one in 750 live births) per year are born in the United States with auditory impairment caused by CMV. At least half of these infants (those with bilateral, moderate to profound hearing losses) will be significantly, if not grossly, handicapped by these defects; the others (those with unilateral or lesser forms of bilateral disease) will undoubtedly experience increased difficulty in achieving their social potential. These figures should likely be doubled for low socioeconomic groups in whom the frequency of congenital CMV [syndrome] may be as high as 2%, as documented by our population."[7]

In this and other studies, CMV infections also caused eye disorders as well as the same array of congenital birth defects caused by *in utero* rubella infections. This combination of learning handicaps makes CMV, like rubella, a major cause of behavioral and mental retardation.

Given these effects, many laboratories around the world started to work on vaccines against CMV infections more than twenty years ago. The development of a good vaccine against the virus proved to be far more difficult than measuring its damaging effects on the developing fetus. For one thing, CMV grows very slowly in tissue cultures and cannot be grown in animals. Even if one wanted to make a killed-virus vaccine, it would be all but impossible to grow it in the amounts needed for inactivated virus vaccines. Live vaccines require far smaller starting quantities of virus.

By the mid-1960s, however, evidence suggesting that the entire family of animal and human herpesviruses might be oncogenic or cancer causing began to put a damper on CMV vaccine projects. There was not a whisper of evidence indicating that the CMV virus might be oncogenic, but cancer is never a threat to take lightly. There was even, as in the case of a poultry infection called Marek's disease, some reason to believe that a vaccine against CMV in time might help in the development of a vaccine against some forms of human cancers.

Marek's disease is a lymphoproliferative, neoplastic disease of chickens, often called chicken lymphoma or chicken leukemia. Before the development of a live, attenuated virus vaccine against the avian herpesvirus that causes it, Marek's disease was the most important cause of poultry losses and condemnations in the world. Today all commercially hatched chicks in the United States are routinely vaccinated against Marek's disease, and it is no longer endemic in American flocks.[8]

After the development of the vaccine against the neoplastic disease caused by avian herpesviruses, some but far from all fears of cancers caused by a vaccine against any human herpesvirus disease were mitigated. In 1973–1974 two live virus CMV vaccines were developed, one in England by S. D. Elek and H. Stern, the other by Dr. Stanley Plotkin at Children's Hospital in Philadelphia. Each vaccine was tested in a few hundred volunteers. Both produced

CMV antibodies without causing cancer or other catastrophic effects in the volunteers. Mass clinical trials, however, do not seem to be in the offing because of the still sticky question of the established oncogenicity of other herpesviruses, and the hypothetical but extremely remote possibility that CMV might be as closely related to some forms of cancer as are other herpesviruses.

Recently in a chapter of a British book on advances in clinical virology, Elek suggested that "a subunit vaccine containing the surface protein antigens of the virus, without the [virus] nucleic acid, would be the ideal solution but the effectiveness and durability of immunity produced by such vaccines, as well as their economic feasibility, remains to be proved. In man, only live vaccines have proved their worth."[9]

"Chemical vaccines" that are analogous to the successful bacterial capsular polysaccharide vaccines developed against pneumococcal pneumonia already exist against influenza and serum hepatitis and, experimentally, against other virus diseases. It is quite likely that such subunit vaccines, compounded of antigen proteins split off from the glycoprotein coats of the CMV virions, and free of the core DNA that constitutes the infective part of the virus itself, might in time prove to be the safe CMV vaccines needed to immunize women before pregnancy to protect their children *in utero*. Experimental chemical vaccines made of synthetic viral structures are also now in development. Meanwhile, maternal CMV infections continue to damage the brains, eyes, limbs, and organs for all the days of our lives.

The varicella-zoster—i.e., chicken pox-shingles virus—which infects nine out of every ten American children younger than ten, like the CMV, is a DNA herpesvirus. In children the virus causes chicken pox, the most infectious of all virus diseases, marked by a fever and a short-lived itchy rash. Most children become totally immune to a second attack, but in many who are immunized against the disease by a natural infection, the virus persists in a dormant state in the dorsal nerve root, or the cranial ganglion cells. There the varicella-zoster virus sits inertly for many years, much like the viral prophages in lysogenic bacterial cells. In most people the dormant varicella-zoster viruses remain harmless for life. In certain people, however, the traumas of later life—the loss of a job, an election, a loved one; or a severe illness, a physically abusive husband, a nagging wife, a sudden change—can reactivate the dormant varicella-zoster viruses. This time they cause not chicken pox but herpes zoster, or shingles, a very painful and often disabling condition.

Michiaki Takahashi, a virologist at Osaka University, Japan, in 1974 isolated a varicella-zoster virus from the chicken-pox skin vesicles of a little boy named Oka. Takahashi cultured the Oka strain in human embryonic lung tissues, and then in successive passages through human diploid cells. These repeated passages ultimately attenuated the Oka chicken-pox virus to the point where it lost virulence but retained its immunogenicity.

324

Since then, the experimental Oka vaccine has been tested in over six hundred children in Japan, with results that led Takahashi to declare, in 1980, that the "potential benefits of varicella-zoster vaccine outweigh the potential risks." If it is eventually licensed and routinely administered to all children, the Oka vaccine could not only reduce or even eradicate chicken pox but also protect adults from the much more traumatic herpes zoster. Not enough clinical data exist, as yet, to make the Oka-strain live varicella-zoster virus vaccine a candidate for imminent licensing for routine use in children. However, it is possible that long before such data are generated, the vaccine will be licensed for the routine protection of immune-deficient children—such as children with leukemia or other cancers treated with immunosuppressive drugs. "It is a particular tragedy that in childhood-cancer treatment, with its increasing cure rates, so many—7%—die of varicella-zoster infection," laments Dr. John A. Zais, a research pediatrician at the Sidney Farber Cancer Institute in Boston. Various institutions around the world are now injecting nonimmune child cancer patients with the Oka vaccine in the hope it will prevent such deaths.

Because of the fears that even the attenuated live viruses in experimental herpes vaccines will remain in a dormant state in the bodies of immunized people, most of the current crop of experimental vaccines against herpesvirus infections are not made of attenuated or even killed whole herpesvirus particles, but rather of subunits of the DNA-free virus coats on which the viral antigen proteins are found. If indeed it does transpire that the DNA of any or all of the herpesviruses is in any way, alone or in tandem with other entities, responsible for causing some forms of cancer in human beings, the new subunit antiviral vaccines would present no oncogenic threats.

In England, Dr. Gordon R. B. Skinner and his colleagues at the University of Birmingham have for the past two years been testing a subunit herpes simplex Types I and II (HSV-1, HSV-2) vaccine they developed in a group of nearly four hundred male and female volunteers. This vaccine is made of surface antigens that are separated from intact herpesvirus particles by ultrasonic disruption, and then chemically treated to both sterilize and purify them. The test population includes people who never had genital herpesvirus infections and their regular sexual partners, and individuals who had primary genital herpes infections before being vaccinated with the experimental subunit HSV-1 and HSV-2 vaccine.

None of the people who had never had a genital herpes virus infection developed one during the two years after being vaccinated, although they continued their normal sex lives during these years. In the other volunteers, Dr. Skinner revealed in the summer of 1982, "patients who have had their first attack of herpes genitalis have a major modification of the likelihood of recurrence. To date 3 of 30 patients have had one recurrence while the expectation in six months following the first infection would be approximately

325

90% of patients. In patients with the established infection approximately 60–70% have improved, but of course this requires a very strict double-blind placebo trial. Approximately 1200 vaccinations have been given to over 400 patients to date without significant or local general side-effect."

More extensive placebo-controlled double-blind clinical trials of the very promising Skinner vaccine are now being arranged.

Maurice Hilleman and his colleagues at the Merck Institute have been working on an equally DNA-free herpes simplex vaccine. They describe it as a "purified glycoprotein in subunit vaccine prepared using chick embryo fibroblasts infected with Type 2 herpes simplex virus as the source of the antigen. The process for preparation included destruction or elimination of all detectable DNA and final treatment with formaldehyde." Tested in mice, the split virus vaccine caused a 60 percent reduction in mortality. This was less effective than the 72 percent reduction when equal doses of a killed whole-virus vaccine were given to other mice, who were then challenged with wild Type II herpes simplex viruses, but it represented an encouraging beginning.

The experimental subunit herpes simplex vaccine evoked antibody production in human volunteers, and Hilleman believes "the vaccine shows fair promise for ability to limit or prevent primary herpesvirus infection" in people.[10]

The most controversial and possibly the most important herpesvirus is the Epstein-Barr virus (EBV). The EBV is the agent of infectious mononucleosis (IM), the debilitating and troublesome "kissing disease" that seizes over 100,000 young Americans each year. Infectious mononucleosis is not in itself a killing disease; during the ten years ending in 1976, only 195 fatal cases were reported to the CDC. It is not a notifiable disease, but some states voluntarily report their cases to the CDC; in 1979 in less than half of all the states, a total of 18,019 cases of infectious mononucleosis were reported. While up to 3 percent of the population will have frank (and medically diagnosed) infectious mononucleosis during their lifetimes, it is estimated that up to 90 percent of all children will have mild or inapparent IM infections before reaching puberty.

"In its classical form infectious mononucleosis causes fever, tonsillitis, swollen lymph nodes and an enlarged liver and spleen. . . . The majority of patients are young adults, and uncomplicated cases run their course in from one week to four weeks with complete recovery. Fewer than 1 percent of the patients have complications (such as encephalitis, pneumonia and kidney failure) and fatal cases are very rare."[11] In half of all those who are treated for IM, doctors report spleen enlargement as a symptom. Usually, the spleen reverts to normal size as the infection ends, but rupture of the spleen is occasionally responsible for IM deaths. Dr. David T. Purtillo, professor of pediatrics and pathology at the University of Massachusetts, puts the current United States death rate for IM at thirty to thirty-five a year.

More ominously, infectious mononucleosis is a known lympho-proliferative disorder, a disease marked by accelerated growth of the lymphoid tissues. Such disorders, including IM, at times develop into lymphoma, a usually malignant growth of any of the lymphoid tissues, such as lymphocytic leukemia, Hodgkin's disease, and lymphosarcoma. Werner and Gertrude Henle, the noted University of Pennsylvania virologists, observe that some clinicians describe infectious mononucleosis as a self-limited form (or precursor) of leukemia.[12] In this concept, it is hypothesized that infectious mononucleosis, if not self-terminated after a few weeks, then develops into a full-blown case of leukemia. Patients with IM show a marked increase in their number of white blood cells, which are often abnormally shaped. "In patients with mononucleosis the abnormal proliferation of lymphocytes subsides; in leukemia," write the Henles, "the [white blood] cells continue to multiply out of control."[13] Because of the huge concentration of white blood cells in people with splenomyelogenous and lymphatic forms of leukemia, Rudolf Virchow, in 1845, named the disorder "weisses Blut" (white blood).

Although IM was not one of their research interests, the Henles's profound involvement in the search for tumor viruses would lead to their largely serendipitous discovery that the Epstein-Barr virus is the causal agent of infectious mononucleosis.

During the late 1950s, Denis Burkitt, a surgeon at the Makerere University Hospital in Uganda, discovered great clusters of young children with particularly deforming and lethal tumors of the jaws. At first, there was little he could do for these children other than to study the tumors, which proved to be lymphomas. Later, with the aid and cooperation of the National Cancer Institute in Bethesda, Maryland, and other national and international agencies, he was able to save the lives of some of the children with anticancer drugs and other aids.

The manner in which the family, neighborhood, and village clusters in which this swiftly killing cancer—soon to be named Burkitt's lymphoma by the duly accredited taxonomic commissions—proliferated in Africa reminded Burkitt of the epidemiological patterns that prevailed in diphtheria and paralytic polio before vaccines to control them were widely available in his native England. Burkitt began to make field trips to various parts of Africa to study the clinical and epidemiological patterns of Burkitt's lymphoma. He found that cancer of the jaw was most prevalent in children between the ages of six and eight who lived in regions where malaria was endemic. By 1958 these studies led Burkitt to suggest that this cancer was caused in whole or in part by an infectious agent, probably a virus, transmitted to people by the same mosquitoes that delivered the larger parasites of malaria.

Burkitt lacked the technological resources to hunt for these postulated tumor viruses, and he sent biopsy tissues from patients with the lymphoma to doctors around the world who offered to help in the quest. In 1964 at London's Middlesex Hospital, Dr. M. Anthony Epstein found, under the electron microscope, what seemed to be herpeslike virus particles in such pathology tissues. Epstein and his coworkers, B. G. Achong and Y. M. Barr, then isolated, cultured, and studied these particles, which they identified as viruses and which were soon named the Epstein-Barr virus (EBV). Epstein sent viral cultures to the Henles, who confirmed the fact that the EBV was a DNA herpesvirus.

The Henles did what any good virologists do when a new disease virus is isolated: They cultured it in tissue flasks and started to test its ability to react with antibodies to it which might be present in samples of blood from many different populations in many cities, states, and countries. To their great surprise, the Henles found that antibodies to the new Epstein-Barr virus were not only circulating in the blood of children with Burkitt's lymphoma, but also in the blood of most African children tested, as well as in large samples of the sera of healthy children around the world. Since as usual such tests begin close to home, the Henles also looked for and found antibodies to EBV in most of the people in their laboratories at Children's Hospital in Philadelphia.

As with the poliovirus, so with the Epstein-Barr virus, "It soon became evident that the age at which antibodies to the virus are acquired depends on the prevailing living conditions. Under the conditions of crowding and poor hygiene prevalent in the developing [i.e., nonindustrial and poor] countries practically all children manufacture antibodies to the [EBV] virus by the age of three or four. In the more advanced [i.e., industrial and higher-family-income] countries the acquisition of antibodies to the EB virus is often delayed until adolescence or adulthood."[14]

While these findings in healthy populations in which Burkitt's lymphomas were unknown were leading the Henles to suspect that the EBV was probably the cause of a common, self-limited illness in most populations, as well as of Burkitt's lymphoma in the malaria-ridden sections of Africa, other workers were making other discoveries. At the Memorial Sloan-Kettering Cancer Center in New York, a group of investigators headed by Lloyd J. Old published findings that indicated the EBV was also involved in causing nasopharyngeal carcinoma. This devastating tumor develops in the space behind the nose and can travel from the nose to the brain.[15] It hits adults in southern China at the rate of ten cases per 100,000 population annually, and at much smaller rates in Tunisia and East Africa, and in Alaskan Eskimos.

The Henles went on looking for the common, self-limited disease they believed was also caused by the EBV. The answer came late in 1967. It turned up in their own laboratory when "one of our young technicians developed classic symptoms of infectious mononucleosis: sore throat, fever and enlarged lymph nodes in the neck. Before her illness she had shown no antibodies to the Epstein-Barr virus, but with the onset of the disease [anti-EBV] antibodies appeared in her serum."[16] Here was a very obvious candidate for the other disease caused by the EBV. With the aid of other investigators who had been studying infectious mononucleosis itself since 1958, and collecting blood samples from college students before and after they had IM, the Henles were able definitely to establish the Epstein-Barr virus as the causal agent of IM.

Subsequently, various researchers used the EBV to cause lymphomas in marmosets and other New World monkeys. These animal lymphomas, while equally malignant and lethal, were very similar to but not quite identical with Burkitt's lymphomas, but then again even New World monkeys are not quite identical with people.

While the mass media described the EBV as the sole cause of at least two human cancers, responsible virologists and cancer workers tried valiantly to make responsible laymen more aware of possible cofactors in EBV-associated Burkitt's lymphoma. The fact that Burkitt's lymphoma was so widespread in (and, in fact, confined to) regions where malaria was endemic did not—despite the obvious model of mosquitoes as carriers of the yellow fever virus—necessarily mean that mosquitoes also carried the virus agent of Burkitt's lymphoma. Malaria both enhances the proliferation of lymphocytes and acts as an immune suppressor which reduces a body's capacity to produce antibody, complement, interferon, and other natural host defenses against viruses and other immunologically "foreign" antigens.

In 1973 D. Kufe and other workers in Sol Spiegelman's cancer research group at Columbia University found that RNA was related to the murine leukemia viruses in both Burkitt's lymphomas and nasopharyngeal carcinomas.[17] This indicated the possible presence of a two-virus carcinogenic system, such as that previously discovered by Harry Rubin in the Rous sarcoma virus-Rous helper virus (RSV-RHV) synergistic collaboration in inducing cancer in chickens.

There were also other possible cofactors in the causation of Burkitt's lymphomas, including severe malnutrition (as common as malaria in most of Africa, Asia, and Latin America), hormonal imbalances caused by various diseases and disorders, and alterations in the nature of bodily tissues caused by malaria and other endemic diseases.

Possibly the most important cofactors in virus-associated cancers are genetic, caused by the chromosomal damage experienced *in utero* or throughout the natural life of a person. They are also the least understood, since many tend to confuse truly hereditary diseases, like hemophilia and phenylketonuria, with nonhereditary but fully genetic disorders like the largest single cause of congenital mental retardation, Down's syndrome.

Hereditary diseases are handed down directly, from parents to children, via the sperm or the ova of both male and female germ cells.

Genetic diseases, on the other hand, are caused by damages to the twenty-three pairs of matched chromosomes in the nucleus of every human cell. The chromosomes contain the genes of heredity. Such genetic damages are caused by many things, including ionizing radiations, viruses, and mutagenic chemical pollutants in the environment. Sometimes these genetic damages cause translocations in which the chromosomes that should be at one of the twenty-three locations appear in each other's spot. At other times, one of a matched pair of chromosomes is too short. The Philadelphia chromosome, in which one of the two chromosomes number 21 is deleted, usually proves to be a marker for chronic lymphocytic leukemia. When one extra chromosome appears at locus number 21, the genetic disorder called trisomy-21, or Down's syndrome, develops.

Because the biological insults that alter the chromosomes of healthy fetuses occur after they or their parents were conceived, they explain why most children with congenital Down's syndrome are born to normal parents. (Another reason is that all males with Down's syndrome, and to all intents and purposes all Down's syndrome females, are born sterile as well as brain-damaged.)[18] The exogenous and nonhereditary causes of genetic defects also help explain why Japanese individuals, who were children or young people living in or near Hiroshima and Nagasaki at the time history's only atom bombs used in anger exposed them to mutagenic and carcinogenic radiations, grew up to have more birth-deformed children and to suffer more cases of leukemia and other cancers than other Japanese, European, and American people of the same age two decades later.

In 1980 Werner Henle confirmed that in all cases of Burkitt's lymphoma associated with the EBV, the chromosomes also had undergone translocations of numbers 8 and 14. "The chromosomal translocation probably takes place after the viral infection," he observed. "In the case of African Burkitt's lymphoma it could be triggered by the malaria that is endemic in those areas. But the 8:14 chromosomal translocation is not EBV-specific. It is also present in B-cell leukemias, as well as in Burkitt's lymphomas that do not contain Epstein-Barr Virus."[19]

Henle says, "We think there may also be a genetic co-factor" in nasopharyngeal carcinomas associated with the EBV. He believes such cofactors might be found in the regional diets, local herbal folk remedies, and other cultural elements in the lives of specific southern Chinese people most prone to this cancer.

All these demonstrable and postulated cofactors led to the prudent scientific and clinical consensus that Burkitt's lymphoma and nasopharyngeal carcinoma have at least two causes, and one of them is the Epstein-Barr virus. Even this is hypothesis. However, as Epstein wrote in 1978, "Direct proof that Epstein-Barr virus causes Burkitt's lymphoma can only be obtained by showing that vaccination against the virus decreases tumor incidence. The new data lend added support to this proposal and to attempts to control by vaccination the numerically more important Epstein-Barr virus associated human tumor, nasopharyngeal carcinoma."[20]

Even if the EBV is only a cofactor in these two human cancers, neutralizing the virus by vaccination would break an essential link in the chain of biological, chemical, and immunological events leading to the onset of the two human cancers. This in itself would be reason enough to mount the considerable effort required to develop a subunit split antigen vaccine, and/or wholly synthetic chemical vaccines, against EBV: Even if either vaccine failed to produce antibodies, they would not, being free of infective nucleic acid, cause either of the two EBV-associated cancers or the milder disease commonly associated with the same virus, infectious mononucleosis. Either vaccine might, in fact, even succeed in preventing IM even if they failed to decrease tumor incidence.

In 1979, supported by a modest NIH grant, Dr. David A. Thorley-Lawson at the Sidney Farber Cancer Institute in Boston developed such a vaccine from partially purified plasma cell membranes of tissue-culture-maintained lines of lymphoblastoid cells that produce EBV antibodies. This vaccine was used to immunize rabbits against the Epstein-Barr virus. Other DNA-free subunit vaccines against the EBVs are being developed in other laboratories, including that of Gary B. Pearson at the Mayo Clinic.

The virus capsid or subunit experimental vaccines against the EBV are not the only possible safe and effective anticancer vaccines. Another frequently and prematurely designated anticancer vaccine is the new and widely tested hepatitis B vaccine, which in recent years gathered considerable publicity because since serum hepatitis is often a common venereal disease of homosexual males, gay communities in New York and other American cities were asked to furnish volunteers for large-scale clinical testing of the new vaccine.

Of course, the virus of serum hepatitis does not differentiate between heterosexuals and homosexuals. It has also been widely reported in the medical and lay press that serum hepatitis is or can be the precursor of hepatocarcinoma, or liver cancer. This temporal relationship to date has been established only statistically. Nobody has come up with an explanation of the carcinogenic mechanisms that might possibly be involved, although the vast numbers of liver cancer cases that are preceded by bouts of serum hepatitis can hardly be ignored.

Certain facts about hepatitis B or serum hepatitis are less ambiguous than the postulated link of the hepatitis B virus (HBV) to liver cancer. As of 1980, hepatitis B was the fifth most frequently reported infectious disease in the United States, exceeded only by the reported cases of gonorrhea, syphilis, chicken pox, and—surprisingly, in view of the availability of the mumps vaccine since 1968—mumps. The actual number of cases, in contrast to the reported serum hepatitis cases in this country is not known, but they certainly outnumbered by eight to ten times the 15,060 cases reported in 1979, given the $650 million estimate of the annual economic costs of hepatitis B injections projected by many authorities.

Yellow jaundice, which Hippocrates named *icterus* from the Greek word for yellow, has been an epidemic by-product of war and overcrowding for millennia. During World War II, there were slightly more than 150,000 cases of jaundice or infectious hepatitis in the United States armed forces, a mere drop in the bucket compared with the more than five million hepatitis cases that plagued German servicemen and civilians. Most of these cases are believed now to have been caused by the hepatitis A virus (HAV), the cause of the infectious hepatitis transmitted via the fecal-oral route to food and drinking water, and to those in contact with carriers of the virus in crowded army barracks, slum tenements, and less structured urban hovels. The HAV has an incubation period of ten days to two weeks, and active cases of debilitating yellow jaundice break out shortly after contaminated food or water are ingested, or when sick or healthy HAV carriers share crowded quarters.

Curiously, it took unexpectedly adverse experiences with two effective live virus vaccines to help doctors differentiate between the types of hepatitis caused, on the one hand, by the short-term-incubation hepatitis A virus and, on the other hand, by the long-term-incubation hepatitis B virus. Late in the nineteenth century, some communities in Germany had still not switched from human arm-to-arm lymph to glycerinated calf lymph for smallpox vaccines. An outbreak of jaundice in German shipyard workers that started three weeks to six months after they were vaccinated with human lymph preparations suggested that there were at least two forms of hepatitis, one of which took months to develop. In World War II, live virus yellow fever vaccines prepared from viruses cultured and maintained in a medium containing human serum caused delayed outbreaks of what quickly became known as serum hepatitis (or, initially, the Rockefeller Institute disease) in servicemen and civilians. In recent years a third type of virus, designated as non-A non-B (NANB), which some now term hepatitis C, has been isolated from patients.

The hunt for the agent(s) of hepatitis started in the nineteenth century, when most investigators were sure they would prove to be bacteria. In Nazi Germany doctors searching for these agents succeeded in transmitting hepatitis to concentration camp prisoners and other "human volunteers" to whom they fed materials dug out from the duodenums of patients with severe cases of jaundice. After World War II, when medical virology began to come of age, hepatitis research provided good evidence that the agent(s) of both infectious and serum hepatitis would prove to be particularly small viruses measuring less than 300 angstroms. However, none of the early attempts to isolate the hepatitis viruses succeeded.

Blood transfusions were and still are a common cause of hepatitis. At the NIH a team of investigators headed by a geneticist, Baruch S. Blumberg, undertook a large study of blood samples from surgical patients, hemophiliacs, and other individuals who had had many transfusions. These blood samples were tested against the antibodies circulating in the blood of people who had recovered from various diseases, including hepatitis. In 1961 Blumberg found blood from a hemophiliac that reacted with the antibodies in the blood serum of an Australian aborigine. Blumberg named the unknown antigen that had caused this reaction the Australian Antigen (AuAg), and then undertook a worldwide search for the presumed virus on whose coat this antigen would be found in nature. He was anxious to find out what, if any, human diseases this virus might cause.

Because blood banks are vitally interested in hepatitis as a possible contaminant of blood used in transfusions, the virologist at the New York City Blood Center's laboratory, Dr. Alfred Prince, was happy to study the clinical materials containing AuAg that Blumberg brought to him late in 1966. Blumberg was sure that it came from a virus. He was right. Prince found the virus in the blood of people who had been getting multiple transfusions, and, as Blumberg had hoped, the Australia antigen was located on the glycoprotein coat of the virus. As other workers had predicted earlier, it was indeed a very small virus, in the 200-angstrom range.

In 1970 in England D. S. Dane discovered the hepatitis B virus in the blood of healthy carriers, and carefully isolated the viruses from the blood plasma of these donors. Some 5 percent to 10 percent of all those who recover from serum hepatitis become chronic carriers of the heptatitis B virus (also known as the Dane particle).

The problems of making a vaccine against this virus, which could not be grown in either animals or tissue cultures or hatching eggs, seemed at the outset to be insurmountable. In 1961 Dr. Saul Krugman, at New York University, showed that when a dilution of one part of hepatitis B infective serum to ten parts of water was boiled for only one minute, its viruses lost the ability to cause hepatitis, while at the same time the viruses' surface antigens retained their immunogenicity, or the capacity to cause the production of anti-HBV antibodies when injected into nonimmune people.

The work of Krugman and Dane became the basis for the hepatitis B vaccine developed by Hilleman and his coworkers at the Merck Institute, and tested with the cooperation of the New York City Blood Center. The tests were organized by the Center's chief of epidemiology and professor of epidemiology at the Columbia University School of Public Health, Dr. Wolf Szmuness (1919–1982), a newcomer to the American medical and research communities. A native of Warsaw, Poland, and trained in the Soviet Union, Dr. Szmuness was already a veteran research worker in viral hepatitis when the Polish communist government in 1968 suddenly started to drive those of its few Jews who had survived the Holocaust out of Poland. Szmuness joined the New York City Blood Center in 1969.

The Hilleman laboratory went to work on the hepatitis B vaccine in 1970. The starting materials were hepatitis vaccine B surface antigens derived from the blood plasma of healthy carriers of the hepatitis B virus. First, the crude plasma antigens were inactivated with formalin to kill any infective virus nucleic acids present. Then they were sterilized to kill any bacterial or other pathogenic organisms that survived the formalin. The formalinized and sterilized virus surface antigens were then highly purified and finally combined with an aluminum hydroxide adjuvant to boost the immune response to these multiprocessed antigens and therefore increase the production of anti-HBV antibodies. It is a complex process that, at this writing, takes sixty-five weeks of intensive work between the arrival of the blood plasma from healthy HBV carriers and the release of the packaged vials of vaccine.

The federally mandated preliminary animal and human tests of the experimental vaccine were not completed until mid-1978, three years after the vaccine itself was ready for testing. After the earlier animal and human tests for safety and antibody production and when hepatitis B vaccine was ready for the large-scale clinical trials that must now be run before a new vaccine can be licensed, Szmuness and his collaborators were faced with a dilemma. "Such a trial," they wrote, "required a population with a high risk of infection with hepatitis B virus (HBV). A trial in a low-risk popultion would require a large number of participants (as many as 40,000 to 50,000) to prove efficacy and would be inordinately difficult and expensive. In addition, it seemed more appropriate for ethical reasons to immunize a high-risk population that could benefit most from an effective vaccine."[21]

Since male homosexuals constitute precisely such a group at high risk for serum hepatitis, and because numerous gay organizations had been very cooperative in earlier hepatitis studies, their cooperation was again sought and received. This meant that only about 1,000 homosexual men would provide the same amount of clinical information that could be derived from 40,000 to 50,000 heterosexuals at lower risk of serum hepatitis.

The New York City Blood Center trials, conducted in 1,083 male homosexuals, began in November 1978. They were placebo-controlled, double-blind, and randomized tests, in which the vials containing the placebos and those containing the vaccines were packed under code numbers so that neither the doctors nor the volunteers knew which were which. "The randomization procedure allocated 549 to the vaccine group and 534 to the placebo group. In May 1980, eight months after the last participant was enrolled, all trial events were reviewed and classified by an expert panel appointed by the trial's advisory committee. In June 1980 the code of vaccine and placebo allocation was broken."

Base-line studies of the volunteers made when they registered for the study showed that over 85 percent were white, most were in their early thirties, and over 30 percent were college graduates. They had an average of ten years of homosexual activity, and during the six months before the vaccine trials, they had had an average of around twenty sexual partners. Their normal patterns of sexual activity were maintained during the twenty months of the vaccine trials.

For the first fifteen months of the follow-up clinical studies, "Hepatitis B or subclinical infection developed in only 1.4 to 3.4 percent of the vaccine recipients as compared with 18 to 27 percent of the placebo recipients. The reduction of [hepatitis B] incidence in the vaccinees was as high as 92.3 percent."[22] There could be no doubt that the vaccine worked very effectively to prevent serum hepatitis.

The results were of immediate significance to many people. Those individuals at greatest risk of catching hepatitis from jaundiced patients include doctors, dentists, and other health professionals who treat patients with either type of hepatitis, handle their blood and urine and fecal specimens, and work in blood banks, where different batches of stored blood might be contaminated with serum hepatitis or infectious hepatitis viruses. Patients who receive many blood transfusions are at high risk of serum hepatitis. Environmental filth and intimate contact with healthy carriers spread hepatitis. It is estimated that in this country the population at high risk of serum hepatitis adds up to at least sixteen million people, of whom from 80,000 to 100,000 contract it annually.

While the trials of the new hepatitis B vaccine were being conducted in New York, Szmuness and his team ran similar trials of the same subunit vaccine in 800 renal-dialysis patients and 1,000 renal-dialysis-unit staff members in forty cooperating centers around the country. The hepatitis division of the federal Centers for Disease Control (CDC) started trials of the Merck vaccine in 1,000 selected individuals in Chicago, Los Angeles, San Francisco, St. Louis, and Denver. Altogether by the end of 1980, close to 5,000 people were vaccinated with the surface antigen vaccine against serum hepatitis.

Szmuness et al. were ecstatic in their final report on the New York trials. They observed that the total number of healthy carriers of the serum hepatitis virus is around 800,000 in this country and 200 million throughout the world, where serum hepatitis is two to ten times as prevalent. Their report concluded on a note that seemed to promise a vaccine against a human cancer:

"Although most carriers of HBsAg [hepatitis B virus surface antigen] are asymptomatic, a substantial proportion do eventually develop chronic active hepatitis and cirrhosis. There is also overwhelming evidence that the hepatitis B virus is the single most important causative factor of hepatocellular carcinoma, an extremely widespread cancer among middle-aged men in Asia and Africa. Thus, mass immunization programs against HBV infection may ultimately affect not only the incidence of acute hepatitis B and the pool of chronic carriers but may also reduce the morbidity and mortality from chronic active hepatitis, cirrhosis and hepatocellular carcinoma."[23]

If, indeed, all that is necessary to prove the role of the hepatitis B virus in causing the liver cancers that often follow bouts of HBV hepatitis is a mass immunization campaign with the new anti-HBV vaccine—particularly among middle-aged men in Asia and Africa—it might be many generations before such proof would be forthcoming. At present prices, it would cost from $75 to $120 for the three-dose regimen of these vaccines needed to immunize people against HBV infection. This is more than an average middle-aged man in Asia and Africa earns in a year.

The sheer labor costs of the technology required to produce the new successful HBsAg vaccine against serum hepatitis have not been ignored by public health and vaccine researchers. For some years many investigators in England and the United States have been trying new ways of growing hepatitis B viruses and splitting off their antigens. Some of their work might well result in less expensive ways to produce vaccines against serum hepatitis.[24]

Professor Arie Zuckerman, at the London School of Hygiene and Tropical Medicine, is working on a new technique of isolating viral-type proteins from the cell surfaces of hepatocarcinoma tumors removed from liver cancer patients who are also HBV carriers. Experimental vaccines made with these antigens are now being tested. While it is still beyond the skills of any laboratory to grow serum hepatitis viruses directly in tissue cultures, Zuckerman has shown that hepatocarcinoma tumors which produce these hepatitis B antigens can be maintained very well in laboratory nutrients, and can even continue to grow and produce viral antigens when they are frozen and stored.

In Edinburgh Professor Ken Murray and his coworkers are trying to transfer what they believe are the genes that code for producing of HBV core and surface antigens from the viral nucleic acid inside the hepatitis B virions themselves to the gene-carrying plasmids in the cytoplasms of the ubiquitous gut bacteria *Escherichia coli*. Their hope is that these delicately transplated virus genes will instruct the *E. coli* organisms henceforth to start producing HBV antigens in their coopted single cells—and that the genetically engineered *E. coli* will then duly cooperate and obey these sophisticated biochemical instructions in high style.

Some researchers, including Zuckerman and Richard Lerner in California, believe that these genetic-recombination maneuvers—which are based on first isolating and then chemically characterizing these segments of the viral genomes that code for producing antigens but not for causing viral diseases—will open a considerably simpler route to developing safe, effective, and much cheaper vaccines than drafting brainwashed *E. coli* to serve humanity by turning themselves into viral antigen factories. They believe that once the specific viral (or bacterial) genes that code for antigen production are isolated and subjected to chemical analyses, it might then become possible to synthesize equally active copies of these gene segments out of ordinary, off-the-shelf chemicals, and use the synthetics as the bases of inexpensive vaccines.

Although hepatitis A is not as severe as hepatitis B, it attacks more than twice as many in the course of an average year. The hepatitis cases reported to local health departments in 1979 probably represent about 10 percent of the actual cases, but even in this small sample, 30,407 cases of hepatitis A and 15,352 cases of hepatitis B were reported. Hepatitis A is often called the food handlers' disease because outbreaks are often traced to infected cooks in restaurants and large institutions; it is a classic disease of overcrowding.

After the hepatitis B antigen and its virus were isolated, it was only a matter of time before new techniques such as immunoelectronmicroscopy (IEM) would enable investigators to find the hepatitis A virus. Late in 1972 at the National Institute of Allergy and Infectious Diseases (NIAID) Stephen M. Feinstone and coworkers used IEM and other techniques to isolate, photograph, and test virus particles found in the stools of patients during the acute phase of infectious hepatitis. They were quickly able to prove that these particles were indeed hepatitis A viruses. Thus were provided not only the virus needed for a serological technique of detecting a serum antibody and "for the first time, a means of diagnosing and studying hepatitis A,"[25] but also the essential raw material for developing a vaccine against hepatitis A.

Unlike the hepatitis B virus, the hepatitis A virus can be grown in tissue cultures. It would be easier and less costly to develop vaccines against HAV than against serum hepatitis. "Virtually everyone is at risk for hepatitis A, since it is easily transmitted by the fecal-oral route and often results in outbreaks and epidemics," Hilleman observed at a 1980 virus meeting.

To date, the Hilleman group has made a formalin-inactivated HAV vaccine which in animal tests proved 100 percent effective. However, the principal goal is the early development of a live, oral one-dose vaccine against hepatitis A, which Hilleman feels should be included among the vaccines routinely given infants and children in this and other affluent countries. He also feels that once a vaccine against HAV is licensed, it should be distributed without charge by world health agencies for mass use in the world's poorer countries, where infectious hepatitis is rampant.

However, hepatitis A, like so many major infectious diseases a measurably social one, is not solely an affliction of poverty. It is also in this country a disease of growing importance to home-owning, two-car, two-salary, solvent families. In the United States, changes in family life-styles have accelerated the spread of infectious hepatitis in many ways. The decades of burgeoning and continuous inflation that followed the American military involvement in the war in Vietnam, and the OPEC oil cartel's sudden vast increases in world oil prices starting in 1973–1974 made it necessary for millions of American mothers to take full-time jobs to help keep their families viable.

To help solve the maternal problems of holding a job and raising children at the same time, thousands of day-care centers were opened by private entrepreneurs and nonprofit community agencies to feed and shelter the children of mothers economically forced to go to work. As of 1980, some eleven million preschool children were receiving some form of nonfamily day care, with close to two million attending full-time day-care centers sheltering twelve or more children.[26]

Clinically, these day-care centers "represent a fertile environment for the spread of communicable diseases, and especially enterically transmitted infections," warns the CDC, which lists hepatitis A, shigellosis, giardiasis, and probably viral gastroenteritis among the infections frequently reported as breaking out in the children sheltered in the centers daily. In all these reported hepatitis A outbreaks "infection characteristically has spread not only among children, but also to the adults who take care of them, both within the center and at home. The spread of infection beyond the day-care centers into the families and then into the general community represents a major potential problem in public health."[27]

A series of epidemiological studies made by the CDC around the nation in 1976–1978 showed that between 6 percent and 8 percent of all reported hepatitis A cases were associated with day-care centers. In 1980 a CDC study of all hepatitis A cases in a single community, Maricopa County, Arizona, revealed that at least 30 percent of all infectious hepatitis cases reported in the total population originated in the county's twenty-eight day-care centers.

From these centers, the CDC learned, the hepatitis A viruses spread to the centers' employees, particularly those who change the infants' and children's diapers and dispose of their feces, clean them, dress them, feed them, and maintain close contact with the preschoolers for forty hours each week. From the adults at these day-care centers, as well as from the children, the hepatitis A viruses then spread to the parents, older siblings, parents' employers, and other family contacts.

Now, as in Jenner's day, human disease viruses draw no distinctions of age, sex, race, or socioeconomic status; their only requirement is that the organisms they infect (and sometimes kill) must be human.

C H A P T E R

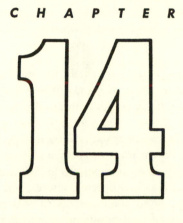

THE STILL ELUSIVE COMMON
COLD VACCINE

When one considers the forceful approach that was used for the development of a vaccine for poliomyelitis, a very minor problem as compared to upper respiratory illnesses, it becomes evident that the whole impact of these infections is not generally realized. Tremendous benefit will accrue to patients with pulmonary and heart disease when multivalent respiratory disease vaccines are available. Complications of respiratory infections, sinusitis, otitis media, bronchitis, pneumonia and meningitis will be greatly reduced. Most of the sicknesses of childhood will be elminated.

—WILLIAM J. MOGABGAB, M.D., "Upper Respiratory Illness Vaccines—Perspectives and Trials," *Annals of Internal Medicine,* October 1962, p. 526

Of the two hundred and more infectious disorders caused by nearly as many different families of viruses, few are more devastating than the most ubiquitous, the various families of viruses that cause respiratory diseases. Consider only four groups: the viruses that cause influenza; the respiratory syncitial virus that causes havoc and death in infants and young children, most of them under two years old; the adenoviruses; and the hundreds of antigenically different strains of rhinoviruses, Coxsackie viruses, ECHO viruses, coronaviruses, and others making up the complex which, alone or in combinations of two or more, are agents of the loose confederation of viral respiratory disorders traditionally designated as the common cold.

Each of the respiratory viruses is dangerous to human health not only because of the diseases it can cause by itself, but also because it can be a precursor to an even more damaging and deadly infection bacteria and other agents, such as the pneumococcal, staphylococcal, and *H. influenzae* pneumonias, bacterial meningitis, and streptococcal pharyngitis, the latter the all too frequent precursor of rheumatic fever and rheumatic heart disease, post-streptococcal nephritis, and inflammation of the middle ear (otitis media).[1] In World War I the great influenza pandemic that in less than one year killed upward of 25 million people around the world was in itself not the prime killer. Bacterial pneumonias secondary to influenza infection killed most of the people who died after catching the Spanish flu. More of the deaths were actually due to pneumonia caused by Pfeiffer's bacillus, which was discovered in 1892 by Richard Pfeiffer in Germany, and which could easily be recovered from the lungs of influenza victims, that it became known as the influenza bacillus and later as *Haemophilus influenzae*. In 1918 in his special bulletin setting forth the facts concerning influenza, United States Surgeon General Rupert Blue named "the bacillus influenza of Pfeiffer" as the sole infectious agent of Spanish influenza.[2] This was a logical mistake, in the absence of the knowledge or even the serious suspicion that influenza was not a bacterial but a viral infection. Not until 1933 would the human influenza virus be isolated; and the *H. influenzae* bacillus in at least a severe influenza infection would play a significant role in what followed.

During the second wave of the 1918 flu pandemic, a U.S. Department of Agriculture veterinarian, J. S. Koen of Fort Dodge, Iowa, observed a disease never before seen in American pigs. He studied it, saw that it was identical to what was then still called Spanish influenza, and published his findings. He was naturally immediately subjected to the kind of abuse from meat-packers, hog growers, and butchers that in our times is directed by cigarette companies and tobacco state senators at doctors who issue studies of the causal links between smoking and lung cancer. Koen refused to retract either his scientific observations or his conclusions. In 1919 he again summed them up for all who could read.

"Last fall and winter we were confronted," he wrote, "with a new condition, if not a new disease. I believe I have as much to support this diagnosis in pigs as the physicians have to support a similar diagnosis in man. The similarity of the epidemic among people and the epidemic among pigs was so close, the reports so frequent, that an outbreak in the family would be followed immediately by an outbreak among the hogs, and *vice versa,* as to present a most striking coincidence if not suggesting a close relation between the two conditions. It looked like 'flu,' and until proved it was not 'flu,' I shall stand by that diagnosis."[3]

Here it was, plainly stated: The great influenza pandemic of 1918 had finally spread from people to pigs, and possibly to other animals. (Contrary to the costly influenza myth of 1976, which held that the flu had spread from swine to Spaniards to Americans.) Koen's loudest detractors could not continue to deny that swine caught flu as year after year following the end of World War I, influenza broke out every autumn with the onset of cold weather in the pig-raising prairie states.

Swine influenza became a growing concern of the U.S. Department of Agriculture, whose responsibilities were to keep farm animals healthy and not to deny that they could get flu. In 1928, ten years after Koen first described swine influenza, C. N. McBryde and a group of other USDA veterinarians transmitted influenza from sick pigs to healthy pigs by inoculating nose and throat washings from the infected to the noninfected swine. However, after filtering these respiratory washings from pigs with influenza, they were unable to induce the disease in other pigs with the filtrates.

That same year, however, Richard Shope, working under the supervision of Theobald Smith at the Rockefeller Institute for Comparative Pathology at Princeton, succeeded where McBryde had failed. The filtrates of respiratory-tract mucus from pigs with influenza he used did cause influenza when inoculated into healthy pigs. What was more, the disease could be transferred repeatedly in pigs by inoculations of the same cell- and bacterial-free filtrates. Of course, this pointed to an as yet not isolated virus as the probable cause of influenza in swine, and possibly in people as well.

Shope continued his studies of swine influenza. In time he was able to isolate the swine influenza virus, but his continuing research in severe and fatal cases of swine influenza also led him to the recovery of a bacterium familiar to influenza pathologists. It was a strain of *H. influenzae* (*suis*), Pfeiffer's old influenza bacillus, that was found in the lungs of so many people who had died of influenza during the 1918 pandemic. Shope observed that when this bacterium was not present, influenza in pigs was always very mild and self-terminating. On the other hand, when the disease turned severe and usually fatal, then vast quantities of *H. influenzae* (*suis*) were found in the lungs and respiratory tissues of the dead pigs.

In 1933 an influenza epidemic caused three fine scientists in England, Wilson Smith, Christopher Andrewes, and Patrick Laidlaw, to undertake their own studies of the causes and nature of influenza at the National Institute for Medical Research Farm Laboratories, Mill Hill.[4] Shope generously sent them samples of the swine virus influenza and cultures of *H. influenzae* (*suis*). Thanks to Shope, the team knew that the etiological "agent of influenza was probably a filtrable virus," but what they wanted to know was if the filtered throat washings of people with influenza—which presumably contained this virus—could cause the disease in animals. Here, using mice, rats, cats, dogs, chickens, rabbits, guinea pigs, and other small and easily manageable animals, Smith and his coworkers tried to transmit influenza from people to other species. "All such attempts, " they admitted, "were entirely unsuccessful until the ferret was used, and the first success was only secured toward the close of the epidemic."

Shortly after they had proved, repeatedly, that human influenza viruses can transmit a respiratory disease in which the flu virus-inoculated "animal sneezes frequently, yawns repeatedly, and in many cases breathes partly through the mouth with wheezy or stertorous sounds which clearly indicate a considerable degree of nasal obstruction," the Smith group fell heir to an unexpected informational bonanza. One of the flu-stricken ferrets sneezed directly into the face of one of the project's young coworkers, Charles H. Stuart-Harris who, after the normal incubation period, came down with a typical case of influenza.

Smith and his coworkers found that three different types of *H. influenzae* "administered along with the virus produced only at most minor variations in symptoms." They did find that there was a high degree of cross-immunity between the virus they had isolated in people with influenza and that which Shope had recovered from sick pigs. "Ferrets after recovery from disease caused by the swine virus proved to be solidly immune to the human strain of virus." But, they continued, "ferrets convalescent from the human [influenza] virus disease were not completely immune to the pig strain of virus."

Their investigation demonstrated that "human sera, particularly from influenza convalescents, were found to contain antibodies capable of neutralizing the virus of the ferret diseases." An attack of influenza conferred active immunity on ferrets, but Smith and his coworkers also reported that "no means of securing an active immunity apart from giving the disease itself have yet been found." This apparently referred to one or more unsuccessful attempts to develop a good influenza vaccine.

Smith, Andrewes, and Laidlaw concluded that their results with ferrets, although limited to very few experiments, "are consistent with the view that epidemic infuenza in man is caused primarily by a virus infection. It is probable that in certain cases this infection facilitates the invasion of the body by visible bacteria, giving rise to various complications," such as staphylococcal, pneumococcal, and *H. influenzae* pneumonia secondary to viral influenza.

Over the next decade, at various times each of these three investigators would try his hand at turning out an acceptable influenza vaccine. Not until 1943, when the formalin-inactivated influenza virus vaccine made for the United States armed forces by Thomas Francis, Jr., assisted by Fred Davenport and Jonas Salk, was put into production, was an even fairly effective flu vaccine available. It offered a fair amount of protection against the vaccine strain of flu for upward of six months.

Since then, various killed whole-virus vaccines and subunit vaccines made of antigens chemically split off from the flu virus capsids (outer coats) have been introduced around the world. Some work is being done in the Soviet Union and other countries on attenuated live virus vaccines. None seems to offer protection against influenza for longer than six months.

All the different kinds of influenza vaccines are handicapped by one predictable factor: Every so often, the viruses go through what is called an antigenic shift. This is probably due more to natural selection than to actual changes in the nature of the viruses themselves. What happens is that no sooner is a vaccine used successfully against the strain or strains of viruses responsible for the latest outbreak of influenza than an apparently totally new virus strain appears that is completely resistant to the vaccine. It might really be a new strain; at times it might also be one that was always present but was so vastly outnumbered by the predominant virus as to have been innocuous until naturally acquired immunity or vaccines killed off the "master race." Whatever its origins, this new strain starts causing a different kind of flu and rules the roost until it too is isolated, cultured, and used in new and effective flu vaccines.

For want of a better term to describe this process, it has been called the antigenic shift of the flu viruses. Until it is better understood, and for that matter until the virus itself is better understood, the chances of our having a vaccine that will induce lifelong or even reasonably long-term protection against this very common respiratory infection are close to nil.

* * *

343

Beween August 1978 and early 1979, what the Naples press labeled *il male oscuro*—the mystery disease—ravaged the ancient Italian port city, killing more than sixty children. One of the reasons for the mystery about this fatal disease was that the hospital to which all the victims had been taken to die had neglected to perform any autopsies on them until six months after the outbreak began. By December 1978 proper pathological examination revealed that the children, who came from overcrowded homes in Naples's poorest neighborhoods, had died of very common respiratory diseases of overcrowding. In the youngest victims, most of the deaths were caused by the respiratory syncytial virus (RSV).

This was a newly discovered virus. Not until 1956 had it been found—in chimpanzees; and a year later, Robert Chanock and Leonard Finberg, of the National Institute for Allergy and Infectious Diseases (NIAID), recovered the same virus from infants with respiratory diseases of unknown etiology. From that time forward, Chanock would play a major part in the world's efforts to study the RSV. The RSV is one of the small members of the paramyxovirus family, which includes the agents of mumps, measles, and parainfluenza, and of three important animal diseases—Newcastle disease of chickens, rinderpest, and distemper. It has a short incubation period of four to five days. Epidemiological studies here and in England have shown that about half of all two-year-old children possess circulating antibodies against RSV, and that upward of 93 percent of all adults now have antibodies testifying to prior and rarely remembered RSV infections.

A prospective study, conducted for thirteen years by the NIAID, of infants and young children admitted to the Children's Hospital of Washington, D.C., with lower respiratory tract infectious diseases showed that "RSV is the major cause of bronchiolitis of early infancy. In addition, the virus is a major cause of pneumonia during the first few years of life."[5]

Since 1957 Chanock and other laboratory workers have been trying to develop a safe and effective vaccine against RSV. Various killed-virus and live virus vaccines have been compounded and tested, but none has worked. At the Merck Institute, Eugene Buynack and his colleagues have developed a live attenuated RSV vaccine that, unlike most other live vaccines, is administered by injection.

The vaccine was tested in 106 children who were seronegative for RSV antibody, and it caused nearly all of them to develop antibody following vaccination. But maternal antibody that is passed transplacentally to fetuses, and via colostrum in mothers' milk to nursing children, as well as naturally acquired postnatal immunity to the RSV, can prevent the proliferation of the vaccine's virus and thus limit the number of RSV antibodies that the viral antigens might cause the children's lymphocytes to produce.

The Merck vaccine against RSV therefore "remains a vaccine in search of an evaluation,"[6] and still requires testing in two-year-old children who have no maternal antibody and also have managed to escape one of the most frequent of all natural infections.

Like the RSV, the family of adenoviruses that are clinically grouped among the respiratory viruses were not discovered until after World War II. Wallace Rowe of the NIAID found them in 1953 in adenoids removed from children during tonsillar surgery. They were soon demonstrated to be the causal agents of what military doctors had named acute respiratory disease (ARD), and which even then was classified as a virus disease. This disorder had been peculiar to military basic training camps since the American Civil War. "Typical ARD is a febrile respiratory disease with symptoms of sore throat and cough, sometimes coryza [running nose], headache and chest pain. Malaise is characteristic, and the illness lasts for approximately 10 days."[7] This clinical description of ARD also describes the common cold rather well.

Because of the obvious economic and training-schedule costs of ARD to the armed forces, the virus laboratories of the Walter Reed Army Institute of Research (WRAIR), then directed by the formidably gifted Maurice Hilleman, got into the picture. "In the short interval of time between 1953 and 1956," Hilleman wrote in 1966, "the adenoviruses were discovered, methods for laboratory diagnosis and serotyping [there are now thirty-one known separate types of human adenoviruses] were established, epidemiology was clarified, and a highly effective vaccine was developed and proved."[8]

This formalin-inactivated vaccine was immediately put to use in the armed forces and, shortly thereafter, was licensed for general civilian uses. The Hilleman vaccine against adenoviruses was marketed by the firm of Parke-Davis as the common cold vaccine. The marketing data submitted by Parke-Davis to the federal government on this common cold vaccine stated that "some millions of doses of vaccine were sold between 1957 and 1964, and no untoward reactions were reported."[9]

In 1959 the same company, in order "to immunize against epidemic influenza and the more common adenovirus infections," brought out a duly licensed product in which killed influenza viruses and killed adenoviruses, identical to those used in the common cold vaccine, were combined in another parenteral vaccine.

Several million doses of this combined-virus vaccine were sold and presumably used in 1959–1965, and "very few complaints" of adverse side effects were received.

Although, for reasons which will be described shortly, both vaccines were voluntarily taken off the market around 1966 and were never manufactured again, it was not until April 1980 that the Bureau of Biologics got around to revoking the licenses for these vaccines "because there are compelling reasons to assume a lack of safety or effectiveness and an unsatisfactory benefit-risk ratio for this product(s)."

Like the respiratory syncytial virus (RSV), the thirty-one known types of human adenovirus are largely the cause of infant and early childhood diseases, and are more apt to infect poor children in crowded quarters, or children in orphanages and day-care centers, than more fortunate children. In some countries, such as Japan and Taiwan, nearly all children have antibodies to different strains of adenoviruses. In New Orleans 80 percent of all one-year-old children tested had circulating antibodies against adenoviruses. About 5 percent of all respiratory disorders in American children are caused by adenoviruses, with the most common symptoms being a cough and a stuffy nose. Adenovirus infections in children often mimic streptococcal pharyngitis. Type 7 adenovirus is a cause of viral pneumonia in children. Various hospital studies show that 2 percent to 7 percent of lower-respiratory-tract diseases in children are due to adenoviruses.

Most children have been exposed to many endemic types of adenovirus by the time they enter school. In later life children and adults are sometimes subject to pharyngoconjunctival fever (PCF), or swimming-pool conjunctivitis, which is believed to be transmitted to the eyes by adenoviruses in small lakes and improperly chlorinated swimming pools. The infection hits the eyes and throat. Adenoviruses also cause epidemic keratoconjunctivitis (EKC), or "shipyard eye," which used to follow in the wake of minor eye injuries to shipyard workers. This is usually an iatrogenic, or doctor-caused, disease, since it is transmitted to the eyes and ears by inadequately sterilized medical instruments, eyewash solutions, and eye ointments, as well as by the hands of doctors and nurses. In recent years there have been some reports of outbreaks originating in ophthalmologists' offices. Severe cases can cause permanent eye damage.

In adults, adenovirus infections are generally experienced by military recruits during their first weeks of training. Most of these young men arrive at the basic training camps with naturally acquired immunity to adenoviruses. But, as we have seen earlier, some enter military life still susceptible to many childhood infections as well as ARD due to adenoviruses. If a recruit catches one or more of the common viral or bacterial diseases, he promptly passes it on to all the other susceptible recruits, and one of the most prevalent of these diseases is ARD.

Before the adenoviruses were isolated, and Hilleman's WRAIR laboratories made the first killed-virus vaccines against the three adenovirus types most responsible for ARD, it was not unusual for hospitals in large basic training camps such as Fort Dix, New Jersey, to admit upward of two hundred recruits daily for acute respiratory disease. Colonel Franklin H. Top, Jr., now deputy director of WRAIR, recalls that these ARD admissions were at "an incredible hospital cost. Many people were needed to man the wards that were set up exclusively for ARD as well as those for convalescence."[10]

Training time was also squandered by ARD. "Many recruits developed adenovirus disease during their third or fourth week in training. It got to the point where company commanders were training two sets of recruits, the second group for those recruits who had to make up for lost time."[11]

For a time the "Salk-type" formalin-inactivated vaccines Hilleman had developed against the three types of adenoviruses most common in ARD all but eliminated the disease in all basic training camps. At Fort Dix, for example, the bivalent vaccine against Types 4 and 7 adenoviruses, made in the WRAIR laboratories and used during a 1956 military ARD epidemic, "was remarkably effective, and brought about a 98% reduction in hospitalized cases of ARD caused by these agents. The vaccine became effective seven days following a single one-milliliter dose."[12]

Like many viruses, the adenoviruses have the ability to hybridize with other strains of the same family, as well as with nonrelated viruses. The military and civilian stocks of the vaccine were in wide use in 1963, when it was discovered that the Types 4 and 7 adenoviruses used to seed the cultures for the bivalent "common cold" vaccines were contaminated with a monkey virus of the papova family. The papovaviruses, like the adenoviruses, are DNA viruses. The genome (the acid-bearing nucleus) of one, simian virus 40 (SV-40), was found incorporated in the two adenoviruses' capsids—the protein envelopes that surround the nucleic acid.

Such hybrid viruses, in which in effect the outer coat is the coat of Jacob while the message is contained in the DNA of Esau, are not unusual. Unfortunately, the papovaviruses are notoriously oncogenic (tumor-causing) agents—in animals.

The SV-40 viruses had already been proven to cause cancers in hamsters and rats; and at about the time they were discovered hiding in adenovirus capsids in the Hilleman vaccines, some cancer researchers started to examine new evidence suggesting that Type 7 adenovirus, along with nonvaccine Types 3, 12, 16, 18, and 31, were also oncogenic in animals. It was never proven that either the SV-40 monkey viruses, or any of the adenovirus types oncogenic in animals, had ever caused anything remotely resembling cancer in people or had even transformed human cells growing in tissue cultures. However, prudence cause the armed forces to stop using the Hilleman bivalent adenovirus vaccine, and commercial manufacturers stopped turning out both versions of their common cold vaccine.

As early as 1962, it had been shown that while Type 12 human adenovirus induced cancer in hamsters, "it is yet to be determined what tumors, if any, may be produced by Type 12 adenovirus in humans."[13] This study, conducted at the M. D. Anderson and Tumor Institute in Houston, Texas, by John J. Trentin, Grant Taylor, and Yoshiro Yabe, a visiting professor from the Okayama University medical school, Japan, also showed that "the possibility that contamination with polyoma virus and simian virus 40 [SV-40] might be responsible for the tumors induced was specifically excluded by a variety of tests."

Further studies in many countries showed that many strains of human, chicken, bovine, canine, and monkey adenoviruses could cause cancers in hamsters, mice, rats, and other animals. Work with human cell cultures in two laboratories suggested that Type 12 human adenovirus caused alterations in these cells, but "neither group of investigators was able to establish continuous lines of adenovirus transformed cells due to the continued production of infectious virus which destroyed the cells."

The National Cancer Institute organized a collaborative study of sera from cancer patients in which no antibodies to the T antigens of human and animal oncogenic adenoviruses could be found. A collaborative study of adenoviruses in human cancer, published by R. M. McAllister, R. V. Gilden, and M. Green in 1972[14] concluded that "the negative results obtained in serological, biochemical, and biological tests suggest that adenoviruses are unlikely to be important causes of human cancer; if they are, the mechanisms involved are different from those of adenovirus carcinogenesis in hamsters."

The authors also pointed to work by Robert Mannaker and John Landon, who, during a two-to-seven-year observation period, found that "adenovirus types 2, 7, and 12 did not induce tumors in 40 cynamolgus or rhesus monkeys." However striking the similarities, the differences between the species are often more significant. Aspirin, for over a century one of humankind's safest and most useful drugs, can blind any type of dog from Chihuahua to Great Dane. The fact that adenoviruses that easily cause cancers in rats, mice, and hamsters completely fail to do so in primates, which are a good deal closer to people on the evolutionary tree than canines, is of possibly seminal importance.

Whereas these and many other studies led the National Cancer Institute to conclude that "adenoviruses were eliminated as causative agents in human cancer," work in Chanock's laboratory at NIAID was clearing the way for the development of live adenovirus vaccines. It had long been known that "commonly thought of as respiratory viruses, adenoviruses almost invariably infect the alimentary tract,"[15] even though the gut adenovirus infections were usually free of symptoms. Chanock, Robert Couch, and their coworkers hit upon the idea of developing an enteric-coated, Sabin-type oral adenovirus vaccine which, after producing an asymptomatic infection confined to the gastrointestinal tract, induce type-specific immune reactions that would cause the production of secretory and circulating antibodies against the vaccine's viruses.

After years of careful development and testing, in 1970 live vaccines against Types 4 and 7 adenoviruses began to be administered to recruits in selected basic training camps. They were (and are) administered orally, in two monovalent pills taken at the same time.

In 1971 Types 4 and 7 oral adenovirus vaccines began to be given routinely to all incoming recruits at *all* military basic training camps in the United States. Prior to that time, in northern posts during the cold months from December to March, six out of every one hundred recruits per week had been hospitalized for acute respiratory infections, two thirds of which were caused by either Type 4 or Type 7 adenovirus. In southern camps, due to the recruits having had a much greater childhood exposure to the same adenoviruses, the ARD hospitalizations were fewer, averaging three to four per hundred recruits per week, and in two thirds of these cases, as in northern camps, the infections were caused by the same two types of adenovirus. By 1980 the average United States military basic training camp reported only two ARD hospitalizations per week, only 2 percent of which were caused by either Type 4 or Type 7 adenovirus.

Two years after the start of this routine immunization program, Peter B. Collis of WRAIR and his coworkers made a cost-benefit study of the two military vaccines and of the entire adenovirus surveillance program. With the aid of modern computers, they estimated that between 1966 and 1971, the total cost of the surveillance program—which included the development of the vaccines, the purchases of vaccine doses made by outside contractors, and the administration of the vaccines to all recruits—came to $4.83 million. Collis et al. estimated that between 1970 and 1971, the vaccines had prevented about 27,000 military ARD hospitalizations at an average cost of $279 per hospital stay. This meant that in dollars alone, "the dollar estimates of benefits derived from vaccine use was $7.53 million (in 1971 dollars)." Thus, the dollar benefits derived during the first two years of the routine use of the NIH-WRAIR vaccine in basic training camps came to nearly twice what the federal treasury had spent on developing and testing the live oral adenovirus vaccines over a five-year period.[16]

Successful as they have proven to be, sooner rather than later—depending how intelligently further research and development efforts are supported by this and other governments—these live adenovirus vaccines will very likely be replaced by DNA-free split antigen or even synthetic antigen vaccines offering the same degree of protection but with none of the potential, however remote, of altered foreign (viral) DNA to mutate and wreak deadly mischief in human bodies.

The adenoviruses are among many now known to be capable of causing the constellation of symptoms which, more for convenience than for any other reason, are called the common cold. Sometimes these cold symptoms are accompanied by high or low fever, while at other times they are afebrile. Usually, they include one or more of the following: stuffy nose, sore throat, cough, sneezing, myalgia (muscular pain), and general malaise. Sometimes more serious respiratory infections develop, such as pneumonia, pharyngitis, bronchiolitis, and bronchitis.

Often when these life-threatening complications develop, they prove to be not primary viral but secondary bacterial infections, from streptococcal pharyngitis secondary to a mild and even afebrile respiratory infection (particularly in children) to bacterial pneumonias and chronic bronchitis. This also means that the well-known side effects of a strep throat (streptococcal pharyngitis), like otitis media, rheumatic fever, rheumatic heart disease, and poststreptococcal nephritis, are not merely the end products of bacterial infections but also of the mild viral respiratory infections that preceded them. Until antibiotics became available, these bacterial infections were incurable; in the absence of good vaccines, most of them are still not preventable.

Recent studies of the effects of naturally acquired and laboratory-induced acute respiratory illness in human volunteers at Baylor University, Texas, suggest that mucosal cell changes caused by these viral infections lead in turn to the increased adherence of pneumonia-causing bacteria. Bacterial adherence to human cells is the first stage in the process of bacterial infection.

The common cold is at least as old as the history of medicine. From the very beginnings of medicine, sufferers from the common cold had their miseries compounded by greedy quacks and self-deluded healers, as witnessed today by the worthless cures huckstered at astronomical expense on commercial television. Hippocrates in 400 B.C. heaped scorn upon those august and ethical practitioners who held that bleeding was the best cure for the common cold.

In the first century A.D., Pliny the Younger had a somewhat more exotic cure. It involved merely "kissing the hairy muzzle of a mouse," a regimen far less traumatic and debilitating than bleeding.[17] Kissing a mouse's whiskers was infinitely less addictive than the "tonics" made of opium and/or alcohol plus colored sugar water peddled by traveling medicine shows and sold over the counter in all American drugstores after the American Civil War. Pliny's cure was also much cheaper than the considerably less effective assortments of every known vitamin, kelp, vinegar, and rutins engorged today by true-believing, and often college-educated, health faddists at the first hint of a sniffle.

The fact is that the only sure cure for a common cold (one that is mild enough to be self-terminating) is to go to bed and give the body's inborn and interacting immune systems time to assemble and deploy the interferons, antibodies, phagocytes, complements, and properdins which, since the creation of our species, have always neutralized the viruses causing common colds. Some good physicians recommend that during the period of bed rest, the patients (including themselves and their loved ones) should be given ample quantities of chicken soup, or Coney-Island clam chowder, or good Scotch or

350

Irish whiskey, but such remedies have more to do with atavism than medicine.

Walther Kruse's demonstration that inoculations of cell-free filtrates made from the nasal secretions of people with colds induced the common cold in healthy volunteers was unfortunately made in 1914, the year his native Germany and other European nations embarked upon World War I. By the time the German and other European laboratories that were shattered, both during the war and in the violence and chaos that followed, were reestablished, the Great Depression—a slightly delayed but entirely predictable sequel to World War I—was raging in America, England, France, Germany, Austria, and other countries.

In 1930 at the outset of the Great Depression, Alphonse Raymond Dochez and his coworkers in New York completed four years of studies, which produced the same information that Kruse reported in 1914: Common colds were probably caused by one or more types of virus. The remainder of the Great Depression, and the six-year Second World War it helped generate, intervened before the development of the electron microscope and the birth of modern virology gave people the insights and the advanced technology required to isolate the viruses responsible for the common cold and attempt to make good vaccines against them.

In 1931, before he became one of the discoverers of the human influenza virus, Christopher Andrewes repeated Dochez's work in medical student volunteers at St. Bartholomew's Hospital in London. When World War II ended, Andrewes convinced the British government's Medical Research Council (MRS), as well as England's three largest drug companies, Glaxo, Pfizer, and Wellcome, to organize the Common Cold Research Unit. This unit was opened in 1961 under Andrewes's direction, and was set up in the former American Hospital built at Salisbury and staffed by the Harvard University medical school during the Second World War.[18]

The hunt for the viruses of the common cold was accelerated after Wilson Smith and his colleagues isolated the influenza agent believed to be one of these viruses, and Dochez transmitted influenza from one human volunteer to another by inoculations of nasopharyngeal filtrates bearing yet another but still not isolated virus. The search was aided greatly by the tissue-culture techniques improved by Enders and his group. Before the Second World War, Dochez had grown some cold viruses in hatching-egg cultures, but they died out after ten or twelve passages. After the war the Salisbury researchers tried repeatedly to grow candidate cold viruses in chick-embryo cultures in hatching eggs, but did not succeed.

Tissue cultures of human and monkey cells were more amenable to growing any viruses that might be present in cell-free filtrates from the nose and throat washings of people with colds. In the fall of 1954, at the Great Lake, Illinois, naval training camp, a group of U.S. Navy doctors headed by

W. Pelon and William J. Mogabgab isolated a cytopathogenic agent from naval recruits with mild respiratory disease. They subsequently found that this agent, GL 2060, was also present in the nose and throat washings of new naval recruits during similar outbreaks in 1955 and again in 1956.

By then, GL 2060—which was consistently found in monkey kidney cultures seeded with cell-free filtrates made from the nose and throat washings of sailors with mild respiratory disease—had been proven impervious to enough different antibiotics to suggest that it was not a bacterium. It failed to react with antibodies of known respiratory viruses or common disease viruses, but like all viruses, GL 2060 was small enough to pass through fine filters that held back even the smallest of known bacterial cells. When living monkey kidney cells in tissue cultures were exposed to GL 2060, they were damaged and fragmented in a manner characteristic of the cytopathogenic effects (CPE) of viruses on cells maintained in laboratory cultures.

There was no doubt that GL 2060 was a virus. Since it came from nasal washings, the name rhinovirus (from the Greek for nose) was proposed, although for years Mogabgab held out for murivirus, since GL 2060 had been isolated from mouse (murine) cell cultures. With the isolation of the rhinovirus at the Great Lake camp, research workers in Salisbury, Bethesda (the NIAID and other institutes of the NIH), and elsewhere started scores of rhinovirus vaccine projects. Few viruses were easier to isolate than the rhinoviruses, and if in the beginning there seemed to be one antigenically specific type of rhinovirus for every living virologist, there was no question about where they came from and what they could do in tissue cultures and human volunteers.

"Rhinoviruses can be isolated from 20 to 30 percent of adults with common colds, and therefore a successful rhinovirus vaccine would be a significant means of protection against this disease," stated a 1965 report by the Scientific Committee on Common Cold Vaccines headed by Andrewes. "As there are many strains of rhinoviruses which are serologically distinct, a polyvalent vaccine would be necessary to insure protection against these viruses."[19]

Mogabgab, who had taken a position at Tulane University School of Medicine, New Orleans, when his naval service was over, felt that vaccines made of a few known respiratory viruses would be cross-reactive enough to protect against much larger numbers of related viruses causing respiratory diseases. That is, he believed that a good vaccine against one strain of rhinovirus would produce antibodies effective against other strains. One reason for advancing this concept was the growing volume of good reports on the effects of the combined adenovirus-influenza virus/common cold vaccine then being marketed. Mogabgab felt that adenovirus vaccines containing the nonmilitary-population Types 1, 2, 5, and 8 "or strains with heterotypic immunizing potentialities would have a place in civilian groups, especially young children.'

In 1958 Mogabgab formulated a number of experimental vaccines against colds. One was a monovalent type made of the formalin-inactivated GL 2060 rhinovirus, which not only was found in "as much as a third of mild upper respiratory illness in some populations," but Mogabgab believed could also "produce heterotypic antibody that reacts with other respiroviruses." Another was a formalinized four-virus vaccine containing the GL 2060 rhinovirus, plus inactivated influenza, parainfluenza, and Coxsackie viruses. These vaccines were tested in various student and industrial populations in Louisiana.

The multivalent four-virus vaccine containing influenza, RSV, adenovirus, and rhinovirus, when tested in the industrial population, induced antibodies that gave protection against a third of the illnesses the influenza vaccine by itself did not prevent. Mogabgab felt that the results of his experimental trials demonstrated the feasibility of "several multivalent respiratory vaccines tailored for different populations, seasons or age groups." He knew that the costs of developing such custom-made vaccines would be staggering, but better than most of his contemporaries, Mogabgab also understood that the human and dollar costs of not having such protection against the common cold were far greater. His description of the needs for a common cold vaccine or vaccines, although written in 1962, remains a succinct and accurate statement of a still unfilled need.

"When one considers the forceful approach that was used for the development of a vaccine for poliomyelitis, a very minor problem as compared to upper respiratory illnesses, it becomes evident that the whole impact of these infections is not generally realized," Mogabgab wrote in the October 1962 issue of the *Annals of Internal Medicine.* "Tremendous benefit will accrue to patients with pulmonary and heart disease when multivalent respiratory disease vaccines are available. Complications of respiratory infections, sinusitis, otitis media, bronchitis, pneumonia and meningitis will be greatly reduced.

"Most of the sicknesses of childhood will be eliminated. Accordingly," Mogabgab continued, "the practice of medicine will be modified to a large extent, especially in the specialties of pediatrics and otolaryngology, and in the management of chronic lung and heart disease. Also, the use of antibiotics will be greatly reduced as evidenced by comparisons of amounts of antibiotics used in this country during years of high incidence of respiratory diseases with those used in years of low incidence. Now that sufficient information is available to make an effective start toward these goals, unnecessary delay certainly is unjustified."

This was an accurate statement of how most medical virologists and infectious disease investigators felt at the time. At Salisbury when the rhinovirus vaccine developed in 1965 was tested in human volunteers, it failed to show any cross-reactive immunological activities. The vaccine protected only against colds induced by rhinoviruses in the vaccine strain and not against other wild types let alone the viruses of influenza, RSV, or other respiratory infections.

As new vaccines were developed for known strains, dozens of new types and strains of rhinovirus were isolated. By 1967 an international cooperative study organized by the NIAID listed fifty-six antigenically distinct types. The next report of this collaborative study, completed in 1971, listed eighty-nine. As of this writing, there are now well over 120 known antigenically distinct types of rhinovirus alone, among the thirty-one known human adenoviruses, respiratory syncytial viruses, notoriously polyvalent Coxsackie and ECHO viruses, and coronaviruses—known to cause colds and suspected of playing a role in multiple sclerosis—influenza viruses, and a few others known or thought to cause mild upper respiratory diseases.

In fact, it was the exponentially increasing number of serologically distinct viruses of many families that in the end led to the closing down of the Common Cold Research Unit at Salisbury in 1970.

There, as in the United States and other countries, scientists had to face the reality that while the development of a good vaccine against the common cold was theoretically not impossible, it was hopelessly premature to work on such a vaccine in the absence of infinitely more knowledge about the immunochemistry, genetics, and biology of all human viruses. To proceed any further without this missing basic knowledge would repeat, with common cold vaccines, the mistake made by Park, Brodie, and Kolmer with their premature polio vaccines in 1935.

The continuing accumulation of evidence underscoring the roles of the common cold and other respiratory virus infections in the processes of bacterial adherence and other stages of major bacterial infections only adds to the urgency of the need for considerably more basic information on the nature of viruses and their interactions with healthy human cells.

If and when such information results in new vaccines to protect people against the common cold, they may yet turn out to be the most clinically important ones—in terms of organs, limbs, and lives saved—since Jenner gave humankind the smallpox vaccine.

One thing is apparent: The story of vaccines against the scores of diseases, many of them fatal, now known to be caused by viruses has barely begun. As with the work on bacterial vaccines, this effort will—just as Pasteur predicted a century ago—bring us closer to the era of what he termed "chemical vaccines."

Pasteur's prescience was, however, the product of and limited by his actual knowledge and observations. He could foresee only the very early forms of what he called chemical vaccines, the preparations made of chemical substances found on, in, or produced by the microbial agents of human diseases. These would include the fragments of protein antigens chemically split off the outer coats (capsids) of whole viruses used in subunit vaccines against hepatitis B, influenza, and other preparations. They would include the bacterial capsular polysaccharides used in making vaccines against pneumococcal pneumonias and bacterial meningitis. They would also include the diphtheria and tetanus vaccines made of the chemically treated toxins produced by the bacteria themselves.

For all his acute insights, the true gift of genius, Pasteur lacked the hard knowledge that would have permitted him even to fantasize about what many laboratories around the world are now working on: vaccines made from off-the-shelf chemicals which, while wholly synthetic, are exact replicas of the biological chemicals that constitute the active immunizing principles of the protein and carbohydrate antigens found on or inside viruses, bacteria, and other microbial parasites.

Before we reach the era of fully synthetic vaccines, another development of potentially great prophylactic importance is the advent of monoclonal antibodies. One of the new characteristics a healthy cell acquires when it is transformed into a cancer cell is immortality. "A tumor is itself an immortal clone of cells descended from a single progenitor."[20] Since many malignant tumors also produce immunologically active tumor antigens, the host immune systems recognize them as "foreign" or "nonself" antigens and program their lymphocytes to manufacture immunoglobulins or antibodies against the tumor cells.

In 1975 the Argentine-born Cesar Milstein and his colleagues at the British Medical Research Council Laboratory of Molecular Biology at Cambridge learned how to fuse the cells of an antibody-producing mouse myeloma tumor with lymphocytes from the spleen of a mouse immunized with a specific antigen. The products of such fusion, called hybridomas, had both the lymphocytes' capacity to produce specific antibodies and the immortality of the myeloma tumors.

It was not long before the Cambridge research workers were able to fuse tumor cells with lymphocytes that produced antibodies against specific antigens, and to isolate clones of these hybridomas which could be grown continuously in tissue cultures. "We had for the first time," Milstein wrote, "developed continuous cultures of fused cells secreting a monoclonal antibody of predefined specificity."[21]

Clinically, this could provide almost inexhaustible sources of specific antibodies for passive immunization for the treatment and temporary prevention of infections, as was first done with antitoxic antibodies in the sera of previously immunized animals in patients with diphtheria, tetanus, and pneumonia. Monoclonal antibodies produced by hybridoma can be made safe to use in people by treating them with the enzymes that break down both types of nucleic acids, along with formaldehyde and other agents that kill viruses and living cells.

In cancer therapy Milstein suggests that "two kinds of role are foreseen for monoclonal antibodies. One role is the targeting of toxic drugs: antibodies to the tissues of a particular organ or to specific tumor antigens could be attached to drug molecules to concentrate the drug's effect. Alternatively it may be possible to produce antitumor antibodies that will themselves find and attack tumor cells."[22]

Monoclonal antibodies in research might also lead to insights resulting in vaccines against presently nonpreventable diseases, starting with malaria—the world's single leading cause of death. Ruth Nussenzweig and her colleagues at New York University recently completed a series of experiments with monoclonal antibodies and the agents of malaria in mice, whose results, as of 1980, "are encouraging for the prospect of developing a malaria vaccine . . ."[23]

The multimillionaire oil man Armand Hammer, a medical school graduate who never practiced medicine, was so taken with what he perceived were the anticancer potentials of monoclonal antibodies that in 1982 he offered a prize of a million dollars to anyone who came up with a cure for cancer. Whether or not monoclonal antibodies, by themselves or in combination with drugs, radiations, surgery, and other anticancer modalities, actually do have such anticancer potentials is yet to be determined. About the only thing certain is that Hammer's prize money will stimulate extended studies of monoclonal antibodies that might have a bearing on the prevention and treatment of many diseases, including possibly cancer.

Hybridomas do not exist in nature. They are laboratory artifacts. The "antibody factories" in which they are produced still require manipulations of their living materials. On the other hand, what is happening now in various laboratories, such as Richard A. Lerner's at the Research Institute of the Scripps Clinic in La Jolla, California, might advance the synthesis of antibodies from living hybridomas to more prosaic antigen factories built and run by living people.

Lerner and his colleagues found that a specific sequence of the single-stranded RNA genome of the Moloney murine (mouse) leukemia virus coded for an unknown protein, which they termed the R protein. They "chemically synthesized part of the R. protein, raised antibodies to the synthetic peptides, and detected immunologically cross-reactive material in infected cells."[24]

The antibodies to the synthetic peptide—a peptide is a compound containing two or more amino acids—were detected by injecting it into the bodies of mice and rabbits. What was important here was the demonstration that it is possible to produce protective and cross-reacting antibodies with only a small, chemically well-defined segment of the nucleic acid in the Moloney murine leukemia virus. The same techniques for mapping the chemical sequences of viral nucleic acids could also be used to help establish the stage preliminary to the chemical synthesis of the segments of viral, bacterial, and protozoan peptides coded for antigen production.

Lerner and his team are currently working on developing the chemical knowledge of the specific viral nucleic acids that are needed to synthesize the segments coded for antigen production, and that they plan to use in wholly synthetic vaccines against influenza and hepatitis. Because the replicas of the viral nucleic-acid segments required for these vaccines, synthesized of stock chemicals, would be very inexpensive to make, sell, and use, they could accomplish many goals.

One of the benefits of such inexpensive synthetic vaccines would be in the possible prevention of some cancers. It is known, for example, that hepatitis B is a frequent precursor of hepatocellular carcinoma (liver cancer). It is equally well known that the presently available hepatitis B vaccine costs $75 to $120 (in 1981 dollars) for the three doses required to immunize a single individual—a guarantee against the mass immunization tests required to determine whether a vaccine against hepatitis B also acts against liver cancer. A synthetic vaccine against hepatitis B would probably cost pennies per dose to produce and would make such trials feasible. Similarly, a synthetic vaccine against the Epstein-Barr virus known to cause infectious mononucleosis, and quite possibly involved as a major cofactor in Burkitt's lymphomas and nasopharyngeal cancers, might prove to block both these cancers if it were put to mass trials in people at greatest risk.

It is not known how many other laboratories around the world are now working on synthetic antigen nucleotide vaccines, and against what infectious diseases. What is known is that the huge health industry corporation Johnson and Johnson has helped support the work of Lerner's laboratory, and has already obtained an exclusive license to make new vaccines by the methods that laboratory is developing. This suggests that Johnson and Johnson's high-priced and knowledgeable staff and contract scientists have enough faith in the clinical and economic prospects of completely synthetic chemical vaccines to put their own jobs on the line. Giant conglomerates do not squander corporate dollars gladly.

The relative costs of the chemical synthesis of organic or living substances from nonliving and biologically inert inorganic materials have not increased substantially since 1828 in Germany, when a young high school teacher, Friedrich Wohler (1800–1882), discovered by combining the inorganic substance potassium cyanate with an equally inorganic substance, ammonium sulfate, that he was able to synthesize urea, an organic compound that in nature is found only in urine. Wohler, who some years later would be Robert Koch's professor of chemistry at Göttingen, may be called the intellectual father of the array of good vaccines that will eventually be made of immunogens as synthetic and as inexpensive as the organic urea he synthesized from coal and ammonia.

The speed at which these inevitable laboratory-synthesized immunogens are developed and put to clinical uses will depend almost entirely on the levels at which the United States and other countries with the required scientific and monetary resources—particularly Canada, England, Australia, France, Germany, the Soviet Union, the Scandinavian nations, Japan, and China—fund and stimulate the education, training, and postdoctoral research of at least a generation of biologists, biochemists, biophysicists, and clinical scientists. Such people are not born; they are made by intelligent and concerned national governments.

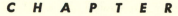

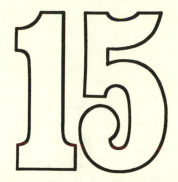

THE REDISCOVERY OF CHEMICAL VACCINES AGAINST PNEUMONIA AND MENINGITIS

Although the last quarter century has seen remarkable advances in the prophylaxis and treatment of respiratory infection, pneumonia remains among the leading causes of death in this country. Since the introduction of penicillin, reports of the mortality from pneumococcal bacteremia have varied but have placed it as high as 25 percent.... It appears unlikely that the prognosis in pneumococcal infections can be improved further by antimicrobial therapy ... prophylactic measures would appear to offer the most likely means of reducing further the mortality from pneumococcal bacteremia and from pneumococcal infection.... Purified pneumococcal capsular polysaccharides are excellent antigens in man.

—ROBERT AUSTRIAN, M.D., in "The Current Status of Bacteremic Pneumococcal Pneumonia. Re-Evaluation of an Underemphasized Clinical Problem," *Transactions of the Association of American Physicians,* 76, 1963, pp. 117–125

As the twentieth century opened, two by-products of industrialization, its instant urbanization, and the low wages that prevailed at the turn of the century, helped make pneumonia the leading cause of all deaths in this and most other industrial countries. These classic by-products were overcrowding and malnutrition.

The bacteria and viruses that cause pneumonia are transmitted from person to person by droplets in the breaths, coughs, and sneezes of sick and healthy people who are carriers of these microbial disease agents. In the absence of adequate living space and adequately ventilated work space, the droplet-borne agents of diseases, ranging from pneumonia and other respiratory infections to diphtheria, meningitis, and the streptococcal infections that cause rheumatic fever and poststreptococcal nephritis, reach far more people per cough or sneeze than they do in less crowded situations. Droplet infections are, for this reason, more prevalent in urban centers than in sparsely populated rural areas.

More than 80 percent of all bacterial pneumonias acquired by people outside of hospitals are caused by the pneumococci, the bacteria first found in the normal sputum flora of healthy people in 1880 by Louis Pasteur in France and, at about the same time, by George Sternberg in the United States. Although they drew and described the bacteria quite accurately, neither Pasteur nor Sternberg realized that these lancet-shaped bacteria caused any diseases in people. It was not until 1884 that Albert Fraenkel, in Berlin, demonstrated that the microbes caused lobar pneumonia in humans. Two years earlier, Carl Friedlander discovered that the bacilli now named after him (but originally isolated by Edwin Klebs in Switzerland in 1875 and known as the *Klebsiella*) also caused human lobar pneumonia.

In 1886 Anton Weichselbaum, a Viennese bacteriologist and pathologist and the discoverer a decade earlier of the meningococci, proposed the name *Diplococcus pneumoniae* for the encapsulated bacteria first described by Fraenkel. Sternberg objected later to this designation, in an article in the *National Medical Review,* writing that "I object to the name 'diplococcus pneumoniae' because this micrococcus in certain culture media forms longer or shorter chains and it is, in fact, a streptococcus." Despite this, the name proposed by Weichselbaum remained the official name of these pneumonia organisms in the United States until 1976, when America's taxonomists rechristened them *Streptococcus pneumoniae,* which is what they had long been called in England.

Since Pasteur's day we have learned that just about any pathogenic bacteria, if enough of them get into the human lungs, can cause pneumonia. Prominent among the more serious causes of bacterial pneumonia are the hemolytic staphylococci, *Haemophilus influenzae type b* (formerly called Pfeiffer's bacillus), the newly isolated *Legionella,* the once rare and exotic but now commonplace blue-pus bacteria, *Pseudomonas aeruginosa,* the venerable *Klebsiella,* and out-of-bounds and normally benign enteric bacteria, such as *Escherichia coli* and *Serratia marcescens,* the latter a coliform bacillus that in its long history as a factor in human affairs has caused not only lethal pneumonias but also, over many centuries, was often the cause of violent massacres of Jews.

While the overcrowding in the dwelling places of the urban poor helped facilitate the dissemination of the saliva droplets that carry pneumonia-causing germs to far greater numbers of people, and in much larger quantities, than were the norm before the vast environmental changes of the Industrial Revolution, the undernutrition common to families unable to afford adequate foodstuffs, which compromised their inborn or genetic host defenses against pneumonia-causing bacteria in crowded dwellings and workplaces, contributed to the rise in pneumonia and other respiratory infections.

It took millions of years for the mammalian inborn host defense or immune systems to evolve and eventually to protect the human species from most common microbial disease agents. These innate systems of cellular and circulating biological and chemical destroyers of invading microbial parasites depend, in turn, on the general health of human beings at risk of infections. The healthier the human body, the more effective its interacting networks of phagocytes, immunoglobulins (antibodies), complements, properdin, and interferons that help comprise the immune system.

The more invasive the pneumonia bacteria the human host defense systems have to attack and neutralize, the greater the body's need for adequate nutrition. This does not call for huge amounts of food, merely for the very modest amounts of proteins, minerals, fats, carbohydrates, vitamins, and trace elements biologically required for growth and development, and the maintenance of human health.

Exactly how much food is enough to keep all bodily systems in good working order is still subject to learned disagreement, but the rule of thumb published by the London family doctor Charles Hall in 1805 is still a very practical one. "It would be difficult," Hall wrote at the dawn of the Industrial Revolution, "to discover whether the poor have a sufficiency of animal and vegetable food by any other method than by considering the quantity of each sort which their nature requires; and their means of obtaining that quantity; or, in other words, what their earnings are, and what a quantity of food such earnings could procure."[1]

This is still one of the most practical medical measurements ever devised. It should come as no surprise that more than two centuries later, when the Surgeon General of the United States appointed Dr. Joseph Goldberger to set up a task force to ascertain the cause of pellagra—then widely believed to be an infectious disease of poor southern white people—Goldberger's first action was to assign the Public Health Service statistician Edgar Sydenstricker to determine how much the poor white millworkers of the South were paid, and how much food of what categories these wages could buy for the families in which pellagra was rife.[2]

In 1900 in the United States, as in 1805 in London, people who could not afford to buy adequate quantities of food were the same people in whom infectious diseases were more prevalent and considerably more deadly than in more properly nourished classes of society. The poor were not the only people to suffer pneumonia in the pre-World War I years when this lung infection was the leading cause of death in the United States. They were, however, the primary focus of community infections, the main reservoir of pneumonia bacteria in this country. As servants, cooks, train conductors, trolley motormen, draymen, foodstore clerks, waiters, barbers, employees in industry and commerce, and in many other capacities, they delivered pneumococci as well as goods and services. Bacterial pneumonia therefore was far from uncommon and killed many people in more affluent families as well as poor ones.

Between 1900 and 1940, pneumonia gradually declined in incidence, slipping from first place to fifth place in the roster of the ten leading causes of all deaths in the United States. In 1900 the single statistical category of pneumonia and influenza killed 203 in every 100,000 Americans; 175 of the deaths were from pneumonia and 27 from influenza. By 1940—as the sulfonamides, the first modern antibacterial drugs, became available—the pneumonia/influenza death rate had been cut by 63 percent, or from 203 deaths per 100,000 population in 1900 to 75 deaths per 100,000 population in 1940. Of these latter deaths, 59 per 100,000 population were from all forms of pneumonia, and 14 per 100,000 population were due to influenza. However, many influenza deaths are caused not by the influenza virus, but by bacterial pneumonias secondary to the primary viral infection.

During the four decades between 1900 and 1940, no systemic drugs or antisera had been developed to neutralize or destroy the influenza virus. The 39 percent reduction in influenza deaths since 1900 was in all likelihood due almost entirely to immunity acquired from the pandemic of 1918, followed by gradual increases in the average American family income, which led to more living space and more food for families at highest risk of contracting influenza. However, after 1910 serotherapy began to play an interesting but very minor role in the reduction of deaths from bacterial pneumonias, which in eight cases out of ten proved to be caused by one of the over eighty infective types of pneumococci.

Prior to 1940 at least three pneumococcal vaccines had been reported in the bacteriological and the medical literature. The first, in 1891, was developed in Germany by George and Felix Klemperer. It was made of live pneumococci, and the two doctors used it to immunize rabbits against pneumococci. The second, the killed whole pneumococcal vaccine of Sir Almroth Wright, was safe enough in all people into whom it was injected. However, it was only sporadically effective when tested in 50,000 black miners in the gold and diamond mines of the South African Rand in 1911–1913.

The third pneumococcal pneumonia vaccine, created by accident in 1926 in Berlin when Wolfgang Casper determined that the purified material derived from the slimy capsules surrounding virulent pneumococci, when injected into mice, immunized them against infection from the same types of pneumococci. Later Casper's mouse experiments were extrapolated to people at Rockefeller Institute and at Harvard University by Lloyd D. Felton. The result was a pneumococcal capsular polysaccharide vaccine, which was tested by the U.S. Public Health Service in over 100,000 males in the CCC camps between 1933 and 1940, with very encouraging results.

One of the major reasons for the failure of Wright's killed whole-organism vaccine in 1911–1912 was the lack of general knowledge that there is more than one capsular type of pneumococcus, and that antibodies against the pneumococci are exquisitely type-specific. First of all, the doses of bacteria in Wright's vaccine were much too low, and when by happy coincidence the pneumococci in a given batch of his 1911 pneumonia vaccines happened to be the same type or types as the pneumococci that caused specific outbreaks of pneumonia at a specific mining camp on the Rand, the antibodies induced in the vaccinated miners by the serendipitously type-matched bacteria in the vaccine did not always protect against these pneumococci.

Prior to Wright's experiments in South Africa, many European and American doctors had tried to adapt the principles of serotherapy to the treatment of pneumonia. Serotherapy involved injecting specific disease bacteria in gradually increasing but sublethal doses into healthy animals until they developed enough immunity to resist lethal doses. The blood sera of the immunized animals contained antitoxic antibodies to the poisons or toxins elaborated by the diphtheria and tetanus bacilli, and injections of the antitoxic animal sera were used to treat patients with diphtheria or lockjaw, as well as to provide temporary immunity to members of the patients' immediate families. The passive immunity provided by these transferred antibodies (immunoglobulins) persisted for as long as the antibodies lasted, or about two weeks.

The early pneumococcal antisera did not usually work as well in sick people as did the serum antitoxins against diphtheria and tetanus. In 1909 and 1910 two investigators at the Koch Institute, Franz Neufeld and Ludwig Handel, showed the reason for the many treatment failures of pneumococcal antisera. They were able to divide pneumococci into three immunologically distinct types. Pneumococcal sera that worked well against one type invariably failed against organisms of the other pneumococcal type.

Although Neufeld was one of the world's leading bacteriologists, Wright apparently chose not to consider the implications of this finding to his experimental pneumococcal vaccine. If he had, the nature of the vaccines he tested in 6,000 people in South Africa, and the results of these mass trials, might have been very different—as also would have been the subsequent history of vaccines against pneumococcal pneumonia. Considerably more attention to the published work of Neufeld on the polyvalent nature of the pneumococci was paid by the Rockefeller Institute and its hospital in New York. After all, pneumonia was a leading cause of all deaths in the United States, and the Institute was committed to curing and/or preventing the nation's major diseases. The doctors at the Rockefeller Hospital began to develop type-specific antisera against the major pneumococci and, in the absence of commercial sources of correctly typed pneumococcal antisera, started to produce large lots for their own and other hospitals' uses.

Serum treatment became a standard therapy for pneumococcal pneumonia in many hospitals. If given early enough in the course of a pneumococcal infection, the antisera were very effective. While doctors gained more experience in the diagnosis and specific serotherapy of pneumococcal pneumonia during the next thirty years, medical bacteriologists around the world went on discovering many new types of pneumococci.

The antisera did not cure every case of pneumonia in which they were tried, and many patients developed serum sickness—a form of severe allergic reaction to the foreign proteins in horse sera. In the mid-1930s, Frank Horsfal and Kenneth Goodner at Rockefeller, and Michael Heidelberger developed a technique for making the clinical antisera in rabbits, and this proved somewhat less likely to cause serum sickness than horse sera.[3] Dubos cites the 1936–1937 annual report of the Rockefeller Hospital, which showed that in patients treated with rabbit antiserum, "Among more than 50 patients with lobar pneumonias due to pneumococcus Types I, II, V, VI, VII, XIV, XVIII there has been but one death. . . . In untreated patients with similar [pneumococcal] type distribution the death rate would have amounted to about 34%."[4]

At the Rockefeller Hospital, where the antisera were of excellent quality, such clinical results were not surprising. But even there Type III pneumococcal antiserum did not produce such good results, just as today penicillin is far less effective against Type III infection than against those caused by all other types of pneumococci.

With the advent of antibacterial drugs, particularly antibiotics, many doctors were convinced that the new wonder drugs would soon eradicate all bacterial pneumonias in this country. As the spectrum of bacterial families sensitive to the antibiotics kept expanding, nearly all the bacterial pneumonias—whether caused by pneumococci or less common microbes—proved quickly curable by drug therapy. The two fine six-type, polyvalent pneumococcal capsular polysaccharide vaccines sold for use in adults and children immediately after the end of World War II by E. R. Squibb and Sons, Inc., had to be taken off the market for want of medical interest in the prevention of pneumococcal pneumonia. Doctors and lay journalists alike hailed the new antibiotics as miracle drugs that would render most major bacterial diseases extinct within the first postwar decade.

During World War II, the virologist Monroe Eaton and his other colleagues who were called in to cope with contagions in the armed forces had isolated and grown, in chick embryos and later in tissue cultures, the submicroscopic agents of atypical or "walking pneumonia," and had characterized them as viruses. In time, other workers showed that this agent of "virus pneumonia" could be killed by tetracyclines and other antibiotics that acted on the nucleus.[5]

In 1961 Leonard Hayflick at the Wistar Institute in Philadelphia, and Michael Barile and Robert Chanock at the National Institutes of Health in Bethesda, grew the Eaton agent in an artificial nutrient medium, as bacteria are grown, and showed that the Eaton agent is not a virus but a mycoplasma, a bacteria-like organism that is the smallest independent form of life yet discovered. Viruses are obligate intracellular parasites and cannot function or replicate except in the cell cytoplasms of their living hosts.[6]

At that time, the mycoplasma species were still popularly called PPLO, standing for pleuropneumonia-like organisms. The pleuropneumonia organisms (PPO) had originally been isolated from the lungs of cattle suffering from bovine pneumonia in 1898 by Edmond Nocard and Émile Roux of the Pasteur Institute. The official name for the PPO type of organisms was later changed to *Mycoplasma,* from the Greek words for fungus and something formed (*plasma*). Unlike true bacteria, which can live in rigid cell-wall growth forms, or cell-wall-deficient forms, or even cell-wall-free forms—which, under the electron microscope, are virtually indistinguishable from the naturally cell-wall-free mycoplasma—the mycoplasma-genus organisms have never been shown to revert to the classic or rigid cell-wall forms. Such reversions can be controlled at will, in the microbiology laboratories, by manipulation of the nutrients and other growth or environmental conditions in which variant cell-wall-free bacteria cultures are maintained.

The Eaton agent—now *Mycoplasma pneumoniae*—was the first mycoplasma proven to cause diseases in humans. It is a major cause of pneumonia in young people (for example, college freshmen and military recruits). To date, all efforts to develop a vaccine against mycoplasmal pneumonia have proven fruitless.

In the post-World War II ambience, when the astonishing ease with which the antibiotics swiftly ended pneumonia infections brought tears of gratitude to the eyes of older physicians, as well as to the eyes of families of patients who recalled the bad old preantibiotic days when bacterial pneumonia was virtually tantamount to a death sentence, it was easy to understand many of the mistakes the medical community began to make in relation to the continuing dangers of pneumococcal pneumonia. Around the nation, major hospital after major hospital gradually abandoned the established custom of routinely isolating and typing the bacteria circulating in the blood of newly admitted pneumonia patients. Here and there, where a hospital chief of medicine or infectious diseases was himself or herself involved in special research or simply reluctant to change, the typing of all bacteria found in pneumonia patients was continued.

By 1952 when the thirty-six-year-old Dr. Robert Austrian accepted a faculty post at the Downstate Medical Center in Brooklyn, New York, pneumonia deaths were down to 26.1 per 100,000 Americans, and most doctors were agreed that bacterial pneumonia was patently on the road to extinction. Nevertheless, pneumonia was still the fifth leading cause of death in the United States, and the 41,134 deaths caused by pneumonia of all forms in 1952 could hardly be ignored.

As a second-generation specialist in pulmonary diseases, Austrian knew that the deaths caused by pneumonia were far from the full sum of the costly effects of all forms of the disease. Nearly thirty years later, he was still in awe of the damages pneumonia could cause. "The greatest number of hospital admissions for pneumonia are of people in the most productive period of their lives," he observed in 1978, when 237,000 people—60 percent of them between fifteen and sixty-four years old and another 25 percent under fifteen—were hospitalized for all forms of pneumonia. "We still haven't the foggiest notion of what the pneumococcus does to the human organism," he maintained. "It is possible, in one sense, to cure the patient by killing the pneumococci with antibiotics, even though the same patient goes on to die of damage caused while the infecting pneumococci were still alive. Since we often cannot reverse the damage caused by the pneumococcal infections—prior to their treatment with antibacterial drugs—it is far wiser to prevent pneumococcal infections in the first place."

This was, if anything, a studied understatement of the grim constellation of biological insults the pneumococci inflict on our species. For lobar pneumonia is only one of the killing and crippling diseases they cause. Next to *Haemophilus influenzae type b* bacteria, the pneumococci are the second most common cause of bacterial meningitis, presently one of the leading causes of acquired mental retardation because of the damage it causes to the brain and the central nervous system. The pneumococci, particularly eight of the types among those most often responsible for pneumonia in this country, are the principal agents of otitis media—inflammation of the middle ear secondary to bacterial infection—which may cause long-term and even permanent hearing losses that are quite possibly the leading single cause of mental maldevelopment in the United States. In our times, the pneumococci are responsible for well over one million cases of bacterial otitis media annually, most of them in preschool children. All these and other damages are in addition to the half million cases of pneumococcal pneumonia they cause yearly in the United States.

Robert Austrian entered his college years with his medical insights and social values greatly influenced by his father, Professor Charles R. Austrian, who had spent his entire professional career as student, teacher, and practitioner at the medical school and the hospital of Johns Hopkins University in Baltimore. Born in 1885, Charles Austrian had entered medical school in 1904 when he was nineteen, but he did not graduate with his class. A year of his career as a medical student was lost to a siege of typhoid fever—then a major disease but now a nearly extinct water-borne infection in the United States. When he recovered from typhoid, Charles Austrian spent the rest of the lost academic year working with Walter Jones on nucleic-acid chemistry at Hopkins. After graduation, he interned at the Hopkins hospital and received his first faculty appointment.

"He was," says his son, "a superb diagnostician. In fact, he was such a good doctor that I really had a problem until I made up my mind that I couldn't compete with him. I knew that I was hopelessly outclassed." Robert Austrian also remembers that "My father always used to say that it's fortunate for physicians that most people get well in spite of doctors, rather than because of them."

As an impressionable young person growing up under his father's loving guidance, it was inevitable that Robert Austrian would come to maturity convinced that if major diseases can possibly be prevented, then it is always much better to prevent than to cure them. Like his father, he too went to Hopkins, and after graduating started his academic career at the same school as an assistant in medicine in 1942. The following year he was promoted to instructor in medicine, but his teaching career was soon interrupted by military service in World War II, in which he served as a medical officer, and in 1945 as a member of the field party of the Typhus Commission in the China-Burma-India theater.

Austrian was always most fortunate in his mentors. After the war he spent a very instructive year as a research associate in microbiology at the New York University School of Medicine, under Colin MacLeod. This was only three years after Avery, MacLeod, and McCarty published their classic paper,

"Studies on the chemical nature of the substance inducing transformation of pneumococcal types," in which the role of DNA in heredity was first revealed—and the nature of all the life sciences transformed for the better.

MacLeod was then attempting to clarify further the role of the nucleic acid DNA. Austrian, working with him, was mindful of the fact that some forty years after his father had assisted one fine scientist (Walter Jones) in nucleic-acid studies, he was doing the same thing under MacLeod. He also learned a great deal from MacLeod about the immunologic properties of pneumococcal capsular polysaccharides when used as vaccines to prevent pneumococcal pneumonia. It was MacLeod who had, as Heidelberger wrote, "so beautifully organized and monitored in the field" the historic trials of the polyvalent capsular polysaccharide vaccines in a South Dakota military air base in 1944 that "showed that epidemics of pneumococcal pneumonia in closed populations could be terminated within two weeks after vaccination with the polysaccharides of the causative types."[7]

Austrian returned to the Hopkins faculty in 1949, completed his residency at the Hopkins hospital, and was certified as a diplomate of the American Board of Internal Medicine before moving to Downstate as associate professor of medicine in 1952. His university connection also included an appointment as visiting physician on the university division of the huge Kings County Hospital across the street from the medical school. There, as far as Austrian could see, pneumonia was still a major cause of hospital admissions, and he had no good reason to believe in 1952, as in 1932, that the pneumococci were not still responsible for 80 percent of all bacterial pneumonias. There was no way Austrian could immediately prove this, however, since Kings County Hospital, like most other American hospitals, had long since stopped isolating and typing the microbial pathogens found in the blood and sputum of pneumonia patients.

According to the reports of his colleagues, he was informed that at this large New York City municipal hospital in 1952, there were only three or four admissions per year for pneumococcal pneumonia, although there were many admissions for pneumonia. The bulk of all hospitalized pneumonia cases, the hospital staff doctors told Austrian, were people with virus pneumonia. The reason for this diagnosis, they told him, was that antibiotics and sulfa drugs do not work against viruses, and that the wonder drugs had virtually eradicated all bacteria which caused pneumonia in Brooklyn.

Austrian found this comfortable belief impossible to accept and undertook a project akin to the reinvention of the wheel: He set up a prospective study in which he screened the sputum and blood of more than 2,500 patients admitted to the Kings County Hospital with pneumonias of all forms during the next ten years, and typed all the pneumococci he isolated from these patients.

In a total of 529, "incontrovertible evidence of pneumococcal infection was provided in each instance by isolation of pneumococci from the patients' blood . . ." Moreover, Austrian was able to type 99 percent of the clinical isolates of the pneumococci that, as of 1952–1962, were supposed to have been eradicated by antibiotics.[8]

There were all kinds of pneumococcal infections in this patient population, from local infections to disseminated or bacteremic pneumonias in which the pneumococci spread from the infected lungs to the bloodstream and circulated throughout the body. Austrian classified these bacteremic patients into three groups. "There were 455 patients with pneumonia, 47 patients with pneumonia and an extrapulmonary focus of pneumococcal infection, and 27 with meningitis secondary to sinusitis or otitis. The overall mortality for the three groups was 25 percent. . . .

"Bacteremic pneumococcal pneumonia resulted in the death of one of every five persons afflicted . . .

"In the 438 patients who received antimicrobial therapy, the mortality was 17 percent. The majority received penicillin, a small number tetracycline, and the remainder a variety of [antibacterial] drugs."

When compared with the preantibiotic-era pneumococcal pneumonia fatality levels of 82 percent reported by two scientists at Boston City Hospital in 1937,[9] the 17 percent fatality rate at Kings County Hospital in 1952–1962 looked very good. However, the young professor who made these comparisons was also acutely aware of a number of clinical realities concerning pneumonia. The first was that "it appears unlikely that the prognosis in microbial infection can be improved further by antimicrobial [largely antibiotic] therapy."

In uncomplicated cases of bacteremic pneumococcal pneumonia treated with penicillin and other antibiotics, the death rates ran between 17 percent and 18 percent. In other pneumococcal pneumonia cases, particularly in patients over fifty who also had underlying heart, circulatory, cancerous, and other systemic disorders, the death rates—despite antibiotic treatments—were more than 25 percent. In the Kings County patient population, "More than half of all deaths from pneumococcal bacteremia were caused by pneumococcus types I, III, IV, VIII, and XII. Two thirds of these deaths occur in persons 50 years of age or older with complicating illness. If bacteremic infections with any of the same six types in persons under 50 with complicating illness, and in those 50 or older with or without complicating disease are combined, these categories account for nearly three-fifths of all deaths from pneumococcal bacteremia."

A year later Austrian and his colleague, Dr. Jerome Gold, showed that when Types II and V were added to the above six pneumococcal types, they "accounted for two thirds of the cases of pneumococcal disease with bacteremia. Types XII, XIV, XVIII, XIX, and XX were also recovered with relative frequency from the blood."[10] This suggested to Austrian that what would protect most people would be a pneumococcal capsular polysaccharide vaccine containing the purified subunit carbohydrates of the dozen or so types of pneumococci which, combined, caused most bacterial pneumonias diagnosed in hospitals.

In 1963 in the first report on his ten-year clinical study of the specific causes and effects of pneumococcal pneumonias, Austrian concluded that a more favorable outcome of postantibiotic treatment "can be anticipated only when the physiologic derangements brought about by [pneumococcal] infection are better understood, and specific measures are devised to correct them." This was a plea for more research into the actual nature of the damages pneumococci cause in human bodies, and which three decades later were still barely known or understood. In the continued absence of such knowledge, he wrote, "Prophylactic measures would appear to offer the most likely means of reducing further the mortality from pneumococcal bacteremia and from pneumococcal infections."

On the basis of these and collaborative studies in various other hospitals, such as the one run later by Dr. Martin A. Fried of the Kaiser Permanente Medical Center in San Francisco, it became evident to Austrian "that endemic pneumonia was still prevalent in the United States and that, even with penicillin therapy, the mortality rate from bacteremic infection, which exceeded 25% in those over 50 years of age and in those with a variety of chronic illnesses, was unacceptably high." He proposed that the only logical means of reducing such an unacceptably high mortality rate was to prevent pneumococcal pneumonias by redeveloping and relicensing the multitypic or polyvalent pneumococcal capsular polysaccharide vaccines that had proved themselves so well in the very recent past.

In his 1963 article on the results of his decade-long study at Kings County Hospital, Austrian cited the polyvalent pneumococcal polysaccharide vaccine. developed by Michael Heidelberger and used in 1944 by Colin MacLeod to end a pneumonia epidemic at a wartime army air base in South Dakota. He had also cited the little-remembered work of Dr. Paul Kaufman at another New York municipal health-care facility, the Goldwater Memorial Hospital. Kaufman had developed a vaccine containing the purified capsular polysaccharides of three common types of pneumococci. During six years starting in 1937, Kaufman and his collaborators had used this cell-surface carbohydrate vaccine to reduce the incidence of pneumonias due to any of the three types of pneumococci to a low 17.2 per 1,000 population in an experimental cohort of 5,750 people over fifty years old. At the same time, in a matched group of nonimmunized people over fifty years old, the case incidence of pneumonias caused by pneumococci of the vaccine's types came to 44 per 1,000 population or 60 percent higher than in the vaccinated population of the same age range.[11]

Austrian knew, at the conclusion of his Brooklyn study, that his task had become primarily one of education, not merely the education of doctors who treated patients but, equally important, of the scientists and laymen who determined the priorities and the budgets of public health research and policies. He concluded his 1963 report with an appeal to medical reason and societal self-interest.

The death rate from pneumonia and influenza, he wrote, was "more than 100 times that from poliomyelitis. The Bureau of Vital Statistics projects an increase in the number of persons over 55 years of age [the population at greatest risk of bacteremic pneumonias] from 28,500,000 in 1955 to 46,000,000 in 1980. If it is worthwhile to invest large sums in the palliation and cure of neoplastic and of cardiovascular diseases, which affect most heavily this segment of the population, it seems reasonable to utilize available knowledge to reduce the morbidity and mortality resulting from one of the most common bacterial infections in our society. To provide essential epidemiologic data, it will be necessary to make pneumococcal typing sera available once again and to reinstitute the diagnostic bacteriologic techniques which have been all but completely abandoned by the medical profession. With these measures and the utilization of knowledge already extant concerning immunization, it should be possible to prevent 10,000 to 15,000 deaths a year from pneumococcal infection."

Austrian's powerful and subsequently often reiterated arguments for the resumption of prewar diagnostic bacteriologic techniques in all American hospitals were, with some notable exceptions, resoundingly ignored from Maine to California. He kept at his task, however, in the laboratory as well as on the rostrum. "No matter how unproductive the day," Austrian said more than a decade after his Kings County Hospital pneumonia investigation ended, "I feel it hasn't been entirely wasted if I have typed a pneumococcus." Most other doctors did not share this value judgment. In his 1975 Maxwell Finland Lecture, Austrian observed that "whenever routine typing of pneumococci has been reintroduced, there has been a two- to 10-fold increase in the recognition of the organism in the institution concerned. Until physicians can be reconditioned to obtain routinely cultures of blood and respiratory secretions before antimicrobial therapy, and until laboratories return to optimal procedures for isolating and typing pneumococci, the true magnitude of illness caused by this organism will continue to be underestimated."[12]

On the other hand, the power of his scientific findings and his arguments based on hard facts found more receptive ears at the federal government's National Institute for Allergy and Infectious Diseases (NIAID), whose funding officers in 1967 provided Austrian with a first "baby grant" for the redevelopment of an improved polyvalent capsular polysaccharide vaccine against pneumococcal pneumonia. Larger grants were to follow from NIAID to expand and continue this line of experimental research.

By 1967, Austrian had become professor and chairman of the department of research medicine at the University of Pennsylvania. As he saw the problem, if he made a vaccine containing the capsular sugars of twelve major types of pneumococci, it would probably protect people against the most common causes of pneumococcal pneumonia in this country. Around 1970, when Austrian had a candidate vaccine in hand, Maurice Hilleman and his colleagues at the Merck Laboratories, who were working in close collaboration with Robert Austrian on the pure cultures of the pneumococcal types Austrian had isolated and typed, went to work at the formidable continuum of challenges involved in developing the techniques of producing this twelve-antigen vaccine in huge quantities.

Both the Austrian and the Hilleman laboratories mounted a number of small-scale tests of the two polyvalent vaccines' safety and immunogenicity in people. Given the previous history of polyvalent pneumococcal capsular saccharide vaccines, neither Austrian nor Hilleman were surprised by the fine results of these limited trials. Hilleman had been with E. R. Squibb and Sons, Inc., as a virologist, when Squibb made the bacterial capsular polysaccharide MacLeod had used in South Dakota in 1944. After the war the company had lost a fortune in its failing attempt to market similar chemical vaccines against six types of pneumococci, but Hilleman had not been professionally involved in either Squibb project, although he was well aware of the great clinical potentials of the vaccines.

Austrian and Hilleman were both "looking for populations in which to test the efficacy" of their reborn and expanded pneumonia vaccine, when a historically very apt trial population was unexpectedly made available. "Sir Charles Stuart-Harris of Sheffield University in England was visiting Philadelphia and told of his trip to South Africa in 1966 to discuss respiratory disease on the mines. There was still much pneumonia among the miners, he reported. At that time, Professor James H. S. Gear, Director of the South African Institute for Medical Research, was on sabbatical at Harvard University. Through his good offices," Austrian reveals, "I was put in touch with the chief medical officers of three of South Africa's largest gold mining companies; and, as a result of these contacts, a trip was made to Johannesburg in September, 1970, to determine the feasibility of conducting vaccine trials at the mines."[13]

Although there had been some improvements in the South African gold mining compounds, little had changed in relation to the prevalence of pneumococcal pneumonia in the miners on the Rand since 1913, when Gorgas gave the mineowners his recommendations concerning the qualities of the housing, family life, food and medical care of the native African gold miners—and which most mineowners promptly ignored.

The first outcome of Austrian's site visit in 1970 "was the establishment of bacteriologic surveillance of pneumonia at several mines through the cooperation of the Mine Medical Officers' Association, the South African Institute for Medical Research, and the Chamber of Mines of South Africa. With the reinstitution of capsular typing at the Institute, it became quickly apparent that pneumococcal pneumonia, though infrequently fatal, was still rife, subsequent data demonstrating an attack rate of approximately 100 per 1000 per annum among African males coming to work for the first time on the mines."[14]

When Austrian returned to South Africa in 1972 to conduct the first clinical trials of two polyvalent capsular polysaccharide vaccines against pneumococcal pneumonia at the East Rand Preparatory Mine (ERPM) in a town fifteen miles away from Johannesburg, he was acutely sensitive to the historical and social aspects of this essentially clinical study. "The gold mine itself," he noted, "is one of the oldest and deepest mines on the Reef, having been established in 1893. It is an unforgettable experience to descend to the deepest workings of the mine two miles below the earth's surface, and a mile below sea level, where the rock temperatures are 125 °F. . . . The mean temperature in the mine is 80 °F, and the humidity holds at 100% . . . The mine's labor force, derived largely from Malawi (formerly Nyasa) and Mozambique, varied during the four and a half years of the trials, from 6450 to 14,000 men, who were housed in barracks in four compounds. . . . Participation [in the vaccine trials] was limited to men coming to work for the first time at any time, but no miner was required to take part and a small number declined to do so. Pneumonia is not a new problem at this mine, an epidemic there having been described by Ordman in 1937."[15]

As in the years before Gorgas conquered pneumonia in the Canal Zone by ending the billeting in fetid, crowded quarters of the black workers building the Canal, and by improving their sanitary, nutritional, and family living conditions, the crowded barracks in which the Transvaal miners slept after a day's toil in the hot, humid mine shafts were highly conducive to the inception of pneumococcal pneumonia, which was found in a hundred out of every one thousand new native African miners.

As in 1910 the deep mine shafts were highly conducive to the proliferation and transmission of pneumococci, even though Austrian notes, "The disease is a recruitment phenomenon that has nothing to do with poor housing. Actually, these people are not housed any differently than soldiers in American military barracks, although perhaps the miners are more crowded. African miners today live under conditions not very different from the American military recruits who got meningitis in basic training camps during the Vietnam War. The immediate cause of the outbreaks of pneumonia in the mining camps, however, is the bringing of immunologically naive individuals into a crowded environment. You see the same thing now in all the large African cities as people move in from the bush—and in the cities pneumonia becomes a very major problem. This is exactly the same kind of thing that goes on in South Africa. So that it can happen here as well as there."

While Austrian tested his vaccine, Hilleman arranged for separate trials of the Merck versions of the pneumococcal vaccines. In 1972, 983 African miners were inoculated with a vaccine containing the purified polysaccharides of six capsular types of pneumococci, and another 2,036 miners participating in the trials served as unimmunized controls. The six-antigen vaccine caused a 76 percent reduction in pneumonias due to the six pneumococcal capsular types in the vaccine.

This trial was followed by one of a twelve-capsular-type pneumococcal polysaccharide vaccine, which was given to 540 miners while another 1,135 miners served as controls. The second polyvalent capsular-sugar vaccine induced a 92 percent reduction in the numbers of pneumococcal infections caused by the twelve-capsular types of pneumococci whose cell-surface carbohydrates were in the vaccine.

More tests and more changes in the vaccine followed. The new vaccines were tested in Australian miners, and in different populations in Chile and New Guinea. In the United States, as of 1977, the polyvalent pneumococcal capsular polysaccharide vaccine had been tested in well over 10,000 adults and children. By the time Merck applied for a federal license to market its version, the vaccine had been developed into a fourteen-antigen preparation designed to protect people against the fourteen capsular types of pneumococci that cause 80 percent of all hospital-treated pneumococcal pneumonias in this country. (The vaccines prepared for use in other countries, such as South Africa—where two of the locally most common infective types of pneumococci proved to be very rare in the United States—are often formulated to include the strains that are most prevalent in given nations.)

The reborn and greatly improved pneumococcal capsular polysaccharide vaccine was licensed for general clinical use by the Food and Drug Administration (FDA) early in November 1977 and released in February 1978—a year in which pneumonia and influenza combined killed an estimated 52,500 Americans. Of this number, 48,000 were pneumonia deaths. Of the 4,500 deaths attributed to influenza, the majority were caused by bacterial pneumonia secondary to influenza infection.

At that time, Austrian estimated that at least 17,000 of the annual toll of pneumonia and influenza deaths could have been prevented by using the effective vaccine that he and Hilleman and their collaborators had revived, improved, and reintroduced into world medicine.

Three years before Austrian's capsular polysaccharide vaccine against pneumococcal pneumonia was licensed, the FDA issued a license for another cell-surface carbohydrate vaccine against another major infectious disease, meningococcal meningitis. Like the pneumonia vaccine, this one also had to be reclaimed from stillborn or aborted chemical vaccines; enormously improved and redeveloped; and created originally to protect immunologically susceptible military recruits in basic training camps.

By the time this monovalent vaccine, or vaccines (there were actually two), was licensed in 1975, it had already been used to immunize all of Finland and Brazil against epidemics of meningococcal meningitis caused in one instance by Group A meningococci and in the other by Group C meningococci. In those hurriedly mounted vaccination efforts, four major American and European pharmaceutical companies produced enough meningococcal vaccines to immunize 130 million men, women (including pregnant women), and children over two years old. The vaccines caused not a single death, nor any serious adverse side effects; no damages of any sort to the fetuses of pregnant women carrying them; and, being merely chemical subunits of the capsules surrounding the meningococci, the purified capsular sugars caused no meningitis or any other infectious diseases. The absence of any serious side effects to one bacterial capsular polysaccharide vaccine made it easier for the FDA to satisfy itself that such chemical vaccines could, as claimed, be safe for people when Merck applied for a license to market the fourteen-antigen vaccine.

Bacterial meningitis, or cerebrospinal meningitis as it is also known around the world, is an infection-generated inflammation of the meninges, the membranes enclosing the brain and the spinal cord. Meningitis is caused by viruses and by bacteria. Viral meningitis, whose causal agents cannot be destroyed or neutralized by antibacterial drugs, is a comparatively benign and self-limiting disease. Bacterial meningitis is a more serious disorder.

Once the meninges of the brain and spinal cord are inflamed by bacterial infection, the inflammations cause multiple symptoms and complications. These range from excruciatingly severe headaches to vomiting, stiffness in the muscles of the neck and back, photophobia (morbid fear of light), constipation, skin eruptions, delirium, paralysis, convulsions, and death. Before antibiotics, cerebrospinal meningitis was an often lethal disease. Some forms, such as tuberculous meningitis and the meningitis caused by the fungus *Cryptococcus,* were invariably fatal during the centuries before systemic antibacterial drugs were developed to treat and cure them.

Nevertheless, "Despite the widespread use of antibiotics the frequency of encapsulated bacterial diseases remains the same or, possibly, may have increased. Thus," write John Robbins, Rachel Schneerson, Carl Frasch, and other colleagues, "endemic meningitis in infants and adults due to pneumococcus and to *Haemophilus influenzae type b* occurs with the same frequency in the 1960's and 70's, as in the pre-antibiotic 1930's. Neonatal meningitis due to Group B *Streptococcus* type 3 may have increased in frequency in nurseries in the U.S. during the past decade."[16]

375

Bacterial meningitis can be treated and generally cured with antibiotics, although the death rates of various types of the disease are still formidable. People who are treated and cured of severe bacterial meningitis episodes are, though saved from death, still susceptible to the classic permanent damages caused by the inflammations of their brains and spinal cords. These end effects of bacterial meningitis appear in the upward of one third of the patients who, thanks to antibiotics, survive the disease itself. They include blindness, deafness, recurrent seizures, paralysis, and behavioral disorders.

Although nearly all known pathogenic bacteria can attack the meninges and cause meningitis, there are three primary groups of meningitis bacteria. They are *N. meningitidis,* the most common cause of cerebrospinal meningitis worldwide; the pneumococci, particularly any one of the fourteen types contained in the polyvalent vaccine, that cause most laboratory-diagnosed bacterial pneumonias; and *H. influenzae* (HI) *type b,* the leading cause of bacterial meningitis in the United States. *H. influenzae* (formerly Pfeiffer's bacillus) does not cause influenza, as we learned earlier; it can indeed cause meningitis, pneumonia (generally secondary to an influenza infection), and other serious infections in people, including subacute bacterial endocarditis, or inflammation of the lining membrane of the heart.

Bacterial meningitis affects people of all ages, but most of all children under six; and among children, by far the greatest proportion of cases involve those under two years old. In the United States and other industrialized countries, bacterial meningitis is much more prevalent among the poor and those just above the poverty line than among the more affluent. Children of the poorer, more crowded, less nourished segments of industrialized societies, when they reach adolescence, show far higher counts of antimeningococcal antibodies than do young people who have had far healthier childhoods. The high costs of acquiring immunity to major bacterial and viral infective agents the natural way, by getting meningitis, or rubella, or polio and other infections, can hardly be recommended as the price of later immunity—since these costs not only include blindness, deafness, and paralysis but also the higher infant and child death rates of the poor.

The social or environmental causes of the lower rates of natural infections among more fortunate children are not an unmixed blessing. They also mean that when young people previously unexposed or barely exposed to common microbial disease agents of bacterial meningitis and other major infections leave home at eighteen for college or to serve a hitch in the armed services, they arrive at the campus dormitories or the military barracks as individuals at high risk of bacterial meningitis, adenoviral acute respiratory infections, and the other common communicable diseases of the poor. Let just one nonimmune college freshman or raw recruit contract one or more of these infections by simple exposure to sick or healthy carriers of their bacterial or viral agents, and he or she becomes a walking focus of infection for all the other susceptible young people in the same closed academic or military subpopulation. As a general rule, to infect just one of these young adult nonimmune susceptibles in a closed population of nonimmune susceptibles is to start a mini-epidemic on a campus or in a basic training camp.

For many wholly explicable demographic, socioeconomic, and bacteriologic reasons, epidemic cerebrospinal meningitis has been on the increase in some areas of the globe since the end of World War II. In the poor (and before World War II, often colonial) countries of Asia, Africa, and Latin America, poverty among the rural populations has led to mass migrations to cities in search of jobs. Then, urban poverty, overcrowding in makeshift hovels, chronic hunger, and the near-total lack of even the rudiments of medical care combine to make millions of rural migrants subject to major killing and crippling bacterial, virus, and other parasitic diseases—including all forms of meningitis—and some of their survivors may become carriers of these diseases to the more comfortable residents of those cities.

In the United States the rising divorce rates since 1945 and the swiftly spiraling fiscal inflation since 1964 have forced many divorced or still married women to take full-time jobs that compel them to place their infants and preschool children in day-care centers that feed, clean, and shelter children of working two-parent and single-parent families.

These child-care centers are at high risk of enteric, droplet, and fecal-oral diseases ranging from infectious hepatitis (hepatitis A), shigellosis, salmonellosis, giardiasis, and rotovirus infections to streptococcal and staphylococcal diseases and, above all else, to meningitis caused by H. influenzae type b. This very common bacterium, by far the leading cause of bacterial meningitis in children under two years old, is, by virtue of the brain damage it causes in young children, one of the leading causes of acquired mental retardation in this country. Four of the five HI meningitis outbreaks between 1975–1979 were in day-care centers. The average mortality runs between 5 percent and 10 percent of all children affected, but 50 percent of them have some form of neurologic sequelae. The CDC believes that not more than 30 percent of all cases of H. influenzae type b meningitis are reported to local health agencies.

In 1944 after the Heidelberger-MacLeod polyvalent capsular polysaccharide vaccine stopped a military air-base pneumonia epidemic, Elvin A. Kabat, the first investigator to earn a doctorate in immunochemistry under Michael Heidelberger at Columbia, was inspired to try to duplicate this work with a vaccine made of the capsular polysaccharides of Group A meningococci. His efforts, funded largely by the army's commission on meningococcal infections, were far from a resounding success. However, the partially purified capsular polysaccharides Kabat used as an experimental vaccine did induce antibodies to Group A meningococci in four of the thirty-three human volunteers in whom it was tested.

The Kabat preparation worked, as the French say, *en principe,* if not in 88 percent of the human volunteers in whom it was tested. What it did prove was that in 12 percent of the volunteers tested, this chemical vaccine was indeed immunogenic. This clearly suggested that improved techniques of extracting and purifying the capsular polysaccharides of meningococci might in time lead to a much more effective vaccine. Kabat was well aware that once Heidelberger originally isolated and purified the capsular polysaccharides of the pneumococci in 1923, it had taken nearly a decade of further improvements in chemical and physical purifying techniques before a pneumococcal capsular polysaccharide was developed of sufficient size and purity to be immunogenic enough to act as a vaccine in human beings. The capsular polysaccharide molecules of bacteria, as Kabat himself had helped demonstrate, had to have a molecular weight of at least 50,000 daltons before they could act as immunogens—and this called for a molecule more than twice as large as the polysaccharide molecules in Kabat's first meningococcal vaccine.

Kabat's attempts to develop techniques of purifying meningococcal capsular polysaccharides so that they would be larger than 50,000 daltons was abandoned shortly after the war, as he later explained, "Because of the enormous strides in the treatment of bacterial infections with antibiotics." These strides had, in fact, witnessed the inception of the use of the antibacterial sulfa drugs for the chemoprophylaxis as well as the treatment of meningococcal meningitis.

The major users of these sulfonamides were the United States armed forces. During and after World War II, every new recruit arriving at his first basic training camp was routinely given one or more sulfonamide tablets to keep him from catching meningococcal meningitis.

In due time, as in the earlier instance of the gonococci during World War II, the sulfonamides inevitably killed off the infective strains of meningococci susceptible to their antibacterial blandishments, and thereby selected out for proliferation the previously very low aberrant subpopulations of equally infectious but naturally highly sulfa-resistant strains of meningococci. Suddenly, despite the sulfa drugs, outbreaks of meningococcal meningitis began to be reported from many training camps. This was in 1963, early in the course of the Vietnam War, which grew less and less popular with the parents of drafted servicemen as the scale of our military involvements and our military casualty lists escalated along with the estimates of enemy "body counts" for over a decade of famous victories.

If there is one thing the military establishment of every country abhors it is an outbreak of visits by angry national legislators to top civilian and military officials on behalf of angry—and often politically potent—constituents whose children are felled by nasty diseases, or killed in training mishaps, in home-country or stateside training camps. The sudden rise in meningococcal meningitis in United States military recruits caused many articulate parents to flood the offices of their current congressmen, senators, and President with angry phone calls and letters of protest.

Unfortunately, there was no good vaccine against meningococcal meningitis. A killed whole-organism meningococcal vaccine had been developed and tested overseas in 1963, but had proven to be a gross failure. What added to the pressures on the military top brass was the fact that there was a major war going on, 8,000 miles from our shores, and the outbreaks of Group C meningococcal meningitis inflicted delays in the military training of raw recruits for combat overseas.

The armed services responded in many ways, one of which was to call up the most talented draft-eligible young research physicians, immunochemists, microbiologists, and other professionals working in or close to fields that might touch on some better way to protect new recruits from meningococcal meningitis, and to spare the military the wrath of the recruits' parents.

The draft claimed many talented young men, among them Emil Gotschlich. Like Robert Austrian, Gotschlich was born to a medical family, but in Bangkok, Siam, in 1935. His grandfather, the first Emil Gotschlich, was born and educated in Germany, and after qualifying as a physician took a position as a sanitation officer in Alexandria, Egypt. He put his younger brother, Felix, through medical school in Germany, and then brought Felix to a post in Egypt where in 1905 he discovered the El Tor strain of the cholera vibrio.

Emil's son, also named Emil, was born in Egypt and sent back to Germany to study medicine. He graduated in 1932, at the nadir of the Great Depression, and took a job as a ship's doctor on a steamer sailing from Hamburg through the Orient to Vladivostock. He fell in love with the East on this voyage, and the following year sailed to Bangkok and went into private practice. There he married another German physician, and they produced the third Emil Gotschlich in 1935.

The family was in Switzerland on vacation when World War I broke out. The father went back to Bangkok at once, and Emil remained in Switzerland with his mother. His parents were divorced during the war, and after Gotschlich's mother remarried, the new family emigrated to the United States. There Emil completed his secondary-school education at Forest Hills High School, a fine public high school with excellent science departments. He entered New York University for his undergraduate and medical education, taking his M.D. in 1959.

At the New York University medical school, Gotschlich came under the influence and personal guidance of two great teachers, Drs. Lewis Thomas and Chandler A. Stetson, both pathologists and microbiologists. Thomas's primary research interest was cancer, while Stetson had worked for many years on the hemolytic streptococci, which are sensitive to penicillin and yet continue to be major causes of diseases and disorders. Thomas and Stetson encouraged Gotschlich's interest in immunochemistry, and were both very instrumental in his next move after completing his internship at Bellevue Hospital. That move was to proceed thirty-three blocks farther north along the East River, from Bellevue Hospital to the Rockefeller Institute (now Rockefeller University).

After Gotschlich entered the Institute as a guest investigator and associate physician, his research for the next five years concentrated on the C-reactive proteins. These are very heavy serum globulins which are found in the presence of inflammations, and which under certain chemical conditions precipitate the cell-wall polysaccharides of some pathogenic bacteria, including those of pneumococci and gonococci.

Gotschlich's interest in the capsular polysaccharides of the meningococci was, as he describes it, "draft induced." It started in 1966, when he was called up by the army, commissioned as a captain, and detailed to work under Dr. Malcolm Artenstein at the Walter Reed Army Institute of Research [WRAIR] in Washington, D.C. Along with Artenstein and the newly drafted Dr. Irving Goldschneider, Gotschlich went to work on some of the problems created by the sulfa-induced natural selection of drug-resistant but infective Group C meningococci, the bacteria responsible for outbreaks in American basic training camps.

Thanks to their own research interests, as well as to the articles and lectures of Robert Austrian, Gotschlich and his new WRAIR colleagues were aware of the prophylactic potentials of bacterial subunit vaccines and of Kabat's early attempts to make a vaccine from the capsules of Group A meningococci. They reviewed Kabat's old journal papers. Kabat himself, still at the Columbia University College of Physicians and Surgeons, was available to answer any questions about his earlier findings.

The capsular sugars of the meningococci, however, existed only in the journal literature. Nobody had even an ounce of these polysaccharides anywhere. Nor had anyone, while they did exist, ever completely elucidated their chemistry.

The young WRAIR research team set out to culture Groups A, B, and C meningococci, strip them of their capsules, and devise better methods of standardizing and testing the white powders to which the bacterial capsules were chemically reduced. These various tasks were completed in a few weeks' time.

Of the three serogroups of meningococci, Group A, a major pathogen abroad, rarely produced disease in this country; Group B was often a serious cause of meningitis here; and Group C was often responsible for epidemic meningitis in the United States, including the basic training camp outbreaks.

In preclinical trials the capsular sugars of Groups A and C meningococci seemed sufficiently immunogenic to be tested clinically. The capsules of the epidemiologically important Group B meningococci proved to be composed of a carbohydrate antigen that was too weakly immunogenic to amount to much (at least by itself) as a vaccine against meningitis caused by this group of *N. meningitidis.*

One of the major accomplishments of the early phase of this work at WRAIR was Gotschlich's development of a very effective and technologically simple method of producing high-molecular-weight capsular polysaccharide molecules. This method could easily be scaled up for commercial levels of production when and if the two antibody-inducing or immunogenic groups of meningococci proved themselves clinically as vaccine materials.

In November 1967 Gotschlich became the first to be inoculated with the new Group C meningococcus vaccine. In April 1968 five more officer-investigators were immunized with the experimental vaccine, and started to produce antibodies to Group C meningococci. These encouraging results showed that the new vaccine was safe and effective. Accordingly, in April 1968 the army tested the vaccine in a few hundred military volunteers, with excellent results. The army then funded E. R. Squibb and Sons, Inc., to produce enough of the new meningococcal subunit carbohydrate vaccines for the large-scale military-population field trials that were run, on schedule, in 1969 and 1970.

During these field trials, the vaccine proved quite capable of protecting new recruits at various basic training camps. Starting in 1971 each of the armed services began routinely to inject the vaccine against Group C meningococci into every new recruit at his or her first basic training camp. The angry letters from parents stopped pouring into Washington. Thanks to the new capsular polysaccharide vaccine, the camps were again and have remained since then free of epidemic Group C meningococcal meningitis.[17]

The testing of the Group A meningococcal capsular polysaccharide vaccine developed at WRAIR originally presented more of a problem, since this group was rare in the United States. A fairly good-sized test was run, with excellent results, in selected samplings of schoolchildren in Egypt, where Group A meningitis was endemic. In 1973 a nationwide epidemic, in which 90 percent of all cases were caused by Group A meningococci, broke out in Finland. At around the same time, resistance to the sulfas manifested themselves in both strains of Group A meningococci involved in the Finnish epidemic.

The WRAIR Group A vaccine was rushed to Finland and administered to the entire population. During that epidemic, under the direction of the bacterial geneticist and physician Helen Mäkelä, a special study was conducted in a cohort of 130,000 Finnish children between the ages of three months and five years. In this study two meningitis vaccines were tested. The

WRAIR Group A vaccine was given to 49,000 of these children. An experimental capsular polysaccharide *H. influenzae type b* vaccine, developed at the University of Rochester, New York, by Drs. Porter Anderson and David H. Smith, was administered to an equal number of children. The 32,000 remaining members of this group were not inoculated with either meningitis vaccine but, like the others, were followed clinically and treated immediately if any meningitis symptoms appeared.

In a second trial, conducted by Mäkelä et al. in children between three months and five years old, 21,007 Finnish children received the Group A vaccine.

After one year, "No cases of meningitis or sepsis caused by Group A meningococci were seen ... among the children vaccinated with meningococcal vaccine; six [cases of Group A meningococcal disease] occurred among those vaccinated with the *H. influenzae* vaccine; and 13 among those not vaccinated."[18] In the second trial, of the WRAIR vaccine alone, "No cases caused by Group A occurred among those vaccinated, although five to seven would have been expected within the year. Meningococcus Group A vaccine appears efficacious in young infants and children."

This level of vaccine efficacy may well have been enhanced by the herd immunity created during the same 1973 epidemic, when the entire population of Finland was immunized with the new Group A meningococcal vaccine that terminated the epidemic. In their full report of the vaccine trials in infants and young children, the Mäkelä group revealed that "a weak anti-Group A meningococcal antibody response could already be seen in many infants of the group three to five months of age, and the response above two years of age (mean of 15 to 20 micrograms [of antibodies] per milliliter) was close to the adult value of 20 micrograms per liter obtained with the same vaccine lot."[19]

In 1975 during the epidemic caused by Group C meningococci in Brazil, when one French and three American pharmaceutical manufacturers produced enough of the WRAIR-developed vaccine to inoculate that entire nation, the mass immunizations stopped the meningitis epidemic in its tracks. However, it was also shown that "although most infants respond to Group C vaccine as early as three months of age, protective antibody levels are not reached until 18 to 24 months of age."[20]

The still experimental capsular polysaccharide vaccine against *H. influenzae type b*, meanwhile, was shown to be ineffective against HI meningitis in children under eighteen months old, although very protective against HI meningitis in children over eighteen months old and in adults.

The present pneumococcal capsular polysaccharide vaccine, whose fourteen capsular types of pneumococci are also most frequently responsible for pneumococcal meningitis, was also demonstrated to be ineffective in children under two years old.

When it came to bacterial meningitis, a disease found primarily in children under six years old, with most under two years old, the failure to date of the new capsular polysaccharide vaccines to protect the infants and children at highest risk tempered much of the joy they brought to those who developed them.

The three groups of causal organisms were each responsive to various antibiotics, and for this reason bacterial meningitis became less lethal than it had been prior to World War II. A study by Dr. Maxwell Finland and Mildred W. Barnes of acute bacterial meningitis at Boston City Hospital during twelve selected years between 1935 and 1972 showed that during these twelve years, only 50.5 percent of all bacterial meningitis patients survived these infections. The three most frequent causative organisms, which together caused 66 percent of all bacterial meningitis cases, were *S. pneumoniae* (33.7 percent of all cases), *N. meningitidis* (17.5 percent), and *H. influenzae* (14.3 percent). Of the three leading causes of bacterial meningitis in this Boston municipal hospital, *S. pneumoniae* was the most deadly, having killed 68.4 percent of all bacterial meningitis patients; *N. meningitidis* killed 17 percent, and *H. influenzae* killed 13.4 percent of all bacterial meningitis patients.

At Boston City Hospital, a staggering 63 percent of all cases of acute bacterial meningitis during the twelve selected years between 1935 and 1972 were nosocomial (hospital acquired). These nosocomial meningococcal infections were in turn responsible for 30 percent of all deaths from bacterial meningitis at this large city hospital during this same period.

Among the forty-one patients with pneumococcal meningitis admitted to Boston City Hospital "in the two years before penicillin became available, only three (7%) survived; after that the rate of survival in different years ranged between 18 and 66%."[21]

Fatalities are not the only major damages inflicted by the agents of bacterial meningitis. *S. pneumoniae,* for example, is by far the most frequent cause of otitis media, one of the leading causes of acquired, recurring, and permanent hearing losses in preschool children. Nor does the lower case-fatality rate (CFR) of *H. influenzae* (HI) *type b* meningitis even begin to compensate for the permanent damages it inflicts on children, most frequently before they are two years old.

In 1972 a follow-up study was published by Dr. Sarah W. Sell and her collaborators at the Vanderbilt University Hospital in Nashvville, Tennessee, of the long-term effects of HI meningitis in eighty-six children who were treated with acceptable antibiotic therapy during an acute HI meningitis outbreak from 1950 to 1964. This study showed that of the eighty-six children, eleven (13 percent) were dead, twenty-six (29 percent) of the survivors had severe handicaps, twelve (14 percent) had possible residual damages, and thirty-seven (43 percent) were free of detectable handicaps.[22]

The defects these doctors found in the children who survived HI meningitis with the aid of antibiotic drugs included hearing losses, partial blindness, speech and behavioral difficulties and temper tantrums, which all combined to cause very low IQ test scores in the 50- to 69-point range, seizures requiring medical treatment and medications, and left spastic hemiplegia. The Vanderbilt group reported that "antibiotic therapy, while greatly reducing mortality, has not reduced the incidence of *H. influenzae* meningitis which, in fact, is reported to be on the increase in several centers in the U.S." Sell and her collaborators concluded that in HI meningitis, "prevention rather than cure should now be a prime goal for the future."

Five years later, another follow-up study of the long-term outcomes of antibiotic-treated cases of HI meningitis was published in an American pediatrics journal by Johan Lindberg and three collaborating physicians of Göteborg, Sweden, where "HI meningitis is the most common type of purulent meningitis and has shown an increasing incidence." They found that of eighty-two Swedish children treated with antibiotics between 1968 and 1975, "a total of 22 (26.8%) showed both neurologic or psychologic sequelae, or both." Hearing loss, the most common long-term damage found, occurred in fifteen patients, one of whom also "showed hydrocephalus ['water on the brain'], mental retardation and motor deficiency."

The four Swedish doctors reported that three (4 percent) of the eighty-two children treated for HI meningitis died of the disease or its complications, while two "had paraplegia and mental retardation without hearing loss. Among the patients who showed only hearing loss, the course of the meningitis had been complicated by subdural effusions in two patients, bacteriologic relapse in one patient, paralysis of the sixth cranial nerve in three patients, and temporary ataxia in three more patients. One girl and one boy, aged 2 and 13 months respectively, showed delayed intellectual development with an IQ between 70 and 80. [IQ tests vary from test publisher to test publisher in the United States and, of course, from country to country, so that no comparisons can be made between the IQ test scores obtained by Sell et al. in Nashville and Lindberg et al. in Göteborg.] Both children had had a complicated course of temporary signs of hydrocephalus at echoencephalography. Three boys, one aged 2 months and two aged 5 years, had behavior problems with pronounced difficulties at school, but the results of their intelligence tests were within normal limits. The course of the disease had been complicated for only one of these patients, with a prolonged coma that lasted six days."

Clearly, bacterial meningitis remains a major health problem when none of the new vaccines that act against its three major pathogens offer protection against them to neonates, infants, and children at great risk of infection, and no available vaccine at all exists against the epidemiologically important Group B *N. meningitidis* bacteria. There is also an important fifth pathogen, Group B *Streptococcus,* which, while responsible for only 3 percent of all cases of meningitis reported to the CDC by thirty-eight states in 1978, is nevertheless a major pathogen. The reason is that most patients with Group B streptococcal disease are infants less than three months old. Group B *Streptococcus* is one of the primary causes of neonatal (birth to one month of life) bacterial meningitis, with an estimated case-fatality ratio (CFR) of 30 percent to 50 percent.

GROUP B STREPTOCOCCUS AND OTHER BABY KILLERS— AND NEW BACTERIAL SUBUNITS TO BLOCK THEM

Since [Rebecca] Lancefield's classification of beta-hemo-lytic Streptococcus in 1933, organisms designated as Group B have been reported as a cause of human disease. Their emergence as frequent neonatal pathogens, however, is an event of this decade. Two distinct types of illness that are related to age at onset are described for neonates with infections due to Group B Streptococcus. The "early-onset type" of infection occurs in neonates 5 days of age or less, results from intrapartum transmission of organisms from the maternal genital tract, and causes a mortality rate in excess of 50%. "Late-onset type" infections, in contrast, are characterized by onset beyond the 10th day of life and are associated with purulent leptomeningitis, significantly lower mortality rates, and modes of transmission in addition to the mother-to-infant route.

—DRS. CAROL J. BAKER, DENNIS L. KASPER, AND CHARLES E. DAVIS, 1976[1]

For all the historic health gains of new licensed bacterial capsular polysaccharide vaccines against pneumococcal pneumonia and the deadly cerebrospinal meningitis caused by the pneumococci, and the equally effective Group A and Group C meningococcal vaccines against meningitis, there remain some very tragic shortcomings in these vaccines. Most cerebral meningitis strikes, cripples, and often kills children under two years old, with the greatest morbidity and mortality occurring in those under three months old. The Group A meningococcal vaccine does not work in children under three months old; the Group C meningococcal vaccine and the fourteen-antigen pneumococcal pneumonia vaccine do not protect children under eighteen months old.

In these otherwise good new bacterial subunit vaccines, the reason for their ineffectiveness in the above age groups lies quite probably in the immunological immaturity of infants and very young children, rather than in the immunogenic properties of the cell-surface carbohydrates of the subunit vaccines—and of the experimental capsular polysaccharide vaccine against *Haemophilus influenzae type b.*

On the other hand, the capsules of the highly pathogenic Group B meningococci are composed of only weakly immunogenic polysaccharide molecules. They do induce a little immunization, but not enough protection to meet the needs of any children or adults exposed to Group B meningococci.

Finally, there has been the very recent emergence of formerly innocuous bacteria as savage killers. Group B *Streptococcus,* for example, has become a significant cause of neonatal meningitis, which kills 22 percent of its victims—and in many centers they are now the organism associated most frequently with neonatal septicemia.

Group B *Streptococcus* was not always a major clinical pathogen. Until 1964 hemolytic Group B streptococci had been much better known as the agents of a common cattle disease called bovine mastitis than as a significant pathogen in people.

It is quite possible that the passage of the Social Security Act of 1965, whose Medicaid portions made nonemergency hospital care available to millions of rural and urban families who could not otherwise afford such medical services, helped broaden the spectrum of Group B infections from adults to newborn infants. The increase in human Group B strep infections began to be noticed in burgeoning numbers once the Medicaid provisions of the Social Security Act became operative after January 1, 1966. This increase was particularly acute in hundreds of hospital nurseries in this country.

According to the National Center for Health Statistics' bicentennial review of the nation's health from 1776 to 1976, "In 1950 little more than half of all births occurred in hospitals"; but by the two hundredth anniversary of this nation's birth, "Of all the babies now born in this country, 99% of them are delivered in hospitals."[2] Nationally, the Group B streptococcal disease attack rate is now about 200 per 100,000 live births, with a mortality rate of 30 percent to 50 percent.

In neonates there are two types of Group B streptococcal disease. There is the early-onset form, in which the infected mother's causal bacteria attack her child in her vaginal canal during the act of birth. Early-onset Group B strep is characterized by severe overwhelming sepsis with a poor prognosis. The other form, late-onset disease, occurs within one to three weeks after birth, during which period hospital nurses, doctors, and visitors can also, like the mothers, transmit Group B streptococci to newborn children in the hospital nurseries, corridors, and wards.

During our bicentennial year, physicians participating in a National Institutes of Health (NIH) workshop on Group B streptococcal infections agreed that this bacterium is now the leading cause of bacterial meningitis during the first two months of life in several regions of this country. They felt that they could then "conservatively estimate that between 12,000 and 15,000 babies will develop this disease during the next year; approximately 50% of these infants will die; and up to 50% of these infants will develop neurologic sequelae."[3]

Another group of clinical specialists in Washington estimated that for every 100,000 newborns, 100 to 200 would develop neonatal meningitis caused, in most cases, either by Group B streptococci or *Escherichia coli;* 380 children would develop *Haemophilus influenzae* meningitis; and an additional 100 children would have endemic bacterial meningitis during their lives. Of these victims of bacterial meningitis, it was estimated that one hundred would die of it and two hundred would survive but with severe neurological damages, such as hearing and vision losses and central nervous system defects.[4]

The pediatrician Carol J. Baker has written that a number of recent American clinical studies have demonstrated that most early-onset Group B strep infections in newborns "can be related to intrapartum [occurring during labor and delivery] transmission from the maternal genital tract, and since the sexual partners of vaginally colonized parturients often have identical strains isolated from their urethral cultures, the Group B Streptococcus has been assumed to be one of several sexually transmitted agents."[5]

In 1973 Baker and her colleagues at Brown and Harvard Universities ran a study of vaginal colonization with Group B *Streptococcus* in 499 college women.[6] The women, with a mean age of 20.6 years, attended colleges in the Boston and Providence areas. Baker and her coworkers found Group B *Streptococcus* in vaginal swabs taken from ninety (18 percent) of these young college women.

Race was not a factor. Some 89 percent of the participating subjects were white, 9 percent were black, and 2 percent were Oriental. While none had ever had syphilis, and other venereal diseases had no apparent bearing on the presence or absence of the Group B streptococci, it is of more than passing epidemiological interest to note that eleven of these 499 college women gave a previous history of having had gonorrhea. Only four (1 percent) of the participating college women who had vaginal colonization of Group B *Streptococcus* gave a history of never having had sexual intercourse, while the remaining eighty-six (17 percent) with vaginal colonies of Group B strep gave histories of sexual intercourse with one to six partners.

In this study population, students who were under twenty tended to have more vaginal colonies of Group B strep than older women, as did girls who wore implanted intrauterine contraceptive devices (IUDs) in comparison with other students who relied on hormone pills and other noninvasive systems of contraception. Baker and her colleagues concluded that "sexual intercourse is an important factor related to the acquisition and transmission of Group B Streptococci."

Newborns do not acquire this sexually transmitted streptococcus during the nine months they are growing and developing from zygote to fetus to child in their mothers' wombs, since the Group B streptococci do not pass through the placental barriers to the womb women are genetically programmed to grow to protect their developing children during pregnancy. Like the equally large maternal gonococci that cause blinding infections in the eyes of newborn infants of mothers with gonorrhea, the Group B streptococci infect neonates when they emerge from the womb into the vaginal canal during birth.

With this mechanism of transmission in mind, Dr. Dennis L. Kasper and Dr. Carol Baker developed and have been testing, in adults, a good Group B *Streptococcus* capsular polysaccharide vaccine, and propose that it be used in pregnant women. In this way, they suggest, the vaccine will instruct the mothers' lymphocytes to produce anti-Group B strep antibodies to these bacteria in the vaginal canal before and during birth. This would not only keep the newborns from being infected at the moment of birth, but since antibodies may pass the placentas, vaccines given during the last trimester of pregnancy would probably also offer the developing fetuses a meaningful measure of passive immunity that would help protect neonates from early-onset Group B strep infections acquired in the birth canal, and from late-onset infections acquired from hospital nursery personnel, hospital visitors, and other potential carriers of Group B streptococci—the agent of an important, new sexually transmitted disease in adults.

If this procedure of maternal vaccination during pregnancy succeeds against Group B streptococcal infections in neonates, it could result in similar uses of the vaccines that protect older children and adults against pneumococci, meningococci, and *H. influenzae.*

This would still leave unresolved the major current problems of how to block the same leading agents of bacterial meningitis in children older than neonates and younger than toddlers, in whom most of the new capsular polysaccharide vaccines do not seem to work well.

What is most needed to protect infants and young children against bacterial meningitis and other killing and crippling infectious diseases is a very detailed body of knowledge that we do not yet have on the precise array and nature of the important differences between the immunologic systems of children and adults. Biologically, chemically, neurologically, and above all immunologically, children are not miniature adults, differing only in size from their parents and all other adults.

Chemically, in fact, the already documented differences between a mother and her newborn infant are so profound, so striking, that the act of birth itself has been compared by many life scientists to what is called in immunology a host versus graft rejection, in which a healthy body expels or sloughs off newly acquired foreign material ranging from transfusions of mismatched blood, to transplants of immunologically "nonself" or foreign skin, organs, and limbs from biologically nonrelated donors, to inhaled plant proteins.

Someday, when and if our educational systems—from kindergarten to and after graduate school—are developed qualitatively and quantitatively to the point where it is possible to acquire enough of this life-enhancing knowledge, and where enough young life scientists can be trained to make the maximum clinical utilization of such vital knowledge, we will probably be able to immunize safely newborns and very young infants against any major vaccine-preventable infectious diseases.[7] Until then, we will have to make the most intelligent uses of what we can presently document about the biology and chemistry of newborns, infants, and very young children.

For example, we know that all but a few desperately sick and doomed children are born with all the inherited capacity to develop presently known cellular and humoral components of a human immune (host defense) system.

We also know that it is at least three to six months before the bodies of healthy infants begin to develop their genetic capacity or immunocompetence to employ their inborn host defense systems to produce antibodies when microbial pathogens appear in their bodies. At first, they do not produce enough antibodies to be fully protected, but as they grow older and more developed, their ability to do so grows apace.

Fortunately, some maternal antibodies do pass the placental walls with ease. Many types of specific immunoglobulins or antibodies donated by pregnant women to the new lives growing in their wombs give their newborns temporary or passive immunity against many common bacterial, viral, and other microbial disease agents.

As these congenitally acquired antibodies expire, nature provides a postnatal source of maternal antibodies in the colostrum in mothers' milk. During the first few weeks after women given birth, their milk is rich in this colostrum, a milky fluid that contains secretory IgA antibodies and other immunoglobulins which help protect infants against respiratory disease and other ailments. The presence of colostrum in mothers' milk is one of the major reasons pediatricians encourage new mothers to nurse their children.

This passive congenital and colostrum-mediated immunity lasts in infants until, in gradual stages, the immune systems in their bodies become mature enough to instruct their own lymphocytes to produce specific antibodies (immunoglobulins) against specific disease agents. By the time an infant is six months old, his or her immune system has become reasonably active, but normally at least another four to six years of additional growth and development are required before a child becomes fully immunocompetent and able to produce enough antibodies, following natural infection or medical vaccination, to develop long-term protection (active immunity mediated by his or her own antibodies) against major infectious diseases.

In pediatric medicine this means that the more new types of vaccines are developed, the greater the chances are that better vaccines for infants and young children will be developed. This is more a matter of empiricism or trial-and-error than the much better method of basing vaccines on new knowledge of the immunocompetence of infants, but it has been known to work.

For example, in 1906 Jules Bordet, the director of the Pasteur Institute of Brussels, and his brother-in-law, Octave Gengou, succeeded in growing in artificial media the pertussis (whooping cough) bacterium, now called *Bordetella pertussis,* they had isolated from a child with whooping cough six years earlier. Prior to that time, in 1897 Almroth Wright had developed the first killed whole bacterial vaccine for use in people, his typhoid fever vaccine. Once Bordet and Gengou published their technique of growing laboratory colonies of *Bordetella,* many researchers around the world began to experiment with vaccines of killed whole-organism whooping cough vaccines. "As typhoid vaccine had long been accepted as a valuable immunizing agent against typhoid fever, the same general principles were followed" against *Bordetella* by an American pediatrician and vaccine developer, Louis Sauer of the Northwestern University medical school.[8]

Killed whole-organism vaccines against whooping cough were developed and used in children by Charles Nicolle (like Bordet a future Nobel Prize winner), at the Pasteur Institute in Tunis in 1913; by T. Madsen, director of the Danish State Serum Institute, a year or so later; and by Pearl Kendrick, of the State of Michigan Health Department, in the 1930s, the 1940s, and after World War II, when she combined her improved killed pertussis bacterial vaccine with the toxoids of diphtheria and tetanus to produce the familiar DTP vaccine that now protects children against all three diseases with one injection.

Perfected and improved over the years since 1913, the killed whole-organism *Bordetella* vaccines have all but eradicated whooping cough in some economically advanced nations—but not without exceedingly rare but nonetheless terrifying side effects, such as screaming syndrome, convulsions, and even neurological damage. These rare side effects are not produced by the modal typhoid vaccine. Empiricism makes no allowances for the differences as well as the similarities between different bacterial disease agents.

In recent years, workers in Japan and other countries have cooperated in developing new experimental whooping cough vaccines, made of complexes of noncapsular antigenic protein subunits on the surface structures of the *Bordetella* bacilli. These high-molecular-weight proteins include two *Bordetella* hemaglutinins, antibodies that cause the agglutination or clumping of certain red blood cells, as well as the fimbrae (or pili), hairlike proteins on the surfaces of Gram-negative bacteria, which attach the disease agents to the cells of people and other animals in the first step of a bacterial infection. The aim is to afford equal protection against pertussis bacilli, but without the adverse (if reversible) side effects the killed whole-organism *Bordetella* vaccines have caused—in England, for example—in one out of every 50,000 vaccinated children.

One of the newly recognized cell-surface proteins that now seems an excellent candidate to help improve the potency of many new subunit chemical vaccines goes by the name of POMP, an acronym for the principal outer-membrane proteins of Gram-negative bacterial cells. POMP was discovered in 1969 by Carl Frasch, then a graduate student in medical microbiology under Drs. Steven Chapman and Lewis Wannamaker at the medical school of the University of Minnesota, Minneapolis. Frasch, the son of a professional army man and the first person in his family to go to college, had qualified as a clinical microbiologist while still an undergraduate at the University of Washington, Seattle, and had worked in clinical diagnostic laboratories in Seattle before he was able to put aside enough money to attend graduate school.

Wannamaker is one of the world's leading researchers in streptococci. When Frasch arrived on the scene, Wannamaker and Chapman were involved in typing, by the method of Lancefield, different strains of Group A hemolytic *Streptococcus* on the basis of the M proteins found on the bacterial cell surfaces. These organisms are responsible for a wide array of human diseases and disorders, including streptococcal pharyngitis ("strep throat") and the demonic battalions of more serious and often fatal disorders that follow untreated or improperly treated strep throats, ranging from rheumatic fever and rheumatic heart disease to poststreptococcal glomerulonephritis, each a major cause of death prior to penicillin, and many still widespread if on the whole less lethal.

This work, Frasch remembers, "gave me the idea that maybe the meningococci could also be subdivided or typed in a similar manner, by the immunological specificity of their surface proteins. I started doing the acid-extraction procedures that worked so well with streptococcal M proteins. This got me nowhere. Then I started doing some other extraction procedures that were much milder than these, and it was not long before I came up with some interesting results." These results included the discovery, in 1969, that the serological types of meningococci could be determined by testing the reactions of their outer-membrane proteins to specific meningococcal antibodies in standard typing sera. The outer membrane is found only in Gram-negative bacteria, and comprises the exterior surface of the cell envelope on the Gram-negative bacterial cell wall.

These outer membranes of bacterial cells contain different proteins, which are found only in specific types of bacteria so that their presence signifies that the bacteria belong to the specific type in which these and only these proteins are found. The outer-membrane proteins are called serotype proteins, since they can be used to identify the different serological types of bacteria.

Frasch was unable to publish any of his work on serotype proteins until after he got his doctorate in medical microbiology, because a university rule forbade the use of any of a doctoral candidate's published work in a dissertation. At that point, while Frasch knew that these cell-surface chemicals were type-specific antigens, he did not yet know that they were proteins. Although the work was not published, Frasch's mentors in Wannamaker's laboratory went out of their way to make it known to major scientists working in related areas. One was the noted bacteriologist, the late Dr. Rebecca Lancefield, who for more than a half-century at Rockefeller Institute (which later became Rockefeller University) had led the world in the typing and characterization of the hemolytic streptococci.

What Lancefield saw of Frasch's work, and of the young graduate student himself, made her insist that when he did get his degree he should work in Gotschlich's Rockefeller University laboratory as a postdoctoral Fellow. She also made this feeling known at Rockefeller, and in 1972 Frasch moved to Gotschlich's laboratory.

"When I began working in Gotschlich's laboratory, I knew that these were surface antigens," Frasch says. "But working there I was able to prove that they were not only proteins but also that they were the principal outer membrane proteins of *Neisseria meningitidis.*" This work was published in 1974. Kenneth Johnston at Rockefeller University and others found similar antigenic proteins in the outer-cell membranes of *N. gonorrhoeae,* and in *H. influenzae* and other pathogenic bacteria not in the *Neisseria* family.

One of the major disappointments experienced by Gotschlich, Goldschneider, and others working on meningococcal vaccines both at Artenstein's laboratories at WRAIR and, later, at their old civilian laboratories, had been the failure of the capsular sugars of Group B meningococci to induce enough antibodies, when used as a vaccine, to protect people against Group B meningococcal meningitis. Like other bacterial capsules, those found on Group B meningococci were serologically active, and even specific enough to serve as typing antigens. However, while all immunogens are antigens, not all antigens are effective immunogens in human beings.

Frasch worked with Gotschlich and others at Rockefeller on developing a vaccine made from the principal outer-membrane proteins of Group B meningococci. The work was funded by both the U.S. Army and NIAID. They had previously determined that "the majority of both Group B and Group C disease is caused by a single serotype, type 2 [and that] the type 2 antigens of Groups B and C are chemically and serologically identical. Antibodies against the serotype antigens are bactericidal in the presence of complement."

It was decided to use Group B meningococcal serotype 2 POMP in the experimental vaccine. Most animals cannot be infected with meningococci, but "the developing chicken embryo is one of the few laboratory animals readily susceptible to meningococcal infection." In this model the experimental POMP vaccine proved to be immunogenic enough to protect chick embryos.[9]

A more important finding, reported in the same article in the *Journal of Experimental Medicine* in 1976, was that when combined with the weakly immunogenic capsular polysaccharides of Group B meningococci, there was a significant cooperative, or synergistic, effect between antibodies against the capsular polysaccharides and the serotype protein antibodies. Synergy is compounding rather than additive. As Frasch explains it, "We noted that if you have antibody to the outer membrane proteins plus antibody to the capsular polysaccharide of the same bacterium, then immunologically they do not add up to $1 + 1 = 2$ in terms of inducing the production of protective antibodies, but, figuratively, to $1 + 1 = 7$ or 8. Another way of putting it is to say that while antibody to serotype protein and antibody to capsular polysaccharides might each be weakly protective, when you put them both together you get a vaccine that is strongly effective."

Prior to this time, when people talked of purified bacterial subunit vaccines they had generally meant toxoids made from toxins of diphtheria or tetanus bacteria, or purified capsular polysaccharides. The work with serotype proteins, Frasch believes, told people that there were other alternatives to whole organisms for much needed vaccines.

When this paper was published, Frasch had already taken his present position in John Robbins's laboratories at the Food and Drug Administration's Bureau of Biologics in Bethesda on the sprawling NIH campus. There he made up a vaccine against Group B meningococci based solely on their serotype proteins. When tested in human volunteers, this POMP vaccine was not a resounding success. Improved vaccines followed, some of them made with Group B serotype proteins combined with capsular carbohydrates of the same organism. These POMP-capsular polysaccharide vaccines worked much better—in animals and eventually in small numbers of human volunteers around the nation.

Other research workers, most notably Wendell D. Zollinger at WRAIR, developed and tested subunit meningococcal vaccines made up of Type 2 serotype proteins and purified Group C meningococcus capsular polysaccharides. When first tested in five human volunteers in 1977, the two variants of this meningitis vaccine "were well tolerated and induced significant increases in serum bactericidal activity against both Group C and Group B strains" of meningococci. Two years later Zollinger and his WRAIR coworkers made up a vaccine based on a "complex of meningococcal Group B polysaccharide and type 2 outer membrane protein" and tested it in eight volunteers. The results led them to "conclude that both the Group B polysaccharide and the outer membrane protein are immunogenic in man when presented as a complex, and that the complex warrants further testing and development as a vaccine against Group B meningococcal disease."[10]

John Robbins and his coworkers at the Bureau of Biologics are presently working on vaccines against HI meningitis in which *Haemophilus influenzae* outer-membrane (serotype) proteins are combined with the purified HI capsular polysaccharides now in the Robbins vaccine. The hope is that the synergistic effects of this complex of carbohydrate and protein immunogens might result in making the Robbins HI meningitis vaccine as effective in infants as it is now in children over eighteen months old.

By 1980 Frasch had developed better methods of extracting the serotype proteins of bacteria, and had tested both improved POMP vaccines as well as vaccines made of complexes of POMP and capsular polysaccharides, which each induced bactericidal antibodies against Group B meningococci in human volunteers. He reported, at an International Symposium on Bacterial Vaccines held at NIH in 1980, that laboratory studies were in progress to evaluate both improved serotype-protein and protein-carbohydrate-complex vaccines in children aged three months and older to determine their safety and efficacy in infants and very young children.[11] By 1981 Frasch and his colleagues were in the early stages of a long-range trial of a Group B meningococcal POMP-capsular polysaccharide vaccine in South Africa that involved 15,000 children.

Shortly before this, Zollinger reported that in tests conducted in over twenty-five consenting military recruits, the complexing of meningococcal

Group B polysaccharide and outer-membrane proteins had resulted in many synergistic gains. These included "an increase in the apparent molecular size of the polysaccharide, increased antigenicity of both components, and greatly enhanced immunogenicity of both components."[12]

Dr. Michael Apicella, at the University of Nevada medical school in Reno, combined the serotype proteins (POMP) of a major pathogen in the *Neisseria* family—*N. gonorrhoeae*, the germ of gonorrhea—with another non-capsular surface antigen of the bacterium in what promises to be a vaccine of considerable potential. In many laboratories scientists were encouraged by such early work to start experimenting with different complexes and conjugates of surface and subsurface cellular subunits, toxoids, and other antigenic materials. It was hoped, and in some quarters loudly proclaimed, that out of these combinations of antigens and coantigens would come new chemical vaccines—many of them cross-protective—against several currently nonpreventable bacterial, mycoplasmal, viral, fungal, and other microbial infectious diseases.

Nowhere would this work become more intense than in the quest for a safe and effective vaccine against gonorrhea, one of the first previously incurable major infectious diseases to be made completely and quickly curable by the new antibacterial drugs. Now, as always, the most urgent current health needs establish the priorities for vaccine research. The years after 1940 saw not only the rise of the sulfas and the antibiotics, used successfully against hitherto incurable or hard-to-cure bacterial diseases, but gonorrhea, one of those antibiotic-tamed disorders that went on to become the most frequently reported communicable disease in the United States today.

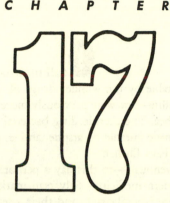

THE OLD GONORRHEA VACCINES
AND OTHER DOCTORS' DELUSIONS

To prevent diseases must be of more importance than to cure them. Little attention, however, has been paid to this branch of the medical art, especially with regard to the venereal disease. Her prophylaxis has generally been left to quacks.... That both clap and pox [syphilis] may often be prevented ... does not admit of doubt ...

—WILLIAM BUCHAN, M.D., in *Observations Concerning the Prevention of the Venereal Disease,* 1796

Of all the major infectious diseases to be rendered swiftly curable by the wonder drugs of World War II—chiefly sulfonamide and penicillin—few were previously more impervious to medical treatment than gonorrhea. The then leading bacterial venereal disease, syphilis, had in 1910 been made curable by arsphenamine, or Salvarsan, by the father of chemotherapy, Paul Ehrlich.

Injected intravenously—to this day a perilous medication route not used very often in modern medicine—Salvarsan marked the world debut of chemotherapy. Salvarsan, Neosalvarsan, and their arsenical successors also inflicted so many agonizing side effects (as many of them due to shooting potent drugs directly into the veins as to the chemical Magic Bullets themselves) on people whose lives they saved that many became instant converts to the concept that syphilis is much better prevented than cured. Unlike the modern, one-injection penicillin treatment of gonorrhea and incipient syphilis, Salvarsan treatment required many painful intravenous shots, administered over a period of at least two years punctuated by equally painful injections of bismuth and/or mercury and, often, by severe side effects.

Once sulfa and antibiotic drugs became available, doctors quickly abandoned the very toxic arsenicals for the far less toxic new antibacterial drugs that represented the next stage of chemotherapy. There had not been a Magic Bullet of any sort against gonorrhea before a single injection of penicillin proved a quick, often overnight, cure. This did not mean that there had ever been any shortage of widely used cures and treatments for gonorrhea, most of them medical modalities that made Ehrlich's painful arsenicals seem blessings. Unlike his chemical cure for syphilis, each of the standard medical treatments for gonorrhea over the centuries had always failed to cure this venereal infection. Moreover, many of the standard treatments that survived into the middle of the twentieth century more often than not succeeded in seriously exacerbating the disease and converted what was in 95 percent of all cases an annoying but self-terminating local disorder into a systemic, agonizing, and even fatal iatrogenic disease.

By 1939, only two years after the introduction of the sulfa drugs, the world's medical journals were carrying euphoric articles about the impending

90 percent cure of gonorrhea. The early wonder drug sulfonamide was employed on a mass scale in the United States armed forces after the Japanese bombed us into World War II at Pearl Harbor. It worked so well against most strains of gonococci, which were those susceptible to the sulfa drugs, that in a very short time it wiped them out of the military-base environments. This led to joyous and true reports of great reductions in syphilis, gonorrhea, and other bacterial venereal diseases. Then the rare, naturally sulfa-resistant but infective strains of gonococci, which survived the massacre of their drug-susceptible relatives, soon became as numerous as the drug-sensitive strains they had replaced.

As a result, the sulfas became less and less effective in the cure of gonorrhea, and were gradually abandoned as useless. At about that time, however, penicillin proved equally effective against gonorrhea. The wartime production and wide uses of penicillin against gonorrhea and other bacterial infections soon revived the deflated dream of a wonder drug that in one dose would eradicate clap and other venereal diseases from the armed forces by war's end; of course, when peace came, penicillin would rid whole nations of sexually transmitted diseases.

On the eve of the war in 1941, syphilis and gonorrhea were the second and third most often reported communicable diseases in the nation. Only measles, with a total of 594,134 cases reported, for a case rate of 443 per 100,000 population, exceeded them in reported incidence. Syphilis, with 485,560 cases of all stages of the disease reported, for a case rate of 368 per 100,000 population, and gonorrhea, with 193,468 cases reported, for an attack rate of 147 cases per 100,000 population, were—like measles—massively underreported. These U.S. Public Health Service cases were exclusive of the known military cases.

By 1946, our first full year of peace, penicillin was the drug of choice for treating gonorrhea and syphilis (and other bacterial venereal diseases like nongonococcal urethritis). Measles was still the most frequently reported notifiable disease, with 695,843 cases reported, for an attack rate of 490 per 100,000 population. (Antibiotic drugs do not work on viruses, and the new live virus vaccine against measles would not be licensed until 1963.) Reported gonorrhea cases in 1946 came to 368,020 and all stages of syphilis to 363,467; 94,957 primary and secondary syphilis cases were reported in 1946, for an attack rate of 71 per 100,000 population.

During the first decade of antibiotic drugs, reported cases of gonorrhea and of all stages of syphilis declined at a very steep rate. After that, things began to change for the worse. All stages of syphilis continued to decline, so that by 1980 the disease was down to 68,832 cases, for an attack rate of 38 per 100,000 population. New cases of syphilis, however, had had a fourfold increase since 1957, with 24,874 primary and secondary cases reported for 1979, for a nearly quadrupled attack rate of 11.4 per 100,000 population. Syphilis of all stages was now the third leading reported infectious disease in the United States, after gonorrhea and chicken pox. Overall, however, syphilis of all stages had declined 88 percent since 1943, from 575,593 to 67,049 cases per year in the thirty-six years since penicillin had been introduced.

On the other hand, gonorrhea, for over a decade the most frequently reported notifiable disease in the United States, had a new high of 1,003,958 cases reported in 1980. This number, however, represented only about one quarter of the estimated actual gonorrheal infections suffered in the United States in 1979.

What these lively and/or dull figures all added up to was that nearly forty years after the advent of the sulfas and the antibiotic drugs, the annual reported civilian cases of gonorrhea had soared from under 200,000 to over one million. The gonorrhea attack rate, 214 per 100,000 population in 1943, the year penicillin went into mass military use, had leaped by 117 percent to an attack rate of 465 per 100,000 by 1979.

Historically, gonorrhea did not really become a pandemic until safe, inexpensive, and very effective antibacterial drugs had, in locker-room semantics, turned the disease into an event "no worse than a bad cold." A few other factors also made social and clinical history during the years in which, despite penicillin, gonorrhea became our leading reported communicable disease.

Between 1946 and today, we engaged in two major foreign wars. During the Korean War of 1950–1953, 5,764,000 individuals served for an average of nineteen months each, and 3,227,840 of them saw service overseas. The matching data on the Vietnam War are not quite as complete, for though some 15,000 Americans were sent into Indochina and saw combat during the Kennedy administration, the war really began to escalate in scope and geography during the Johnson and Nixon administrations. The government's *Statistical Abstract of the United States* shows only that 8,982,000 veterans were discharged from the armed forces between 1965 and 1977, and that 2,894,000 of them—or 32.2 percent of the total—served in Vietnam. The median period spent in the armed forces during those years was thirty-four months.

To specialists in communicable diseases, the contribution of both these presidential wars to the spread of gonorrhea was no mystery. Professor Wesley M. Spink observed that "one important factor was a succession of major wars during this period. Herding healthy young males into the armed services and then sending them to foreign shores where the only relaxation with the opposite sex was with prostitutes resulted in an alarming dissemination of venereal diseases."[1]

There were other factors that contributed their mite to the rise of gonorrhea during the same decades. One was the new birth-control technologies, such as the hormonal birth-control pills, the venerable but newly institutionalized rhythm method, and the implanted intrauterine devices (IUDs), which did away with earlier antibacterial barrier birth-control devices including condoms and diaphragms, and the spermicidal foams and jellies used in conjunction with the diaphragms. Spink, with these new birth-control methods in mind, added the scholarly observation that "in the civilian population the fear of pregnancy had been a major deterrent against sexual promiscuity, but with the advent of highly publicized birth control measures and available abortions this fear was greatly reduced."

Greatly reduced, also, were the moral and social constraints that had survived the Great Depression much better than they had the three major foreign wars that followed. During the Depression decade of 1930 to 1939, for example, families tended to hold together. In that traumatic period, the divorce rate averaged 165 divorces per 100,000 population, just about what it had been between 1920 and 1929. By 1940 the winds and fears of war had pushed the divorce rate up to 200 divorces per 100,000 population. This was merely the start of a swift rise to an all-time high of 430 divorces per 100,000 population by the first full year of peace in 1946. By 1979 the American divorce rate had climbed to 530 divorces per 100,000 population, and it is still climbing. In 1979 there were 1,170,000 divorces to 2,359,000 marriages in this country, for a ratio of one divorce to every two marriages. Divorced people living alone are statistically at much greater risk of getting venereal diseases than are married people of the same ages and social classes.

Wars break down more than the morals and values of healthy young servicemen and servicewomen; they also directly affect the wives and children of families at war. To Professor Spink, a lifelong specialist in communicable (and in considerable measure societal) diseases, it came as no great surprise in 1978 to learn from the Centers for Disease Control (CDC) that among American teenagers from fifteen to nineteen, between 1956 and 1978 the total number of reported cases of gonorrhea rose from 45,161 per year to 254,928 per year, with the annual attack rates in these youngsters rising from 416 to 1,229 per 100,000 population. However, Spink was as shocked and dismayed as any parent and grandparent when he learned, also from the CDC, that in American children between the ages of ten and fourteen, most of them girls, the number of reported cases of gonorrhea rose from 2,431 per year in 1956 to 9,518 in 1978, for an attack rate of 49 per 100,000 population.

The post-World War II changes in sex-behavior patterns shattered social class as well as age and regional lines; they were neither racial, nor economic, nor sectional. They were not even national. In this country, instant typewriter and microphone sociologists dubbed these behavioral changes part and parcel of what they instantly termed "The Sexual Revolution," and there was almost nothing our somewhat more professionally qualified sociologists, historians, and anthropologists could do to make literate people see this glib catchphrase in terms of the striking complex of catastrophic social changes it so gaily masks from the civic consciousness. To call any historical cataclysm as profound as the one whose incidental by-products currently include the hypersexuality of schoolchildren, adolescents, and adults merely "The Sexual Revolution" is literally the equivalent of describing the decline and fall of the Roman Empire as "The Table Manners Revolution."

In hucksterized, public-relations-manipulated societies, unfortunately, simplistic catchphrases emerge as functional equivalents of serious thought. Therefore, instead of reading about the rising clinical and economic costs of venereal diseases, more educated people now seem to prefer to read the latest best-selling books on how to copulate, fornicate, and pontificate on human sexuality, seated comfortably in their deck chairs aboard the *S.S. Titanic* as the great ship steers toward the Arctic route to the Nirvana called Perfect Orgasm. Nevertheless, to the at least four million American adults, adolescents, and schoolchildren who get gonorrhea each year, to their families, and to the government agencies who have to pay most of the tax-dollar costs of treating the victims, the differences between the cure and the prevention of gonorrhea have been made abundantly apparent.

Gonococcal resistance to penicillin started to show up in some Asian countries by the time of the Korean War. Returning servicemen from Korea, Vietnam, and the Philippines over the course of more than two decades unwittingly became carriers of various innately resistant strains of gonococci. This did not, as in the earlier instance of the sulfa drugs, lead to the necessary abandonment of penicillin and alternate antibiotics as the drugs of choice against gonorrhea. For one thing, the naturally drug-resistant strains of gonococci never became as numerous in bacterial populations as did the innately sulfa-resistant strains during the first years of World War II. For another, it was found that gradual increases in the normal doses of antibiotics used to treat gonorrhea, when generically antibiotic-resistant strains in patient populations of gonococci reduced the effectiveness of penicillin against gonorrhea, restored penicillin's original (c. 1943) capacity to cure it.

Although gradual, these increases in antibacterial drug dosages have not been minor. Whereas it took injections of 300,000 to 400,000 units of penicillin to cure gonorrhea in the 1940s, by 1979 the officially recommended dose was 4.8 million units—an increase of 1,100 percent over the original amount of penicillin needed to cure gonorrhea when the antibiotic was first available. To date, these megadoses of penicillin (and the alternate antibiotics for people allergic to this drug) have worked. There is no guarantee that the antibiotic-induced processes that selected out the once innocuous minorities of hereditarily resistant gonococcus strains and saw them proliferate to clinically meaningful proportions will not in time terminate the effectiveness of penicillin and other antibiotics as they had earlier nullified the effects of sulfas against gonorrhea.

While new antibiotics other than penicillin continue to cure gonorrhea caused by penicillin-resistant (PPNG) strains of *Neisseria gonorrhoeae,* the CDC, in a 1982 report on the world distribution of drug-resistant gonorrhea agents, observed that "alternative regimens for effective treatment may be difficult to identify and may result in increased treatment costs to the point where many governments or patients can no longer afford such treatment."

All patents on penicillin having expired, it is now a very inexpensive drug; the fine new antibiotics that do provide effective alternative treatments for penicillin-resistant gonococci are still patented and still very high-priced. Therefore, the CDC cautions, "Because alternative [antibiotic] therapies are expensive, less effective treatments such as penicillins continue to be used [against penicillin-resistant gonococci]. This further selects for drug resistance and extends the infectious period for patients. Thus gonorrhea transmission may be expected to continue, and the proportion of infected patients who develop complications may be expected to rise."

Other clinical problems associated with antibiotic-cured cases of gonorrhea present more pressing medical urgencies. Consider, for example, only one side effect of gonorrhea, ascending pelvic inflammatory disease (PID), or acute salpingitis. In gonorrheal PID infections, which develop when the gonococci of local infections in women are disseminated from the cervix through the endometrium to the Fallopian tubes, the resulting complications usually require hospitalization.

Two years after the sulfa drugs began to be used against gonorrhea in 1927, Wolfgang Casper wrote that "50% of all gynecological operations are a consequence of gonorrhea."[2] More than thirty years after penicillin made gonorrhea a 100 percent curable disease, Professor King K. Holmes, a noted expert on sexually transmitted diseases (STD), conducted a study which revealed that in 1975 "in Seattle, 50% of a series of 204 consecutive cases of pelvic inflammatory disease were associated with gonococcal infection."[3]

There was one difference between the gynecological surgery patients Casper referred to in 1939 and those Holmes studied in 1975: All the Seattle women with gonorrheal PID had been treated and cured of gonorrhea with antibiotics prior to their PID complications. Antibiotics can cure severe infections but cannot prevent the lasting damages the cured infections inflict on human bodies.

The federal Centers for Disease Control, reviewing PID complications that developed after women were cured of gonorrhea by penicillin, estimated that PID develops in 17 percent of all women known to have gonorrhea, for a total of 220,000 to 270,000 reported cases of acute salpingitis a year. "Complications of gonorrhea in women," the CDC reported, "account for 78,000 to 97,200 hospital admissions, totaling 518,200 to 645,600 hospital days annually," at an estimated cost of at least $1.26 billion annually.

Gonorrhea is also a major cause of ectopic pregnancies, which in turn cause over 17 percent of all deaths from pregnancy and childbirth. Blockage of the Fallopian tubes from a single case of adequately treated gonorrhea results in sterility in 15 percent to 40 percent of cases in which antibiotic drugs cured the gonococcal infection itself. "This means," according to the CDC, "that in the United States 34,000 to 92,000 women annually are involuntarily sterilized due to tubal damage from PID as a result of gonorrhea."

American women are not the only women to be involuntarily sterilized by gonorrhea. A study made in 1978 by the International Planned Parenthood Federation in eight central African nations found that 30 percent of married couples were unable to conceive, and that the major cause of this infertility was PID due to gonorrhea. Although in central Africa, as in the United States, gonorrhea had long been primarily an urban disease, the study revealed that "gonorrhea has begun to intrude into the village, too, carried by traders and disillusioned youngsters returning home from the cities."[4]

The U.S. costs of treating the complications of gonorrhea in women, in and out of hospitals, is estimated now by the CDC to be over $500 million every year. Women, however, get only 40 percent of all gonorrhea infections annually. The costs of treating all local and systematic gonorrhea infections and their complications are now estimated at well over one billion dollars a year. This includes treatment of adults and adolescents and also schoolchildren, who now lose over one million school days each year because of gonorrhea and its complications. Of all the newly reported cases, 10 percent of those that occur in men, and 15 percent of those reported in women, are reinfections. It is as easy to catch gonorrhea again and again as it is to cure it with appropriate antibiotics each time reinfection occurs.

The chief generator of gonococcal and other venereal infections in this country remains the prostitution industry. A 1982 epidemiological survey by New York City Health Department inspectors of known houses of prostitution revealed that "about 40 percent of the women tested turned out to have gonorrhea or to be carriers." The gonorrhea infections acquired in New York's brothels are carried throughout the nation by business visitors, convention delegates, and tourists, as are the venereal diseases contracted in equally virulent brothels in all other major port cities.

All data on gonorrhea and other venereal diseases are subject to an important caveat. While the laws that make it mandatory for doctors to report all cases of legally notifiable diseases are well known, they are more noted for being ignored than obeyed. Most of the gonorrhea cases reported to local health departments are in clinic patients, whose costs of treatment are funded by local and national health agencies. "A little more than half of all Americans with gonorrhea are treated by private physicians in non-institutional settings," notes Dr. Richard Roberts, head of the division of infectious diseases at the Cornell University Medical Center in New York. "These private physicians, in turn, report only from 18 to 30% of all the cases of gonorrhea they treat."[5]

In most cities when a case of gonorrhea or syphilis is reported to the local health department by the treating physician, the department has a venereal disease contact-tracing staff who are supposed to visit the patient, get the name and address of the individual from whom the disease was contracted, and the names and addresses of all of both parties' subsequent sexual contacts. Each individual at risk is traced and visited by health department workers who take blood and smear cultures, and then start the individuals on antibiotic treatments.

There are a number of well-known reasons why doctors who treat patients with venereal disease in their private practices are loath to obey the notifiable disease reporting laws. Once a VD case is reported to the local health department, as the law requires, the case ceases to be private. The patient is visited by strangers from the health department and generally talked into revealing the source of the infection and his or her subsequent sexual contacts—touching off chain reactions of chagrin and fury that last for years and often bring such complications as divorces in their wake. These in turn make the patients furious enough at their old doctors to seek new physicians who "can be depended upon to keep their mouths shut."

Some doctors feel, in addition, that what passes between doctor and patient in the privacy of the examining room must remain privileged information. Whatever their reasons for not complying with reporting laws, the doctors who do not report all new cases of gonorrhea, syphilis, and other venereal diseases have created a curious situation in which the families and subsequent sexual contacts of poor or medically indigent people with VD are made safer against infection than the families and subsequent sexual partners of those who can afford to get private medical care.

Failure to report all private VD cases has also led to the permanent skewing of available statistical data. For many years after World War II, publication of raw government data on sexually transmitted diseases resulted in the cozy conventional wisdom that gonorrhea was primarily an affliction of the medically indigent poor, and in large measure, the nonwhite and Hispanic poor at that.

Until about 1970 our most influential citizens tended to ignore the astonishing rise in gonorrhea cases reported annually in the mass media as soon as the government released the figures. Even after that, if this rise was noted it was not often viewed with alarm. One of the nation's leading professors and practitioners of obstetrics and gynecology was far from alone in his conviction, which he still frequently expresses to his staff and students, that gonorrhea is not a completely bad disease, since by sexually sterilizing women with PID it serves the socially useful purposes of (a) slowing the "population explosion" abroad, and (b) gonorrhea helps ameliorate the "welfare mess" at home by reducing the birthrates of what he chooses to describe as the class of "hereditary welfare clients."

By 1970 something new had been added to the commonly perceived aspects of gonorrhea, and that was the reluctant acknowledgment that the clap had not all that suddenly become most upwardly mobile, socially. The still rising divorce-to-marriage ratio then stood at roughly one divorce to every three marriages. What with many concurrent cofactors—among them the lasting behavioral effects of three major foreign wars, new nonbarrier birth-control methods, the rise of soft pornography to the status of a principal component of both the entertainment *and* the commercials on network television, the rise of hard pornography to a multibillion-dollar industry, and other well-defined historical developments, such as the explosive rise in alcohol consumption since 1946—gonorrhea had made the leap from the boondocks to the Buena Vistas of America. Traditionally ignored as a plague of the poor, gonorrhea was now a major health problem in middle- and upper-class families, causing particular havoc in children, adolescents, and young adults.

The explosive upward social mobility of gonorrhea gave rise to a readiness to talk quite openly about it as a problem of familial and national concern. Like the earlier social intrusion of marijuana smoking, the appearance of the gonorrhea epidemic in the higher and better-educated classes led to its acceptability as a subject fit for polite discussion. Unlike marijuana, which was coopted to become reborn in the conventional wisdom as a perfectly safe, respectable, and socially proper recreational mind-affecting drug in a class with alcohol and tobacco when it achieved a higher social status, gonorrhea remained repugnant. Marijuana gave only innocent pleasure (except, of course, to people killed or crippled by automobiles driven by people on marijuana highs) and therefore had to be legalized. Gonorrhea, although acquired with great pleasure, delivered dysuria at best, and gonorrheal heart disease, arthritis, and PID at worst. So gonorrhea had to be eradicated, as smallpox and diphtheria had been eradicated.

Reports in the mass media on new cases of antibiotic-resistant gonorrhea continued to alert and alarm articulate Americans even further. Community leaders who participated in the political processes and contributed regularly to the campaign chests of their state and federal representatives began to write impassioned letters to Washington. These letters demanded that their elected leaders do something about preventing gonorrhea as, during the post-World War II era, "American know-how" had come through with vaccines that prevented polio, measles, mumps, and rubella. The executive and legislative branches of the national government endorsed and passed these demands from the taxpayers and voters on to the government's own National Institute for Allergy and Infectious Diseases (NIAID) in 1971.

This presented quite a bouncy gift porcupine to the principal scientists of the NIAID, since they themselves did not think that gonorrhea vaccines were remotely near the realm of possibility.

In the NIAID handbook, *Immunology: Its Role in Disease and Health*, was a table on the 1972 status of available, experimental, potential, and other needed vaccines. The seventh and last category, titled "No vaccine available, current prospects remote," put the gonococcus at the head of the list. Under the heading of needs that had to be met before a gonorrhea vaccine could be developed, the text read, "Basic microbiological research." Even syphilis, in this carefully reasoned NIAID table, was given a better chance of prophylaxis by vaccine than gonorrhea.

Nevertheless, in 1971 the NIAID authorized the chief of its bacteriology and virology branch, Dr. Milton Puziss, to release $100,000 in grants to support research in the immunobiology and immunochemistry of *Neisseria gonorrhoeae*. Subsequent seed money and more substantial grants helped broaden the NIAID gonorrhea research program, and eventually the federal funds allotted to such research climbed to over seven million dollars.

That initial NIAID grant bundle also proved to be the major turning point in the world history of gonorrhea research. Dr. John Swanson, then professor of pathology and microbiology at the University of Utah in Salt Lake City, went into gonorrhea research then, as did many other talented young investigators. "Milt Puziss was far-sighted. He pumped a lot of seed money in and people jumped aboard. Myself included. We did it because there was easy money involved. It was a case of Sutton's Law in action.[6] But then," Swanson recalls, "I discovered the gonococci, and I've been hooked since. In all of nature I don't think that anyone will ever find a more unusual and fascinating bacterium.

"But the scientific payoff of that 1971 NIAID gamble has been even more fascinating," Swanson says now. "Because of the well-known rapid technological advances after World War II, people had all hopped from doing standard kinds of mundane bacteriology to molecular biology and virology. Those were the hot fields, and for many reasons. Now you could see viruses under the electron microscope, and work with automatic DNA analyzers, and ultra-centrifuges, and even make good vaccines against major virus diseases. The antibiotics took us all off guard because they were so damned effective. It was years before it dawned on any of us that we still had a lot of bacterial disease problems that were not being looked at with any sophisticated methodology. Gradually, and I think it really started with the capsular bacterial polysaccharide vaccines against meningococcal meningitis and pneumococcal pneumonia that were still 'experimental' in '71, the whole area of pathogenic bacteriology has really taken off again."[7]

Precisely a decade after the NIAID grants, and after three years of large-scale tests for safety and antigenicity, a sophisticated vaccine made not of whole gonococci but of subunits from their surfaces, was scheduled to be put into large-scale clinical trials in military posts around the world by the NIAID in conjunction with the Walter Reed Army Institute of Research (WRAIR).

Other gonorrhea vaccines that also grew out of the initial NIAID grant of 1971 were in active states of development and testing. They, too, were not whole-organism vaccines but were made of one or more immunologically active subunits of bacteria found on their cell surfaces.

Whatever the outcome of the major clinical trial of the first of the "Class of '71" vaccines to get this far, it appears as if we shall, in this decade, have available more than one inexpensive, safe, and effective vaccine against gonorrhea. Along with them, unfortunately, will also come a Pandora's box full of social, political, and clinical problems that for wholly explicable reasons have until now been overlooked or ignored.

That these predictable adverse effects of the advent of a safe and effective vaccine or vaccines against gonorrhea continue to be ignored is mute testimony to the fact that although gonorrhea has for over a decade continued to be our leading reported infectious disease, too little is known, by too many people who should know, about the epidemiology, geography, biology, and above all else history of gonorrhea in its millennia of interactions with our species.

A usually self-terminating disease found only in people and no other animals, gonorrhea is at least as old as the first written languages. In the Old Testament, the fifteenth chapter of Leviticus deals with what to do about the social health hazards that ensue "When any man hath a running issue out of his flesh, and because of this issue he is unclean." Many doctors believe this refers to the pus-filled exudates that issue from the urethra at the start of gonorrheal infections. In this chapter the Lord advises Moses that every bed in which the running exudates are found, the clothing of the men and women from whom such materials flow, and even such fomites (nonliving carriers) as earthen jugs touched by unclean individuals must be washed or destroyed. Nor, the Lord commands, must anyone touch the unclean people until they are cleansed—that is, until their gonorrhea is cured by these measures plus the healing passage of time.

There is some dispute among medical anthropologists as to whether the "running issue" refers to gonorrhea or to various other diseases including leprosy. However, among all doctors there is no disagreement about this entire regimen being one of the least damaging and therefore safest gonorrhea cures ever prescribed prior to penicillin.

The Chinese emperor Huang Ti is cited by E. B. Crabtree as writing about gonorrhea (c. 2337 B.C.) that "among the external diseases is one that is different from all others, the symptoms of which are easy to recognize: They are (1) affections of the urethra and vagina at the same time as the bladder. (2) Drainage of corrupt materials white or red by the urethra or vagina." Hippocrates gave a description of gonorrhea in 400 B.C. that remains rewardingly up to date. Rosebury mentions references to what might have been gonorrhea found in ancient Japanese and Vedic writings, as well as on an Assyrian cuneiform tablet. The medical historian Victor Robinson described the Persian physician Rhazes (850–923 A.D.) as having been "so sagacious in this field [gonorrhea] that he may be considered a genitourinary specialist. He gave a detailed description of strictures [narrowing or blockage of urethral canals], and if they produced any retention of urine he at once introduced a catheter. It seems that a gonorrheic was as safe in his hands as in our own."[8]

Unwittingly, Dr. Robinson, a New York physician, was also declaring in this passage that no real progress had been made in the treatment of gonorrhea between the ninth century and 1931, when his book was published. What had followed Rhazes's use of a catheter generally did not improve matters, as witnessed by Robinson's description of the contribution of the equally famous Persian physician Avicenna, or Ibn Sina (980–1037 A.D.). "In treating gonorrhea, Avicenna was probably the first person to use catheters made of the skin of various animals," Robinson wrote, "and he mentions intravesical [into the bladder] injections by means of a silver syringe. That he advised a louse to be inserted into the meatus [the opening, in the penis, of the urethral canal] of persons suffering from retention of urine, is simply additional evidence of the easy capacity of the Arabians to mix absurdities with their rational procedures." Rosebury notes that "Avicenna's louse frequently reappears in the later literature of gonorrhea, sometimes transformed into a bug or a flea."

Live fleas, lice, and other insects were the least of the hundreds upon hundreds of irrigants, herbal extracts, astringents, botanicals, acids, mercurials, and other outright poisons that during the next millennium would be injected and syringed into the urethras of patients with gonorrhea by doctors who were completely *au courant* with the latest in medical concepts of gonorrhea, its causes and its cures.

Whether Rhazes was or was not the first physician to insert a catheter or a syringe into the urethra of a patient with early symptoms of gonorrhea will never be known. What is well established is that from that first doctor-invasive instrument-patient encounter onward, gonorrhea was transformed from a painful but almost always self-terminating disorder into one that often became, when medically treated, a much more disseminated and complicated disease, as much iatrogenic as bacterial in origins.

Some of the most dangerous treatments for gonorrhea, and disastrous misconceptions about the actual nature of the disease itself, came from some of the most talented people in medical history. Consider, for example, Aureolus Theoprastus von Hohenheim, better known as Paracelsus (1493–1541), who started out as an alchemist and who is considered today by some authorities to be "the greatest medical figure of the sixteenth century."[9] It was Paracelsus who finally destroyed the humoral theory of diseases proposed by Galen (130–201 A.D.) in Rome and accepted as dogma in Europe for the next 1,500 years.

Long before medical microbiologists learned that syphilis spirochetes are so tiny they can pass through the placenta that protects developing fetuses from foreign pathogens, Paracelsus concluded that syphilis was transmitted *in utero* from diseased mothers to their fetuses. Of course, the germs of syphilis are most often transmitted venereally from adults to adults. Parcelsus saw syphilis as only a congenital disease and recommended that mercury be taken internally to treat all cases in adults, children and newborns.

By the time the London anatomist and surgeon John Hunter (1728–1793) rose to his golden opportunity to prove that—at least where gonorrhea was concerned—the greatest doctors could be counted upon to make the greatest mistakes, the concept of syphilis and gonorrhea being phases of a single disease had become unquestioned clinical dogma, not as hoary as the Galenic theorems perhaps but equally mind-binding. In 1767, the year Hunter was elected a Fellow of the Royal Society, he was supposed to marry Ann Home, but the wedding had to be postponed following what he described in his monograph *Experiments Made to Ascertain the Progress and Effects of the Venereal Poison.* The experiments, performed upon himself, were to last three years.[10]

In May 1767 Hunter dipped a clean lancet into the urethral discharge of a patient with gonorrhea. He then punctured both the glans and the foreskin of his penis with the tip of this contaminated knife. In due time, syphilitic chancres appeared at the two puncture sites. Hunter would write in his 1786 *Treatise on the Venereal Disease* that this proved that "matter from a gonorrhea will produce chancres [syphilis]," and that therefore gonorrhea and syphilis were once again proven to be one and the same. Obviously, Hunter's syphilitic chancres proved nothing of the sort. What they did prove was that the gonorrhea patient whose exudate had been inoculated into Hunter's organ had also had a bacteriologically productive, asymptomatic incipient or latent stage of a concurrent but separate venereal disease called syphilis.

It took Hunter three miserable years to cure his self-inoculated syphilis infection by swallowing near-fatal doses of mercury, as well as by supplementary applications of mercurial plasters and ointments (which have no effect whatever upon syphilis) to his private parts. Mercury, which is a deadly poison, did cure him, but Hunter was never again a well man. By the time he married Ann Home in 1771, he was suffering frequent attacks of dizziness, possibly caused by chronic mercurial poisoning, as well as chest pains (angina) from the syphilis-caused heart disease that would ultimately kill him in 1793.

Hunter's painful self-experiment helped sustain the power of the dogma of a single venereal disease. The many doctors who agreed with this dogma included William Buchan, Fellow of the Royal College of Physicians, Edinburgh, a private practitioner and the author of *Domestic Medicine,* the most widely sold—and most frequently pirated—medical text of the late eighteenth and early nineteenth centuries.

Buchan wrote his textbook for private practitioners and people living far from easy access to medical care, as in the then sparsely populated new

American republic. Here, every new revised edition of *Domestic Medicine* was reprinted in New York, Philadelphia, Boston, and other cities, and widely used by professors, physicians, and purchasers of medical care, as well as by preachers who had to provide medical care in many remote communities and by parents concerned for family health. American editions continued to be reprinted until well into the 1830s, and helped establish in the New World the medical concepts that dominated medical practice in the British Isles and the Continent, where an authorized French version had been issued in five volumes.

Essentially a practitioner rather than a medical innovator, Buchan was not alone in the medical community in his conclusions and recommendations. For example, he said nothing new when he wrote of both gonorrhea and syphilis as being caused by the same "venereal poison," with each disease entity as separate stages of a single disease. What Buchan wrote represented a consensus of European medical thought. It explains why for centuries poor people who could not afford any medical care had a much easier time with gonorrhea than others—particularly those solvent patients whose physicians earnestly kept up with the medical literature. The invasive treatment strategies Buchan prescribed remained little changed until antibiotics rendered them obsolete after World War II.

Buchan observed that "though the Venereal Disease is generally the fruit of unlawful embraces, it may be communicated to the innocent as well as the guilty. Infants, nurses, midwives, and married women whose husbands lead dissolute lives are often infected with it, and frequently lose their lives by not being aware of their danger in due time. The unhappy condition with such persons will certainly plead our excuse, if any be necessary, for endeavoring to point out the symptoms and the cure of this all too common disease."

Buchan cautioned that when anyone has reason to "suspect that he has caught the Venereal Disease, he ought most strictly to observe a cooling regimen." This meant the patient "had to avoid everything of a heating nature, as wines, spiritous liquors, rich sauces, spices, salt, high-seasons, and smoke-dried provisions, as also all aromatic and stimulating vegetables, such as onions, garlic, shallots, nutmeg, mustard, cinnamon, mace, ginger and the like. His food ought to consist chiefly of mild vegetables, milk, broth, light pudding, panado [a fruit-enriched boiled bread pudding], gruels, etc. His drink may be barley water, milk-and-water, decoction of marshmallows and liquorice, linseed tea, or clear whey. Violent exercises of all kinds, especially riding on horseback and venereal pleasures, are to be avoided. The Patient must be aware of colds, and when the inflammation is violent he ought to keep to his bed."

Nothing in this regimen would exacerbate any patient's clap, and the advice on avoiding venereal pleasures would certainly, particularly in women with gonorrhea, keep the local infections from disseminating to other regions. A most prudent man, Buchan cautioned that "a virulent gonorrhea cannot always be cured speedily and effectually at the same time." Weeks would often be required, although "sometimes, indeed, a slight infection may be carried off in a few days by bathing the parts in milk and warm water, and injecting frequently up the urethra a little sweet oil or linseed tea about the warmth of new milk."

Like most of his responsible and conservative medical peers, Buchan was a great believer in injections for the cure of gonorrhea. These were really invasive irrigations, in which a syringe full of one or more acids, astringents, emollients, botanicals, and chemicals, diluted in plain or rose water, were emptied into the urethra. Unless the clap had caused urethral strictures that had to be treated surgically, the "injection" passed from the urethral canal into the bladder or the prostate or the endocervical canal, usually taking with it the quiescent colonies of gonococci, which, having induced the early gonorrheal symptoms, were perfectly content to settle down to a state of submucosal *détente* during which their human hosts would provide them with food and shelter, and the contented bacteria would not in effect bite the warm bodies that sheltered and fed them. Once rudely transported to the Fallopian tubes and the lining of the heart and other touchy sites, the injection-dislodged gonorrhea agents, alone or in synergistic collaboration with other bacteria already present, often caused salpingitis, arthritis, heart disease, and other systemic complications.

Buchan favored an injection made of one drachm (⅛ ounce, or 60 grams) of white vitriol—zinc sulfate, a compound of sulfuric acid—"diluted in 8 or 9 oz of common or rose water, and an ordinary syringe full of it thrown up [injected into the urethra] 3 or 4 times a day."

Again with his peers, Buchan believed that "cooling purges are always proper in the gonorrhea. Ideally, they should produce 2 or 3 stools a day for the first fortnight, which would be generally sufficient to remove the inflammatory symptoms, to diminish the running [the gonorrheal exudate], and to change the color and consistence of this matter. It gradually becomes more white and ropy as the virulence abates. When the inflammatory symptoms run high, bleeding is always necessary at the beginning."

Bleeding, then a standard procedure in gonorrhea and most other diseases, also diminished the human body's supply of the complex of antibodies, complements, phagocytes, and properdins that interact to make blood serum vital to our inborn defenses against bacteria, viruses, and other disease-causing parasites. In all good conscience, Buchan wrote that in gonorrhea, as in other "topical inflammations," bleeding must be repeated "according to the strength and constitution of the patients and the vehemence and urgency of the symptoms."

Buchan also recommended, along with abstinence, injections, purging and bleeding, the use of diuretics in the treatment of gonorrhea. His own favorite diuretic was "an ounce of nitre [potassium nitrate, or saltpeter] and two ozs of gum arabic, pounded together, divided into 24 doses, one of which may be taken frequently in a cup of the Patient's drink."

When the catheters and the syringes of Rhazes and Avicenna failed to cure gonorrhea, there was always the therapeutic legacy of Paracelsus to save the day. Buchan was by professional choice a therapeutic moderate, but when he felt that the time for heroic measures had arrived, he did not flinch. "When everything else fails," he wrote, "there is the great remedy—mercury."

The prudent Buchan held that many doctors "on the first appearance of a gonorrhea, fly to the use of mercury. This is a bad trend. Mercury is often not at all necessary in a gonorrhea; when taken too early it does mischief. Mercury may be necessary to complete the cure, but it can never be proper at the commencement of it. When bleeding, purging, fomentations, and the other things recommended above have eased the pain, softened the pulse, relieved the heat of urine, and rendered the involuntary erections less frequent, the patient may begin to use mercury in any form that is least disagreeable to him."

Buchan's favored forms of mercury in gonorrhea therapy included "the common mercurial pill, two at night and one in the morning would be a sufficient dose." He also recommended calomel (mercurous chloride), corrosive sublimate of mercuric salts, combining quicksilver (liquid mercury) and gum arabic and suspending the mixture in a watery vehicle to be swallowed at regular intervals, and "for those who cannot take mercury inwardly, the common mercurial or blue ointment will answer very well. That which is made by rubbing together equal quantities of hog's lard and quicksilver, about a drachm may be used at a time. The best time for rubbing it on is at night, and the most popular place is in the inner side of the thighs. The patient should stand before the fire when he rubs, and should wear flannel drawers next to his skin, at the time he is using the ointment."

Along with mercury, there remained one last group of standard treatments. These were the suppurating candles, or bougies, prepared of cloth or paper soaked in various medicaments, including many combinations of mercury, herbal astringents, acids, and vegetable extracts. "Before a bougie may be introduced into the urethra, however," Buchan cautioned, "it should be smeared all over with sweet oil to prevent it from stimulating too suddenly. It may be suffered to continue in for from one to eight hours, in accordance with how long the patient can bear it." Patients were urged to put up with the annoyance of such foreign bodies in their urethral canals, since he assured them that "obstruction of the urinary passages, tumors, and execrescences may all be taken away by means of bougies."

In 1796 Buchan wrote a new book, *Observations Concerning the Prevention and Cure of the Venereal Disease.* His great preventive measure was simply a thorough washing, with plain soap and water, after having sexual intercourse. Buchan described various expensive "secret washes," which he said contained mercury, lead, quicklime, and other ingredients, and which were sold at vastly inflated prices. None of them, he wrote, were any better than plain soap and water. Unfortunately, Buchan's own modestly priced modality did not exactly prove very effective in prophylaxis against gonorrhea.

In 1792 Benjamin Bell, a practitioner and a member of the Royal College of Surgeons of Ireland and Edinburgh, published *A Treatise on Gonorrhea Virulents and Lues Venera* [syphilis]. The book sought to differentiate between both major plagues of Venus as separate disease entities. In the absence of germ theory, Bell's case had to rest on such entirely empirical observations as that while mercury completely cured syphilis, it did not cure and often exacerbated gonorrhea. Bell also reminded his professional peers that "no stage of pox [syphilis] has ever been known to induce gonorrhea, which surely would occasionally happen if the two diseases were of the same nature."

Bell was a very shrewd clinical observer. Every doctor knew, he wrote, "that gonorrhea will often terminate whether any remedy be employed or not, merely by moderate living and keeping the parts regularly cleaned. In most cases the disease by this manner will become gradually milder, so at last it will disappear entirely. No such thing, however, happens with syphilis. In this even the mildest symptoms will become daily worse, unless mercury be employed."

To the intelligent doctor, the reactions of patients to medications and other treatments can reveal as much about the nature of a disease as about the prognosis of the individual patient. Bell noted, for example, that in gonorrhea cases, "For years mercury was chiefly relied upon, employed on the supposition that gonorrhea was a symptom. . . . Lues Venera [syphilis] was, for the most part, easily cured by mercury, but no advantage was derived from this remedy in gonorrhea." In fact, he wrote, the mercury "employed in gonorrhea, instead of proving useful, rather did harm."

Unlike John Hunter, Bell concluded that gonorrhea and syphilis were produced by "two different kinds of contagion; and when pox [syphilis] has appeared as a sudden termination of gonorrhea that the two kinds of infection had either been communicated together, or what may more frequently perhaps be the case, the patient may be found to have received a pocky [syphilitic] contagion by communication with a diseased woman at the very time that he labored under gonorrhea."

In 1793 William Cockburn, a medical contemporary of Bell's, took a whack at defining the gonorrheal contagion in the fourth edition of his book *The Symptoms, Nature, Cause and Cure of Gonorrhea.*

According to Cockburn, "The real and true cause of a Gonorrhea is a corruption of the natural liquor, separated from the Blood and contained in the Lacunae, the Sharpness of which Corruption stimulates the Lacunae, and excites the Running." Therefore, "The cure of a Gonorrhea must be obtained by destroying the Corruption in this natural liquor; helping it to run off in the way it sometimes does, when the disease cures of itself." Whatever else these sentences meant, they also indicated that Cockburn, like other medical authors, knew that gonorrhea sometimes or oftener is a disease that "cures of itself."

Cockburn's only cure for the disease was the endless array of urethral injections described by Buchan, Bell, and other busy practitioners.

The medical history of James Boswell (1740–1795), lawyer, heir, diarist, and biographer of Samuel Johnson, epitomizes in microcosm what intractable womanizers who could afford the best available medical care during the second half of the eighteenth century received for their money when "Signor Gonorrhea came a-calling."

Like many of his titled and equally affluent friends, Boswell was an avid collector of venereal diseases. His diaries show that between March 1760, when he was nineteen years old, and 1790, when the great biographer was fifty, he suffered at least nineteen claps bothersome enough to be recorded. Boswell was also a well-traveled collector of gonorrheal infections who caught claps in Edinburgh, London, Dublin, Rome, and Venice.

The roster of distinguished doctors who treated Boswell for gonorrhea included Sir Percival Pott, the surgeon of St. Bartholomew's Hospital in London, and Giovanni Battista Morgagni, founder of modern pathology and professor of anatomy at the University of Padua.[11] In April 1765 young Boswell contracted gonorrhea from an unknown donor in Rome, and after two months of treatment by Dr. Murray, a prominent physician who attended the British colony in the Eternal City, left Rome for the next stop on the proverbial Grand Tour. En route to Venice, Boswell stopped off in Padua for a consultation with the eighty-three-year-old and still active Professor Morgagni. Once he reached Venice, Boswell lost no time in catching a new dose from a charming dancer; he convalesced from this poignant episode in the villa of a British general.

In the end, as described in a fascinating study, "Boswell's Gonorrhea," by the New York pathologist William B. Ober in 1969, Samuel Johnson's famous biographer "probably died of complications of that disease."[12]

Most of Boswell's claps were acquired from prostitutes. At times, he tried to protect himself by wearing armours during intercourse. These devices were penis sheaths made of the dried intestines of sheep, lambs, goats, and calves, the precursors of modern condoms. Worn by cautious amorists as prophylactics rather than contraceptives, they were brittle unless stored in water until immediately prior to use. Army officers carried and deployed armours decorated with their regimental colors.[13] When these armours worked, they often could protect a prostitute's customers from her venereal disease agents, but more often than not they cracked, ripped, and became otherwise penetrable by *N. gonorrhoeae* and *Treponema pallidum,* the syphilis spirochete.

Prior to his marriage in Edinburgh to Margaret Montgomery in 1769, Boswell returned from Scotland to London to take the most fashionable gonorrhea cure of the moment, a course of treatments based on drinking one pint daily of Dr. Gilbert Kennedy's Lisbon Diet Drink (at, Boswell did not fail to record, a half-guinea per pint bottle). The formula for the expensive Lisbon Diet Drink included the then reigning multidisease wonder remedy, sarsaparilla, as well as sassafras, licorice, and guiac wood; it also had the added negative virtue of being entirely free of the deadly poison mercury.

During this cure, Drs. Duncan Forbes and Percival Pott convinced Boswell to have minor surgery for gonorrheal paraphimosis, an infection-associated and extremely painful immobile retraction of an inflamed foreskin. The usual surgical relief of a phimosed foreskin was to remove it by circumcision.

Of the standard mix of therapeutic regimens under which, over a quarter of the eighteenth century, Boswell was treated for repeated gonorrheal infections, Ober writes that "one can only imagine the discomfort caused by instilling acid into an already inflamed, pus-producing urethra. If purulent exudate or coagula blocked the urethra, surgeons were accustomed to maintain its patency by inserting bougies and cannulas. Not uncommonly such instillations and instrumentation succeeded in forcing infected material from the anterior urethra into the posterior segment, thence into the prostate. One can scarcely be astonished at the frequency with which chronic prostatitis developed or at the high rate of urethral stricture. (A century later, Louis Napoleon died of uremia, the result of urinary calculi [kidney stones] which formed as a complication of gonorrheal stricture of the urethra with urinary tract outflow-tract obstruction and secondary infection.) If all went well, the acute infection would subside, usually in four to six weeks, but an appalling number of cases became chronic."

Boswell was also an inveterate self-medicator and frequently engorged the favorite street remedies—mercury pills, sold everywhere for a mere sixpence a packet, and the more expensive (two shillings, eight pence) "sulphurated pills."

These mercury pills and the mercuric irrigations, ointments, and potions in standard medical treatments of gonorrhea may well have cured Boswell of many an incipient syphilis infection acquired simultaneously with the claps that tormented him for most of his life. The germs of gonorrhea mature and start to cause dysuria and other symptoms two to seven days after they are acquired. On the other hand, *T. pallidum,* the syphilis spirochete, has an incubation period that runs an average of three to six weeks before the spirochetes mature and soft chancres appear at the sites of infection. If they are killed by mercury, the arsenicals, bismuth, or penicillin during their periods of incubation, the immature syphilis microorganisms fail to cause any symptoms—and their human hosts remain happily ignorant that they had ever had incipient syphilis. People are not, however, immunized against syphilis by immature spirochetes.

Boswell experienced a number of urethral strictures or blockages that required medical instrumental treatment over the years. Nor did he always seek medically qualified healers: On July 4, 1790, for example, Boswell had a London barber-surgeon operate on him for a sore on his penis. Ultimately, his oft-repeated gonorrheal infections took their toll. By the time of Boswell's nineteenth recorded clap, in 1790, the complications were, according to Ober, "consistent with the ascending infection of the urinary tract with prostatic or renal involvement." Boswell died on May 19, 1795, at the early age of fifty-five of, Ober believes, "uremia, the result of acute and chronic urinary tract infection, secondary to post-gonorrheal urethral stricture."

Although he caught most of his venereal infections from professional and semiprofessional part-time prostitutes, Boswell contracted one of his most severe bouts of gonorrhea from a twenty-four-year-old actress of good family and a member of the company at Covent Garden Theatre. Boswell gave her the pseudonym of "Louisa" in his diary. Her real name was Anne Lewis, and she was separated from her actor husband, Charles Stander. Louisa—whom Boswell in a subsequent literate moment of self-derision would aptly term his Dulcinea—was a very genteel creature with whom Boswell took tea, read French, discussed religion, literature, and moral philosophy, and to whom he delivered the solemn promise to support any child that might come of their passion. Louisa did not fall in love with Boswell at once. When she did, the affair began on January 11, 1763, in an upstairs room engaged at Hayward's Inn under a suitable false name.

"That Ceres and Bacchus might in moderation lend their assistance to Venus," Boswell wrote in his diary the next night, "I ordered a genteel supper and some wine." What followed this repast was a night of ecstasy, with Louisa's passion more than matching his lust. "A more voluptuous night," he wrote, "I never enjoyed."[14]

A few equally passionate sexual congresses followed until the night of January 19, after an evening at the theater with old friends, when Boswell got home, "came sorrow. Too, too plain was Signor Gonorrhea," whom he had encountered at least twice before.

The next morning Boswell "rose very disconsolate, having rested very ill by the poisonous infection raging in my veins and anxiety and vexation boiling in my breast. I could scarcely credit my own senses. What! thought I, can this beautiful, this sensible, and this agreeable woman be so sadly defiled? Can corruption lodge beneath so fair a form? Can she who professed delicacy of sentiment and sincere regard for me, use me so very basely and so cruelly?"

What added fury to Boswell's ire was that along with this infection born of Louisa's love he had, possibly for the second time in his young life, also been afflicted with one of gonorrhea's most painful side effects—epididymitis. Epididymitis is an inflammation of the epididymis, the excretory duct of the testes, and can cause the testicles to swell to the proportions of oranges.

Confronted with this development, the lady was visibly shocked and surprised. She confessed to Boswell that she had indeed had a bad clap some three years earlier, when she was twenty-one. "But for these fifteen months I have been quite well," she protested. "I appeal to God Almighty that I am speaking true; and for these six months I have had to do with no man but yourself." She was probably telling the gospel truth; gonorrhea in women is often asymptomatic.

Boswell however chose not to believe her and peevishly demanded the return of the two guineas he had, in a moment of sheer rutting madness, lent her some weeks earlier. She sent the two guineas to his rooms a few days later.

Dr. Andrew Douglas, who had probably treated Boswell's first clap in 1760, and would treat his eleventh dose in 1776, resorted to the standard therapeutic regimen of urethral irrigants containing acids, mercury, and astringents, bloodletting, starving, and purging. Fortunately, the epididymitis was of the transient variety that responded well to standard treatment. Boswell did not describe his treatment for this complication, but Buchan described it carefully in a subchapter titled "Of the Swelled Testicle," in his chapter on The Venereal Disease. Treatment called for bleeding and for a light diet.

"Poultices of bread and milk, softened with fresh butter or oil, are likewise very proper," Buchan wrote, "and ought to be applied when the patient is in bed: when he is up, the testicles should be kept warm, and supported by a bag or truss, which may easily be contrived in such a manner as to prevent the weight of the testicle from having any effect." In a footnote Buchan informed his readers that "I have been accustomed for some time past to apply leeches to inflamed testicles, which practice has always been followed with the most happy effects." Whether Dr. Douglas also applied leeches to Boswell is not known, but the practice was quite common at the time.

A little over two centuries after Boswell wrote in his diary about the etiological and temporal links between ecstasy and epididymitis, two physicians at the Royal Victoria Hospital in Bournemouth, England, S. M. Laird and R. M. Roy, sent a pertinent communication on the same general subject to the *British Medical Journal*. They wrote, "In women, the gonococcus remains superficial and readily found on bacteriological investigation for only a short time after infection; it rapidly 'digs in' in the deeper recesses of the mucous glands of the cervix and becomes superficial again only during menstruation or after sufficient sexual stimulation for the woman to approach or actually achieve orgasm. Given that both have gonorrhea, 'the enthusiastic amateur' may thus be more infectious than the prostitute with her numerous but entirely commercial consorts."[15]

Had Boswell contracted his gonorrheal infections a century later, the only real change in medical treatment would have been in the variety of irrigants introduced into his urethral canal by his physicians. What had changed was the nature of the passing medical fads. For example, in the mid-nineteenth century there were such cults as Eclectic Medicine and the closely related organic-therapy movements based on the uses of "natural" remedies, such as essences of herbs, flowers, berries, and other botanicals. These cults relied on "organic" urethral irrigants made of "natural" ingredients instead of chemicals like the mercury, vitriols, saltpeter, and acids that figured so prominently in Boswell's gonorrhea treatments.

The "organic" irrigants, intrinsically less toxic and damaging than the eighteenth-century chemicals, were syringed into the male and female urethras just as often (daily) as the "injections" pumped into Boswell every time he had dealings with his Signor Gonorrhea. These "organic" irrigants were therefore as responsible as the chemical irrigants for flushing out and transporting the gonococci from the mucosal membranes of the urethra into the bladder and other organs, the synovial joints, and the bloodstream, turning mild and transient local infections into disseminated serious complications.

In 1879 Albert Neisser, professor of dermatology at the University of Breslau, East Prussia (now Wroclaw, Poland), isolated from the urethral discharge of a patient the paired cocci that cause gonorrhea. Neisser described, drew, and could isolate at will the gonococci in his patients, but he was unable to grow them outside of the human body. It was not until 1885, at the Charity Hospital in Berlin, that the gynecologist Ernst von Bumm, director of the hospital's women's clinic, succeeded in growing *N. gonorrhoeae* in nutrient media in laboratory flasks and dishes.

Prior to Neisser's isolation of the gonococci, Carl Franz Credé, professor of obstetrics at the University of Leipzig and at that city's Charity Hospital, had long been concerned about the children of mothers with gonorrhea. The babies were often born with a serious eye infection that seemed to flare up a few days after birth, causing often permanently blinding lesions. Credé experimented with different drugs to cure this eye infection but found none that worked, until he turned to a solution of nitrate of silver as a last resort. Nitrate of silver, while bactericidal, is also a caustic, and were it not for the fact that it seemed to cure the infected children's eyes overnight, Credé would never have dared to use it. The benefits seemed to so far exceed the real risks that for the next six years he used it on all children born with gonorrheal ophthalmia neonatorum at the Charity Hospital—with invariably excellent therapeutic results. Some children did develop very painful chemical conjunctivitis (eye inflammation) from the caustic silver-nitrate-solution drops that protected them from blindnness, but the inflammations were short-lived as a rule.

When Neisser isolated the causal germs of gonorrhea and published his findings, Credé and other concerned obstetricians and gynecologists began looking for gonococci in their pregnant patients. It was not long before they isolated gonococci growing in measurable numbers in the vaginas of pregnant women. In 1873 before the gonococci were isolated, Credé had reported finding frank gonorrheal infections in forty-five out of 323 pregnant women who delivered (13.6 percent), but these were all overt infections diagnosed by their clinical signs and symptoms. After 1879 when he started looking for gonococci themselves, Credé most probably found that the numbers of asymptomatic or healthy carriers of virulent gonococci came close to equaling the numbers of pregnant women with overt gonococcal infections. It was then that Credé began to employ silver-nitrate dilution drops prophylactically on all newborn babies at the Leipzig Charity Hospital. By 1884 he had succeeded in reducing the incidence of gonococcal opathalmia neonatorum to just about zero.

In the more prosperous countries around the world, this soon became the routine clinical practice in all babies during the first hours of life, with results similar to those reported by Credé a year before anyone had even succeeded in culturing the gonococci *in vitro* (outside of human or animal bodies, in laboratory nutrient media). Until noncaustic antibiotic drops and ointments came along to replace silver nitrate drops, all newborn children in the United States and other affluent countries were routinely subjected to the "Credé maneuver." Since World War II, there has been a slow but inexorable change from silver-nitrate dilutions to antibiotic drops in hospital nurseries here and abroad.[16]

In 1885 when the gonococci were first cultured *in vitro,* the only available vaccines—Jenner's cowpox virus against smallpox, and Pasteur's attenuated bacterial and viral vaccines against chicken cholera, anthrax, and rabies—were all live pathogen vaccines. Few physicians were reckless enough even to dream of a live gonococcus vaccine against gonorrhea. Even had they wanted to experiment with an attenuated but live whole bacterial organism vaccine, they were hampered by not being able to use a live animal model in testing it. Only people get gonorrhea.

Not until 1896, after Almroth Wright developed the first clinical killed-bacterium vaccine, his dead *Salmonella typhi* vaccine against typhoid fever, did doctors, led by Wright himself, start to work on killed gonorrhea vaccines. Subsequently, as we shall soon see, new vaccines began to proliferate at the speed of light, and were shot into vast numbers of patients in Europe, North America, Australia, and elsewhere.

Even before the era of killed whole-organism vaccines, the isolation and laboratory culturing of the gonococci helped demonstrate that germ theory was as subject to misinterpretation and abuse by doctors with particular axes to grind as was any other great advance in medical science. A classic case of the misuse of germ theory to prove medical analogs of the flat-earth and phlogiston theories was Dr. John Buchanan's massive *Encyclopedia of the Practice of Medicine Based on Bacteriology,* published in New York in 1890.

On page 1174 under "Venereal Diseases," Buchanan wrote, "Whenever sexual intercourse is loose and varied, few women among many men, there takes place a change, an alteration or degradation of the living elements concerned in the nutrition of the genital organs of both sexes into a diseased germ. This change in the embryonic cell or primary elements of nutrition is the direct result of a violation of natural and divine law. This degradation of biophasm may result in the evolution of an immature or perfect germ." The immature germ caused gonorrhea; a germ that "never enters the blood, even if the individual has it [gonorrhea] a thousand times [and] if it is not interfered with will die out in a few weeks." The mature form of the same germ was "the microbe of syphilis, the perfectly developed germ that invariably enters the blood."

Not only did Buchanan take his peers back to the unitary venereal disease dogma Benjamin Bell had tried to shatter in 1792, he also incorporated the vitalist and miscegenation phobias of the era's leading pseudoscientific prophets. Hence: "The growth of the true syphilitis germ in the blood depends altogether on the degree of vital force he [the patient] possesses; if the vital force is good, its fecundation and growth may be retarded—that is, it will remain latent; but if the vital force be slightly deteriorated, it will grow; and if vigor be low, it will grow with rapidity. Nothing can be more disastrous than the contraction of the disease from an opposite and distinct race of men or women."

These verbose concepts of a mystic "vital force" and the health perils of race mixing were not unique to Buchanan. The vital force was soon to emerge as Bernard Shaw's "life force" in *Man and Superman,* and the eugenic miscegenation bit was then being solemnly taught as biology in most American universities.

Buchanan illustrated this chapter with very impressive-looking light-microscope drawings of "The Micrococcus of Gonorrhea," and a mixed culture he described as "the gonococcus and the germ syphilitic in the same patient." The bacteria he called the "germ syphilitic" turned out to be comparatively huge segmented rods as unlike the very small corkscrew-shaped and exceptionally tiny spirochetes of syphilis as they were to the face of the moon.

Buchanan was evidently an experienced clinician, as witnessed by his excellent descriptions of the symptoms and prognoses of clap. "The act of micturition is described [by patients] as if molten lead was passing," he wrote. "In four or five weeks, without treatment, there is a gradual subsidence of acute symptoms."

On the other hand, Buchanan added, although "as a rule, the gono-coccus dies in from five to six weeks in an acute attack of gonorrhea without treatment; with treatment, of a germicidal kind, a few days, or at least from a week to ten days, should be ample time to kill the germ and cure the patient."

This was particularly true, Buchanan advised, when concentrated or-ganic or botanical medicines, alone or in therapeutic combinations, were used as urethral irrigants. "Injections [irrigants] are usually divided into irritating, sedative, emollient, and astringent, and we have these qualities in a pre-emi-nent degree in these concentrated remedies. Indeed, the introduction of these agents marks a new era in the treatment of diseases."

James Boswell would have recognized Buchanan's treatment imme-diately, even though the 1890 chapters on treatment began with the brave new words: "Since the recent discovery of the germ origin of gonorrhea, the treatment has been somewhat modified." These modifications proved to con-sist of teaching the gonorrhea patients how to irrigate their urethras after every urination with "the ozonized distillation of eucalyptus." Buchanan as-sured his readers that "if this is performed early enough, the gonococcus is killed; even if it is the true syphilitic germ, it is likely to be sterilized [killed]." The clap patients also had to be irrigated with "large quantities of a tepid so-lution of boroglyceride or creolin," repeating the procedure three times a day. These solutions were to be delivered to the urethral canal from a fountain sy-ringe bag "elevated four feet above the pelvis."

Buchanan's treatment regimens included the familiar mix of purga-tive and laxatives to "keep the bowels open," as well as to "keep the urine al-kaline to obviate the presence of an overloaded rectum, overcome the local congestion, and to lessen the pain in urinating." The formulas for the re-quired urethral irrigants and local poultices that would kill the gonococci in-cluded the then standard dilutions of nitrate of silver, permanganate of potash, sulfate of zinc, chloride of lime, bismuth, and iron—as well as more advanced and more organic urethral irrigants and ointments, such as tincture of kalmia, balsam capaiba, oil of sandalwood, sweet spirits of niter, mucilage of acacia, tinctures of opium, iodine, and lavender, and kavakava paste. "The use of gelatinized urethral bougies, highly ozonized, is to be recommended in all cases." Buchanan was a particularly keen believer in the curative potentials of both kavakava and ozone.

It was not, one shudders to admit, until the enlightened twentieth century that medical treatments for gonorrhea became so painful, so danger-ous, and so bloody that Boswell and any of his fellow gonorrheics, risen from the dead and allowed to watch these regimens in action at our best hospitals, would not have been able to do so without flinching, gagging, and fleeing the premises. Again, as in Buchanan's 1890 medical encyclopedia, the power of reigning fads on clinical thinking—doctors are as subject to the lure of brain-bending panaceas as anyone else—inflicted needless agonies on gonorrheic patients. In our century the fad-based regimens were far more perilous to human life than the mercury, vitriol, and ozonized kavakava remedies of yesteryear.

Consider, to cite a few examples, the array of heroic treatments offered in the *Oxford System of Medicine* in 1926; in the first edition of R. L. Cecil's now standard *Textbook of Medicine* in 1927; and in the second edition of the British textbooks Topley and Wilson's standard *Principles of Bacteriology and Immunology* in 1936. Any single one of three modalities described in these standard clinical textbooks would have staggered a Hercules or a Wotan; the combination of two or more would quite easily have terminated more than *Ein Heldenleben.* Professor George Blumer of Yale, who wrote the chapters on gonorrhea for the Oxford and the Cecil texts, described two little-remembered standard treatments: (1) protein shock therapy, and (2) eradication by surgery of the primary focus—the focal infection—of disease. Topley and Wilson described the third then fashionable treatment for gonorrhea: artificial pyrotherapy.

In Cecil's *Textbook of Medicine,* Blumer wrote that "a form of treatment which has come into vogue in recent years is 'protein shock therapy.' This is based on the principle that the introduction of an alien protein into the system causes a non-specific reaction which stimulates the body processes concerned in the production of immunity. The technic of treatment consists in intramuscular or intravenous injections of pure albumose, or of sterilized milk or bacteria (typhoid vaccine) into the patient." This referred to the Wright-type killed-bacteria vaccine. In clinical practice, doctors also injected live cultures of *S. typhi,* the typhoid fever bacteria, into gonorrhea patients. The function of the live typhoid germs was a dual one: to create the desired protein shock, and also to give the gonorrhea patient typhoid, whose high fevers would help kill the gonococci in patients who survived the protein shock.

Blumer observed that in protein shock therapy, "the foreign protein reaction is characterized usually by a severe chill, headache, and general aching lasting a half hour or longer. The reaction is accompanied by a leukocytosis [an abnormal rise in the number of white cells in the blood] and a rise in blood pressure. . . . A few deaths have been reported. . . . Some patients refuse to continue the treatment for more than a few doses on account of severe reactions."

The surgical and medical craze for removing what were (mistakenly) labeled as the foci of infections in people with gonorrhea and many other diseases, from arthritis to sore arms, was not the work of a scientifically illiterate crackpot but of two of the most honored and responsible men in American medicine and medical bacteriology, Frank Billings (1854–1932) and Edward C. Rosenow (1875–?). Billings, who had studied in Vienna, London, and Paris after graduating from the medical school of Northwestern University in

1881, served as professor of medicine and dean of the medical schools at both Northwestern and the University of Chicago. He was a noted teacher and practitioner who, in 1902, had been selected to deliver the very prestigious Shattuck Lecture (on "The Changes in the Spinal Cord and the Medulla in Pernicious Anemia"). Billings served as president of the American Medical Association in 1902–1904.

In 1915 Billings delivered the coveted Lane Medical Lectures at Stanford University; the title was "Focal Infection." During the same year, his work in this and other areas of medicine caused Harvard University to award him an honorary doctorate in science. Rosenow, a bacteriologist at the Mayo Clinic, made many contributions to medical bacteriology, including the Rosenow stain for making bacterial capsules visible.

The basic principle of focal infection was that a primary or focal infection could cause many pathological side effects in other locations in the body. A baseball pitcher's suddenly bad throwing arm, for example, could be a side effect of abscessed teeth—and could therefore be restored only by extracting all his teeth. In 1912 Billings published a historic article, "Chronic Focal Infections and Their Etiologic Relations to Arthritis and Nephritis," in which he described the great improvements he had found in the general health of patients with these rheumatoid and kidney conditions after surgical or dental removal of what he termed "foci of infection."[17] Shortly after that, Rosenow, who was soon to announce his discovery of a special kind of streptococci that he identified as the real cause of poliomyelitis, began to collaborate with Billings in bacteriologically documenting the concept of focal infection.

"Rosenow claimed he had found proof in experimental studies of elective lodgment of bacteria in certain organs, and published evidence that certain organisms, especially different strains of streptococci, could frequently be isolated simultaneously from a focus of infection and from a distant organ," writes Dr. Paul Beeson, coeditor of the venerable Cecil-Loeb *Textbook of Medicine* and former professor of medicine at Yale and Oxford. "In 1915 Rosenow reported a series of experiments with 800 strains of streptococci isolated from such lesions as appendicitis, cholecystitis, herpes zoster, and mumps. When the bacteria were injected into rabbits there appeared to be a tendency for them to localize in the same tissue as that from which they had originated in man."

Beeson notes that "Billings described acute appendicitis as a focal infection caused by germs originating in the nose and throat, and gave illustrations of streptococci from human peptic ulcer which were said to have an affinity for stomach tissues when injected intravenously into animals. With regard to treatment, he advocated surgical removal of foci of infection as well as the administration of autogenous vaccines."[18] Autogenous vaccines were custom-made from the bacterial flora isolated from the patients themselves, and until the antibiotic era were extensively used to cure and prevent infectious diseases.

"American doctors," Beeson continues, "with few exceptions, suddenly became adherents of the whole [focal infection] thesis, and their example was followed in many parts of the world. Over a thirty-year period literally millions of unnecessary surgical and dental procedures were carried out in vain efforts to alleviate a large variety of disorders."[19]

The massacres of tonsils, teeth, sinuses, appendixes, gallbladders, spleens suffered by people in all walks of life—from baseball pitchers seeking to revive their lame pitching arms to overworked mothers with aching backs, to politicians getting in top shape for grueling political campaigns—were probably without parallel in the histories of medicine, surgery, and dentistry. Gonorrhea patients were in the foremost ranks of those to be cut and butchered by medical true believers in the doctrine of focal infection.

In the 1927 first edition of Cecil's textbook, under treatment of gonorrhea, George Blumer wrote, "In all forms of metastatic [disseminated] gonorrheal infection the first essential is *the eradication of the primary focus of the disease.*" [Blumer's italics] On the next page he wrote, "Destructive lesions, such as the phlegmonous [inflamed] type of [gonococcal] arthritis, call for prompt and often radical surgical intervention, with removal of necrotic tissues, free drainage, and the use of antiseptics."

Until the focal infection concept was proven to be totally without foundation in 1940, thousands of people with lesions of disseminated or systematic gonorrhea were subjected to unnecessary, costly, and highly traumatic surgery.

For gonorrheic patients who were afraid to endure such operations, and who also were deathly afraid of the splitting headaches and other pains, chills, and discomforts produced by protein shock therapy—let alone the wracking high fevers that followed injections of live typhoid fever vaccines—Topley and Wilson had good news in 1936.

"Of recent years," they wrote in the second edition of their textbook on bacteriology and immunology, "a method of treatment by artificial pyrotherapy has been introduced, depending on the fact that in [laboratory] culture the gonococcus is almost completely destroyed by exposure for two hours to a temperature of 41.5–42° Centigrade [106° F–107.6° F]. The patient's temperature is raised by placing him in a special cabinet heated with carbon filament lamps, or by passing high-frequency currents through his trunk. The aim is to keep his temperature at a sufficiently high level for a sufficient length of time to bring about *in vivo* sterilization of the gonococci."

This technique of treatment by artificial high heat was put to extraordinarily wide use in many countries, not only to kill gonococci but also other germs, including the syphilis spirochetes. In at least one major city, Chicago, the syphilis control program was based on the use of special pyrotherapy cabinets in which people were installed, as a friend who interned at Cook County Hospital at that time liked to say, to determine "whether the heat or the syphilis would kill them first." Not since European Christians of most denominations stopped burning dissenting Christians and Jews at the stake for heresy had so much heat been deliberately applied to so many people in the western world until liberation came in the form of the sulfas and the antibiotic drugs.

The one thing the post-germ-therapy world never lacked, particularly between around 1900 and the post-World War II mass marketing of cheap, safe, and effective penicillin and other antibiotics, were gonorrhea vaccines.

Unlike all our modern licensed vaccines against a dozen infectious diseases, the gonorrhea vaccines of the first half of the twentieth century were administered more to cure than to prevent gonorrhea. Unlike the earlier "injections" forced into the urethral canals of affected men and women, the twentieth century's first massive wave of gonorrhea vaccines were injected under the skin of the arms, legs, and buttocks. For this reason, whether or not the old gonorrhea vaccines were employed as total alternatives to the standard and invasive medical treatments for the disease, the vaccine-treated patients generally had fewer iatrogenic gonorrheal complications.

The popularity of killed whole-organism vaccines against every bacterial infection but tuberculosis and syphilis was due entirely to the work and the charismatic personality of Almroth Wright (1861–1947), whose killed-bacterium typhoid fever vaccine opened the era of bacterial vaccines in British clinical medicine. Wright was a man of extremely forceful convictions, a good scientist, and a great self-advertiser who made up in Paracelsan bombast what he very often lacked in the way of valid, replicable scientific proofs of his frequently unveiled new hypotheses. As every first-year bacteriology student is still taught, Wright was also his good friend Bernard Shaw's model for the insufferable Sir Colenso Ridgeon in *The Doctor's Dilemma.*

Wright's great contribution to human immunizations was not his typhoid vaccine, which was of very limited effectiveness. He was, however, the pathologist who, on the heels of the earlier work along the same lines by his chief, the British army pathologist William Boog Leishman, nailed down the fact that certain discrete substances circulating in human blood play a definite role in immunity. With the aid of his assistant at the Royal Army Medical School, Captain Stewart Douglas, Wright succeeded in showing that certain substances in the blood fluids coat the surfaces of pathogenic bacteria, and thus make them infinitely more subject than otherwise to be phagocytized (engulfed and destroyed) by the white blood cells—the leukocytes—when the bacteria enter the bloodstream. Wright named this the "opsonic effect," from the Greek word *opsono,* meaning "I cater for; I prepare victuals for." He therefore proposed the term "opsonins to designate the elements in the blood fluids which produce this effect."

The different opsonins are highly specific for particular bacteria, and for no other germs. This is very logical because they happen to be very special types of immunoglobulins or antibodies—the opsonic antibodies. Wright's discovery of their immunological functions helped explain the clearly interacting relationships between humoral (or circulating) immunity and phagocytic (or cellular) immunity. This made the opsonins (or opsonic antibodies) essential elements in one unified immune system.

Wright developed his system for determining what he called the "opsonic index" of people, and based his subsequent vaccine therapy for bacterial diseases on this index. The opsonic index was derived from counting the numbers of specific bacterial pathogens found in the phagocytic white blood cells in sick and healthy individuals before and after the bacteria were combined with samples of blood from each group of people, incubated for fifteen minutes, and then examined under the microscope. The greater the number of bacteria found within the leukocytes of the tested bloods, the higher the opsonic index, and vice versa. Therefore, vaccine therapy had to be based on the opsonic index: The higher or lower the levels of opsonized and phagocytized bacteria, the lower or higher were the amounts of killed-bacterial cultures in the vaccines used to stimulate enough phagocytes in patients' blood fluids to kill the same bacteria in their bodies.

Wright's killed-organism vaccines were administered subcutaneously, and different bacteria called for varying amounts of killed organisms. In 1910, according to Drs. Nathaniel Bowditch Potter and Oswald Avery, the dosage ranges in local gonorrheal infections averaged from five million to 500 million killed gonococci per vaccination. The vaccine dosages for general gonorrheal infections ranged from five million to 100 million killed gonococci per shot.[20]

Opsonic or killed-organism vaccine therapy was a very logical plan. Unfortunately, like Wright's equally logical killed-organism typhoid fever vaccine, the whole-bacterium gonorrhea vaccine was marginally effective at best. Generally, it lacked any effect at all on the patients' disease.

Wright believed further that since bacteria came in many types and strains, the best way to assure that the killed-organism vaccines contained the specific bacteria that made a patient sick was to isolate that patient's own infecting bacteria and then use them to make up an autogenous or self-vaccine. Pending the isolation, culturing, and processing of the specific organisms needed for these autogenous vaccines, stock vaccines made up of one or more strains of the bacterial pathogens of specific diseases were prepared and kept on hospital and neighborhood pharmacy shelves. These stock vaccines were used until the more favored autogenous ones were available to cure gonorrhea and other bacterial infections.

Between 1905 and 1945, vaccine therapy became an important medical modality in the treatment and prevention of gonorrhea. If one goes through the old issues of such standard medical journals as *Lancet* and the *British Medical Journal* in England, and the *Journal of the American Medical As-*

427

sociation in this country, and similar publications in France, Germany, Italy, and Austria, many articles appear on gonorrhea vaccines. The articles were written as a rule by the people who developed the vaccines, as well as by the physicians who first used them on their patients. These 1905–1945 articles each share two conditions: (1) As described by their authors, they were marvelously effective; and (2) the same gonorrhea vaccines were rarely heard from again in the world's medical journals.

For example, A. P. Ohlmacher, M.D., read a paper before the Chicago Medical Society on January 16, 1907, called "A Series of Medical and Surgical Affections Treated by Artificial Autoinoculation According to Wright's Theory of Opsonins," which was printed in the *Journal of the American Medical Association* the following month. Ohlmacher described a whole series of great successes of his killed-whole-organism vaccine against complicated gonococcal infections.[21] Ohlmacher felt that his experiences with gonorrhea vaccines were unique, because while "Wright has steadily predicted that gonorrheal infection would yield to opsonic therapy, because of the difficulty in making a suitable vaccine he had not advanced in this line of work. Perhaps, with some element of chance, it has been my fortune to obtain a strain of gonococcus from which a standard or stock vaccine was prepared," and which produced virtually miraculous cures.

The first test of this killed-whole-organism vaccine was in a patient with "gonorrheal urethritis of eight months' duration, with the usual picture of an immensely swollen and phimosed foreskin and a thick scar-like preputial orifice. On the second day following an injection of the gonococcus preparation the swelling began rapidly to subside and by afternoon the patient reported with the foreskin retreated, the glans clean and free from redness or pus, and the urethral discharge much diminished. He stated that this was the first glimpse of the glans penis that he had had for eight months. Four succeeding injections brought a check to the urethritis and at last account the patient was well."

A young patient of Ohlmacher's with double epididymitis, proctitis, and periurethral abscess not only had these gonorrheal complications cleared up with a few subcutaneous vaccine injections, but this young man's "appetite returned and he began a gain in the flesh" that increased his weight by nine pounds since he was put on Wright's opsonic killed-organism vaccine therapy. Ohlmacher declared: "That a further field of great usefulness is in store for opsonic therapy is my belief from my experience in treating two cases of gonococcal polyarthritis, or so-called gonorrheal rheumatism. In one of these patients the infection had existed four months and involved several joints. Progressive betterment of the arthritis with the departure of the swelling, pain, and immobility was effected by four injections when the patient considered himself cured and he no longer reported."

At the Annual Meeting of the American Medical Association in 1910

Benjamin A. Thomas, M.D., of the University of Pennsylvania, delivered a paper on the "Status of Therapy by Antigonococcus Serum, Gonococcus Bacterin [killed gonococcus vaccine], and Pyocyaneous [now *Pseudomonas aeruginosa*] Bacterin,"[22] in which he observed that while passive immunization serotherapy (treatment with antigonococcus serum from rams) worked well against gonococcal arthritis, "Wright, Pardoe, Douglass, Freeman, Wells, Fleming [Wright's assistant at St. Mary's Hospital, London, and future discoverer of the antibiotic effects of the common mold *Penicillium notatum*], Cole, Meakins, Irons, Hamilton and Cooke have apparently justified the belief that by active immunization—injection of bacterin or killed gonococcus vaccine—a much larger sphere of gonorrheal affections is afforded for treatment." Thomas added that the killed whole-organism vaccines were better for the treatment than for the prevention of gonorrhea, and that "permanent immunization must be accomplished solely by living [gonorrhea] organisms."

In Paris in 1913, Drs. Dopter and Pauron told a meeting of the Medical Society of the Hospitals that, as reported by the special correspondent to the *British Medical Journal,* "they had obtained excellent results by adopting Cruveilhier's method of treating gonorrheal rheumatism with a sensitized vaccine. In one case in which the joint affected was the knee, the swelling, pain and stiffness before treatment were marked. The first injection of the vaccine produced a marked general reaction, but on the following day the pain in the joint had ceased and the swelling around it greatly diminished."[23] A second injection cured this patient. The *BMJ* dispatch reported that the two French doctors "had also adopted the treatment in cases of gonorrheal orchitis [epididymitis], and had obtained corresponding results. In about 24 hours pain disappeared and swelling diminished, and in three or four days the patient could go about without discomfort, and was speedily and completely cured."[24]

During World War I, extensive uses of ordinary or stock killed whole-organism gonococcal vaccines were made by the British armed forces both to treat and prevent gonorrhea. How many vaccine doses were used is not known, but a hint of their volume can be gleaned from an article, "Detoxicated Vaccines, with Special Reference to Gonorrhoeae, Nasal and Bronchial Catarrh, and Influenza," published in *The Lancet* on June 28, 1919. The author, David Thomson, O.B.E., M.B. Ch.B.Edin., D.P.H. Camb., was a temporary captain, Royal Army Medical Corps, and a pathologist at the Military Hospital, Rochester Row, London.

Thomson's article opened with the information that "early in 1917 Brevet Colonel L. W. Harrison, K.H.P., D.S.O., asked me to make up a large amount of ordinary [i.e., stock killed whole gonococcus] gonococcal vaccine for use in the army. He stated that his experience with the ordinary [stock] vaccine had been very promising and he thought it deserved an extensive trial on a large number of patients. Since that time about one million doses have been sent out from the laboratory, and injected into soldiers. In those cases where the stock killed-organism gonorrhea vaccines were used instead of urethral irrigants and all the other standard medical treatments that helped convert local, transient doses into disseminated infections which, in turn, became chronic symptomatic gonorrhea, the soldiers who received the vaccines escaped such iatrogenic complications—and the vaccines were duly credited with their improved conditions. Clean tap water, or sterile dilutions of chicken soup, injected into the same soldiers would have produced the same fine results.

Thomson's work with these vaccines led him to what he firmly believed was the revolutionary finding that "the gonococcus and indeed all germs consist of stroma [the framework, usually connective tissues, of an organ or gland] and toxin." The immunogenic antigens of bacteria were, he believed, contained in the stroma, and caused the body to produce antibodies against the toxin. Thomson found a simple way of removing a bacterium's toxin by precipitating out the stroma with a little alkali, and "simply washing the precipitate repeatedly with a weak acid." The pure and "detoxicated" stroma were then used as the active ingredients in "detoxicated vaccines." Thomson wrote, in *Lancet,* that "this is obviously a discovery of great importance and I feel confident that it will mark a great advance in the science of vaccine therapy."

Since his vaccines were toxin-free, greater amounts of gonorrhea antigens could be shot into people. As Thomson explained, "Each species of germ, alive or dead, is a specific antigen. The greater the amount of antigen injected into the tissues, the greater is the quantity of the antisubstance [antibody] produced." Army tests of these "detoxicated" killed whole-organism gonorrhea vaccines produced glowing testimonials to their worth.

Like Thomson's revolutionary stroma-toxin hypothesis, his "detoxicated" gonorrhea vaccines soon vanished from the medical and scientific literature and from clinical practice. Almroth Wright's stock and autogenous killed-gonococci vaccines did survive the post-World War I era, as witnessed by medical textbooks of the period. The eighth edition of William Osler's *Principles and Practice of Medicine,* published in 1913 while the great generalist was still living, said only that "the use of antigonococcus serum and vaccine treatment are worthy of trial." The eleventh edition, revised by Johns Hopkins University Professor Thomas McCrae after Osler died in 1919, and published in 1930, said, "Of special measures, the use of foreign protein injection and vaccine treatment are worthy of trial; either helps some cases, both fail in many."

In the *Oxford System of Medicine* in 1926, George Blumer recommended vaccine therapy for gonorrhea but observed that "it is now generally conceded that autogenous vaccines are not necessary." A year later, in Cecil's *Textbook of Medicine,* Professor Blumer declared that "vaccine therapy has a definite place, especially in the subacute and chronic stages of local gonorrheal processes. The vaccines now in use are generally polyvalent and are made from several strains of gonococci. The dosage depends on the patient's reaction and varies from 5,000,000 to 500,000,000 micro-organisms."

By 1936 Topley and Wilson's *Principles of Bacteriology and Immunology* said only that "opinions as to the value of vaccine treatment differ considerably. The evidence available does not lend itself to statistical analysis." This was a gentle way of saying that anecdotal accounts of great successes which for some reason could not be replicated by most doctors were not very solid clinical data.

There was good reason for the faith many clinicians—particularly older practitioners—continued to place in the killed whole-organism gonorrhea vaccines until well into the antibiotic era. Until the Wright-type gonorrhea vaccines came along, they had treated gonorrheal infections as they had been taught in medical school: by urethral irrigations, medicated bougies, and other modalities that exacerbated local gonorrheal infections into disseminated infections causing sterility in women, epididymitis in men, and arthritis and heart disease in men and women.

Now, with the Wright-type gonorrhea vaccines, doctors no longer had to flush irrigants and shove instruments into human urethras. The new opsonic therapy vaccines were injected subcutaneously in the limbs, the backsides, and anywhere but the genitalia. Whatever the microbiologists said to demean the old gonorrhea vaccines, clinical statistics showed that in every medical practice where the killed whole-gonococcal vaccines replaced the older treatments, the rates of systemic gonorrheas and their complications dropped significantly—and in clinical practice it is tangible results that count the most. There was no way of convincing the doctors that these clinical gains had nothing to do with the vaccines themselves, and only concerned their abandonment of the older invasive and iatrogenic treatments.

By World War II, the United States armed forces—which had the greatest stake in curing and preventing gonorrhea—elected not to use the opsonic therapy, killed whole-organism vaccines for either purpose. However, as a good friend who was a medical officer in the U.S. Army's 77th Infantry Battalion discovered at first hand in the South Pacific, every captured Japanese base on the island route to Japan yielded thousands of vials of killed-organism gonorrhea vaccines.

Curiously, the printed labels on each vial, which read, "Gonorrhea Vaccine, Made in the Imperial University, Tokyo," were printed in English rather than Japanese. Whether this was done to hide their function from Japanese soldiers with gonorrhea, or as a humanitarian gesture to the incoming American troops, or because the Japanese had learned by then that the Wright-type gonorrhea vaccines were worthless and hoped to slow the American military advance by tricking American military doctors into using them on the troops, is one of the remaining mysteries of the war.

* * *

The saga of the killed whole-organism gonorrhea vaccines persisted long after World War II, particularly when it became painfully evident that antibiotics could cure but not prevent either the side effects of ascending pelvic inflammatory diseases (PID) or subsequent reinfections of gonorrhea.

The last and, one hopes, final chapter of the killed-bacterium vaccine story was unfolded in Inuvik, an Eskimo village on the Mackenzie River in the Northwest Territories of Canada. This is a very poor, simple settlement with no television, libraries, museums, concert halls, golf courses or tennis courts, Disneylands, movie houses, bingo emporia, and, in fact, none but the most ancient and basic forms of amusement and pleasure.

Into this Eskimo village, in the winter of 1972–1973, came a covey of Canadian government physicians and paramedical assistants to conduct a trial of a killed-gonococcus vaccine for the prevention of gonorrhea, developed from three strains of gonococci isolated from patients in Ottawa and Toronto. Their killed whole-organism vaccine was a very elegant one, lyophilized (freeze-dried) into a fine white powder sealed in vacuum glass capsules and reconstituted at Inuvik with a little distilled water. Essentially, the vaccine tested at Inuvik was the original killed whole-organism gonorrhea vaccine, made into a powder for ease of storage and travel.[25]

The vaccine field tests were run in a population of sixty-two men and women, slightly less than half of whom were under twenty. Following inoculations of each of these Inuvik Eskimos with either the killed-bacteria vaccine or with an inert placebo, or mock vaccine, both the vaccinated and control groups pursued their normal, active sex lives.

In due time gonorrhea developed in ten (30 percent) of the thirty-three Eskimos vaccinated with the killed-gonococcus preparation, and in seven (24 percent) of the twenty-nine who had been injected with the placebo. The vaccinated cohort proved to be more prone to catching gonorrhea than the nonvaccinated Eskimos.

These disastrous Inuvik results were not devoid of benefits. For one thing, they caused the cancellation of the much larger and already funded and scheduled World Health Organization field trials in Uganda, which was then governed by the irascible mass murderer Idi Amin.

The negative results of the Inuvik trial also, as Dr. Stephen J. Kraus of the CDC's venereal diseases control division remarked, "terminated the Dark Ages of gonorrhea vaccine research." There would be later gonorrhea vaccines, but they would be made of neither killed nor living whole gonococci nor, indeed, of any manner of whole gonococcal organisms.

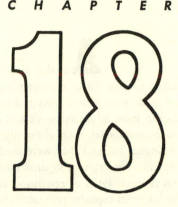

THE NEW GONORRHEA VACCINES: BOON, BUST, OR TIME BOMB?

I have never given up hope that one of these days the urologists would recognize the fact that the faster we treat gonorrhea, the faster we would get back the newly infected. Even the therapeutic results with penicillin will make no exception. I still believe gonorrhea is a preventable disease.

—WOLFGANG A. CASPER, M.D., in a letter to
Professor P. S. Palouze, March 30, 1944

At the time of the Inuvik killed whole-organism gonorrhea vaccine fiasco, the main currents of bacterial vaccine research no longer dealt with whole bacterial organisms live, dead, or skewered. For over a decade, most advanced work had involved immunogenic subunits of the bacterial disease agents, such as the sugars from the capsules of the pneumonia and meningitis bacteria that were used as active principles in the new safe and highly effective vaccines against two types of bacterial meningococci and fourteen capsular types of pneumococci.

The first of the bacterial capsular polysaccharide vaccines reported in the medical literature was one serendipitously used to protect mice from a strain of highly virulent pneumococci in 1926. Subsequently, chemists and physicians in the United States repeated Casper's and Schiemann's work in animals, and extrapolated their results into vaccines against pneumococcal pneumonia in people.

Young Casper had moved from work on a pneumonia vaccine to something closer to his immediate clinical interests: a safe and effective vaccine against gonorrhea. At the Virchow, Casper had trained under and by 1929 was assistant chief of dermatology under Professor Abraham Buschke—who himself had trained under the discoverer of the gonococcus, Albert Neisser, at Breslau. The venereal diseases were, for the pre-antibiotic century, the province of dermatologists.

The Virchow wards were an inexhaustible source of fresh clinical cultures of gonococci. To Casper, the most interesting thing about these gonococci was that when anyone put a smear of freshly isolated gonorrhea germs from infected patients under a good light microscope, it was usually possible to see that they were surrounded with structures that appeared to be quite similar to the capsules of virulent pneumococci. Clearly, these bacterial capsules might well yield the sugars (polysaccharides) which could be purified, reduced to fine white powder, and used to immunize people against gonorrhea.[1]

There was only one hitch. When Casper tried to produce the gonococcal capsular polysaccharides by the method Michael Heidelberger and Oswald Avery used that had been so successful with the pneumococcal subunit sugars, the method failed to work with the gonorrhea bacteria. He tried a number of variations of the Heidelberger precipitation technique, and in the end succeeded in precipitating from materials on the cell surfaces of fresh clinical cultures of gonococci a supply of carbohydrates very similar in character to the capsular polysaccharides of the pneumococci. Casper later (1937) published these methods in detail in the American *Journal of Immunology.*[2]

Before he could try these polysaccharides as a vaccine—since gonococci infect only people, there were no animal models in which an experimental vaccine could be tested—it was necessary first to determine if Casper's carbohydrate precipitates were safe in humans. He began by injecting minute quantities of the gonococcal cell surfaces into his own body. They were safe enough, but since Casper had never suffered from gonorrhea, these self-inoculations did not tell him if the dilutions of white sugar powders were immunologically active. He made up some dilutions containing as little as 8/10,000 of a milligram of the purified cell-surface gonococcal carbohydrates, and he injected them into present and former gonorrhea patients who volunteered to be tested at the hospital.

In these volunteers, Casper found that in people with active cases of gonorrhea, the bacterial capsular or cell-surface antigens caused skin reactions demonstrating the presence of gonococci in their bodies. More than that, Casper soon reported, the same minute quantities of gonococcal cell-surface sugars were also capable of "detecting infections when bacteria could no longer be found, and also aided in determining the serological type of gonococcus responsible for the individual's gonorrhea."[3]

These findings impressed Casper's clinical colleagues as a possible basis for a good test for the detection and diagnosis of gonorrhea, particularly in the symptom-free carriers who unknowingly spread this venereal infection to healthy people. Casper recognized this potential, but the very acute immunological sensitivity of the purified gonococcal cell-surface sugars suggested something far more important: The carbohydrates he had isolated from the cell surfaces of gonorrhea germs possibly were as likely to induce the human production of protective antibodies as were the capsular polysaccharides of the pneumococci in mice.

Since a vaccine made of the gonococcal cell-surface polysaccharides could be tested only in human beings, much would depend on the confidence any human volunteers had in the competence and motives of doctors looking for human bodies in which to test experimental vaccines. Casper had a good relationship with the hundreds of male and female gonorrhea patients on his wards at the Virchow. Since he was acutely sensitive to the iatrogenic potentials of standard medical treatments for gonorrhea, he spared all but the patients with disseminated gonorrheal complications any treatment except a week or so of bed rest, three square meals a day, daily baths, and perhaps a game or two of chess. Left alone, the average local gonococcal urethritis cleared up by itself in two weeks or less.

The world economic depression had by 1929 turned prostitution into

Berlin's leading growth industry. Most of the women on the gonorrhea ward were people newly forced into the industry to stay alive. The majority of the male gonorrhea patients were Berliners rendered jobless and in many instances homeless by the Great Depression, members of the marginal working classes who were the first to suffer economically in any fiscal crisis. Many of them were, in addition, very vocal communists, and took pleasure in good-naturedly chaffing the young doctor on what would happen to him come their revolution.

After Casper had precipitated enough of his antigenically active carbohydrates from fresh gonococcal cultures to make up five doses of an experimental vaccine against gonorrhea, he asked for ten volunteer males and one female to help him test the vaccine. He explained his experimental protocol to each of the people whose cooperation he sought. It was a very simple one. He proposed to move ten men into one ward, and to inject five of them with the vaccine and five with an inert placebo. After that, he would move the female volunteer, a prostitute with an active case of gonorrhea, in with the men, along with a barrel of beer. The eleven volunteers would be encouraged to drink as much beer as they wished during the night that followed their being locked into this ward together.

Casper had no trouble in getting ten destitute Berliners he had previously treated for gonorrhea to risk getting the clap again for science, if it also assured them of a few weeks of hospital shelter, meals, baths, clean linen, and, as a bonus, all the beer they could drink. The lady volunteered to participate in this experiment for similar motives.

Within a week of this one-night stand, four of the men who had not been vaccinated with the polysaccharide preparation woke up with new doses of clap. None of the five homeless men who had been vaccinated with the gonococcal polysaccharides caught gonorrhea, although each had also had intercourse with the prostitute.

Although still in his twenties, Casper was by family heritage (he was a member of the fourth generation in his family to become physicians) and training too responsible a clinical investigator to publish these results immediately. The total number of individuals involved was much too small to prove anything other than that larger clinical trials of this candidate vaccine were possibly justified. What were needed now were huge amounts of the gonococcal cell-surface polysaccharides in order to prepare enough vaccines for larger trials in many types of populations.

Neither the Virchow Hospital nor the Robert Koch Institute for Infectious Diseases had the technological resources to precipitate and purify these raw vaccine materials in the vast quantities called for. Only the pharmaceutical industry had such resources. Accordingly, in October 1929 Casper obtained a German patent on a gonococcal capsular polysaccharide vaccine and assigned it to the firm of Schering-Kahlbaum in Berlin for development.

When Schering failed to get moving after the promising Virchow trials, the impatient young dermatologist transferred the assignment of the patent to the I. G. Farben company. The widening world economic crisis not only stopped Farben from making any of Casper's gonorrhea vaccines, but it also brought the Nazi regime to power.

Within weeks, this political revolution affected Casper in a number of ways. For one, a few days after Hitler took over Germany, Schiemann told Casper that the new regime had ordered him to notify Casper that he was no longer permitted to work—even as an unpaid volunteer—at the Koch Institute. Casper was a Jew. His chief, Buschke, also Jewish, was forced to take early retirement from the Virchow Hospital staff, and Casper was appointed to succeed him.[4] Finally, many of Casper's former communist patients, on whom he had performed circumcisions to relieve gonorrheal paraphimosis of the foreskin, now came around to the hospital for duly notarized medical certificates assuring the masters of the new *nordische Seele* regime that their circumcisions had been performed solely for medical and not religious reasons. A few days after Casper signed these certificates of racial integrity, the same men were back, former communists now, and sporting the jackboots and brown uniforms of Hitler's *Sturmabteilung,* the notorious Storm Troops. They assured Casper that they still held him in high and even affectionate regard, but Herr Professor must understand that people had to bend with the wind of the new order to survive.

Early in 1934 some of the newly converted Nazis came to the Virchow Hospital to warn the thirty-three-year-old Casper to get out of town: His name had just appeared on the Gestapo's latest list of Jewish doctors, lawyers, and university professors scheduled to be rounded up and herded into extermination (race purification) camps. The brownshirts told him to hide until it was safe to return. He and his wife, Annaliese, also a physician, left Berlin in their sailboat, and their Nazi-cum-communist friends arranged to signal them from different lakeshore sites when it would be safe for them to put ashore again.

It would never again be safe for the Caspers while Hitler ruled. With the aid of friends—some of whom were personal physicians to the new Nazi elite—the Caspers escaped from Germany.

They arrived in New York during the Depression winter of 1934. Relatives helped them open offices for the private practice of their medical specialties, Annaliese in allergy and Wolf in dermatology. The depth of the Great Depression was hardly the time to start new private medical practices. At Rockefeller Institute, to which Avery had invited Casper in 1927, the job of developing a human analog of Casper's pneumococcal polysaccharide vaccine for mice had long since been completed by other research workers. Casper's friends at Rockefeller got him a job at NYU-Bellevue medical center. He worked as a urologist at Bellevue Hospital and taught the sections on the "diplococci" (pneumococci, gonococci, and meningococci) in Thomas Francis, Jr.'s bacteriology courses at the New York University medical school. He was also given his own laboratory, but was not provided with any funds for an assistant (*Diener*) to wash his glassware and perform other housekeeping tasks. Between his clinical duties at Bellevue and his housekeeping chores in his laboratory, Casper was unable to repeat any of his basic or clinical work on the gonococcal polysaccharides.

At the medical school, the closest Casper ever came to doing any work on gonorrhea was shortly before America was bombed into World War II. At that time a major line of research on poliomyelitis, which had involved the purchase and uses of a large number of macaque rhesus monkeys, was terminated before all the monkeys were utilized. Casper was requested by his academic superiors to determine if he could induce gonorrhea in these monkeys by inoculating them with fresh clinical cultures of gonococci, and he was offered the necessary staff assistance to manage the monkey tests. He protested that the gonorrhea bacteria attacked only people, and that there was "no point in injecting gonococci into the monkeys with pants and shoes and tickets to ball games just to find out what everyone already knew." The medical school brass dangled a gleaming carrot at the end of their stick: Casper was promised extra support to test his polysaccharide vaccine in rhesus monkeys if he somehow managed to get the gonococci to cause clap in the animals.

Reluctantly, Casper agreed to shoot the tiny monkeys full of fresh virulent cultures of gonorrhea germs, which were always in abundant supply in Bellevue. Before he inoculated them, he recalled that "in the old days, at the Virchow, if you wanted to determine whether a gonorrhea patient was really cured, you filled him up with beer to stir up the gonococci. So I made these rhesus monkeys drunk on beer, first. Then I injected them with fresh gonococci from gonorrhea patients. The monkeys, of course, never did get any symptoms of gonorrhea. What they did get were beer hangovers that lasted for days. I couldn't look any of them in the eyes again."

Casper wrote a number of important articles for American journals based largely on his Berlin investigations. There was a paper on the extraction of immunogenic gonococcal polysaccharides in the *Journal of Immunology* in 1937. There was his article "Degeneration and Variation of Gonococci," published in the *Journal of Bacteriology.* In this paper, Casper showed that the known "degeneration" of pneumococci when cultured in laboratory media also occurred in artificially grown gonorrhea germs, and that "this degenerative process, including the decrease of the type-specific carbohydrate [i.e., specific cell-surface polysaccharides], carries with it a decrease of virulence." With this chain of events, Casper continued, "In chronic gonorrhea the gonococcus, by adaptation to human tissues, may undergo the same degenerative processes that occur after prolonged cultivation on artificial media."[5]

In an article in the NYU *Medical Bulletin* in March 1939, Casper suggested that "in this degenerative state the [gonorrhea] organisms even lose their diplo [double] form and may not be recognizable microscopically as gonococci." In the same article Casper listed some of the unresolved problems "which reflect the need for greater research in gonococcal infection before we attempt to establish a specific cure for the disease."

At the invitation of Dr. Thomas M. Parran, the Surgeon General of the United States, Casper wrote a prescient article in 1941 for a Public Health Service publication on "The Biochemistry of the Gonococcus and Its Practical Importance." The article dealt with the role of the gonococcal cell-surface polysaccharides in infection by and prevention of gonorrhea. Published in April 1941, four years after the sulfa drugs had begun to be used against gonorrhea, originally with dramatic therapeutic effects, Casper concluded with a warning that gonorrhea "is not a solved problem, even with new therapeutic discoveries. . . . Just as we could not treat malaria, in spite of our knowledge of quinine, if we did not know the life-cycle of the parasite, so do we need extensive studies of the antigenic structure of the gonococcus and its effects on the human organism to give us a thorough knowledge of gonococcal infection and lead the way to its prevention."[6]

Parran did not disagree with Casper about the need for much more basic knowledge of the gonococcus. However, by the spring of 1941, Parran as a good public health officer felt that Casper's 1929–1930 gonorrhea vaccine had to be further developed and subjected to large-scale clinical trials if only for clearly impending military reasons. Parran tried without success to get the federal health agencies to fund Casper's vaccine work.

After Pearl Harbor, Parran invited Casper, by then a United States citizen, to Washington. The Surgeon General asked Casper to prepare a protocol—a plan of action—for developing a gonococcal cell-surface polysaccharide vaccine against gonorrhea under the auspices of the U.S. Public Health Service. He also commissioned Casper as a surgeon (a rank equivalent to major) in the Service.

It was an auspicious time for Parran to launch the gonorrhea vaccine project, since the sulfa drugs had worked only too well against various types and strains of gonococci in the military camps, wiping out just about all the strains that were naturally sensitive or susceptible to the drugs. This left only the few and hitherto inconsequential infectious strains of gonococci that were naturally resistant to the sulfa drugs, a process in which the antibacterial sulfa drugs acted as efficient agents of natural selection. The resistant strains of gonococci thus selected out for survival now inherited the bodies of American servicemen. Without competition from the formerly more numerous strains of bacteria that were sensitive to the sulfa drugs, the drug-resistant strains began to take over. The faster they proliferated, the more rapidly the sulfas lost their effectiveness as quick cures for gonorrhea.

However, by the time Casper reported for duty, penicillin had been introduced as the possible successor to the sulfas. What drug resistance to penicillin then existed among any gonococcal strains was not evident at the start. Penicillin killed the germs even more efficiently than the sulfas, and it continued to do so for the duration of the war.

The priority of vaccine research and development in the Public Health Service kept falling as the clinical successes of penicillin against gonorrhea made welcome medical history. Penicillin was generally in short supply, and most of it was spoken for by the antibacterial drug needs of combat troops. For those stateside soldiers and civilians not lucky enough to be able to be treated with penicillin, there were doctors, including Casper, to administer the standard medical treatments. A century and a half after the combination of James Boswell's nineteen gonorrheal infections and their medical treatments finally killed him, nothing really much had changed in the clinical management of the disease. Silver-nitrate dilutions (germicidal but caustic) had been substituted for the port wine and mercurials and jalap and herbal essences and kavakava as irrigants injected into human urethras by hand and fountain syringe. The medicated bougies inserted in patients with gonorrhea were now made of metal rather than of bone and cloth or wax. One further modality had been added in male gonorrheas, and that was the prostate massage, which of course helped disseminate the gonococci from the bladder to the rest of the body.

Casper, who by January 1944 had been made chief of the gonorrhea section of the Service's Chicago venereal disease control program, was by then terribly disheartened. Bureaucratic medicine demands standard treatments for all disorders, and the standard treatments were what Casper had been fighting against all his life as a clinician.

He was still fighting against the invasive, aggressive treatment of gonorrhea thirty-five years later and still, as he neared eighty, seeing patients every week. "The first time you see the gonococcus in a male patient it is just at the proximal end of the urethra, the segment of the urethral canal at the outside entrance of the vessel. And only by our miserable treatment do we push it back, further into the body," he noted after more than a half-century of practicing medicine. "The same holds true in a female. The gonococci are in the urethra, first, before they are pushed back into the vagina, the Fallopian tubes, the ovaries. My God! So many of the complications of gonorrhea are iatrogenic—the products of syringes and bougies shoved into the urethra, or of prostate massages."

The first day Casper, just out of medical school, entered Buschke's clinic at the Virchow, the professor showed him a patient with testicles massively swollen from epididymitis. "Professor," the new intern said, "that's not normal. The gonococcus has no feet or fins or wings. It doesn't wander from the urethra to the testes. Somebody put those gonococci in the epididymis, and I'm wondering if that somebody wasn't a doctor."

"Buschke just looked at me and smiled. All he said was, 'Do something to make gonorrhea treatment safer. Invent something.' That was Buschke. He was always saying something like that. Not in anger, no. He wanted young people to question everything, to improve clinical practices.

"So I did something. I 'invented' the gonococcal polysaccharide vaccine. Buschke liked what I did, and he thought it should be developed further. Hitler disinvented it for me, and he nearly disinvented my wife and me. In the end, Hitler killed Buschke. Then Parran came along, and he agreed with Buschke. But not even Parran could make his peers understand that no matter how effective penicillin was and is in curing gonorrhea, the gonorrhea problem can only be solved by prevention."

Parran refused to abandon his plans to have a gonorrhea vaccine developed. Toward the end of 1944, he phoned Casper in Chicago and asked him to present a working paper on his vaccine before the National Postwar Venereal Disease Control Conference held in St. Louis on November 9–11. It was the moment Casper had been waiting for. He prepared a deliberately short paper and a batch of slides, and counted the hours before he set off for St. Louis.

At the conference, no sooner did Casper start presenting his vaccine plans than Dr. J. R. Heller, chief of all venereal disease work in the PHS, interrupted him. "Stop right there, doctor," the chief said. "After the war you'll never see a gonococcus again in your lifetime." Penicillin, as everyone but apparently Casper knew, was totally eradicating gonorrhea. When peace came, and penicillin was available to everyone, gonorrhea would cease to exist.

Casper retorted, "Doctor, the gonococci are smarter than you are, and they'll outlive both of us."

His riposte was a grievous gaffe, and Casper knew it even before his words brought an instant array of new colors to Heller's cheeks. Since Casper had two stripes less on his uniform sleeve than Heller did, he was banished to a venereal treatment center in Jackson, Mississippi, for the duration of hostilities.

Once the war ended, Casper looked for a university appointment that would enable him to teach medicine and work on a gonorrhea vaccine. No medical center was interested in this field of research. He was unable to find such a job. Early in 1946 the gracious Michael Heidelberger, by then professor of immunochemistry at the Columbia University College of Physicians and Surgeons, sent Casper a copy of one of his papers on pneumococcal capsular polysaccharide vaccine field studies at an army air force training base in South Dakota during the winter of 1944–1945. Heidelberger's letter said, in part, "I was sure you would be interested in the polysaccharide work, as you certainly 'started something' years ago. I have had no experience with gonococcus carbohydrates, but if you have a method of preparing active ones, possible T. D. Gerlough of E. R. Squibb and Sons Biological Laboratories in New Brunswick, New Jersey, would be interested in your evidence and in extending it."

By the time Casper saw Gerlough, a week or so later, penicillin had utterly destroyed the market for the fine pneumococcal polysaccharide vaccines Squibb had started to manufacture at war's end to be used in adults and children. Doctors considered that pneumonia, like gonorrhea, was a disease that would shortly be eradicated by penicillin. Squibb was going out of the vaccine business, and was therefore not interested in extending any work on a vaccine against gonorrhea or any other bacterial disease. What was true at Squibb held true at all other pharmaceutical companies here and abroad: There was no future for bacterial vaccines, and therefore no interest in what Casper wanted to develop.

Casper settled down on Staten Island, the least urban of the five boroughs of New York City, and established a very comfortable practice in dermatology and dermatologic surgery. Now out of active research, Casper nevertheless became a familiar and often abrasive figure at postwar medical conferences. When invited to speak, he kept presenting data and arguments for the resumption of work on the polysaccharide vaccine against gonorrhea.

As he had always predicted, penicillin did not eradicate gonorrhea, which by the mid-1950s started its spectacular rise to being the most frequently reported infectious disease in the United States. When he was invited to speak, Casper always put his need to speak bluntly ahead of any local sensitivities. Thus at a medical meeting in Ottawa in 1971, on the eve of the ill-fated Inuvik trials of the killed whole-organism gonorrhea vaccine, when the leaders of the Canadian medical team that had developed the vaccine presented a preliminary report on their work, Casper rose to plead with them to abandon their plans to test it on the Inuvik Eskimos and the Ugandan university students. He reminded his Ottawa peers of the inexplicably forgotten half-century of failures of earlier killed whole-organism gonorrhea vaccines.

"I made a Don Quixote of myself, after World War II, trying to get medical school and other investigators to go back and pick up my work at the stage where it was when Hitler ended my laboratory career in gonorrhea infection and immunity research. I kept telling everyone that none of us knew enough about what happens to the gonococci after they infect human tissues. Nothing came of my pleas. But there were some small compensations. For example, whenever I ran into Rod Heller at a medical meeting, I never once failed to tell him, 'In your lifetime, doctor, you're always going to see millions of gonococci.' He knew I was right, of course. But it made no difference. I was ignored."

In 1953 when Heidelberger received a Lasker Award in basic medical research "for decisive contributions in developing a new sub-science, the precise measuring tool, immunochemistry," he paused at the podium while naming the roster of scientists who used his basic immunochemical findings to create new bacterial capsular polysaccharide vaccines. "Here in the audience is a man who started it all, Dr. Wolfgang Casper. We're all living on his work, and don't look around because you won't recognize him."

Casper was not around to be unrecognized when the then ninety-year-old and still active founder of immunochemistry won his second Lasker. This was the award in clinical medical research that Heidelberger shared with the principal developers of the new capsular polysaccharide vaccines against pneumococcal pneumonia and meningococcal meningitis, Robert Austrian and Emil Gotschlich. Like Heidelberger, who was then still actively engaged in research and teaching at the New York University medical school, the seventy-seven-year-old Casper was still in active medical practice, but he was out of medical research completely. What extra intellectual and physical energies he possessed had long since been lavished on the breeding, showing, and judging of pedigreed Irish setters.

By 1978 many investigators were trying to develop gonorrhea vaccines. When they looked for the gonococci capsules, they were often unable to find them. From the sidelines Casper hectored them to "use fresh clinical cultures! That's the only way you can ever recover the capsules and their polysaccharides. Don't wait until they degenerate and lose their cell walls." By then, however, Casper had become an embarrassing link to the not very inspired medical history of what had reigned for at least a decade as America's most common infectious disease, gonorrhea. It was far easier to ignore Casper than to argue with him, and that was what most—but not all—of the younger generation of investigators proceeded to do during the eighth decade of this century.

In 1971 when Milton Puziss started to award NIAID grants for gonorrhea vaccine research, many people began looking into the immunogenic potentials of the capsules of *Neisseria gonorrhoea*. By that year, the meningitis vaccine developed at WRAIR from the capsular polysaccharides of Group A and Group C *Neisseria meningitidis* were being administered routinely to every new recruit in the basic training camps of the armed services. The capsules of the closely related *N. gonorrhoeae* could be seen and photographed, although none of the postwar workers had yet succeeded in removing and working with the gonococcal capsules.

Not all capsules are immunogenic or at least sufficiently so to serve as vaccines when removed from the outer walls of bacteria and chemically purified into a white powder. This had only recently been proven true of the capsules of Group B *N. meningitidis*, a significant cause of meningococcal meningitis.

In nature, the slimy carbohydrate capsules are believed to have the function of protecting bacteria from being phagocytized and destroyed by the circulating leukocytes of their human hosts. This would make them antiopsonic chemical structures. The microbiologist Walter W. Karakawa, at Penn State University, has demonstrated that pathogenic *Staphylococcus aureus* bacterial cells found in the bodies of sick people have very photogenic outer slimy capsules. However, when the same bacteria are removed from patients' tissues and are cultured for a few bacterial generations in laboratory vessels, their laboratory-cultured direct descendants start to grow without their ancestral slimy capsules. This parallels, in one species of major disease-causing bacteria, the findings Casper reported in the gonococci nearly fifty years ago.

When carbohydrate capsules are needed, quite possibly for protection against destruction by phagocytosis, they are apparently grown by many species of pathogenic bacteria. On the other hand, when colonies of the same bacteria are removed from patients and grown in laboratory vessels filled to the brim with fine nutrients and completely free of phagocytic human white blood cells, the same bacteria will often stop forming the outer capsules, as in Karakawa's *Staphylococcus* cultures.

This is not due to Lamarckian inheritance. These bacteria never lose the capacity to make antiphagocyte capsules, but they merely avoid the effort of synthesizing capsules when there is no evident need for them in laboratory culture flasks and plates. However, when the same capsule-free bacteria are taken from their artificial phagocyte-free laboratory environments and inoculated into healthy animal or human bodies, within a few bacterial generations—a bacterial generation can take as little as twenty minutes under laboratory conditions—the same bacteria's lineal descendants will again start to grow the thick, slimy capsules that they were always capable of growing when these structures are needed for survival.

Not everyone agrees that proof exists that the visible capsule-like structures seen on the cell walls of gonococci are either polysaccharide capsules or have antiphagocytic functions. One of the prominent skeptics, Emil Gotschlich, maintains that "a bacterial capsule is not a capsule until it can be reduced to a fine white powder in a bottle." Without this proof, he maintains, we can only guess at what it is that is actually seen on the gonococci, let alone what its function might be.[7]

Other investigators, among them Jerry Sadoff at Walter Reed Army Institute of Research (WRAIR), and John Swanson, now director of the NIAID Laboratory of Microbial Structure and Function at the Rocky Mountain Laboratories in Montana, insist that what look like capsules on the outer cell walls of the gonococci are in fact just that—fully paid-up, card-carrying capsules. Swanson, an old friend and frequent collaborator of Gotschlich's, has a sneaking suspicion, however, that the capsules of the gonorrhea bacteria, like those of the Group B meningococci, are only weakly immunogenic at best, and therefore of little use by themselves as the raw materials for vaccines.

Whatever the actual nature and potentials of the gonococcal capsules, after the federal grants for gonorrhea vaccine research started to attract good scientists into working on the gonococci, no one seemed able to remove the slimy capsules from the outer cell walls of the gonorrhea organisms, let alone purify them for further analysis and/or uses in experimental vaccines. With the gonococcal capsules apparently unworkable, and the ancient dream of killed whole-organism vaccines having fallen through crevices in the ice of Inuvik, it became apparent that the shortest route to arrive at safe and effective vaccines against gonorrhea lay in studying the natural history of the gonococci, in general, and in investigating, in particular, the cellular and subcellular events that ensue when gonococci invade human mucosal cells.

Not very much had really been learned about gonorrhea since Dr. Benjamin Bell, in London in 1792, tried and failed to make his professional peers realize that gonorrhea and syphilis were two separate "contagions" rather than two forms of the same venereal disease. In 1838 the French surgeon Philippe Ricord defined and described the three essential stages of syphilis, but at the same time he insisted that gonorrhea, while a different disorder than syphilis, was not even a contagious disease.

The dawn of germ theory initiated a universal hunt for the germs of gonorrhea. In 1879 at Breslau, Albert Neisser discovered the gonococcus in the urethral discharge of a gonorrhea patient. Neisser showed that this bacterium caused gonorrhea but definitely not syphilis. Some doctors, in the tradition of those who until well into this century insisted that the cowpox virus was a degenerated form of the smallpox virus, continued to write and teach that gonorrhea and syphilis were one and the same disease, caused by the immature and mature forms, respectively, of Neisser's gonococcus.

Not until 1905, when Fritz Schaudinn and Erich Hoffman isolated the corkscrew-shaped spirochete, *Treponema pallidum,* in syphilis patients, and this smallest of all bacteria was shown to cause syphilis in rabbits and other animals, did all physicians finally agree that gonorrhea was not a junior form of syphilis.

Not until 1885 were bacteriologists able to grow the gonorrhea germs in artificial media. However, since 1905 no microbiologist has to date succeeded in culturing *T. pallidum.* The syphilis spirochete has been isolated from patients, smeared on glass microscope slides, stained for better viewing, photographed, and even inoculated into rabbits and monkeys to cause syphilis as well as to provide laboratories with fresh cultures of the bacterium. However, no laboratory has yet succeeded in growing *T. pallidum* outside of live mammalian bodies. This explains why, in the absence of adequate supplies of syphilis bacteria to work with, there has been little or nothing done on syphilis vaccines made of killed spirochetes, live attenuated spirochetes, altered live spirochetes, or subunits of *T. pallidum,* such as their possible capsular polysaccharides and other cell-surface antigenic structures.

Since Neisser two highly important differences between gonorrhea and syphilis have been defined by work with their respective bacterial agents. The gonococci are a bacterial species with a very short period of incubation. Two to seven days after they enter the urethra, the gonococci mature and cause gonorrheal infection and its first nasty symptoms. The incubation period

445

of the syphilis spirochetes is considerably longer. The primary lesions of the first stage of syphilis, the soft chancres at the site of the original point at which the *T. pallidum* organisms entered the human body, do not appear until the syphilis bacteria complete their period of incubation, which occurs from twenty-one days to six weeks after the sexual transaction in which the germs were transmitted from the infected donor to the healthy individual.

In our times this variance between the effects of the gonococci and the syphilis spirochetes is not unrelated to the different periods of incubation required by each species of bacteria. The gonococci confer no lasting immunity against further gonorrheal infections once a clap is cured. The syphilis spirochetes, on the other hand, once fully matured and able to cause soft chancres and more serious subsequent manifestations of clinical syphilis, can confer long-term or permanent immunity against subsequent infections by *T. pallidum* in people cured of the disease.

Fortunately, reinfections of gonorrhea can be cured as effectively and as quickly with massive and usually single injections of penicillin as can first cases. The systemic penicillin and other antibiotics used to cure gonorrhea (and many other bacterial infections) also nips slowly incubating cases of syphilis in the bud by killing the potentially pathogenic spirochetes before they have time to mature. In these cases, however, the aborted preclinical syphilis infections induce no immunity against subsequent attacks; only fully matured *T. pallidum* organisms in long-standing cases of syphilis can induce enough antibodies to protect people against new syphilis infections. The rule of thumb in clinical practice is that the longer a syphilis infection lasts, the greater the degree of protection it provides against reinfection.

The differences between microbial pathogens can be as striking as their similarities. The great advantage of the "Sabin-type" live virus oral vaccines against polioviruses and typhoid fever bacteria is that once ingested they stimulate the swift production of secretory IgA antibodies by the mucosal cells of the alimentary system. The gonococci also cause the mucosal cells to secrete antigonococcal antibody of the IgA (classes 1 and 2) type. Unfortunately, in 1975 it was discovered that cultures of *N. gonorrhoeae* also secrete an enzyme, IgA-1 protease, which cleaves the human serum and secretory IgA-1 antigonococcal antibodies. IgA class 2 antibodies seem to be enzyme-resistant. However, the findings in IgA-1 suggested that these proteases (enzymes that split proteins, such as the immunoglobulins or antibodies) may be of clinical importance, since "the IgA protease may allow the [gonococcal] organisms to resist immune attack."[8]

In the absence of capsular polysaccharides, the quest for other subunits of the whole gonococci that might also function as immunogens led to many promising vaccine candidates. There are the principal outer-membrane proteins (POMP) of the *N. gonorrhoea* that Kenneth Johnston and his colleagues at Rockefeller University found after Carl Frasch discovered that such proteins in the outer membranes of *N. meningitidis*—the agents of meningococcal meningitis—are, in the presence of complement, immunogenic. They obviously had a role to play as the primary or co-components of experimental vaccines against *N. gonorrhoeae.* There are also the endotoxins, or lipopolysaccharides (LPS), of bacteria. Like the capsules, the LPS structures are also bacterial cell-surface chemical compounds.[9]

The endotoxins (LPS) of the gonococci are found in the outer membrane (OM) of the bacterial cells that also contains the principal outer-membrane proteins (POMP). The gonococcal endotoxins are believed to play contributory roles in the causation and virulence of gonorrhea. They have also been shown to induce the production of anti-LPS antibodies in infected people.

Unlike the often lethal exotoxins released by such bacteria as the tetanus and diphtheria bacilli, the endotoxins, which usually remain attached to the bacterial cell structures, are rarely fatal to people. The LPS compounds do, however, cause severe shock, diarrhea, high fevers, and leukopenia (an abnormally low count of circulating leukocytes), followed by leukocytosis (an abnormally high level of circulating leukocytes). Nevertheless, because the endotoxins or lipopolysaccharides are such excellent immunogens, they have been used as the active principle of experimental vaccines against other bacterial diseases, like the burn-wound infections caused by *Pseudomonas aeruginosa.*

Malcolm B. Perry and his collaborators at the Canadian National Research Council in Ottawa helped determine that of the two principal components of the endotoxin compound, only the lipid (fat) segment was toxic. The remaining polysaccharide portion was as nontoxic and as immunogenic as the bacterial capsular polysaccharides which are the active ingredients of new meningococcal meningitis and pneumococcal pneumonia vaccines now on the market.

Perry and his group applied the Ludwig-Westphal method of detoxifying the LPS by removing the lipid component and retaining the carbohydrate or polysaccharide fraction. They and other workers in the United States and elsewhere have since been working with the detoxified LPS in experimental methods of detecting and diagnosing gonorrhea in people. They have also been investigating experimental vaccines based on detoxified LPS alone and in combination with other bacterial cell-surface materials, like POMP and on the attachment organelles of Gram-negative bacteria, the pili.

The pili are among the major biological fallouts of the electron microscope. Prior to the advent of this microscope, these hairlike or fiberlike protein appendages on the surfaces of pathogenic bacteria were invisible even under the most powerful light microscopes. Once people started to study common bacteria under the greater resolving powers of the new electronic microscopes, it was only a matter of time before they stopped dismissing the pili as dirt or as the debris of specimen preparation for viewing. One such moment arrived at the University of Pittsburgh in 1950, when a young microbiologist, Dr. Charles Brinton, realized that the hairlike fuzz around many species of bacteria was not of laboratory origin but the natural surface structure of the bacterial cells themselves.[10]

These thin, rod-shaped, nonflagellar bacterial surface appendages were clearly more than laboratory curiosities. Brinton named them pili from *pilus,* the Latin word for hair. He understood that nature is too efficient to create normally present biological structures that have no function other than to entertain microbiologists with access to an electron microscope. In time, careful observation of *Escherichia coli* and other piliated bacteria enabled Brinton to demonstrate that bacteria have two types of pili, which he termed the sex pili and the somatic pili.

Depending upon the environment in which they live, bacteria exist in piliated and nonpiliated phases. In human or other mammalian bodies, bacteria usually grow in their piliated phases; once transferred to aerated liquid nutrition media, particularly in small numbers, the bacteria tend to grow in their nonpiliated phases. Both growth phases can be completely reversed by manipulating their environments. When grown on solid media, such as nutrient-enriched agar (a gelatinous material made from certain seaweeds), clones of piliated bacteria, Brinton found, "usually form colonies that are smaller, more opaque and with more sharply defined edges than non-piliated phase clones."

The sex pili, much larger than the somatic pili, have as far as Brinton could observe, two functions in nature. The first is to transfer bacterial virus nucleic acids from one bacterial cell to another during the somewhat rare act of bacterial sexual conjugation (usually, bacteria reproduce by splitting or dividing into two daughter cells). The second function of the sex pili is to transfer plasmids, or paragenes, which are nonchromosomal genes, or episomes, from one bacterial cell to another during sexual conjugation. Since these plasmids at times include the genes that code for resistance to antibiotics and other drugs, the combination of natural selection and these nonchromosomal genes for drug resistance make the sex pili of Gram-negative bacteria potentially important in therapeutics.

Brinton showed that the smaller but far more numerous somatic pili are, among other things, the instruments of the bacterial surface translocations that are variously termed twitching motility, gliding motility, or creeping motility. This mechanism of moving across the outer surfaces of human cells enables the piliated gonococci and other pathogenic Gram-negative bacteria to spread infections to many sites in the body. (Other disease-causing Gram-negative bacteria include the agents of syphilis, *salmonellosis,* typhoid fever, cholera, plague, dysentery, *Haemophilus influenzae,* and the pyelonephritis, meningitis, pneumonia, and septicemia caused by *E. coli, Pseudomonas, Proteus,* and *Klebsiella* species.)

In 1957 and 1958 in Scotland, pili were discovered on sixty-five out of eighty-one strains of *Salmonella,* and on most strains of *Enterobacteriaciae,* by J. P. Duguid and various colleagues. Duguid, who much preferred to call these structures fimbrae—from the Latin word for threads or fibers—described the observed tendency of piliated bacteria "to adhere to intestinal epithelial cells," as well as to bind or agglutinate red blood cells in clumps. At that time the Scottish workers speculated that this pili- or fimbrae-mediated adhesiveness may assist *Salmonella* and other enteric or gut bacteria in the colonization of human intestines. Brinton, who welcomed Duguid's work, also determined that when pili were removed from bacteria, purified, and then inoculated into rabbits, they caused the rabbits to produce an antiserum that prevents this pili-induced agglutination of red blood cells.

Pili were found on the gonococci in 1971 by John Swanson, Stephen Kraus, and Emil Gotschlich at Rockefeller University, and independently by Drs. Jephcott, Birch-Anderson, and Alice Reyn at the State Serum Institute in Copenhagen. Shortly afterward, while investigating the virulent and avirulent colonial forms of cultures of *N. gonorrhoeae,* Swanson and Reyn discovered that gonococci in the virulent colonial forms of the germs were piliated, while the gonococci growing in the avirulent types of colonies were nonpiliated.

Laboratory studies of the role the pili and similar fiberlike cell-surface structures play in helping disease-causing bacteria adhere to human cells and tissues started to proliferate.

Drs. R. J. Gibbons and J. van Houte, at the Forsyth Dental Center in Boston, studied the mechanisms of adherence of cariogenic (cavity-causing) oral streptococci to the surfaces of teeth. Their investigations included electron microscopic studies of the fibrillar coating on the surfaces of these Gram-positive streptococci. "These surface fibrils," they reported, "seem to differ from the pili typical of Gram-negative organisms by being shorter, thinner, and more densely distributed over the bacterial cell surface." Their own and other studies, however, showed that "these fibrils mediate the attachment of" several species of oral streptococci to epithelial cell surfaces, such as the enamel of human teeth.[11]

Shortly after this, Swanson started to explore the ways in which the pili of the gonococci mediated the attachment of gonorrhea bacteria to healthy human cells. The NIH grant program administered by Milton Puziss provided funding for various other studies of the pili's functions in initiating gonorrhea and other bacterial infections.

After Brinton's laboratory found that antibodies to the pili could inhibit such pilus functions as sticking to the blood and epithelial cells, "we made a very simple hypothesis," he states. "To wit, if we were to take the purified somatic pili, and try to immunize with them, the pilus antibodies should neutralize or block whatever functions the somatic pili of bacteria have that contribute to colonization and virulence."

Brinton and his group developed three purified pili vaccines based on this very simple working hypothesis. Two of the vaccines, the first against *P. aeruginosa,* a major cause of burn-wound, lung, and urinary-tract infections, and the second, against certain strains of *E. coli* that cause diarrhea in newborn piglets, could be and were tested successfully in animals in the late 1970s. The third experimental purified pili vaccine, against *N. gonorrhoeae,* had to be tested in the only living species it infects, the human species.

Grant support from governmental and nongovernmental agencies had not been available in any meaningful amounts for the first two decades of Brinton's work. Then by the end of 1971, the Great Awakening to the upward mobility and pandemic spread of gonorrhea in this and many other countries led to serious funding support of research on gonorrhea vaccines.

"Until then," John Swanson now recalls, "even twenty years after Charley Brinton had discovered and described the pili, there was little interest in them, except in a small way for their role as sex factors in bacteria. There was some fragmentary stuff by Duguid in Edinburgh on the role of the pili in the attachment of *Salmonella* [one of the major causes of bacterial diarrhea] to intestinal cells in the late 1950's, and Brinton's early publications. Then the taxpayers began demanding that the government do something about the spread of gonorrhea, and the NIAID set up its granting program. One of the most worthwhile fallouts of the federal granting program became the intensive work in many laboratories on the role of the pili in the cause and potential prevention of gonorrhea."

The NIAID grants enabled Brinton to develop further his purified pili gonorrhea vaccine, but they did not fund or authorize immediate human tests of its safety, antigenicity, and protection against live and active gonococci. Those tests had to be performed by Brinton and whoever volunteered to be tested on their own, and were to be done by using other, nonfederal funds. In 1974 in Brinton's laboratory, he and four other senior investigators, each with an M.D. or a Ph.D. degree and high faculty rank (i.e., no "student volunteers" were either sought or used), assembled to participate in the first human test of the gonorrhea pilus vaccine, a preparation of purified gonococci suspended in a mineral-oil adjuvant. An adjuvant is a substance or a combination of substances—such as the compound of mineral oil and killed tubercle bacilli in Freund's adjuvant—that hopefully increases the antigenicity of a vaccine or increases the therapeutic action of a medicine.

Only two volunteers received the vaccine. Each of the five were then inoculated, via a plastic catheter inserted into their urethral canals, with measured doses of fresh gonococci isolated from patients with clap, a somewhat more impersonal or joyless mechanism of the transmission of gonorrhea germs than the usual method.

Within a few days it was evident that the two men immunized with the purified pili vaccine were protected against gonococci at the normal infective-dose levels. The three unimmunized volunteer controls had each acquired gonococcal urethritis from the catheterized doses of the gonorrhea agents.

The levels of the infective doses of gonococci were then raised, in progressively larger amounts, for follow-up challenges of the two immunized volunteers whose pili antibodies had protected them against the initial doses. With each increase in these challenge doses of gonococci, the antibodies in the pili vaccine continued to protect until the infective doses were large enough to cause gonorrhea. These last doses were in quantities far higher than would ever be encountered during sexual contacts.

One year later a third series of tests of the purified gonococcal pili vaccine in the bodies of the same five doctors produced similar results. The two who were originally vaccinated with the purified pili plus a mineral-oil adjuvant preparation remained immune to normally infective doses of *N. gonorrhoeae*. "And that," Brinton said, "was the first time anybody really knew what the infectious gonococcal dose range for people really was. Nobody had ever done this experiment before."

Because few diseases are easier to cure with antibiotics than gonorrhea, there were no lasting or disseminated gonorrheal infections in any of the five volunteers. However, Brinton later wrote that there were some unpleasant side effects. "Mild transient chills in two human volunteers injected with gonococcal pili was [sic] attributable to the use of mineral oil adjuvant, as was a single sterile abscess at one injection site."[12] This was somewhat of a masterful understatement and merely hinted at another, if negative, beneficial result of this first test of the purified gonococcal pili vaccine: The particular mineral-oil formulation was never again used as an adjuvant in the Brinton vaccine.

In itself, this experiment—like Casper's ten-man, cell-surface gonococcal polysaccharide vaccine experiment of 1929—proved only that further tests were probably justified. However, the NIAID felt that not enough was yet known about the natural history of gonococcal infections to justify such additional tests of the vaccine in any other human beings for a while.

Before the purified pili vaccine could be tested in large numbers of people, some important problems had to be resolved. One was type specificity. As in the cases of the poliovirus and the pneumococcal pneumonia vaccines, this problem was solved (1) by incorporating either killed or attenuated live strains of all three known types of polioviruses in each of the different poliomyelitis vaccines, and (2) by including in the pneumonia vaccine the purified capsular polysaccharides of the fourteen types of pneumococci responsible for over 80 percent of all United States pneumococcal pneumonias.

Resolution of the type-specificity problem called for a closer look at the immunochemistry of the gonococcal pilus itself. As Emil Gotschlich, recognized as the foremost worker in the *Neisseria* species, pointed out a few years ago, "the pilus of any type of *N. gonorrhoeae* has about 165 different amino acids. We have identified about 30 of them, at one end, and these are always identical. The human immune response to pili from all types of gonococci seems to be a slightly cross-reactive response. That is, the purified pili of almost any type of gonococci will, in laboratory tests, react in a minimum degree with blood serum from a person who has been [temporarily] immunized by gonococcal infection. To a major extent, this is a cross-reactive response." Cross-reaction does not necessarily mean cross-protection, but it does suggest—at least in the gonococci—that there could be a common antigen in many types of these organisms.

"The best way to study the common or variable antigens of gonococci is in the order of the sequences in which they appear in nature," Gotschlich believes. "That is not an impossible task, but at the same time it is not going to be accomplished overnight. We've been at it for more than five years in this laboratory [Rockefeller University], and have not gotten very far as yet."

Brinton's studies at the University of Pittsburgh suggested to him that the antigens in the pili of more than fifty strains of gonococci contain certain common sequences that cause them to cross-react with one another. To Brinton, this meant that the common antigen deduced or presumed to be present in the pili of all strains of gonococci could be used as the active principle in a purified gonococcal pili vaccine that would protect against all types of *N. gonorrhoeae.* At first, small-scale tests on a small number of human volunteers seemed to confirm his working hypothesis. He then began to put it to more sweeping tests.

As in the 1974 experiments on himself and four colleagues, the new tests in each of a hundred male volunteers involved infecting the individuals with "calibrated numbers of viable gonococci via intraurethral catheterization . . . instilled using a syringe attached to the catheter. The catheter is held in place for 10 minutes, then removed. Using this method," Brinton and collaborators reported, "we produce infection at predictable levels for a given dosage. The experimental disease closely resembles the natural acute gonococcal urethritis of the male," even though the mode of inoculating the male volunteers with gonococci was quite unlike that experienced in nature for many millennia.

Because of the armed services' vital stake in protecting their personnel of all ranks against gonorrhea, when Brinton was ready for large-scale tests of the safety and antigenicity of his purified pili vaccine, the WRAIR organized a series of such tests in military volunteers at various bases. Starting in 1979 and for the next two years, each volunteer was given a series of three injections of the vaccine alone. These vaccines, made only of the subunit pili—the attachment organelles on the outside of the gonococcal cells—were unable to cause gonorrhea or any other disease.

The safety tests were conducted only to establish if the purified gonococcal pili vaccines caused any adverse side effects when injected into healthy human bodies. After two years of testing, it became clear that the new subunit bacterial vaccines caused no serious side effects.

The antigenicity tests were also quite harmless, since all that was involved was drawing a little blood from each vaccinated volunteer, and then testing these blood samples against laboratory cultures of cells from people with medical histories of gonorrheal infections and/or against cultures of virulent gonorrhea bacteria themselves. If the vaccines caused the volunteers to start producing antibodies against gonococci, these immunoglobulins circulating in their blood would cause both the gonococci and the cells of patients who had once had gonorrhea to agglutinate or clump.

None of the military personnel was subjected to the crude type of challenge, inoculating live gonococci through a plastic intraurethral catheter, that Brinton and his four colleagues and a hundred male volunteers after 1974 had experienced. Actually, in large populations of young people exposed to continuous, statistically predictable and measurable risks of annually contracting gonorrhea, such laboratory challenges of a vaccine's efficiency are not really necessary. Over a two-year period, when enough servicemen and servicewomen have been experimentally immunized with any vaccine against gonorrhea, and an equal number of service people have been followed as unimmunized controls, and if careful medical records of both the immunized and the nonimmunized cohorts are maintained, follow-up studies by military epidemiologists will give a pretty good idea of whether or not any tested vaccine prevents or fails to prevent gonorrhea.

The results of the first two years of large-scale (but happily unpublicized) military service tests of the Brinton vaccine for safety and antigenicity were promising enough to convince the army that the time had arrived to put the purified gonococcal pili vaccine to use tests. These tests also did not involve pumping virulent gonococci or anything else into the urethral canal. Instead, they were based on the laws of probability and averages dealing with the number of cases of gonorrhea that are normally expected to be reported to military clinics annually in posts surrounded by known specific ratios of prostitutes to service personnel.

The first of these large-scale but prudently unpublicized use tests of the Brinton gonococcal pili vaccine were scheduled to start in 1981 on either an aircraft carrier or at carefully chosen foreign and (later) domestic military posts. In these trials half of the service volunteers were to be injected with the harmless and noninfective purified pili vaccine, the other half with a placebo, and neither the doctors nor the military personnel were to know who was injected with what until the trials were completed. If, as now expected, these immunizations do lead to a decline in the expected numbers of gonorrheal infections contracted per cohort, and to a concomitant and measurable immunity against gonorrhea in the vaccinated individuals, then the tests would be broadened to include many other military sites at home and abroad.

Were they to work as well in these camps, then the armed forces would probably start routinely to immunize all new service people against gonorrhea with the purified pili vaccine, as was previously done with the army-developed vaccines against meningococcal meningitis and adenovirus respiratory diseases.

Long before the end of the large-scale military-population trials of Brinton's pili vaccine—whether it worked well, poorly, or not at all—various other gonorrhea vaccines now in development and early testing stages in this country, Canada, and Europe will have been tried in other populations. Like Brinton's vaccine, some of these vaccines will contain purified gonococcal pili alone. Others will be subunit types but combined cell-surface antigen vaccines, such as the one containing both pili and POMP (principal outer-membrane proteins) that Tom Buchanan and his group have been working on at the U.S. Public Health Service laboratories in Seattle for some years. Malcolm Perry in Ottawa, Fred Sparling at the University of North Carolina, and Jerry Sadoff at WRAIR have been working on gonococcal vaccines containing detoxified lipopolysaccharides (LPS) alone or in combination with pili and/or POMP.

Some of the antigens in the new gonorrhea vaccines will be the products of post-World War II research and even of post-1971 research. Some of these new antigens might be the specific proteins that cause gonococci to grow in opaque colonies at certain times and in transparent colony forms at others. Swanson and his coworkers discovered a few years ago that males who are asymptomatic or healthy carriers of gonococci carry these opacity proteins. When they transmit gonococci to a female during coitus, the time of her menstrual cycle will determine whether the same bacteria growing in her body will or will not have those proteins. If she is in midcycle, the gonococci growing in her body will have opacity proteins. As she starts to menstruate, her resident population of gonococci undergo biochemical changes and they lose these opacity proteins. Now, when they are removed from her tissues and cultured in the laboratory, the gonococci grow in the highly virulent transparent forms.

Swanson has observed "a very interesting correlation between the increased virulence of those bacteria during the period of menstruation and the increased incidence of serious gonococcal diseases in females at about the time of menstruation. And then the same gonococci will start cycling back. So that at about the time of ovulation, or mid-cycle, she will have those dark colony gonococcal growth forms again, the opaque forms that have the opacity proteins."

Work by Drs. John James and Geoffrey Brooks at San Francisco

Medical Center suggests that vaccines based at least in part on these gonococcal opacity (and virulence) proteins might find their way into the medical armamentaria in our times.

Some of the new gonorrhea vaccines (or vaccine components) might not only be based on the oldest, and to date rarest, principle in the history of vaccines, but might actually be licensed and used in daily medical practice against other infectious diseases right now. After all, the history of safe and effective vaccines began in 1796 with a preparation in which the antigens of the cowpox virus (vaccinia) cross-reacted with the antigenic determinants of the smallpox virus (variola), and thus protected people against smallpox. In the late 1970s, Malcolm Perry and his coworkers in Ottawa noted a similar cross-reactive relationship "between the Type-14 pneumococcal capsular polysaccharides and the core oligosaccharide moiety of the R-type lipopolysaccharides (LPS) of *Neisseria gonorrhoeae*." They pointed out that their "previous studies have indicated that the R-type LPS of *N. gonorrhoeae* is chemically and immunochemically similar in all strains examined to date, and therefore represents the common antigen of *N. gonorrhoeae*."

The Type XIV pneumococcal polysaccharide that cross-reacts here with all types of gonorrhea bacteria is one of the fourteen capsular antigens present in the pneumococcal polysaccharide vaccines licensed in 1978 and later, and since that time is available in all the United States drug stores. The Type VII pneumococcal polysaccharide antigen is not in the commercial fourteen-antigen vaccines now on the market, but Michael Heidelberger has found it to be as cross-reactive with other pathogenic bacteria as Type XIV pneumococcal capsular polysaccharides, and it is just as easy to find, isolate, and purify for gonococcal vaccine uses if need be.

Perry and his coworkers suggested in 1979 that "the capsular polysaccharide of *Strep. pneumoniae* type 14 be used as a vaccine against *gonorrhoeae*, perhaps in a close population study, on males and females at risk. Such a vaccine has already been licensed and is readily available in the U.S.A., and it is non-toxic and known to be antigenic in man." This suggestion was not lost on at least two giant pharmaceutical companies, which have been quietly exploring the concept since it was published.

In short, it is quite probable that the present fourteen-antigen capsular polysaccharide pneumococcal vaccines, with or without the addition of Type VII and other cross-reacting pneumococcal polysaccharide antigens, or without other cell-surface subunit gonococcal antigens, are even now being quietly tested by manufacturers who know when silence is golden and when the time has come to crow.

At least one other gonorrhea vaccine now in development has its roots in another major episode in the history of vaccines. The cell-surface carbohydrates that Casper precipitated from the fresh clinical cultures of virulent gonococci succeeded in protecting five men against gonorrhea in the first and only test of Casper's gonorrhea vaccine at the Virchow Hospital in Berlin in 1929. Casper published the techniques used to extract or precipitate these cell-surface sugars in the *Journal of Immunology* in 1937.

Nearly forty years later in 1976, a young investigator, who had not yet been born when this was published, read this article. He was Dr. Michael Apicella, then at the medical school of the State University of New York at Buffalo. What had led him to Casper's 1937 paper was that, while studying the gonococci, he had extracted four immunologically distinct acidic polysaccharides from the cell-surface structures of four strains of gonococci. As is routine practice in scientific research, Apicella then undertook a study of the literature of published work on the immunology of the gonococci and the immunogenicity of their cell-surface structures to see if similar findings had been reported before.

Apicella, the cultural heir to the forty-seven years of immunochemistry that followed Casper's gonococcal polysaccharide vaccine of 1929, was struck by the methods Casper had used to precipitate the capsular carbohydrates. On the basis of Casper's accounts, Apicella suspected that what he had really extracted from the gonococci were not the capsular polysaccharides but "the polysaccharide components of the lipopolysaccharide or endotoxins attached to the bacterial cell walls." If this was so, it would mean that Casper had detoxified the LPS compounds and used their polysaccharide components as vaccines against gonorrhea.

Subsequent laboratory studies convinced Apicella, now at the University of Nevada medical school, that this was indeed what had happened in Berlin in 1929: Casper's vaccine worked, Apicella was certain, because it consisted of detoxified LPS—or lipopolysaccharides stripped of their toxic fat or lipid component, leaving only their immunogenic sugars. Apicella is presently developing a gonorrhea vaccine compounded of detoxified or lipid-free gonococcal LPS and of the immunogenic POMP of gonococci.

The chances are that the ultimate gonorrhea vaccines licensed for general use will contain at least two, and possibly three, or even more than three gonococcal cell-surface and outer-membrane antigens. The reasons are clear to many investigators. Purified pili alone, for example, can prevent local gonorrheal infections by preventing the attachment of virulent gonorrhea to the mucosal surfaces of the epithelial cells in the urethra—and 95 percent of all gonorrheal infections are sexually transmitted local infections that never spread beyond these urethral sites. However, as John Swanson observed a few years ago, "it is possible that the loss of pili for attachment to the mucosal and epithelial cells might prove important because it would also send the gonococci sailing past the usual local sites of attachment and cause the clap to go systemic. We have no data on that [this was in 1979] but it is a reasonable possibility."

Shortly afterward, Professor Zell A. McGee and his associates at the

Vanderbilt University School of Medicine in Nashville, Tennessee, provided considerable data on the importance of the pili in attachment of gonorrhea bacteria to human cells, and also on the ability of nonpiliated gonococci to attach themselves to human mucosal and epithelial cells by other and as yet undiscovered mechanisms. They found that piliated gonococci "attached to and damaged the mucosa much more rapidly than did the" nonpiliated strains of gonorrhea bacteria. However, they also learned that the nonpiliated gonococci "do attach to and damage fallopian tube mucosa."[13]

The McGee group's work, most of it done in human Fallopian tubes that were removed during sterilization operations and kept alive in tissue-culture liquid media, also showed that the lipid or toxic segments of lipopolysaccharides on the surfaces of gonococcal cells are one of the major toxic factors.

This would indicate that the ideal gonorrhea vaccine should, at minimum, protect against the attachment of gonococci to urethral and other human cells, and against the toxic damage caused by gonococcal endotoxins, or LPS. It also indicates that antigens against the outer-membrane proteins and against the common antigen of *N. gonorrhoeae* would add to the protective functions of any good gonorrhea vaccine.

There is one thing that seems very probable: Within the next few years there will be available on the market one or more safe and effective gonococcal subunit vaccines for the prevention of gonorrhea. This historic clinical achievement will, unfortunately, create at least twice as many medical and societal problems as it will solve.

Two of these problems had better be faced now, while there is yet time to think about their components without the hysteria that results in expensive and generally disastrous crash programs.

1. Who will be vaccinated?
2. What are we prepared to do about coping with the major health and national budgetary problems that could well escalate even faster than continuing fiscal inflation when the massive prevention of gonorrhea by the new vaccines might conceivably cause the rates of all primary and advanced cases of syphilis to take off with the speed and trajectory of rockets to the moon?

The question of who should be vaccinated is easy to answer. In gonorrhea, as in every other major communicable disease, the public health rule is obvious: The target populations for protection by vaccination (immunization) are those people known to be at the highest risk of getting and transmitting the disease.

In gonorrhea this rule has to be administered to accommodate to the peculiar conditions of the transmission of the disease itself, since "most female cervical infections, and some male urethral infections, are asymptomatic in a situation analogous to the carrier state of other infectious diseases. It is when the gonococci spread from the urethra and cervix that they can cause serious medical problems."[14] This means that "the single most important axiom about the spread of this disease is that gonorrhea is usually spread by carriers who have no symptoms or who have ignored symptoms."[15] Upward of half of all gonococci carriers are possibly and innocently unaware that they harbor and transmit gonorrhea bacteria to their sexual contacts.

In this country the subpopulations at the greatest risk of both contracting and transmitting gonorrhea are well defined. In order of the degree of risk of acquiring and spreading gonorrhea, young adults between the ages of twenty to twenty-four are at the top of the list.

Teenagers between fifteen and nineteen are the second highest risk group in the United States. American schoolchildren miss over one million school days annually because of gonorrhea and its complications.

The population at the third largest risk are men and women in the twenty-five to twenty-nine age group.

In 1977 young adults between twenty and twenty-four accounted for 39 percent of all gonorrhea cases reported in this country, while teenagers between fifteen and nineteen made up 25 percent of the total gonorrhea cases reported.

The actual number of cases annually in the United States is estimated by governmental and academic epidemiologists to be at least two to four times as great as the number of reported cases.

Gonorrhea is very much a young people's disease. It is also, among the world's industrial nations, a very American disease. Holmes observed that as of 1980, "the reported [gonorrhea] incidence rate in the United States is now three times higher than in England and Wales. The true incidence rate is probably ten times higher in the United States, since reporting of gonorrhea is far more complete in the United Kingdom, where most patients with gonorrhea are seen in public clinics for sexually transmitted diseases. Suboptimal clinical practice, including the use of subcurative therapy and especially failure to trace any infected contacts, probably contributes to the higher incidence rate in the United States."[16]

The costs of treating gonorrhea in the United States now come to well over a billion dollars annually, more than half of them federal tax dollars. The dollar costs of vaccinating every American at even remote risk of catching gonorrhea in the course of a year would come to considerably less than a tenth of the gonorrhea treatment and other economic costs per year.

Most Americans (around 90 percent of the population) live in cities, and urban areas account for 75 percent of the nation's total gonorrhea case load. The more densely populated the cities, the higher the rates. Like most other contagious diseases, gonorrhea is also in significant measure a result of crowding.

Federal Centers for Disease Control (CDC) data show that in thirty-seven American cities with populations of over 500,000, the gonorrhea case rate is 920 per 100,000 population. In twenty-six midsized cities of 200,000 to 500,000, the case rate is higher, with 960 per 100,000 population. On the other hand, in 271 small cities with populations of 20,000 to 200,000, the gonorrhea case rate is only 22 percent that of midsized cities, with a still-too-high rate of 209 per 100,000 population; while in all nonurban areas the reported cases also average exactly 209 per 100,000 population.

Changing sexual preferences and customs have also helped expand the range of gonorrheal sites and symptoms. As Dr. Richard B. Roberts at the Cornell University Medical Center observes, "Where in former years localized gonococcal infections were found almost exclusively in the urethras of men and the endocervixes of women, today gonorrhea of the pharynx [throat] and the rectum present as not uncommon products of oral and anal intercourse." Roberts cautions that "any patient who comes to a physician with pharyngitis [sore throat] and is in the sexually most active age group—between 15 and 35—should have a culture for *N. gonorrhoeae.*"[17]

Since gonorrhea is a nationwide health problem that affects all regions, social classes, and racial and ethnic groups, the logical approach to planning for the most sensible utilization of the new safe and effective gonorrhea vaccines would be a national program to mandate equal vaccine protection for the citizens of the poorest states as well as the most affluent states. Historically, of course, this is not about to happen. The prevailing political tendency is to make all major health programs the undertakings of the 50 state governments rather than of the national government.

Turning gonorrhea vaccination over to the fifty states will mean fifty state gonorrhea immunization programs of varying medical worth, from highly effective to totally useless—as in the widely varying state regulations for clinical laboratory testing that in most states offer no assurance at all that those who perform the laboratory tests are even minimally qualified and competent to make bacteriological, viral, and chemical determinations medically ordered in human blood and urine.[18] As a wise but anonymous editorial writer for *The New York Times* observed in 1981, ". . . To say, 'Let the states do it' or, 'Let the private sector do it' is a barely varnished way of saying, 'Don't do it.' "[19]

The crisis atmosphere and professional public relations apparatus hyperbole under which the catastrophic "swine flu" vaccination program that was undertaken by the Ford administration during the great nonepidemic of nonswine influenza of 1976 should serve as a humanly and economically costly reminder of how not to introduce the forthcoming gonorrhea vaccine or vaccines at either national, state, or village levels.[20] What is important is that our doctors and other public health workers, our medical ethicists, our more responsible civic and religious leaders, and our most competent legislators start to examine the clinical, social, and human aspects of this approaching dilemma, and arrive at a published consensus about how to deal with it while there is still time.

In most states, people cannot be issued marriage licenses until they present clinical laboratory certificates showing that they do not have syphilis. Could the same states be persuaded to add a medical certificate of vaccination against gonorrhea as an equally mandatory requirement?

There are certain well-defined high-risk populations that might be considered target groups for vaccination. The men and women in our armed forces constitute one such group, and for good military defense reasons, they will probably be the first American subpopulation to be fully protected by federal programs for making maximum use of the new gonorrhea vaccines in the military services. However, attention should be directed to nonmilitary groups, like food handlers; doctors, nurses, ward clerks, hospital porters, and other occupations and professions that deal with hospital patients; prisoners and prison guards; children's nurses and governesses; college students living away from home; and scores of other specific age and social groups at greater than average risk of getting gonorrhea and carrying and/or transmitting its causal bacteria to others. Do we declare vaccinations against gonorrhea mandatory, or merely advisory but voluntary, or do we rule gonorrhea vaccinations mandatory for these and other demonstrably high-risk subpopulations?

From 10 percent to 15 percent of men and women treated and cured of gonorrhea sooner or later turn up with reinfections. Penicillin can cure but not prevent gonorrhea. It would probably be clinically and socially prudent to vaccinate all people who are medically treated for gonorrhea, whether in free public clinics or in private doctors' offices. An excellent case can be made for the legally mandated immunization of all those with verified gonorrhea. An equally good case can also be made against compulsory vaccination of people who catch the disease because there is no equally binding legislation mandating the compulsory vaccination of all other classes of unimmunized Americans.

Most people would probably have no moral objections to vaccinations against gonorrhea and other venereal diseases. However, there is a large, vocal, and politically very powerful group that sees sexually transmitted diseases as heaven-ordained punishments for the moral transgressions of sinners. During World War II, Winston Churchill and his generals in North Africa had to deal with British representation of this viewpoint in 1943 when penicillin was still scarce, and the moral guardians wondered, in letters to Parliament, "Why were all the gallant wounded men unable to have penicillin, while some scallywags received it to relieve them of the discomforts their own indiscretions had brought on them?"[21]

It is quite possible that in our times, in this country, the well-organized defenders of perceived morality will oppose the waste of government funds because it is immoral to protect those who sin against the consequences of their own indiscretions. Like their zealous forebears in the 1920s who succeeded in some states in making it illegal to teach the Darwinian theory of variation, natural selection, and evolution—the core theory of modern biology

460

and genetics—the politically more potent legatees cannot be ignored in the formation of national and state policies dealing with gonorrhea vaccinations.

The self-annointed guardians of national morality aside, there are some very fundamental moral and civic imperatives involved. For example, is it moral or immoral, fiscally prudent or fiscally reckless, to provide or deny lifelong immunization against gonorrhea to the millions (perhaps the majority)[22] of young people who, before, during, and after marriage, lead very active sex lives that result in upward of four million cases of gonorrhea annually in themselves, their sex partners, and their infants and young children? This is not a question of whether their parents, communities, churches, and peers approve or disapprove of their sexual practices and preferences. In an America where by 1976, "A national survey of college students showed that the rates of premarital coitus were 74% for both sexes," and where in the same year, "The proportion of sexually experienced never-married women who had had more than one sex partner increased from 38.5% in 1971 to 49.9% in 1976,"[23] these realities prevailed despite our personal feeling about their desirability or morality.

What really matters is that since the end of World War II—itself a major cause of current American patterns of behavior, including sexuality—while antibacterial drugs made gonorrhea 100 percent curable, it rose from being the third to the leading reported notifiable disease in the United States. Reported cases showed more than a threefold increase, from 313,363 reported cases in 1945 to 1,003,959 in 1979. Between 1956 and 1979, the case rate of reported gonorrhea cases again rose threefold, from 136 per 100,000 population to 460 per 100,000—and reported cases are estimated by different experts to add up to between one tenth and one half of all actual cases annually.

Given the development of one or more vaccines that can prevent gonorrhea as effectively as earlier vaccines were able to prevent other once major crippling and killing diseases of children and adults, there is no good reason that would interfere with the new gonorrhea vaccines' eradicating the disease in this country within a decade of the start of their intelligent use. Once safe and effective vaccines become available, the only reasons for the persistence of gonorrhea would be societal, not clinical.

The eradication of epidemic and endemic gonorrhea by the subunit and, most probably, the combined antigen vaccines can quite predictably trigger a devastating syphilis epidemic in this and most other technically advanced countries on four continents.

Syphilis is much more damaging and lethal than gonorrhea. In the preantibiotic 1930s and 1940s, United States deaths from syphilis averaged 15,000 to 20,000 per year. Before World War II, there was one death for every five to ten cases reported to local health departments. Thanks solely to antibiotics, syphilis deaths are now down to 300 per year.

Psychoses due to syphilis of the brain (paresis) are down 98 percent

461

since 1942, again thanks to penicillin and other antibiotics. In 1941, 10 percent of all institutionalized mental patients had psychoses due to paresis; in that year there were 8,083 such patients. In 1979 only 162 patients with syphilitic psychoses were admitted to hospitals in this country. Nevertheless, despite the 98 percent reduction in admissions for syphilitic psychoses, the cost of maintaining patients with paresis now comes to over $60 million per year in the United States.

The cruelest of all forms of the disease is congenital syphilis, acquired by the developing fetus in the womb of a gestating mother who is syphilitic. When this venereal infection occurs early in the pregnancy, it usually causes death to the fetus and spontaneous abortion. This occurs in at least 30 percent of cases. When fetuses are well along their genetically programmed development from microscopic zygotes to fully formed infants, and are born with congenital syphilis, many are very lucky: They are born dead or die within a few hours of birth. Children with congenital syphilis enter the postnatal world suffering from a constellation of skin, central nervous system, bone, liver, lung, kidney, and other organic disorders that range from blindness and deafness to brain and severe neurological damages. Few survive the first months of life; those who do enter upon a course of living death that prior to penicillin was a mercifully short one. Before penicillin there was no way to spare the child of a syphilitic mother. Penicillin administered to the infected mother throughout her pregnancy can protect the growing child *in utero* against the syphilis germs she sheds that pass the placental barrier.

In 1941 in this country, 17,600 infants were born with congenital syphilis—at a rate of 13.4 cases per 100,000 live births. By 1979 there were only 331 infants born with congenital syphilis—at a rate of 0.2 cases per 100,000 live births. This was still 331 too many, for each child born with congenital syphilis was tragic testimony to the total lack of medical care during each pregnancy. It was also, however, a 6,600 percent reduction in the yearly incidence of congenital syphilis over a period of thirty-eight years. Trendy people who write didactic books on doctors and medicines being the major causes of all diseases, and on the healthier vistas for humankind beyond the obsolete Magic Bullet barrier, might pause and review abundantly available twentieth-century data on congenital syphilis before they write their next books on modern therapeutics.[24]

In absolute numbers, in the United States reported cases of syphilis of all stages fell from 485,560 (or a rate of 368 per 100,000 population) in 1949 to 67,049 (or 30.7 per 100,000 population). This twelvefold drop since 1941 is completely attributable to the efficacy of antibiotic drugs against the syphilis spirochete.

Despite the well-established fact that syphilis is as much a product of the prostitution industry as gonorrhea, why have reported cases of syphilis of all stages continued to decline since the end of World War II, while reported and actual cases of gonorrhea soared to first place on the official lists of all reported notifiable diseases? The reason is well known to every doctor.

The different strains of *N. gonorrhoeae* have an average incubation period of two to seven days, during which the telltale symptoms of gonorrhea begin to plague the victims. The bacterium of syphilis, *T. pallidum,* requires an average incubation period of twenty-one to forty-two days. Not until this incubation period ends, and the now mature syphilis spirochetes cause the soft chancres that are the first clinical signs of the disease, is the infected individual aware that he or she is harboring a slowly incubating syphilis organism.

Both the gonorrhea and syphilis germs are equally susceptible to being killed by the same antibacterial drugs. In many instances people who get gonorrhea are never aware that during the same sexual encounter they also caught an incipient syphilis infection, which was terminated by the penicillin or other antibiotics used to treat and cure their gonorrhea once the first symptoms of clap appeared. As Dr. Ivan Bennett observed some years ago, "Incipient syphilis is usually aborted in the early stages of the disease by penicillin given for concurrent gonorrhea." Bennett added that the widespread use of antibiotics to treat streptococcal, staphylococcal, and other bacterial infections since 1945 has also aborted incipient cases of syphilis and helped reduce the reported incidence of all forms of that disease.

Even if gonorrhea was eradicated by a sensible and honestly administered national immunization program, people would still continue to use and even overuse antibiotics in huge quantities, and many a case of incipient syphilis would continue to be absorbed by antibacterial drugs taken for concurrent but nongonococcal infections. These antibiotics, for example, are now being administered not only for gonococcal urethritis and more complicated cases of disseminated gonorrhea, but also for nongonococcal urethritis (NGU), and for postgonococcal urethritis (PGU), which "occurs when urethritis recurs after successful treatment for gonorrhea. PGU probably represents co-infection with other organisms at the time gonorrhea is acquired. The micro-organisms that cause both NGU and PGU are resistant to penicillin," advise the federal government's Centers for Disease Control (CDC). These penicillin-resistant bacteria and mycoplasma are treatable with tetracycline, a widely used inexpensive antibiotic that also acts against the syphilis spirochetes.

Unlike gonorrhea and syphilis, neither forms of nongonococcal urethritis are legally notifiable venereal diseases. Therefore, where it is possible to make some fact-based estimates of the number of gonorrhea infections actually contracted in this country every year, at this writing it is quite impossible even to roughly estimate the approximate numbers of NGU and PGU suffered. In fact, reported numbers only add to the confusion.

The 1980 CDC survey of seven selected municipal venereal disease clinics showed that in this cross-sectional sample of 132,777 free-clinical visits in seven different cities, NGU was diagnosed in 19.4 percent of the male patients, and in only 0.3 percent of the female patients, for a grand total of 13.4 percent of all the free-clinic patients examined. By startling contrast, the same federal government's National Center for Health Statistics (NCHS) survey of a large national sample of office visits to private physicians by paying patients showed that in 1975 and 1976, yearly averages of 533,900 male private patients and 715,000 female private patients were described by their physicians as having had NGU during each of those two years. These figures would indicate that in 1976 private, fee-paying patients suffered a total of 1,248,900 cases of nongonococcal urethritis, while during the same year, private and free-clinic patients combined had 1,001,994 reported cases of gonococcal urethritis, or frank gonorrhea.

These differences between free-clinic patients and fee-paying private patients—particularly women—hardly mean that people who can afford to pay for their own medical care are more likely to catch nongonococcal urethritis and other nonnotifiable forms of venereal disease than less affluent fellow citizens treated in the free VD clinics. These differentials possibly have considerably more to do with private patients' fears of the social and personal consequences of having their venereal diseases reported to local health departments than to any evolutionary or biological differences between paying and nonpaying VD patients.

The huge amounts of antibiotics now being used against nonvenereal, venereal, notifiable, and nonnotifiable bacterial infections will abort enough cases of slow-incubating, incipient syphilis to guarantee against a return to the pre-antibiotic-era levels of the disease.

The latest annual government survey of drugs most frequently used in private, office-based medical practice reveals that 13.3 percent of all prescriptions written by nonhospital-based doctors in 1980 were for antibiotic drugs—or an estimated ninety million prescriptions. The majority of all drug prescriptions, however, have for over a decade been written by hospital- and clinic-based physicians. This would bring the total number of antibiotic prescriptions per year to at least 180 million, enough to dose over 85 percent of our entire population. However, not all of the patients for whom these prescriptions were written were sexually active or carriers of occult or asymptomatic incubating syphilis germ colonies.[25]

Nevertheless, should a good gonorrhea vaccine succeed in either eradicating or massively reducing the case rate of gonorrhea in our times, it would be lunacy to ignore the possibility that in the absence of the present levels of antibiotics used to treat gonorrhea, there could be a formidable increase in the new cases of primary, secondary, and end stages of syphilis. This is particularly true of those cases of syphilis acquired from prostitutes along with gonorrhea, but which are terminated before they mature by antibiotics used to cure the much earlier active gonorrhea infection.

There are enough hard epidemiological and bacteriological data now in hand to enable the U.S. Public Health Service and its constituent agencies, as well as cooperating state and municipal health departments, to make some clinically useful projections of just how far-reaching this revival of syphilis as a major health problem might become. Given such base lines, work can begin on the formulation of practical public health policies to cope with the predictable rise in reported and actual cases.

None of these sanitary, treatment, sexual contact tracing, and other public health measures, however, can be lasting substitutes for what is most needed to fight syphilis and a host of other diseases and disorders. That need can be met only by long-range educational and training programs that could lead eventually to highly trained young investigators who can develop still missing basic knowledge about the natural history of *T. pallidum,* required so that at long last syphilis spirochetes can be grown in laboratory cultures and thus probably open the way to vaccines against syphilis.

Some of these trainable young people are presently in college or in medical school. Some are in high school. Most are just entering kindergarten or maybe they are a little older, learning the first rudiments of biology or chemistry or physics or mathematics. It is when these children are very young, during the first six or seven years of schooling, that education counts most. For in those years they are not taught how to become life scientists, or statesmen who can prevent life-destroying and demeaning wars and depressions, or poets and artists who help us know our worlds, or teachers of the young, or lawyers or engineers. Or computer programmers or bus drivers or ditchdiggers. They are taught how to think for themselves, how to use books and libraries, how to pursue the interests that good schools and good teachers help them develop. The special education and training that produce competent professionals are also crucially important, but not nearly as important as the quality of the general elementary education that equips children to learn and introduces them to the world of higher studies.

An education that makes science and all other aspects of our culture the legacy of young people should begin early and must continue through and beyond graduate school. It has to be good, and it has to be availble to all children of all socioeconomic classes. Until the Vietnam War era and the Arab oil boycott, we had a number of such school systems in place, developing talents of young people in several states and cities. The school systems of California, New York, and Tulsa, Oklahoma, come to mind, and I know there were others of equal worth to their pupils and to the nation. The raging fiscal inflation that followed the costly military interventions in Indochina, plus the oil cartel's successful adventure in extortion, bankrupted America's school systems and left them in shambles.

Educational systems from kindergarten through graduate school, eroded by inflation and its political consequences, are being dismembered by government order and government policies, not only for budgetary but also for profoundly ideological reasons. Education, in our angry and malignantly anti-intellectual times, has become expendable. As surely as day follows night, this phase of our republic's history too shall pass, but by then considerable and lasting damage will have been caused, and many lives needlessly ended by ultimately preventable diseases like syphilis.

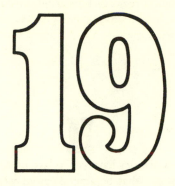

THE FUTURE OF VACCINES: NEVER BRIGHTER, NEVER DARKER

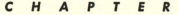

There is a moral obligation to be intelligent. Ignorance is a vice, and when it results in injury to anyone it becomes a crime, a moral if not a statutory one. To infect another with disease, either directly or indirectly, as a result of ignorance, is an immoral act. The purpose of government is to protect its citizens, and a government which fails to shelter its citizens against infections is neither intelligent nor moral.

—Victor C. Vaughan, Ph.D., M.D., President of the American Medical Association, 1915[1]

I don't think people are entitled to any services.

—David A. Stockman, Budget Director of the United States, 1981[2]

Historically, safe and effective vaccines against infectious diseases have yet to live up to the multiple potentials of induced immunizations that became apparent when smallpox variolation was supplanted by safe and effective, cross-reacting live cowpox virsus vaccine. Only about a dozen really useful vaccines against bacterial and viral diseases have been developed and put into general use in the nearly two centuries since Jenner.

Highly lethal mass contagions eradicated by vaccines—such as smallpox the world over, and diphtheria, and paralytic poliomyelitis in this and other rich countries—have a way of receding swiftly from the popular consciousness to the point where they become completely forgotten. There is nothing wrong with this; in fact, it is probably better for people to grow up without ever-present tragic reasons for having morbid fears of such once common major diseases. The danger however is that many people, particularly those who establish our national health and research priorities and government policies, have also forgotten—or worse, have never learned—the history of these mass diseases and of the inexpensive vaccines that rendered them extinct.

Jenner's vaccine converted smallpox from a purely clinical disease (for which in 1798 as today there were no medical cures) to a societal disorder, disseminated and/or prevented largely by the values and actions of certain societies. The smallpox vaccine was introduced early in the period when the Industrial Revolution created, seemingly overnight, high population densities in the new factory and mining towns as well as in rapidly industrializing older cities. This sudden crowding turned smallpox into an urban plague. Overcrowding, particularly where most factory workers and their families lived, became the major vehicle for the massive transmission of smallpox viruses from carriers to noninfected people. This overcrowding persisted for the rest of the nineteenth century, but not until 1871 did Jenner's native land make any serious efforts to introduce and really administer laws mandating the compulsory universal smallpox vaccination and providing free vaccines to accomplish this protection.

Before the vaccine was available, nearly everyone in England had smallpox during their childhood years, upward of half of them died of it, and most adults who survived had faces mildly or grotesquely pitted with permanent telltale pocks. In 1769, in the first edition of his classic *Domestic Medicine,* William Buchan wrote that in England and Scotland one in every two newborn infants failed to survive the first year of life. Smallpox was not the only reason for the 50 percent infant mortality rate in pre-Jennerian England and Scotland; it was simply the most deadly of the major contagions responsible for this carnage.

More than eighty years later, when despite the moral paralysis of Parliament many (but not enough) people in England had been vaccinated against smallpox, Charles Dickens wrote that as of 1852, one in every three coffins in London "was made for a little child: a child that has not yet two figures to its age. Although science had advanced, although [smallpox] vaccination has been discovered and brought into general use [albeit neither universal nor compulsory], although medical knowledge is tenfold greater than it was fifty years ago, we still do not gain more than a diminution of two percent in the terrible mortality among children." Smallpox was still endemic in Dickens's England; two decades later the Manchester physician William Henry Barlow noted that "two out of every three persons applying for relief to the Hospital for the Indigent Blind owed their loss of sight to smallpox."

To one degree or another, similar lags between development and maximum utilization of the essential vaccines that followed Jenner's smallpox vaccine have marked the history of world human health since 1798. To this day, smallpox remains the sole vaccine-preventable major contagion to have been completely eradicated from this planet by the proper universal use of a vaccine. Other equally vaccine-preventable major diseases, such as measles, diphtheria, and paralytic poliomyelitis—while controlled or virtually wiped out by mass vaccination in the United States, England, most European countries and Japan—remain endemic and continue to plague, cripple, and kill millions of children in the poor countries of Asia, Africa, and Latin America, where most of this world's people live.

In the United States—birthplace of the diphtheria, polio, measles, mumps, and rubella vaccines—over one third of our infants and very young children have not been immunized against any of the major infections for which good vaccines are available. Children are at their maximum risk of catching these vaccine-preventable diseases during their first two years of life—and not after they enter school at age six.

Antibacterial drugs have reduced but far from eliminated both the deaths and the permanent brain, lung, heart, eye, ear, kidney and central nervous system damages that are only too often caused by curable infections like pneumococcal pneumonia, strep throat, and cerebrospinal meningitis. We still have no systemic drugs which, like the antibiotics, act against virus diseases from polio and measles to the common cold. The prevention of all serious infectious diseases, by social improvements, by vaccines, or most preferably by combinations of both, would be still better for the human condition—and the federal budget—than curing them by good drugs.

Since the end of World War II, scientific workers here and around the world have launched an exciting new era in vaccine development. The father of all bacterial vaccines, Louis Pasteur, dreamed of what he called "chemical vaccines" made not of whole bacteria but of chemicals found in bacterial cell structures and produced by the bacteria themselves. In our times, this dream is being realized, not only in preparations against bacterial infections but against diseases caused by viruses too small to be seen under the most powerful microscopes of the Pasteur generations.

Although there have been some spectacular exceptions, the thrust has been toward the development of vaccines made only of immunogenic subunits of bacteria and viruses that can cause neither the diseases they contain nor any of the endotoxic, rheumatogenic, nephritogenic, or other adverse side effects which many whole-organism or whole-virion vaccines are theoretically capable of inducing. Some physicians, immunochemists, and medical microbiologists are not afraid to write about a feasible "supervaccine" against all or nearly all infectious diseases. "Theoretically, it should be possible to prepare a multivalent capsular polysaccharide vaccine for all common invasive bacterial organisms," John B. Robbins and an international array of prominent investigators wrote in 1977.[3]

However, these and other vaccine research scientists are more involved in coming to grips with the human and economic consequences of not having any available vaccines to protect against the streptococci, the staphylococci, the principal agents of otitis media and bacterial meningitis in infants and very young children, the bacterial and viral venereal diseases, the bacterial and viral gastrointestinal and diarrheal diseases, and the Gram-negative bacteria, which have emerged fairly recently as major causes of an entirely new major disease category, hospital-acquired, or nosocomial, infections, which presently kill over 100,000 in this country alone.

Many of the major infections for which vaccines are urgently needed, like the Gram-negative diseases, are new to their present eminence in the vital statistics of this and other industrial nations. Others, like the venereal diseases, are older than European and American civilizations. To one degree or another, each of the old and new infections that demand vaccines to prevent them are products of technological, socioeconomic, anthropological, and historical changes that, for known but very ill-conceived reasons, are not normally considered the province of the health community.

The patterns of historical, economic, military, geographic, and political changes that controlled the introduction and spread of smallpox from Asia Minor to Europe, and from Europe to the Western Hemisphere, as well as the patterns of uses and nonuses of Jenner's smallpox vaccine in many nations starting with England, are paralleled by the changing attack rates and controls of major diseases in this country in recent years. Some of the factors that contribute to either the increase or decline of the major infectious diseases are very well known. Many of the more important infectious disease factors or cofactors are not usually perceived in terms of their negative or positive roles in human health.

Consider, for example, only the following three of many recent major environmental and historical changes.

1. The Tandem Rise of Gram-Negative Bacterial Infections and Hospital-Acquired (Nosocomial) Infections

Because of their different cell-wall chemical structures, bacteria have been divided into two easily differentiated groups: the Gram-positive bacteria, which can be stained by using the method developed by the Danish bacteriologist Christian Gram in 1875, and the Gram-negative organisms, whose cell walls do not accept the Gram stains. Both groups cause human diseases.

The Gram-positive bacteria are the agents of gas gangrene and of most but not all bacterial pneumonias, and include the ubiquitous and massively destructive hemolytic streptococci and the even more numerous staphylococci that between them cause many infections and inflammations, some fatal, including septicemia, endocarditis, osteomyelitis, carbuncles, boils, cystitis, pyelitis, post-streptococcal nephritis, St. Vitus' dance, and rheumatic fever.

Many of the Gram-negative bacteria, including the agents of gonorrhea, syphilis, *Haemophilus influenzae* meningitis and otitis, gastroenteritis, dysentery, and whooping cough, have been infecting our species for many years. Some Gram-negative bacteria, such as *Escherichia coli,* historically caused only water-borne diseases until a number of medical and social advances after World War II turned them into major pathogens. These advances included the intravenous blood-pressure monitor, in which a recording catheter inserted and kept for days on end in the veins of patients with hypertension and other conditions provide their nurses and doctors with a means of instantly detecting life-threatening blood-pressure changes in many of the critically ill. Medical advances also included new anticancer drugs, which after about 1960 have routinely been used in the treatment of leukemias, lymphomas, and various other cancers. The drugs kept people from dying of cancer, but they had to be used with immune suppressants, or were themselves immune suppressants, and thus the identical life-saving cancer drugs exposed patients to previously harmless and generally Gram-negative microbial agents which their own immune systems normally cleared from their bodies.

The most important of the changes that significantly altered American infectious disease patterns was congressional passage of the Social Security Act of 1965. Titles XIX (Medicaid, for the medically indigent working and welfare poor) and XX (Medicare, for all people aged sixty-five and over) of that landmark act made hospital care available at little or even no direct cost for millions of poor and near-poor people who could never afford it before. Between 1966 and 1974, United States hospital admissions climbed from a rate of 146 per 1,000 population to 159.2 in 1974, up 9.04 percent. In absolute numbers, total hospital discharges climbed from 29 million in 1965 to 37 million in 1976, a gain of 27.59 percent.

The post-1965 class of new hospital patients were mainly poor people. As the NCHS observed in its first few annual reports to the President and the Congress on the state of the nation's health, "Poor people in families with low incomes are hospitalized more often, and once hospitalized remain in hospital longer than people in families with higher incomes." Historically, the hospitalized and nonhospitalized poor here and in other countries have always been more subject to community- and hospital-acquired infections than the better-fed, better-housed, and better medically cared for subpopulations. The poor have carried larger numbers of community-acquired infectious diseases to the hospitals than more affluent inpatients, and once in the hospitals the poor patients were, in turn, far less resistant to nosocomial (hospital-acquired) infections than the better-nourished patients.

A well-regarded CDC study of infections in the United States, directed by Dr. Richard E. Dixon and published in 1978, disclosed that "each year, over 3 million community-acquired infections require persons to be hospitalized, and over 2 million nosocomial infections are acquired. Approximately 90% of the infections treated in hospitals are bacterial. These infections account for an estimated 29 million days of acute hospital care, which is approximately 10% of the patient days in U.S. acute-care hospitals. The direct hospitalization costs for treating infectious diseases are estimated to be over $4.8 billion."

At $5 billion plus a year, the annual costs of hospital treatments of infectious diseases continue to exceed by far, in a single year, the total educational, laboratory, and clinical expenses of developing a good vaccine over the course of twenty years.

2. The Decline and Decay of Old and New Water Systems

The nineteenth-century epidemics of water-borne diseases, from cholera and typhoid fever to dysentery and other diarrheal disorders, that menaced European and American economic development as much as they decimated human lives, saw every major American city, and many thousands of smaller communities, invest local and regional tax dollars in safe drinking water systems and safe human waste disposal systems. There is no question that had these hygienic necessities not been constructed in Europe and the United States, the Industrial Revolution would have been sunk by fecally contaminated waters.

In this country some of the new drinking water systems were built and operated by private water companies in the nineteenth and early twentieth centuries, and are still in business. Most of them were built by cities, counties, and even states. Many larger systems were built and continue to be operated by government agencies, as were and are all the sewage and waste disposal systems constructed to keep city streets, streams, and drinking water reservoirs free of human and animal fecal matter and other disease-causing contaminants.

Here, as in Europe, these new systems eradicated or nearly eliminated various infectious diseases caused by water-borne pathogens. (The rest of the world is not so fortunate; most people live in countries where diarrhea, caused by *E. coli* delivered via human excrement to streams, rivers, lakes, and other sources of drinking water not protected against such contamination, is a major cause of infant and child deaths, and where typhoid fever, cholera, and bacterial dysentery are still endemic.)

Had American sanitary installations been maintained and expanded, drinking water and sewage systems would still be as effective in the maintenance of good health as when they were constructed generations ago. Time, and various historical cycles of wars, depressions, and inflation, have caused thousands of water systems built before World War II to decay and become wholesale delivery systems for microbial disease agents.

Legislation passed during the environment-conscious 1960s and 1970s set new and medically sensible clean water and clean air standards. Most of the regulatory legislation dealing with the safety of drinking water is now and for some years has been unenforced, owing to inflation-magnified costs and abundantly financed and well-orchestrated crusades against environmental protection and all other regulations dealing with health and human welfare. We were told that once we got the federal government and its regulatory agencies off our backs, the gates of paradise would open for us all. We are now getting the government's environmental safety agencies off our backs, and receiving in return *E. coli, Salmonella, Shigella, Giardia,* and other water-borne pathogens in our guts.

Water-borne infections are coming back in force in a nation where adequate water systems and well-enforced water safety standards had come very close to eradicating them only a few decades ago. Thanks primarily to the spreading physical decline of American urban and regional water systems, salmonellosis—a diarrheal infection caused by some of the nontyphoid *Salmonella* species found in drinking water—has now overtaken tuberculosis as the second most commonly reported bacterial disease in the United States. Only gonorrhea is reported more frequently.[4] However, according to Dr. David

W. Fraser, until recently head of the special pathogens branch of the CDC, "the similarity of rates is largely illusory, since only about one percent of all non-typhoid cases of Salmonellosis are actually reported." This would put the actual cases of salmonellosis in the United States at considerably more than three million per year.

By the time Fraser made these observations in 1980, CDC and foreign field studies were suggesting that another bacterium, Campylobacter jejuni, transmitted in contaminated food and water, is now quite possibly responsible for more enteric infections in this country than either the *Salmonella* species or *Shigella,* the bacteria of shigellosis, or bacillary dysentery. *Campylobacter* are very interesting organisms, which until recently had been known primarily for the multimillion-dollar losses they cause by inducing spontaneous abortions in cattle and sheep. The *Campylobacter jejuni* subspecies causes enteritis marked by explosive diarrhea in people.

In 1977 Dr. M. B. Skirrow, acting director of the Public Health Laboratory in Worcester, England, described *Campylobacter* enteritis as a "new" disease after he isolated *C. jejuni* organisms from the feces of 7.1 percent (fifty-seven) of 803 patients with explosive diarrhea. During the same investigation, his assistants were unable to isolate any *Campylobacter* organisms from 194 healthy community controls. Skirrow's investigation showed that in addition to being transmitted by contaminated water and food, campylobacteriosis was transmitted from children to parents, and from dogs and other pets to whole families.[5]

Skirrow was careful to put quotation marks around the word "new," because he had good historical and epidemiological reasons to suspect what is generally believed today—namely, that enteritis due to *Campylobacter* is neither new nor rare but is actually a newly diagnosed and quite common old disease.

The largest prospective medical study of the prevalence of this water- and food-borne bacterium in the United States, conducted in Denver by Drs. Martin Blaser, Wen-Lan Wang, and their associates, examined the stools of 2,670 healthy adults, starting in 1978. As of 1980 they had isolated *Campylobacter jejuni* from the feces of 4.6 percent of these healthy volunteers, *Salmonella* from 3.5 percent, and *Shigella* from 2.9 percent. During the entire year of 1979, the Mayo Clinic Laboratories in Minnesota examined the stools of 1,953 patients who either had enteric symptoms or who had been traveling abroad. *Campylobacter jejuni* organisms were found in 3.4 percent of all fecal samples cultured, while *Salmonella* and *Shigella* combined were isolated in only 1.3 percent of these close to 2,000 human stools. A more recent joint study of 185 consecutive healthy adult fecal cultures, conducted in San Francisco's Mt. Zion and General Hospitals, isolated *C. jejuni* from 5.4 percent of all samples, *Salmonella* from 2.4 percent, and *Shigella* from 4.3 percent.[6]

Ideally, the best way to prevent *Campylobacter* and other water-borne infections would be to enforce all presently ignored federal, state and local laws and regulations governing the safety of drinking water and human waste disposal systems. Since nothing of the sort is about to happen in this decade, or possibly even in this generation, it becomes incumbent upon all levels of government to develop, and put into clinically indicated uses, good vaccines against campylobacteriosis, *E. coli* enteritis, salmonellosis, and shigellosis.

Live- and killed-organism vaccines against campylobacteriosis in sheep and cattle are presently being used, with mixed results and, at times, no results.[7] A toxic lipopolysaccharide (LPS) from one of the *Campylobacter* subspecies that attack animals was isolated in Australia as long ago as 1959, and it is perhaps theoretically possible that similar endotoxins exist on the surfaces of *Campylobacter jejuni* organisms—and that this LPS can be detoxified to produce a safe and effective vaccine for human immunizations.

One thing is certain: Given the deteriorating state of this country's drinking water systems, water-borne and food-borne bacterial and viral enteritis will grow worse, not better, in the foreseeable future.

3. Fiscal Inflation and Its Continuum of Adverse Health Effects

Vastly increased incidences of venereal diseases are not the only adverse health effects of major wars between nations. There are also the classic wartime plagues, from smallpox and typhus to typhoid and malaria, influenza, pneumonia, and tuberculosis. There was and is still the primary adverse health effect of most wars—fiscal inflation.

The statesmen who make wars the inevitable consequences of their blunders do not lead their nations into military conflagrations in order to create inflation at home, any more than the religious leaders who mounted the four Holy Crusades in the Middle Ages did so in order to make certain that smallpox would be brought back from the Levant in volumes great enough to make it endemic in Europe. Inflation is as devastating to the health of nations as smallpox and any of the other classic plagues exacerbated and disseminated by wars through the centuries.

In affluent industrial nations, inflation broadens the socioeconomic base of preventable diseases, so that the traditional legacy of deficiency and vaccine-preventable infectious diseases of poverty and near-poverty start to make vast inroads into the skilled blue-collar and supervisory white-collar classes, the fixed-income classes (teachers, engineers, lawyers, auditors, and other civil-service professionals), owners of small businesses and others who a generation ago, on the eve of the current fiscal inflation, were termed the middle-class-income population.

Health is the most valuable commodity that family income can buy. As the real purchasing power of the dollar is decreased by inflation, the costs of what the previous century called the necessaries of health—food, housing, clothing, preventive and curative medical care—climb to beyond the ability of more and more putatively middle-class families to pay.

The Consumer Price Index (CPI), compiled by the federal government, measures the purchasing power of the dollar as compared with what it was in an arbitrarily selected base year. The current CPI base year is 1967, a year in which the inflation caused by the economic costs of the Vietnam War was already a half-dozen years old.

To review the rise in the CPI since 1960 is to clarify the reasons why socially and vaccine-preventable infectious diseases have been increasing in middle-class families. What cost $100.00 for an average item in 1967 dollars one could have bought for only $88.70 in 1960, before inflation raised the average cost of all items to $266.60 in 1981. In 1960 the American dollar would have purchased for $79.10 the same amount of medical care that cost $100.00 in 1967. After fourteen more years of continuing fiscal inflation, the purchasing power of the dollar was so eroded that the same amount of medical care costing $79.10 in 1967 cost, as of May 1981, $286.60, an increase of 262 percent since 1960. During the same two decades, the actual costs of food and housing, in constant 1967 dollars, increased by 201 percent and 211 percent respectively.

Prior to this generation of fiscal inflation, the not exactly spontaneous post-World War II abandonment of electrified commuter and street railways[8] left most American families with no alternatives to family cars for their necessary daily transportation. Even before the Arab oil boycott of 1973–1974 quadrupled and, in some cities, quintupled retail gasoline prices, inflation had been making the purchase of a car and car insurance and the maintenance costs of daily automobile use affordable only by reducing family expenditures on necessities like food, housing, and medical care. After the Arab oil boycott, the American family car became, in exponentially growing numbers, an economic incubus.

The sharp increases in food costs, felt only by the very poor at the start of the Vietnam War, were somewhat ameliorated by federal food-stamp and school breakfast and lunch programs, each of which distributed surplus foods to the poor and near poor. In time, as food prices doubled and trebled, family nourishment became increasingly inadequate for millions of American blue-collar and white-collar families whose incomes were too high to make them eligible (or "truly needy") to receive food stamps or school lunches for their children, but at the same time were much too low to meet their minimal nutritional needs. In 1981 these federal food programs were the first to be slashed or abandoned to help pay the costs of the soaring new military expansion budget.

In millions of families who at the start of the decades of fiscal inflation were able to afford regular private family and pediatric medical care, inflation that more than halved the purchasing power of their dollars priced such regular services out of their reach. Historically, one of the first casualties of fiscal inflation is preventive medical care, and our times have proved no exception to this rule.

This was nowhere better demonstrated than in the treatment and prevention of infectious diseases, particularly in children between the ages of one and four, the group at highest risk of contracting otitis media and streptococcal infections—for which no vaccines existed as of 1982—and the seven devastating infections for which good vaccines are now available: diphtheria, tetanus, pertussis (whooping cough), polio, measles, mumps, and rubella.

When diagnosed and treated in time with appropriate and sufficient antibiotics, otitis media, streptococcal infections, and many other bacterial diseases are curable with a minimum of severe and often permanently adverse postinfection damage. The longer the fiscal inflation and its interacting consequences persisted, the more both the start and the duration of medical care for such infections in infants, young children, and adults were delayed and reduced.

The American Academy of Pediatrics (AAP) issues a periodically revised recommended schedule of immunizations. Based on purely clinical reasons, this schedule calls for immunizations with available vaccines to start at the age of two months and within the first six months of an infant's life, to include three doses each of the DTP vaccine (the combined vaccine for diphtheria, tetanus, and pertussis) and the trivalent oral poliovirus vaccine (TOPV). At twelve months, the child should receive immunizations against measles, mumps, and rubella (which are also provided in a single vaccine against all three viruses). Third or fourth booster doses of DTP and TOPV should be given by the time the child is eighteen months old. The AAP schedule calls for children to be fully immunized against all seven diseases by the age of four, with fifth booster shots of DTP and TOPV to be given between the ages of four and six, when the children enter school.[9]

In families who can still afford the fairly low costs of this entire series over the prescribed preschool years, these immunizations are given routinely by pediatricians who attend to their children between birth and puberty.

A measure of how many families can and cannot afford these optimal immunizations courses before their children enter school is provided by the CDC's United States Immunization Survey. This survey reveals that in 1979 in American children at highest risk, 12,386,000 infants and young children between the ages of one and four, only 63.5 percent had been vaccinated against measles, 62.7 percent had been immunized against rubella, 65.4 percent had had the medically recommended three DTP doses, 59.1 percent had had the recommended three doses of polio vaccine, and 55.4 percent had had the mumps vaccine.

This survey, which was based on household interviews, found that measles infections were reported for 3.1 percent (or 383,966) of these infants and young children, and that 7.0 percent (or 867,020) had suffered rubella infections. The effects of these virus-preventable diseases on the children who contract them, in the case of measles, and on the fetuses of pregnant women

477

to whom rubella viruses are transmitted by children, are very well known. The dollar costs to families as well as to government agencies are far higher than the costs of buying and administering vaccines to prevent them.

The diminishing power of the consumer dollar, and the two decades of continually escalating prices of food, shelter, and health care, have had many other health effects. Seemingly endless inflation has forced the mothers of more than half of all children in the United States to take full-time jobs away from home in order to be able to help meet rising family food and clothing costs, home-mortgage payments, quadrupled home heating oil and gasoline costs, and even the costs of already seriously reduced medical and dental services. The stresses of these changes in the fabric of family life have also contributed to increases in the soaring divorce rates.

The entry of millions of mothers of infants and very young children into the job market has also resulted in the rise of multiple foci of infection that barely existed before the Vietnam War. These are the commercial day-care centers whose personnel feed, clean, change diapers, and shelter infants and preschool-age children of working two-parent and single-parent families. As of 1980, about eleven million preschool children were receiving some form of nonfamily day care. Some authorities estimate that an even greater number of children of working mothers are cared for in smaller and less structured groups run in the homes of women who supplement their families' incomes by caring for their neighbors' children. Most day-care centers are known to be at high risk of enteric infections, particularly among the one- and two-year-olds.

Of course, there are far fewer health risks in expensive day-care centers that offer one highly qualified teacher to every three or four infants and toddlers, and provide healthful and mentally stimulating care in safe settings. They are very costly to maintain, can accommodate only limited numbers of children, and of necessity must provide this good care at dollar costs beyond the reach of all but a tiny percentage of working mothers.

Concurrent with the increases in working mothers, the continuing decline in the live birthrate since 1957 has long since led to the abandonment of thousands of unused or underused public elementary and high schools, and to the placement of the remaining pupils in other community public schools. In many cities, these student transfers, plus inflation-caused cutbacks in the ratios of teachers to pupils, have led to much more crowded classrooms. Like the day-care centers, these classrooms become reservoirs of the agents of common infections.

These changes in infant and child environments add to public health pressures for increased research and development on vaccines against the infectious hepatitis virus, *Haemophilus influenzae*—the cause of most day-care-center outbreaks of bacterial meningitis around the nation—and, possibly above all others, the organisms causing Group A hemolytic streptococcal infections for otitis media.

478

The big problem is that the same inflation responsible for the huge increase in these infectious diseases is also in large measure responsible for the massive cutbacks in state and federal support for basic and clinical research necessary to develop such vaccines. These cutbacks in federal and local public funding have slowed vaccine developments since the American participation in the Vietnam War grew from a minor involvement in 1961 into an astronomically costly (in lives and dollars) military intervention by 1965.

Even in the absence of vaccines to prevent Group A streptococcal infections, it was possible during the past century to reduce the astronomical case incidences of these diseases to the merely gigantic case numbers of our times. The most common infection, streptococcal sore throat, is probably acquired more frequently and by more people than is our leading notifiable disease, gonorrhea. The not uncommon medical consequences of common strep throats include rheumatic fever, St. Vitus' dance (Sydenham's chorea), and poststreptococcal nephritis. The consequences of inadequately treated rheumatic fever include such rheumatic heart disorders as bacterial endocarditis, or inflammation of the endocardium and/or membranes of the heart valves, acute myocarditis, and congestive heart failure. Not the least of the clinical consequences of strep throats is that the same streptococci cause between 5 percent and 10 percent of all cases of otitis media in the United States. Surely the human race has few more murderous enemies than the ordinary strep throat and its causal agent.

The mechanisms by which the number of strep throats and their more serious secondary effects were reduced during the past century were not all medical modalities. They were based originally on increases in wages and other sources of family incomes, which in turn resulted in less crowding in family habitations, and in more and better food, clothing, heating, and medical care. Family incomes started to increase gradually for people in industrializing nations around the third quarter of the nineteenth century. In the late 1930s, the sulfa drugs, followed by penicillin and later by the many families of antibiotic drugs since penicillin, helped reduce strep throats, and their rheumatic fever, heart, and end-stage kidney disease consequences, to the point where the category "streptococcal sore throat and scarlet fever" ceased to be a notifiable disease entity in 1969.

In terms of legally and voluntarily reported cases in this century, the actual number of strep throats reported by treating physicians to their local health departments before and after 1969 amounted to no more than 5 percent to 10 percent of all cases. One reason for this has to do with Siltzbach's law: A minimal requirement for the diagnosis of any disease is a patient and a physician. Only physicians report notifiable diseases to their local health departments.[10]

In many countries most strep throats are not treated by physicians. In officially reported numbers, U.S. Public Health Service records show that in

479

1920, when our population was 106 million, 161,432 cases of strep throat and/or scarlet fever were reported, for a rate of 152 per 100,000 population. In 1944 after the sulfas, but a year before antibiotics were available for civilians—200,539 strep throat cases were reported, for a rate of 144 per 100,000 population. In 1945 (that September, antibiotics went civilian) the population was close to 145 million, among whom 185,570 (132 in every 100,000) were reported as having had either strep throats or scarlet fever. Five years later, when the 1950 population stood at 152 million, only 64,494 cases of strep throat and/or scarlet fever were reported, for a rate of 42 per 100,000.

After 1969 some physicians in a shrinking roster of states continued to report voluntarily the strep throats they treated. (By then, scarlet fever, a sequela of streptococcal sore throat, had been virtually eradicated by penicillin in this country.) During the last year of mandatory reporting of the disease, the records show that 450,008 cases of streptococcal sore throat and/or scarlet fever had been reported in the then population of 201 million, for a rate of 238 per 100,000. This increase in reported streptococcal infections was considered the product of better reporting by physicians rather than an increase in the actual number of strep throats. By 1979 physicians in only forty-one states voluntarily reported a total of 465,430 cases of streptococcal sore throat or scarlet fever in their patients, for a rate of 207 per 100,000 population in those forty-one states.

As early as 1930 J. Alison Glover, the chief medical officer of the British Ministry of Health, supported the medical thesis which held "that the incidence of acute rheumatism [acute rheumatic fever] increases directly with poverty, malnutrition, overcrowding, and bad housing.[11] Like all droplet infections, Group A streptococcal infections and their secondary effects became societal diseases, particularly after the development of antibacterial drugs. "In the many developing [poor] countries of this world, and among the poor of our own country, rheumatic fever persists as a major cause of heart disease," observes Dr. Lewis W. Wannamaker of the University of Minnesota. A study published in 1973 by two New York physicians showed that in the city's schools the acute rheumatic fever "incidence in the lowest income area was more than three times that in a high and middle income area" of the same city.[12]

In 1928 Rebecca Lancefield discovered that the surfaces of Group A streptococci were covered with fimbraelike bundles of proteins which she designated the M proteins. Later it was found that these M proteins of Group A streptococci—the organisms responsible for 95 percent of all throat and skin strep infections—are "surface antigens primarily responsible for the virulence of Group A streptococci by virtue of their unique antiphagocytic characteristic."[13] That is, the M proteins inhibit the leukocytes and other circulating phagocytes in the human immune system from engulfing and destroying Group A streptococci. The exact mechanisms by which the M proteins enable these streptococci to resist destruction by phagocytosis is not yet clearly understood. What is known is that, much like the somewhat different pili of the gonococci and other bacteria, the M proteins enable the Group A streptococci to attach and adhere to the human cells they infect.

In 1945 Dr. Philip I. Cavelti, at the University of California, found that the antibodies produced by patients with acute rheumatic fever against the specific antigens of the Group A streptococci involved proved to be antibodies to the human heart as well as to these bacteria. He reported that "these autoantibodies to heart are present during the early and most active stages of the disease and disappear when the rheumatic process becomes inactive.[14] Cavelti reported that in these studies, "The presence of autoantibodies to human heart has been demonstrated in 75% of a group of patients with acute rheumatic fever."

The concept of autoimmunity, in which diseases are caused when people are injured by their own antibodies, was proposed in 1901 by Paul Ehrlich. Ehrlich wrote that the human body is subject to disorders of the immune system to the serious or pathological extent that "one might be justified in speaking of a 'horror autotoxicus' of the organism."

Subsequent studies, by Melvin H. Kaplan at Harvard, by John Zabriskie, Maclyn McCarty, Earl Freimer and Vincent Fischetti at Rockefeller University, and by many other investigators elsewhere, showed that when laboratory animals were inoculated with Group A streptococci, "an antibody appears which binds to heart tissue," and that "this heart-reactive antibody (HRA) will also bind to skeletal muscle of vessel walls as well as preparations of sacrolemmal sheath of cardiac myofibers."[15] Many investigators since Cavelti have reported finding similar HRAs in the blood of patients with acute rheumatic fever.

"The antibodies to heart tissue in the patients with acute rheumatic fever and the detection of deposits of immunoglobulin [antibody] and complement in the myocardium [the cardiac muscle, or middle layer of the heart] of patients with rheumatic carditis suggest a possible autoimmune pathogenesis," Drs. Ivo van de Rijn, Zabriskie, and McCarty reported in 1977.[16] The killing and crippling diseases now classified as possibly immune diseases include—but only among those caused by the heart-reacting and smooth-muscle-reacting antibodies to Group A streptococci—acute rheumatic fever, the constellation of heart diseases caused by rheumatic fever, and poststreptococcal glomerulonephritis.

Reported cases of acute rheumatic fever declined in this country from 6,526 cases in 1956—the first year in which this post-streptococcal disease was made notifiable—to 1,865 cases in 1976, and to 629 cases by 1979. However, the National Center for Health Statistics also shows that in 1978 a total of 6,000 Americans, of whom 2,000 had active cases of rheumatic heart disease, received approximately 40,000 days of hospital care for rheumatic fever during the same year in which only 851 cases were actually reported by their doctors to local health departments. The only thing we really know about the numbers of actual cases of acute rheumatic fever suffered annually in this country is that they are grossly underreported.

In the world's less affluent nations, and particularly in the bone-poor countries of Asia, Latin America, and Africa, the actual numbers of post-streptococcal autoimmune heart and kidney diseases are simply unknown. However, there is no question that rheumatic fever, rheumatic heart disease, and post-streptococcal glomerulonephritis have become epidemics that ravage millions of poor people who, since the end of World War II, have been gravitating to their nations' larger cities in search of jobs and survival.[17]

Rheumatic heart disease "represents the main cause of death among school age children" in the world's poor countries, according to the World Health Organization. The same WHO study also noted that the incidence of rheumatic fever in the "Western [industrial] countries started long before sulfonamides and penicillin were used for the treatment and prevention of these [streptococcal] infections. This decrease has been attributed to improved socioeconomic conditions, elimination of overcrowding, development of physical barriers to the spread of streptococci, and possibly also improved nutrition. Although health policy-makers in developing [poor] countries should keep in mind these factors, for a long time to come they will have to rely on medical approaches in those places associated with a high risk of streptococcal infection and rheumatic fever."[18]

The WHO recommended that medical approaches begin with "preventing the occurrence of first attacks through very large [penicillin] treatment coverage of streptococcal infections, even though only 0.3 to 3.0% of these infections will result in rheumatic fever," and also include the development of "a wide infrastructure for health care delivery and adequate diagnostic facilities for identifying streptococcal throat infections." Both medical recommendations look fine in cold print, but somewhat close to wildly utopian when one thinks of carrying them out in, say, Guatemala, Egypt, Bangladesh, Somalia, and fifty or sixty other poor nations, let alone most American states and major cities in the current post-Vietnam-War-inflation era.

The burgeoning human tragedy of the consequences of not having the economic or professional resources to keep common, easily curable strep throats from being the main cause of death in school-age children in the majority of poor countries is in itself reason enough to speed the development and universal utilization of safe and effective vaccines against Group A streptococci. For those national policymakers who demand more "practical" reasons for such an investment, there is always the historical lesson that such worldwide misery is pathognomonic of the communism against which we are now arming ourselves to the teeth and supporting a massive military build-up at the expense of the billions of dollars formerly allocated to fund health, education, and basic and applied clinical-research programs.

Before the First World War, when nobody was aware that by 1981 over seventy types of Group A streptococci would be identified—and as well as nearly as large a number of discrete but untyped other strains—killed whole-organism vaccines, based on the opsonic therapy concepts of Almroth Wright, were in wide use around the world. These vaccines, made of heat-killed but untyped cultures of streptococci originally isolated from sick people, were used in both opsonic therapy and the prevention of acute rheumatic fever, scarlet fever, and other streptococcal infections and diseases.

Wright was very certain of their value. In 1914 he wrote that just as it was true that "quinine is an effective therapeutic agent in malaria; [and] that salvarsan is effective in syphilis; [killed whole-organism] staphylococcus and streptococcus vaccines are effective in localised staphylococcic and streptococcic infections." Two thirds of this statement has stood the tests of time: Quinine and Salvarsan most certainly did work against malaria and syphilis. Wright was wrong only about the clinical worth of killed whole-organism vaccines against streptococci and staphylococci.

By 1910 these streptococcal vaccines were widely used in the United States when Drs. Nathaniel Bowditch Potter and Oswald Avery, the young associate director for bacteriology at the Hoagland Laboratory in Brooklyn, wrote the chapter on opsonins and vaccine therapy in a standard medical textbook. They described the average therapeutic dose of the streptococcal vaccine as containing from one million to 25 million killed whole organisms for use against general infections, and from five million to 200 million heat-killed streptococci for local infections.

The authors noted that "the prophylactic use of streptococcus vaccine in scarlet fever by Gabritschewsky and other Russian investigators has been brought to more general notice in this country by a recent résumé of their results by Smith. The vaccine employed consists of a concentrated bouillon culture of streptococcus isolated from a case of scarlet fever. The culture is killed by heat at 60° C., and preserved by the addition of 0.5 per cent carbolic acid." They relayed the published information that in this route to prevention of streptococcal infection "over 50,000 vaccinations have been made," usually in three doses, and that "usually after two there is established a complete immunity against scarlet fever."

Potter and Avery called for wider trials of this immunizing vaccine, for use in both healthy people and in presurgical patients. Strep infections, they wrote, were then known to be "one of the chief dangers of operative surgery." If the vaccine worked as well as it seemed to, they suggested that "the preliminary administration of vaccines, either before or after surgical operations, with the intention of protecting the patient against any post-operative infection, is a procedure which may find future application."

These killed whole-organism streptococcal vaccines failed, primarily because what protection they did offer applied only against the type or types of organisms in the vaccine. When they worked, the antibodies they induced vaccinees to produce were, alas, most probably autoimmune, heart-reacting, and smooth-muscle-reacting antibodies, now known to be the cause of rheumatic fever and its cardiac consequences. In any event, they had been long abandoned, if not forgotten, by 1925, when the husband-and-wife team of Drs. George F. and Gladys H. Dick introduced a new vaccine.

Previously, the couple had developed the Dick test for susceptibility or immunity to the toxin of scarlet fever. Like the precursor Schick test for immunity to diphtheria, the Dick test called for injections of the scarlet fever toxin into the surface of the skin.

In 1924 the Dicks "reported a scarlet fever antitoxin produced by immunizing horses with scarlet fever toxin. The antitoxic serum thus obtained was concentrated by the method commonly employed for the concentration of the diphtheria antitoxin." Up to that time, they wrote, "the serums prepared for the treatment of scarlet fever had been produced by immunizing horses with living cultures of hemolytic streptococci." Further experiments led them to conclude, "The fact that scarlet fever antitoxin may be employed in the concentrated form makes its use in the treatment of scarlet fever practical."

Moreover, they felt that "we are dealing with a toxic substance specific for scarlet fever, and that it might be used in the production of active immunity."

In July 1924, with the cooperation of Dr. O. B. Nesbit, medical director of the Gary (Indiana) public schools, the Dicks went to the steel-mill city, read a paper on scarlet fever, and helped launch the immunization of nearly 2,000 children by injecting each child with three doses of their concentrate of antitoxic horse sera. With this, Nesbit wrote in 1925 in the *Journal of the American Medical Association,* "the immunization of the susceptible was commenced."[19]

Nesbit's account of this now-forgotten event stated that "three doses of the scarlet fever toxin [sic] appears to immunize about 65 per cent of the pupils," and concluded that "larger immunizing doses of the scarlet fever toxin such as we have now begun to use, are desirable."

Nesbit's 1925 article is noteworthy also for his use of the hyper-Americanisms of World War I—when sauerkraut was renamed liberty cabbage and frankfurters relabeled hot dogs, and German measles (rubella) rechristened liberty measles, the term this Hoosier school doctor felt it expedient to use in the days when the Ku Klux Klan controlled the state government of Indiana.

The next generation of streptococcal vaccines were created long after World War II, during the capsular polysaccharide vaccine *Zeitgeist.* The Group A streptococci, unlike *Streptococcus pneumoniae* and the Group B streptococci of neonatal meningitis, do not have carbohydrate capsules. For fairly obvious reasons then, the new experimental streptococcal vaccines were made of purified M proteins removed from the surfaces of Group A streptococcal cells.

One of the first of these M-protein vaccines to be tested clinically was developed in the late 1960s by Dr. Benedict F. Massell and his associates at the Harvard medical school. This vaccine, made of purified Type III Group A streptococcal M protein, was injected into twenty-one siblings of patients with rheumatic fever at the House of the Good Samaritan in the Children's Hospital medical center in Boston. All but one of these healthy children started to produce type-specific anti-Group A streptococcal antibodies after they were vaccinated.

However, Massell reported in 1969, "Two cases of definite rheumatic fever and one additional case of probable rheumatic fever"—that is, 14.3 percent of the children vaccinated—developed in this test population. "Our experience," Massell and his collaborators concluded, "indicates the need for extreme caution in the use of streptococcal vaccines in human subjects."[20]

At Rockefeller University, Dr. Vincent Fischetti has been studying the different M proteins of many types of Group A streptococci in search of more specific knowledge of their antiphagocytic mechanisms. His investigations have centered around the structural similarities he found to exist between the alpha-helical molecules of the M proteins and the alpha-helical molecule of mammalian tropomyosin, a component of the thin filament in muscle cells.

Fischetti discovered that the immunodeterminants on the surfaces of the M-protein molecules found on the walls of different types of Group A streptococcal cells were all quite different and presumably type-specific structurally. On the other hand, the consistent similarities between the alpha-helical structures of all M-protein molecules and the tropomyosin molecule were close enough to suggest a tentative molecular basic for the cross-reactivity that prevails between streptococcal heart-reacting antibodies (HRA) and heart tissues.[21]

To Fischetti, this meant two things. First, it was an added reason for more intensive studies of M proteins, as well as of the history of earlier work on streptococcal vaccines. "The kind of response Massell evoked in those three healthy children who developed rheumatic fever after being inoculated with the experimental Group A streptococcal M-protein vaccine was," he says, "probably similar to the effects caused in patients by the pre-World War I killed whole-organism vaccines that were used to both treat and prevent strep infections. Patients were not followed as closely during the first decades of the century as they are now, but it was not necessary to strip the M proteins off the streptococcal cell walls in order for them to induce heart-reacting antibodies. Even in the absence of follow-up data on these patients, we can probably assume that the immune response induced by the whole-organism streptococcal vaccines may have played a role in causing rheumatic fever in some of them."

The second implication of his findings, Fischetti feels, is that they constitute urgent warnings that a great deal remains to be learned about the structures and functions of Group A streptococcal M proteins before they are again shot into people. "In terms of what is now known about this molecule," he states, "if I were handed a consent form saying that you proposed to vaccinate me with a Group A streptococcal M protein shown to be structurally similar to heart muscle tissue, I wouldn't sign it. I'd have to be crazy to let anyone inject me with it until they could prove it had no pathologic significance in any way, shape or form."

Various laboratories around the world are now trying to determine whether altered M-protein preparations that appear to be free of heart-reacting antigens in animal tests will be equally safe in people, and whether or not they can be used in a polyvalent subunit vaccine against Group A streptococcal diseases. Theoretically, it might be possible chemically to alter the M-protein antigens to the stage where they no longer induce heart-reacting antibodies, and this line of research is certainly worth intensive investigations.

Every aspect of the problems of developing safe and effective vaccines against Group A streptococci is of prime importance. With only one exception most of the more serious disorders that follow untreated or improperly treated strep throats are known to be major killers. The exception, however, is one of the most damaging diseases in this country. It is called otitis media, or inflammation of the middle ear, and it is "the most common diagnosis made at office visits to pediatricians." Otitis media is "most prevalent during the first two years of life," writes Dr. Jack L. Paradise of the University of Pittsburgh. "Next to the simple upper respiratory infection, [otitis media] is the most common organic disease confronting the practicing pediatrician."[22]

In 1979 Dr. Jerome O. Klein, professor of pediatrics at Boston University, estimated that of the 3,300,000 babies born during that year, 2.5 million of them—or 75 percent—would suffer otitis media during childhood.[23]

Drs. Robert Austrian, Virgil M. Howie, and John H. Ploussard described otitis media as "one of the commonest infections of early life," and noted that it had been estimated that "between 76% and 95% of all children will have at least one attack of otitis media by the time they reach six years of age." They reported that otitis media caused by only one of the bacteria known to induce it, the pneumococcus, "may infect the middle ear of as many as 20% of children born in the United States during their first two years of life. At the present time, there are approximately six million children two years of age or younger in this country who will experience an estimated 1,200,000 or more attacks of pneumococcal otitis media." Still other children will have attacks of otitis media caused by bacteria other than the ubiquitous pneumococci, including *Haemophilus influenzae,* the even more common Group A streptococci, *Staphylococcus aureus, Neisseria catarrhalis,* and the newly significant Gram-negative bacteria, including *E. coli, Proteus,* and *Pseudomonas aeruginosa.*

Austrian and Howie, in the same article, went on to spell out the primary reason why otitis media, although a nonfatal disease since the availability of antibiotics, is much better prevented than cured. "Any measure that would reduce significantly the burden of this infection would be of appreciable benefit to society, not only in terms of diminished costs for medical care but also in terms of preventing suffering and either temporary or permanent damage to hearing. . . . Otitis media occurs most frequently during a stage of life when development is rapid, and when reduction in auditory acuity has a deleterious effect upon learning. It has been estimated that, in some socioeconomically deprived segments of the population, as many as a third of the children have some impairment of hearing at the time they enter school."[24]

The temporary hearing losses suffered by children with otitis media often inflict permanent damage in mental development. Klein estimated that in 75 percent of the 3.3 million children born in 1978 who would have "at least one episode of otitis media before they are two years old, one-third [about 830,000] will have three or more episodes." This means that at the precise period when hearing is most important in the perception and learning of language, the temporary hearing losses caused by the infection will block or seriously retard development of this essential learning tool.

A well-known study published in 1969 by Drs. Vanja A. Holm and LuVern H. Kunze, of the University of Washington, followed sixteen children, aged five to nine, each with chronic otitis media and with fluctuations in hearing documented by audiograms. The doctors found "that the fluctuating hearing loss accompanying chronic otitis media was the cause of the delay in language development" in these Seattle children.[25]

Most governmental and scientific population surveys generally reveal that children under six will show a 15 percent to 20 percent prevalence of otitis media. All these children show some degree of temporary or permanent hearing loss. Marion P. Downs, at the University of Colorado, as early as 1974 wrote that "definitions of a handicapping hearing loss must be drastically revised in view of recent investigations on the effects of mild hearing impairments on children. Significant language retardation is now shown to result from hearing losses as mild as 15 dB [decibels]. This level, which should be adopted as the lowest limit of a handicapping hearing loss, would increase epidemiologic estimates of the prevalence of hearing loss in children from 2.7% to over 15%."[26]

A study published in 1973 by the National Academy of Sciences showed that in Washington, D.C., 30 percent of all children between the ages of six months and three years had signs and symptoms of otitis media, and that 7 percent of the four-year-olds had hearing losses of fifteen decibels (dB) or greater. The study showed that in this population, hearing losses were highest in those children who had suffered serious ear damage caused by otitis media.[27]

Abroad, similar studies have recently yielded similar findings. The British general practitioner John Fry found a hearing loss of 20 dB or more in 17 percent of children who had had a single case of otitis media five to ten years earlier, in contrast with the 4.5 percent of the matched controls who had suffered similar hearing losses. A ten-year study of Alaskan Eskimo children revealed that a hearing loss of 26 dB or greater was present in 16 percent, and that "children with a history of otitis media prior to two years of age and a hearing loss of 26 decibels or greater had a statistically significant loss of verbal ability, and were behind in total reading, total math, and language. In addition, children who had an early onset of otitis media and had normal hearing with a conductive component [battery-powered hearing aid] were also adversely affected in verbal areas. The number of otitis media episodes was related to tympanic membrane [eardrum] abnormalities, hearing loss, and low verbal and achievement test scores."[28]

The mechanism by which otitis media causes hearing losses has to do primarily with its effects on the Eustachian tube, the auditory canal from the back of the nose to the tympanic membrane in the middle ear. The Eustachian tube is lined with mucosal cells and with thousands of hairlike structures of the mucociliary apparatus, whose normal function is to sweep the auditory canal free of the bacterial flora normally present in healthy people. The functions of the Eustachain tube, write Drs. Charles Bluestone and Paul Shurin, include protection of the middle ear from nasopharyngeal secretions, the drainage of fluid secreted by the middle ear, and the ventilation of the middle ear.[29]

"The lining of the musosa of the middle ear depends for its health on a continuing supply of air, under normal circumstances supplied from the nasopharynx via the Eustachian tube," writes Dr. Paradise.[30] When common colds and other infections cause inflammations of the upper respiratory tract, the entire middle-ear ventilatory system becomes disrupted. Fluids produced in the middle ear and usually eliminated via the Eustachian tube accumulate and block the auditory canal, and the mucociliary transport system becomes unable to sweep the ambient bacteria out. The bacteria start to proliferate, causing both infection and inflammation. This is the onset of otitis media.

When enough fluid accumulates, otitis media is diagnosed as otitis media with effusion, or OME. This is one of the many names by which otitis media is known. There is secretory otitis media and serous otitis media, but the most descriptive name of all is glue ear.

In many children the pain caused by fluid backing up against the tympanic membrane becomes so acute that they have to be treated surgically.

This is an office procedure, seldom performed in hospitals, called a tympanotomy. It involves making an incision in the eardrum itself with a special knife, and then inserting a tube into this cut to drain the middle ear of fluid. Before antibiotics, it was an exceedingly common procedure, and few American children reached school age without having had their tympanic membranes lanced at least once, generally by their family doctor, and often, as in my childhood, while being held down on the kitchen table.

This operation is far less common today, but in health statistics, as in other matters, everything is relative: According to the prominent otolaryngologist Charles Bluestone, at least one million children in this country have the more recently developed tympanotomy tubes inserted into their lanced eardrums each year to relieve the pressure caused by acute or recurrent otitis media with effusion. "Circumcision," he states, "is probably the only minor surgical procedure performed more often in children than the insertion of tympanotomy tubes."[31]

In recent years various doctors have observed that with or without tympanotomies, many children with otitis media continue to experience frequent occurrences of middle-ear effusion after their inflammation has been treated with antibiotics, and the infection itself diagnosed as cured. A follow-up study of 123 children treated with antibiotics and cured of otitis media at Boston City Hospital was recently published by Paul Shurin and other doctors.[32] The average child in this study was observed for fifty days, and some were followed for as long as three months. The Boston doctors observed "persistence of middle-ear effusion for the entire period of observation in 45 of the patients (42.1%), whereas 62 children (57.9%) were considered cured."

They also found that in this cohort, "children who were less than 24 months of age (median, nine months) at initial presentation were 3.8 times more likely to have persistent middle-ear effusion than children who were older (median, 52 months)."

According to the raw data collected by health and hospital agencies, Alaskan Eskimo children are infinitely more prone to have otitis media than most other ethnic groups in North America. A study of native Alaskan Eskimo children by D. D. Beal, published in 1972, showed that "approximately 60% of all native children have at least one episode of acute middle ear infection in the first year of life." However, Beal's study also described how after oil was discovered near an Alaskan native village with this high a rate of otitis, the new incomes brought to the villagers raised the standards of living so steeply that otitis all but disappeared.[33]

Two British doctors, J. H. Kerseley and H. Wickham, published a study of exudative otitis media in two hundred children in which, among other things, they found that "this is a disease associated with poor hygienic conditions and overcrowding." A decade later Dr. R. M. Harvey, in Londonderry, Northern Ireland, published the results of an eight-year study of hearing loss and deafness associated with glue ear in rural and urban Irish children. Harvey found massive evidence to support the links between crowding and OME in children, with the greatest incidence of secretory otitis in the urban areas with the highest population densities and the highest air-pollution levels. Harvey concluded that the considerable decline since 1954 in children arriving at outpatient clinics with purulent otitis media "may well be due, firstly, to adequate treatment of the glue ear, and secondly to the improved housing conditions consequent upon slum clearance schemes."

If otitis, like most other infectious diseases, is societal, it is also insidious, particularly, thinks John D. Nelson, professor of pediatrics at the University of Texas, Dallas, in light of recently discovered and ample evidence of persistent "effusion that remains in the middle ear even after the child has taken a complete course of antibiotic therapy and is assumed well by the physician and the baby's parents. A child suffering from otitis media is almost predestined to have repeat episodes." Nelson is concerned about the obvious danger that infants with almost constant otitis can become accustomed to the fluid in their middle ears, as well as to reduced or fluctuating levels while "no one realizes the seriousness of the problem."

Also there is a clear and present danger that, as happens only too often in understaffed public schools, when such hearing-handicapped children enter school at the age of six, they, like many other children with the same disadvantage, will be treated as slow learners or even as mentally retarded. In many cities in the United States where thanks to inflation entire school systems have been forced to eliminate their doctors and nurses, the actual cause of otitis-damaged children's fluctuating ability to comprehend what their teachers say will be mislabeled as functional retardation due to hereditary factors, rather than as a treatable and reversible infectious disease secondary to the common cold.

It is much easier to blame the hearing and visual losses, the minimal-to-gross brain damage, the days of absence from classrooms due to respiratory and other infectious disorders caused by common and, in the cases of polio, measles, mumps, and rubella, vaccine-preventable infectious diseases of childhood, on parental genes rather than on parental income. This makes it easier to warehouse with a clear conscience the otitis-handicapped children in classes and institutions for the mentally retarded (the feebleminded of yesteryear). It also dooms most of them to become chronic welfare clients rather than self-supporting taxpayers.

Otitis media was not always a nonfatal disease. Before World War II, it was a major cause of brain abscess, an often fatal disorder, as well as of mastoiditis, an inflammation of the antrum, cells, and other areas of the mastoid process, the knob of bone reaching from the skull to the region behind the ear. Prior to the use of antibiotics, when this bony knob was inflamed by otitis media or middle-ear infections, abscesses formed and portions of the bony structure had to be gouged out by life-threatening surgery. The survivors of these mastoidectomies were left with large visible depressions in the bone structure behind their ears. Antibiotics made the brain abscesses and the mastoid complications of otitis media both preventable and curable without either minor or heroic surgery.

New chemotherapeutic conditions also changed the social nature of the disease itself. For the families who could afford regular, periodic, and invariably available pediatric and other medical care, otitis became a quickly diagnosed and easily treated minor ailment with no chronic hearing loss or other complications. This is true even if, as happens in children of all socioeconomic classes, those who are medically well cared for are exposed to and suffer the repeated common colds and less common bacterial upper respiratory infections that can initiate otitis media.

Among families who cannot afford regular private medical care, and who in this age of vanishing mass transit systems lack the private transportation to and from the nearest low-cost or free pediatric clinic (one American in every three does *not* have a car), infants and very young children with otitis media often go untreated. When otitis is finally treated, it is often too late to reverse the permanent damage it has caused in the ears, such as the scars and other pathologies so frequently found during subsequent medical ear examinations some years later. When otitis media infections are recurrent or chronic, they are more often found in the children of poor families.

There is nothing genetic or racial about the higher proportions of hearing loss caused by untreated or inadequately treated otitis in the children of America's more than 30 million poor and near-poor families, the majority of whom are white. Treating otitis properly is very costly for families with low incomes.

A report prepared for the general public by ranking medical specialists in both otitis and pediatrics recommends that "the parent should be asked to call the physician or return to the doctor's office within 48 or 72 hours of the child's initial visit to determine whether the patient is free of pain, fever and complications. Careful follow-up includes a re-examination after completion of therapy and should include pneumatic otoscopy. If the diagnosis of middle ear fluid is equivocal, tympanometry should be performed."[34]

This simple regimen calls for a minimum of three visits to a doctor's office. Pneumatic otoscopy is a fairly inexpensive procedure, performed in the doctor's office or at the patient's home with a flashlight-type instrument carried in a doctor's black bag. Tympanometry, which employs the same principles as sonar, is done with a costly, nontransportable machine that delivers sound to the eardrum through a special probe placed in the ear canal, reflects it back to an amplifier, measures the absorption of energy, and records it on paper as a tympanogram, which helps otolaryngologists make a more precise diagnosis than a pediatrician is trained or instrumentally equipped to make. It is not an inexpensive procedure.

Antibiotics, particularly penicillin, are now very inexpensive. However, private doctors to diagnose otitis media, to write prescriptions for specific antibiotics, and to follow up the results of their use are, for purely economic reasons, not available to over 30 million poor and near-poor American families and their children.

Vaccines protecting children against the bacteria that cause most middle-ear inflammations would, if they were available—and if they worked in infants and children under two years old—fill a very great human and social need. When Robert Austrian was testing his pneumococcal capsular polysaccharide vaccines against pneumonia, one of the doctors who followed his work assiduously was Virgil M. Howie, an otitis specialist in private pediatric practice in Huntsville, Alabama. Howie knew that the pneumococci were one of the commonest bacteria found in the flora of healthy people, and he also knew, from his own clinical isolates, that the pneumococci were also one of the most common bacteria found in the middle-ear fluids of children with exudative otitis media.

Howie sought Austrian out for help in typing the pneumococci he found in his patients with otitis. Austrian offered to type the recovered bacteria for him. Thus, the Alabama pediatrician learned that in his patients four of the pneumococcal types—VI, XIV, XIX, and XXIII—were responsible for 57 percent of all attacks of otitis media, and also that "three of these four capsular types, types 6, 19, and 23, are the ones most commonly isolated from healthy carriers of pneumococcus among pediatric populations."

In 1974 Howie, with the encouragement and help of Austrian, and supported in part by a grant from the National Institute of Allergy and Infectious Diseases (NIAID), made up an octavalent purified pneumococcal capsular polysaccharide vaccine containing the carbohydrate antigens of the eight capsular types of pneumococci most commonly found in middle-ear exudates of children with serous otitis media, or glue ear. Howie administered this vaccine subcutaneously "to 60 infants 2–19 months of age, whose clinical histories were closely followed for an additional year."[35]

Ten of the children who were given this vaccine at the ages of two to five months experienced otitis caused by one or another of the pneumococci represented in the vaccine, as compared with five of eight age-matched children of the same age who had not received this vaccine. However, when the Huntsville pediatrician gave the same experimental vaccine to a group of twenty-six older children, who were originally immunized with the octavalent preparation at the ages of six to nineteen months, only one child came down with otitis due to any of the pneumococcal types in the vaccine.

Howie and his collaborators took this as an indication that the vaccine might possibly protect children older than six months, and started a long series of efficacy trials in other children.

Subsequently, combined trials of the eight-antigen (octavalent) and the commercial fourteen-capsular-type pneumococcal polysaccharide vaccines as potential prophylactic preparations to prevent otitis media in infants and very young children were, with parental consent and active cooperation, held in this country and in Finland. In Huntsville, the eight-antigen pneumococcal capsular polysaccharide vaccine was tested in children between the ages of six months and twenty-four months in the private practices of Drs. Virgil Howie and John Ploussard after the children's first observed episode of otitis media. In Boston children in five health-care centers were observed by staff pediatricians for otitis media from birth or before they were three months old. Those who, between the time they were five months and twenty months old, had three episodes of otitis media were also given the octavalent pneumococcal vaccine.

The Finnish trials were conducted in the cities of Oulu and Tampere in children under seven years old who had been taken to the outpatient otolaryngology or pediatrics departments in local hospitals because of otitis media. In these samplings, randomly selected children from three months to eighty-three months old were given age-adjusted doses of the fourteen-antigen pneumococcal capsular polysaccharide vaccine.

In none of these four American and Finnish centers did either the eight-antigen or the fourteen-antigen vaccines reduce the total otitis media attack rates. The vaccinated children contracted just as much otitis during the next year or more as the nonvaccinated control children in the same cities. The basic immunochemical differences between infants, toddlers, and their parents—in these cases they apparently concerned the maturation of children's inborn immunologic defense potentials—were apparently great enough to render ineffective the presently available pneumococcal capsular polysaccharide vaccines in infants and children under eighteen months old. Unfortunately, these infants and toddlers are precisely those who are at highest risk of catching otitis media.

"We'll just have to develop a new way to fool nature," said Robert Austrian, the "godfather" of the present fourteen-antigen pneumococcal capsular polysaccharide vaccine.

There was clearly much more to learn, starting at the most basic levels, about the mechanisms of immunity in babies before it would be possible to plan any bacterial capsular polysaccharide vaccines as effective against pneumococci and other bacteria that cause otitis media as are other vaccines that protect babies today against paralytic poliomyelitis, whooping cough, diphtheria, tetanus, measles, mumps, and rubella.

Together the chronic and recurring side effects of otitis media that are the primary cause of hearing loss in preschool children, and the Group A streptococcal infections that are a major cause of school absences due to chronic and recurring strep throats, rheumatic fever, and rheumatic heart diseases, rob poor and nonpoor but medically indigent children of their innate capacities to develop mentally and physically to their maximum genetic potentials. They also serve as necessary reminders to health professionals and laymen that the deaths caused by specific diseases are not the only index by which the impact of infectious diseases upon individuals and societies must be measured. Given the known major chronic effects of many infectious diseases, deaths are possibly not even the primary measurement of the human and economic costs of infectious diseases.

As every pediatrician, family doctor, and geriatrician knows, otitis and streptococcal infections are only two of many good reasons to fund and expand research for vaccines still needed against many diseases. The availability of a pediatric vaccine against the pneumococci that cause around half of all cases of otitis media will reduce but not itself eliminate the endemicity of middle-ear infections.

First, there are still other bacteria, such as the many different types of *Haemophilus influenzae* and Group A streptococci which, between them, are responsible for 20 percent to 30 percent of the otitis media infections not caused by the pneumococci—and against which there are still no safe and effective vaccines that will work in infants and very young children. Above all else, there is also the not so small matter of the common cold and other upper respiratory infections that precede the onset of otitis media. Group A streptococci are responsible for a very small proportion of these pre-otitis upper respiratory infections, most of which are caused by a wide array of common cold viruses, which include adenoviruses, rhinoviruses, respiratory syncytial virus, and enteroviruses.

Some of the most intensive studies of the pathology and microbiology of otitis media have been going on for over a decade at the medical school of the University of North Carolina, Chapel Hill.[36] A recent study, conducted by Dr. Margaret A. Sanyal and her colleagues, of the effects of upper respiratory infection on Eustachian tube ventilatory function in Chapel Hill preschool children suggested that once the middle ear becomes blocked by effusions, and the mucociliary clearance mechanisms are compromised by inflammations caused by the upper respiratory (and generally viral) infections, any of the bacteria normally present in the human body can become trapped in this closed space and start to proliferate and cause otitis media.

This also suggested to the North Carolina doctors that intervention strategies [vaccines] designed to control the viral infections that precede all outbreaks of otitis media "will be more likely to effect a decline in O.M.E. [otitis media with effusion] than strategies directed against the bacterial pathogens, pneumococci and Haemophilus influenzae."[37]

Ultimately, this might mean that in order to eradicate otitis media we will have to return to the long-surrendered Square One: the still unrealized dream of a vaccine against the common cold.

Because of advances in basic knowledge of the processes of infection and immunity since British and American efforts to develop a common cold vaccine were abandoned over a decade ago, this problem might prove to be a bit less intractable than it proved to be earlier.

Whatever its immediate effects on vaccines against the common cold and other virus diseases, the vastly increased reservoir of new (and published) basic knowledge, techniques, and strategies of using the knowledge and clinical experience acquired since the end of World War II has yielded, and will continue to produce, vaccines of immense value to all. A most appealing recent example of how this combination of basic knowledge and shared clinical experience was used to create a revolutionary new type of vaccine is the genetically sophisticated new vaccine against typhoid fever, which was developed by Dr. René Germanier of the Serum and Vaccine Institute in Berne, Switzerland.

People in industrial Europe and North America perceive typhoid as a once ubiquitous disease that was eradicated during this century by the building and constant improvement of safe drinking water systems. In a broad sense this is true, but typhoid fever is far from a matter of ancient history in our country. As late as 1930, there were over 27,500 cases of typhoid fever reported in the United States. Environmental controls of water pollution helped reduce the reported numbers of typhoid cases to 9,809 by 1940. However, it was only when antibiotics became available for the early treatment of symptoms that reported typhoid cases fell below 1,000 per year—and that was not until 1959, when reported cases fell to 859.

By 1959, at least half of all typhoid cases were imported, brought into this country by foreign visitors and returning American tourists and businessmen. In 1970 many of the 346 medically reported cases were imported by military servicemen returning from Vietnam; by 1973, the last year of the Vietnam War, reported cases had nearly doubled—to 680. At last count there were 528 reported cases—which represents probably no more than 5 percent of all actual incidences of typhoid fever in this country in 1979.

Typhoid fever is caused by *Salmonella typhi,* one of the many *Salmonella* species of bacteria that are carried by water, ingested by people, and then returned to running water in human excreta. Reported cases of salmonellosis, a diarrheal disease caused by some of the nontyphoid subspecies of *Salmonella,* have recently passed tuberculosis as the second (next to gonorrhea) most frequently reported bacterial disease in this country. Salmonellosis cases are estimated to run as high as three million yearly. The development of a vaccine against any subspecies of *Salmonella* therefore makes a better typhoid vaccine something of more than passing interest.

Although typhoid fever is usually water-borne, its causal agents can be and often are food-borne, transmitted from person to person by the same fecal-oral route through which many serious infections reach human beings. Dr. Charles Haley of the CDC notes that in many restaurants around the world, where salads are mixed by hand, "If someone who prepares food does not wash his hands well after going to the toilet, he or she can become a carrier of the typhoid bacterium—which is exactly why you are advised not to eat lettuce in many countries."

The first human vaccine against *Salmonella typhi* was developed a decade after Dr. Daniel Elmer Salmon (1850–1914), discoverer of the *Salmonella* species of water-borne enterobacteria, and Dr. Theobald Smith, his twenty-seven-year-old assistant in the U.S. Department of Agriculture laboratory in Washington, D.C., had produced the world's first killed whole-organism vaccine, the hog cholera baccillus vaccine, in 1886.[38]

In Koch's laboratories in Berlin, Richard Pfeiffer and, in England, Almroth Wright, then a new professor of pathology at the army medical school in Netley, began working on killed whole-organism vaccines against typhoid around 1895. In the grand tradition, the first people to be vaccinated with the Wright vaccine were Wright himself and his Netley colleagues. By 1897 Pfeiffer announced his vaccine almost simultaneously with Wright's, and then the world had vaccines against an infection much more common in people than rabies and anthrax and, by 1898 in Europe, more common than smallpox.

The Wright and Pfeiffer killed whole-organism vaccines were far from adequate for human needs. Their chief shortcoming was that they protected people against only small numbers of *S. typhi,* and failed to provide any protection against large doses of the enteric or gut bacteria.

"If that vaccine came out today," Haley believes, "we'd never license it in this country, and probably not even allow it to be used in human trials." Because it did offer limited protection, however, the federal Centers for Disease Control, on the principle that half a vaccine is better than none, continued to recommend its forewarned use by Americans who had to visit areas of the world where typhoid fever was and is still endemic.

In most countries, and particularly in poor countries, the need for a safe and highly effective typhoid vaccine is as great as ever. This was what attracted René Germanier to the idea of working on a better typhoid vaccine.

Given the benefits of hindsight, the modern efficacy data on the killed whole-organism vaccine suggested to Germanier that a better typhoid vaccine would have to be either a live organism vaccine or a bacterial subunit chemical vaccine. Guided by the striking example of the Sabin oral live polio vaccine—and the data on the secretory IgA antibodies produced by the mucosal cells of the alimentary system seconds after the attenuated polioviruses in the Sabin vaccine entered the human body by the same portal of entry polioviruses use in nature—Germanier was inclined to look into the practical possibilities of a whole live bacterial vaccine that could also be taken by mouth.

The Sabin live poliovirus vaccine also presented a potential danger, however, that was not present in killed-pathogen vaccines like the Salk formalin-inactivated poliovirus vaccine or the heat-killed whole-bacterium typhoid vaccine. When given in the proper dosages at the proper intervals—the first three doses when a child is two, four, and six months old, a fourth dose at eighteen months, and a fifth dose when the child is between four and six years old—the poliovirus antibodies induced by the live attenuated viruses in the vaccine kill off all the viruses descended from those in the vaccine. The trouble is that too many children fail to receive the proper dosages of the trivalent oral poliovirus vaccine (TOPV). In 1979, for example, of the 12,386,000 children aged one to four in this country, only 59.1 percent had received three or more doses of TOPV by the time they were four years old, 6 percent had received zero doses, and 34.9 percent (4,323,028) had received one or two doses when they should have had three or more.

Although together the Salk and Sabin vaccines had effectively eliminated paralytic poliomyelitis in this country by 1970, a small number of cases—ranging from thirty-one in 1970 to seven in 1974, and then rising to twenty-six in 1979—continued to be reported. An examination of these cases showed the CDC that "of the 187 paralytic cases reported to the poliomyelitis surveillance program between 1969 and 1979, 74 (40%) were classified as vaccine associated. Eliminating the 43 cases that occurred during the poliomyelitis epidemics of 1970, 1972, and 1979, 53% of cases were attributed etiologically to OPV (oral poliovaccine).[39] Vaccine-associated cases constituted 21%–80% of annual cases during the eight years during which no poliomyelitis outbreak occurred. Forty-two percent of vaccine-associated cases occurred in contacts of vaccines; 34% in household contacts; 8% in nonhousehold contacts. The rest (58%) were in OPV recipients."[40]

The millions of children who received TOPV and neither developed nor caused any cases of paralytic polio were proof enough that had all the oral polio vaccines been properly administered in sufficient numbers of doses at the proper times, none of these reported vaccine-associated cases might have occurred. However, when more than one third of all courses of oral poliovaccines are apparently not completed in this country, there is a danger that certain of these courses will turn some recipients into carriers of attenuated polioviruses who can infect and paralyze a handful of immunologically atypical individuals who are susceptible to them.

Ideally, Germanier knew, it would be nice to have a live oral pathogen typhoid vaccine that would protect as efficiently as Sabin's oral poliovaccine and yet be as unlikely to produce typhoid fever as is Wright's killed whole-bacterium vaccine.

Salmonella typhi, is pathogenic only in humans. This meant that basic research for a more efficient vaccine was handicapped by the lack of a suitable animal model in which to test it. There are in the *Salmonella* family many "cousins," or subspecies, that cause typhoid fever in mammals other than people. One of them, the *Salmonella typhimurium* subspecies, which causes typhoid fever in mice, was chosen by Germanier for investigation as a working analogue of *S. typhi*.

Germanier then made a series of highly sophisticated studies of the genetics and biochemistry of *Salmonella typhimurium* and, afterward, of *Salmonella typhi*. Two major findings resulted. The first was that the important prerequisite for a vaccine strain of either of these typhoid bacteria "is that attenuation is not based on a mutation that prevents the synthesis of smooth-type lipopolysaccharide (LPS). Rough strains [of LPS] are ineffective." The LPS compounds are the endotoxins on the surface of *Salmonella* and other bacteria that promote infection and induce the production of antibodies against their own saccharide (carbohydrate) components.

Germanier's second major finding was that this LPS requirement is met by galactose-dependent mutants of *Salmonella typhi*. Galactose, a sugar, is a breakdown product of milk essential for nutrition in these mutant typhoid bacteria. Germanier and his colleagues selected several gal-E (galactose-E) mutants of *S. typhi*, the human typhoid bacterium. After elegant analyses of their chemistry, they selected gal-E mutant strain Ty 21a as their experimental vaccine strain.

The Ty 21a mutant *S. typhi* lacks the enzyme UDP-galactose-epinerase. This enzyme controls the effectiveness of the two other enzymes (galactokinase and galactose-l-phosphate-uridyl-transferase) that normally metabolize or break down galactose. In fact, without the missing enzyme, the other two lose the ability to metabolize 80 percent of the galactose on which they act.

In the Ty 21a mutant human typhoid organism, Germanier reported at a 1980 international symposium on bacterial vaccines, "the galactose taken up by the cell is partly incorporated into the [bacterial] cell wall, allowing synthesis of the smooth type LPS."[41]

The balance of the ingested galactose is accumulated in the *S. typhi* cell's cytoplasm—that is, everything inside the cell but the nucleus. There, the mutant *S. typhi* metabolize, or break down, the galactose, but at only 20 percent of the rate at which it is broken down into nutritionally more essential products by the nonmutant wild strains of *S. typhi*. The unmetabolized (or undigested) galactose continues to be taken into the cell, and four fifths of it continues to accumulate inside the cell, gaining in volume until it finally puts so much pressure on the cell walls that after only two reproductive devisions, they rupture and the bacteria lyse, or disintegrate.

These self-destructing mutant bacteria were used by Germanier as oral vaccines against typhoid fever. Once the vaccines containing these live galactose-dependent mutants of *S. typhi* are swallowed and reach the gut, they start to induce protective antibodies against *S. typhi* immediately, starting with the secretory IgA antibodies produced by the mucosal cells of the alimentary system. Then because of the accumulations of unmetabolized galactose in their cytoplasms, the *S. typhi* cells in the vaccine lyse. After the second reproductive division of the typhoid bacteria cells, they cease to reproduce, having lived only long enough in their human recipients to program their hosts' alimentary-system mucosal cells and circulating lymphocytes to forever after produce antityphoid-bacteria antibodies in the presence of any *S. typhi* strain.

In short, the new mutant live organism typhoid vaccine has all the protective advantages of a live pathogen oral vaccine—and none of the (however remote) theoretical reversion-to-wild-type and other virulence potentials of a live pathogen vaccine.

Germanier's vaccine was tested in over 30,000 schoolchildren in 1979 and 1980, during two typhoid seasons in Alexandria, Egypt, one of the majority of the world's nations in which typhoid fever is endemic and, periodically, epidemic. Not a single case of typhoid fever developed in any of the 16,482 children in the experimental cohort who were given three doses of the new vaccine over a period of four weeks. By contrast, there were fourteen bacteriologically confirmed and seventeen probable typhoid fever cases among the 15,902 children in the control population who had been given either placebos or nothing at all.

"Clearly, this is the way to go," said the CDC's Dr. Haley, "not only for typhoid, but for all the other enteric bacterial and viral infections."

The development of altered live oral bacterial vaccines that, after one replication, will live just long enough to program the immune systems of their vaccinees to make antibodies against the diseases their normal prototypes cause, might be one of the most feasible of the new ways of protecting people against major bacterial diseases.

Among the other new directions of vaccine development are the subunit vaccines, in which single classes of cell-surface carbohydrate or protein antigens are the immunogens used, as in the presently available bacterial capsular polysaccharide pneumococcal and meningococcal vaccines.

There are also the complexes of carbohydrates and proteins, as in the still experimental vaccines in which the antigens of the principal outer-membrane proteins (POMP) are combined with the capsular polysaccharides of Group B meningococci or *Haemophilus influenzae* to prevent bacterial meningitis in infants. Also in this category are the experimental vaccines in which the POMP antigens are combined with the detoxified LPS of gonococci, or with the purified pili or attachment organelles of the gonococci, to prevent gonorrhea.

There is the barely explored field of cross-reacting or common or shared antigens in which injections of vaccines against one disease can protect people against one or more other infectious diseases. Some existing vaccines—such as the polyvalent pneumococcal capsular polysaccharide vaccine—might already be providing their recipients with effective cross-protection against the gonorrhea bacteria, Group B streptococci, *Klebsiella*, and other major pathogens.

There are the antigens common to certain types of *E. coli*, the newly deadly Gram-negative bacteria that cause most hospital-acquired infections, and the antigens of strains of common enterobacteria, such as those of *Salmonella, Shigella,* and *Proteus*.

These shared and combined antigen possibilities in vaccine development might help resolve the clinical problems caused by the sheer multiplicity of bacterial species and the serological and capsular types of subspecies of microbial pathogens that are involved in major infectious diseases of people. Other approaches to the formulation of vaccines that either do not exist yet, or vaccines that could be improved and made at lower than present costs, are based on recombination DNA techniques and/or on wholly synthetic chemical antigens.

The recombination DNA techniques have become so newsworthy of recent years that clever promoters have already reaped fortunes by forming and selling stocks in companies whose announced aims are to use these techniques to produce and mass-market all sorts of clinical products, from insulin and growth hormones to vaccines, interferons, and sexual rejuvenators. The chief assets of some of these new companies are their stock promoters' mailing lists; other companies in the genetic recombination business are scientifically responsible and may yet produce some of the expected miracles.

In vaccines these recombination DNA techniques, many workers now believe, should be able to reduce materially the costs of vaccine production. In the most discussed applications of the genetic recombination techniques to vaccine production, the viral or bacterial genes that code for the making of specific immunogenic segments of microbial proteins will be delicately removed, and then just as delicately inserted, as short segments of the DNA that contain them, into the gene-bearing plasmids or episomes found inside the cytoplasms of the common gut bacteria, *E. coli*. The hope is that these transplanted bacterial and viral genes will instruct the metabolic machinery of the *E. coli* host cells to henceforth start synthesizing replicas of these immunogenic proteins, which in turn will be harvested from the brainwashed *E. coli* and used as vaccines.

Some investigators, including Michael Sela at the Weitzman Institute in Israel, Arie Zuckerman, of the London School of Hygiene and Tropical Medicine, and Richard Lerner, at the Scripps Institute in California, believe that these genetic recombination maneuvers—which begin by isolating and chemically elucidating those segments of viral and bacterial nucleic acids that program for producing immunogenic proteins—will open a considerably simpler pathway to the development of safe, more effective, and much cheaper vaccines than forcing the violated and hoodwinked *E. coli* to turn themselves into vaccine antigen factories.

These investigators believe that once the particular amino acids (the "building blocks" of the nucleic acids) specified by these gene segments when they synthesize or manufacture proteins within living cells are isolated and chemically defined, it might become possible to synthesize chemically equally active replicas of these amino acids out of ordinary, off-the-shelf chemicals. The wholly synthetic copies of nucleic-acid components would be used as the active ingredients of inexpensive vaccines.

More than amino acids can be synthesized by genetic recombination techniques. In 1981 at MIT Drs. Vincent R. Racaniello and David Baltimore employed recombinant DNA techniques to synthesize biologically active poliomyelitis viruses out of common off-the-shelf laboratory chemicals. These artificial polioviruses were capable of infecting human cancer cells and normal monkey cells growing in tissue cultures.

To vaccine workers this suggests that it might now be theoretically feasible to develop synthetic viruses with other altered characteristics, starting with the chemically programmed capacity to immunize but not harm people when these altered viruses are used as "live" virus vaccines against scores of virus diseases.[42]

Finally, there are the adjuvants, which when added to the antigens in any vaccines, amplify their immunogenicity, or their capacity to induce the production of specific protective antibodies by the vaccines' human recipients.

As we saw earlier, in the formulation of their very effective subunit antigen vaccine against the hepatitis B virus, Maurice Hilleman and his Merck Institute associates added aluminum hydroxide as an adjuvant to boost the effectiveness of this fine new vaccine.

The idea that adjuvants, while not antigens themselves, can when combined with proteins and other known antigens increase their known capacities to induce the production of antibodies is not very new. Nearly sixty years ago, Karl Landsteiner introduced the concept of haptens, or nonantigenic substances that acquire antigenicity when combined with proven antigens. Landsteiner was able to show, for example, that ordinary tartaric acid linked to protein became an immunogenic material.

In the early 1930s, the Hungarian American bacteriologist Jules Freund (1890–1960) introduced two haptenic compounds as adjuvants, which have since been widely used in experimental bacteriology and clinical medicine. One of them, the Freund incomplete adjuvant, is simply a mixture of mineral oil and an emulsifying agent, which was combined with vaccines and other antigens (such as those used to desensitize allergic people against specific antigens) both to amplify the immunogenic effects of the vaccines and to remain in the body as depots that would slowly release the immunologically active materials into the circulatory system. The other preparation, Freund's complete adjuvant, consists of the mineral oil-emulsifier mixture plus heat-killed whole tuberculosis bacteria. It has a far more powerful amplifying effect on vaccine antigens than the incomplete adjuvant, but it also causes a few serious side effects, like high fevers and severe abscesses at the injection sites. For this reason, it is as a general rule used only in experimental animals.

In recent times, research demonstrated that the excellent immunogen-amplifying effects of the complete adjuvant are caused by muramyl dipeptide (MDP), a bacterial cell-surface compound of sugars and amino acids. Unlike the heat-killed whole *Mycobacteria* (tuberculosis) organisms on whose cell walls they are found, the muramyl dipeptides are not toxic in people. Since they are simple chemical compounds, variant MDPs with various characteristics are fairly easy to synthesize in chemical laboratories. By 1979 when the NIH sponsored an international symposium on new adjuvants in prophylaxis, nearly a hundred variant forms of MDP—many of them not found in nature—had been synthesized in scholarly, medical, and commercial pharmaceutical laboratories around the world. Certain forward-looking pharmaceutical firms have invested heavily in the development of new adjuvants, which, unlike vaccines, can be patented.

It is expected that nearly all vaccines now used in preventive medicine will be reformulated by their manufacturers to include the addition of at least one new adjuvant. This should add to their protective powers, but it will not begin to meet the most crying need in the entire field of vaccine development: the knowledge we still lack on the basic natures of infection and immunity.

Barely a century has elapsed since 1878 when Louis Pasteur published his memoir *Germ Theory and Its Applications in Medicine and Surgery.* Since that time the knowledge and insights acquired by painstaking research around the world have resulted in our present armament of all vaccines but one (Jenner's smallpox vaccine, perfected twenty-six years before Pasteur was born); immune sera, antibacterial drugs, and our present scientific understanding of the specific causal links between overcrowding, malnutrition, and poverty and infection and impaired immunity.

A century after the blossoming of germ theory, and nearly two centuries after Jenner, we still do not have good vaccines against most major bacterial, viral, and protozoan diseases that continue to infest this earth. This is not a commentary on humankind's intellectual inadequacy, but, rather, on the formidable dimensions of the research that must yet be done before we can really understand the interacting mechanisms of infection and immunity. We do not know how microbial agents actually cause infectious diseases, nor do we even begin to understand the processes in which antibodies that end Group A streptococcal infections can also cause autoimmune diseases, such as fatal rheumatic heart disease and post-streptococcal kidney disease.

However, what we do know very well is how this missing knowledge must be acquired. It is called the education and posteducation training of the people who are needed to acquire and apply this missing knowledge.

* * *

At different times in the history of science, various nations developed and exploited this cultural resource. There was England in the days of Jenner and his mentor, John Hunter. There were France and Germany during the days of Pasteur and Koch and Ehrlich, and the first of the golden decades of bacteriology, immunology, and the birth of chemotherapy. There was also the United States, particularly between World War II and the Vietnam War.

Science is essentially the quest for new truths about the nature of the world into which we are born, a "complex exploratory process which puts a premium on curiosity, skepticism, imagination and scholarship.... After World War II," declared a delegation of distinguished American biomedical scientists, including six Nobel laureates in medicine, physiology, and chemistry, "it became our national policy to nurture this complex exploratory process on a large scale. In what is widely appreciated as one of the most enlightened achievements of any government anywhere, the United States constructed a support system that optimally encouraged science with a minimum of regulatory interference. The result had been a prodigious outpouring of new discoveries and benefits for people. In the biomedical area alone it has been estimated that for every dollar spent in research $15 have been saved in longer life and reduced illness. Furthermore, non-health related commercial exploitation of biomedical discoveries alone is returning $37 billion per year to our economy, one year of which is equal to the nation's total investment in biomedical science."[43]

The era of the prodigious outpouring of new discoveries began to lose momentum when the rising costs of American involvement in the war in Vietnam began to consume ever-escalating millions of the tax dollars which, between 1945 and 1965, had been allocated for education, postgraduate scientific training, and biomedical research. "During the period of rapid growth and development of biomedical research from 1955 to 1967, the need for well-trained scientists was clearly recognized," writes Dr. John A. D. Cooper, president of the Association of American Medical Colleges. "Increased federal support for research was paralleled by increased funds for fellowships and training grants to carry out the research. However, in 1967 the fears of an impending recession, President [Lyndon B.] Johnson's disaffection for the university faculties that vigorously opposed the Vietnam War, and the change in federal emphasis to equality of educational opportunity and access to undergraduate education, effected a leveling off of the National Institute of Health (NIH) budget, which has continued during the subsequent fiscal years in terms of constant [1967] dollars."[44]

The cutbacks in federal support for education and research continued under the Nixon administration, which as Cooper notes, "called for an end to federal research training support." Congress did not agree, and in 1974 passed the National Research Service Award Act, which allocated funds for research training. However, it is the President who controls the disbursement of federal funds Congress allocates for education, training, and research. The act was noted more for its laudable intent than its performance.

The Carter administration (1977–1981) continued the cutbacks begun and extended during the three previous administrations. These cutbacks, however, were not made to meet the combat costs of the Vietnam War, but to cope with the fiscal inflation caused by that war. In his penultimate (fiscal year 1980) proposed federal budget, President Carter made a nearly 50 percent cut in the already reduced federal funding of new investigator-initiated grants for health research. The same White House budget also called for the termination of ongoing federally funded programs for capitation grants to schools of medicine, nursing, allied health, and public health. While the dollar budgets for the eleven NIH institutes remained at their 1979 levels, continuing double-digit inflation turned the Carter FY 1980 budget for them into an at least 10 percent reduction in federal funding.

The mounting erosion of federal investment in scientific education and training during the Vietnam War and the postwar years has made itself felt acutely in industry and enterprises as well as in academia. In 1982, for example, when the stock bubble burst and shares in the new recombinant DNA or biotechnology firms could not be sold at any price, a study published in the financial section of *The New York Times* listed the "shortage of trained manpower" as the leading reason for the virtual collapse of most of the firms in the new "genetic engineering" industry.

"The five leading companies alone are adding more than 400 professionals annually," reported the *Times* writer. "At present, however, American graduate schools are turning out fewer than 100 Ph.D's annually in the necessary microbiological and biochemical disciplines."[45]

Carter's FY 1980 budget was submitted to Congress a few months after the report prepared by the National Science Foundation (NSF), at his order, on "Science and Engineering Education for the 1980's," was completed and released to the White House and the nation. This 230-page report revealed that because of the breakdown of our lower and college educational systems, most Americans were headed "toward virtual scientific and technical illiteracy." It warned that unless the quality of the American educational system was restored to what it had been before the Vietnam War, this nation would be making critical policy decisions on the basis of "ignorance and misunderstanding." The NSF report also spoke of the desperate need to develop courses for nonscience majors in high schools and colleges that would provide them "with a better basis for understanding and dealing with science and technology they encounter as citizens, workers," voters, future judges, legislators, national budget directors—and Presidents.

Two years earlier, on April 29, 1978, in an address to the American Federation for Clinical Research in San Francisco, the Secretary of Health, Education, and Welfare, Joseph Califano, pointed with alarm to the fact that the presence of young scientists on American university faculties had declined from 43 percent in 1968 to 27 percent in 1975. Dr. John Cooper found such facts "ominous and alarming." Jimmy Carter found them embarrassing. Mr. Califano found himself out of Carter's Cabinet.

In 1981 when Carter was succeeded by Ronald Reagan, the new administration's budget proposed to "more than double annual spending for defense in five years, from $174 billion in 1981 to $374 billion in 1986." This would be accomplished by increasing the annual military appropriations by 7 percent after allowing for inflation for the next five years. When the budget was debated in Congress, Representative Ted Weiss (D., New York) observed that "the total over that period, $1,635 trillion, will almost match the $2.3 trillion spent on defense in the last 35 years—including wars in Korea and Vietnam. This huge boost in the Pentagon's budget will far outweigh projected cuts over the same period in non-defense spending, and poses an inflationary threat to our economy as well." At the same time, the new administration proposed an annual across-the-board 10 percent cut in income taxes for all taxpayers, from billionaires to the working poor, for the next three years.

There is no question that the new United States military appropriations frightened the gentlemen of the Kremlin very much. However, the fears they engendered in Moscow were minuscule compared with the nightmares they evoked in American pediatricians, family doctors, obstetricians, nutritionists, infectious disease specialists, and other concerned health professionals. Many health workers were appalled by the administration's announced determination to fund the new military buildup by slashing all social programs, including the decimation and/or termination of all ongoing federal infant, child, nursing mother, family, and senior citizen nutrition and health programs. The American economists who remembered how earlier administrations' failures to raise taxes to fund the Vietnam and Cambodian wars had caused our present fiscal inflation were equally terrified by the tax cuts that accompanied the inflated costs of military hardware and personnel.

The administration also proposed to "essentially eliminate the National Science Foundation's science education activity."[46] When Reagan took office, the NIH, the principal source of funds for physicians who needed training for careers in medical research, had already been forced to reduce its training-support expenditures from 15 percent of its budget in 1970 to 3.5 percent in 1979. The Reagan administration proposed to cut this even more.

While the Vietnam War and its lasting economic consequences were bankrupting the kindergarten-through-graduate-school educational and postgraduate training systems that had given post-World War II America a near-monopoly on all Nobel prizes in science, and had resulted in the historic procession of new vaccines developed in this country—including those against polio, measles, mumps, rubella, and the adenoviruses, pneumococci, and meningococci—various other countries were reconstructing and improving their own systems designed to produce new scientists. Nowhere was this more apparent than in the two giant industrial nations which, after World War II, were relieved of the enormous fiscal and educational burdens of maintaining vast military machines—Japan and Germany.

In other countries, despite the mounting burdens of national defense, from France and England to Israel, Canada, Australia, China, and the Soviet Union, scientific education and training of young people, and support for their independent research, have contributed to the strength and health of their own and all other nations. It is possibly more than a coincidence that the most revolutionary new vaccine to appear since the subunit vaccines against pneumonia and meningitis and serum hepatitis were developed in the United States—Germanier's live oral vaccine against typhoid—was made in Switzerland, a country that has not been a participant in any of this century's wars.

The Reagan administration's stated intentions toward the further diminutions of education and research evoked many protests in the scientific and educational communities. "We confront a major national problem in the disintegration of science education," warned a delegation of internationally famous American scientists, six of them recent Nobel laureates.

By May 1981, when the Delegation for Basic Biomedical Research presented their thoughts to official Washington, it was well known that Japan, Germany, China, and the Soviet Union—the first two our leading economic competitors, the second two our ideological and perceived potential military adversaries—"all provide rigorous training in science and mathematics for all their citizens." The delegation, reviewing the new proposed cutbacks in the funding of education and research, declared that "we confront a major national problem in the disintegration of science education."[47]

These essentially conservative scientists were not unaware of our needs for national defense. They were, however, also acutely aware of the history of modern civilizations, and therefore concluded by declaring that "at a small fraction of the cost of a massive weapons buildup and a swelling 'safety net,' a rebirth of the quest for knowledge across the nation is our best defense against our enemies and the worst in ourselves."

Only one of our one hundred senators, Mark Hatfield of Oregon, a man of the President's own party, voted against the new administration's "massive weapons buildup." His single dissenting vote is an accurate measure of how seriously the advice of our leading life scientists is regarded in the corridors of national power these days, for many reasons ranging from ideology to political opportunism to entropy.

Ours is not the first nation to let its sciences degenerate. In 1893, when he received the Royal Society's Copley Medal in the theater of London University, with Lord Kelvin in the Chair, Rudolf Virchow, the founder of cellular pathology, spoke of how the history of science has always been punctuated by "long periods of stagnation and numerous interruptions experienced owing to erroneous doctrines." Virchow had political as well as scientific errors in mind.

Virchow was a political man, a long-term reformist member of his nation's Reichstag, as well as a pathologist and a medical scientist; he was as immersed in the history of science and civilization as he was in the multiple structures and functions of the human cells in health and disease. "That which has saved science," Virchow said in the same Croonian Lecture to the Royal Society in 1893, "is identically the same; it only appears to be different, because the co-operation of many is necessary to secure its advance; hence, the exalting and consoling thought that one nation after another comes to the front, to take its share in the work. When the star of science becomes dim in one country it rises sooner or later to yet higher glory in another, and thus nation after nation becomes the teacher of the world.

"No science, more often than medicine, has gone through these waxings and wanings of brilliancy; for medicine alone of all the sciences has, for more than 2000 years, found ever new homes in the course of a progress which, though often disturbed, has never been wholly arrested."

New vaccines will continue to be developed and save millions of more lives. However, in growing numbers they will be developed by scientists whose native language is not American English. The advance of medical science, as Virchow observed on the eve of the centenary celebration of Jenner's smallpox vaccine, "though often disturbed, has never been fully arrested." Not in all countries.

Whatever the nationalities of the men and women who will create the century's next wave of important vaccines, there is still no medical or moral justification for this nation's present underuse of the vaccines presently available to fight major infectious diseases of infancy and early childhood. No matter how one manipulates the data, or how cleverly apologists lie about the realities, there is no escaping the fact that more than one third of this country's over 12 million children under the age of four are deprived each year of available immunizations against polio, diphtheria, tetanus, whooping cough, measles, mumps, and rubella.

When the former Secretary of the former Department of Health, Education, and Welfare, Joseph Califano, looked back on what he had learned, he realized that "in addition to the human illness it prevents, dollar for dollar, childhood immunization is a superb health care investment: For every dollar spent on polio vaccine, our society saves $90 in costs, the highest cost-benefit ratio of any public health program. From 1963 to 1978, this nation's investment of $189 million in polio immunization has saved almost $2 billion in health care and rehabilitation costs."[48]

Paralytic poliomyelitis was always a greatly dreaded affliction, but it was never a major epidemic disease in the United States or any other country. In terms of actual numbers infected, paralytic polio was never as widespread a plague as diphtheria, measles, tetanus, and other now vaccine-preventable contagions. During the decade prior to the licensing of the first polio vaccine in 1955, a total of 218,470 cases of acute or paralytic polio were reported by American doctors to their local health departments; during the ten years prior to the licensing of the first measles vaccine in 1963, a total of 5,206,791 cases of measles were reported in this country, nearly twenty-four times the number of polio cases reported here during a comparable decade.

Mass-vaccination programs have considerably reduced the number of reported measles cases—from 481,530 cases reported in 1962 to a gratifying low of 13,406 reported in 1980. Reported cases, unfortunately, represent only a fraction of the actual cases of measles and most other common and usually self-terminating infectious diseases in the United States. Measles is still a major cause of death, impaired vision, and mental retardation among unimmunized poor children around the world.

Given the known data on deaths, major defects, and chronic dependency caused by all six of the other vaccine-preventable major infectious diseases of infancy and childhood, it is apparent that the tax-dollar savings achieved for the U.S. Treasury by available vaccines since 1955 have added up to considerably more than the well over $2 billion that our modest investment in polio vaccinations alone have saved for the people of the United States.

The continued failure to make intelligent and maximum use of available vaccines for people of all ages is therefore not only immoral—and for one third of the nation, it is actually genocidal—but it is also criminally wasteful of the tax monies our government collects from the hard-working people who pay most of those taxes.

Notes and References

CHAPTER 1

1.   John B. Robbins, "Vaccines for the Prevention of Encapsulated Bacterial Diseases: Current Status, Problems and Prospects for the Future," *Immunochemistry,* 15:839–854, 1978, see p. 849.

2.   Oswald T. Avery and Michael Heidelberger, "Soluble Specific Substances of the Pneumococcus," *Journal of Experimental Medicine,* 81:73–79, 1923.

3.   O. Schiemann and W. Casper, "Sind die Spezifische Präcipitablen Substanzen der 3 Pneumokokkentypen Haptene?" *Zeitschrift für Hygiene und Infektionskrankheiten,* 108:220–257, 1927.

4.   Memorandum from Dr. T. J. Bauer, U.S. Public Health Service, Chicago, to Dr. Wolfgang Casper, Re: Assignment, January 6, 1944. Note: For a few years before his death in 1982, Dr. Casper made his files available to me and generously had photocopies made for my use, of this and other documents. These included letters to and from Dr. Casper, patent papers, and reprints of journal articles in German and English. I also taped many hours of interviews with Dr. Casper. These documentary and taped accounts were the primary sources of the materials in this chapter that deal with his contributions to the development of purified bacterial capsular vaccines against bacterial infections.

5.   Michael Heidelberger, "A 'Pure' Organic Chemist's Downward Path: Chapter 2—The Years at P. and S.," *Annual Review of Biochemistry,* 48:1–21, 1979.

6.   Ibid., p. 12.

7.   John V. Bennett, "Human Infections: Economic Implications and Prevention," *Annals of Internal Medicine,* part 2, 89:5, November 1978.

8.   Ibid., pp. 821–825.

9.   Ibid., pp. 761–763.

10.   Allan Chase, "The Fourth Leading Cause of U.S. Deaths," Health News Commentary, *Medical Tribune,* September 12, 1979, pp. 10, 13.

11.   Statistical Abstract of the United States, 99th ed., 1978.

12.   *Morbidity and Mortality Weekly Report (MMWR), Annual Summary 1979,* Centers for Disease Control, 28:54, September 1980, p. 65.

13.   Sarah H. W. Sell et al., "Long-Term Sequellae of Hemophilus [sic] influenzae Meningitis," *Pediatrics,* 49:206–211, 1972. See also J. Lindberg et al., "Long-term Outcome of Haemophilus influenzae type b Meningitis Related to Antibiotic Treatment," *Pediatrics,* 60:1–6, 1977.

14.   René Dubos, *Louis Pasteur, Free Lance of Science* (Boston: Little, Brown, 1950), pp. 355–356. See also René Vallery-Radot, *The Life of Pasteur,* Paris, 1901, tr. by Mrs. R. L. Devonshire, 1902 (Garden City, N.Y.: Garden City Publishing Co., undated), chapters XII and XIII.

CHAPTER 2

1.   H. Thursfield, "Smallpox in the American War of Independence," *Annals of Medical History,* 2:312, 1940. See also Solon S. Bernstein, "Smallpox and Variolation," *Journal of Mt. Sinai Hospital,* vol. 18, 1951, pp. 228–244.

2.   John Baron, *The Life of Dr. Jenner,* 2 vols. (London, 1827, 1838). See also W. R. LeFanu, *A Bio-Bibliography of Edward Jenner, 1749–1823* (London, 1951).

3.   Donald A. Henderson, "The Eradication of Smallpox," *Scientific American,* 235, 4:25–33, October 1976.

4.   John W. Osborne, *The Silent Revolution: The Industrial Revolution in England as a Source of Cultural Change* (New York: Charles Scribner's Sons, 1970), p. 32.

5.   Florence Nightingale, *Notes on Nursing* (London, 1859; New York: Dover replica edition, 1969), pp. 32–33n.

6.   Robert H. Halsey, *How the President* [Jefferson] *Established Vaccination,* New York Academy of Medicine History of Medicine Series, no. 5, 1936.

7.   For more on Galton, see his own writings, principally, *Hereditary Genius* (London, 1869); *Inquiries Into Human Faculty* (London, 1883); and *Memories of My Life* (London, 1908), as well as the hagiographic four-volume *Life, Letters and Labours of Francis Galton* by his disciple and intellectual heir, Karl Pearson (Cambridge, 1914–1940). For a more recent view of Galton and his influence, see Allan Chase, *The Legacy of Malthus* (New York: Alfred A. Knopf, 1977), chapters 1–3, 5–12, 14–16, 20–22. For more on Spencer, see works cited in text pages.

The dogmas of Galton and Spencer permeated the education and the conventional wisdom of the people who controlled American as well as British public health and social policies for a century; Spencer's attacks on free vaccinations, free libraries, and public safety regulations are very clearly reflected in current legislative and administrative programs and policies. The fashionable American neo-conservatism of the 1980s is, in essence, Spencer's New Toryism of 1884.

8.   Wesley W. Spink, *Infectious Diseases, Prevention and Treatment in the Nineteenth and Twentieth Centuries* (Minneapolis: University of Minnesota Press, 1978), Shattuck Report of Massachusetts, 1850, appendix I, pp. 449–454.

9.   John Duffy, *The Healers, A History of American Medicine* (Urbana, Ill., 1979; New York: McGraw-Hill, 1976), p. 202.

10.   Wilson G. Smillie, "The Period of Great Epidemics in the United States (1800–1875)," chapter II in C.E.A. Winslow et al., *The History of American Epidemiology* (St. Louis, Mo.: C. V. Mosby, 1952), pp. 52–73. Professor Smillie, chairman of the Department of Preventive Medicine and Public Health, Cornell University Medical College, wrote in this chapter that "urbanization of the nation without proper understanding of the problems and hazards of crowded community life was one of the most important factors in the high death rate," p. 63. He added that during the years "1800 to 1870, the period of great epidemics" in this country, "the data show that the great proportion of deaths were due to unfavorable environmental factors, to polluted water supplies, indescribable systems of feces disposal, overcrowding, with resultant disreputable housing conditions, bad milk, bad food, flies in millions, poor nutrition, long hours of overwork, and gross ignorance and carelessness," p. 69.

11.   Data from the World Health Organization, 1980.

12.   The Jenner Society, "Antivaccination Propaganda: The Bane and Its Antidote," *British Medical Journal,* July 5, 1902, pp. 50–52.

13.   Anonymous [possibly, E. J. Edwardes, M.D., M.R.C.P.], "Sanitation or Vaccination. Subsection I: Vaccination Without Sanitation," ibid., p. 69.

14.   E. J. Edwardes, "A Century of Vaccination: Small-pox Epidemics and Small-pox Mortality Before and Since Vaccination Came Into Use," ibid., pp. 27–30.

15.   Data from annual reports of the New York City Board of Health; various years starting in 1850.

16.   *British Medical Journal,* July 5, 1902.

17.   Norman Howard-Jones, *The Scientific Background of the International Sanitary Conferences, 1851–1938,* World Health Organization, Geneva, 1975, pp. 97–98.

18.   At the spring meeting of the American Pediatric Society in Philadelphia in 1965, Dr. Kempe presented his suggestions that smallpox vaccinations should not be performed routinely. Kempe and Benenson were not opposed to smallpox vaccination per se. In their *Journal of the American Medical Association* (*JAMA*) article they declared, "When international eradication has been

achieved, there will be no need for smallpox vaccination. Until that time, we are faced with the problem of deciding whether the benefit of protection thus produced outweighs the dangers associated with the procedure." See C. Henry Kempe and Abram S. Benenson, "Smallpox Immunization in the United States," *JAMA,* October 11, 1965, pp. 161-166; and Kempe, "Studies on Smallpox and Complications of Smallpox Vaccination," *Pediatrics,* August 1960, pp. 176-189. See also Anonymous, "Curb on Vaccination Urged. Charging that Smallpox Vaccine Is Responsible for More U.S. Deaths Than It Prevents, Pediatrician Would Stop Routine Immunization Until Better Methods Are Developed," *Medical World News* (*MWN*) June 4, 1965, p. 40. The *MWN* news story quotes the reactions of the doctors present at the Philadelphia meeting, including Dr. Saul Krugman, chairman of pediatrics at New York University, who was quoted as asserting, "If we accept Dr. Kempe's proposal, we are likely to revert to the 1920-1930 prevalence of smallpox." Dr. Margaret H. D. Smith of Tulane University said that she was "in favor of immunizing travelers entering the country—people really at risk. But I agree that universal vaccination of children has not only become obsolete but is reprehensible." Kempe agreed that travelers should be vaccinated.

CHAPTER 3

1.   *Charles Dickens' Uncollected Writings from Household Words,* Harry Stone, ed. (Bloomington: University of Indiana Press, 1968). Henry Morley (1822-1894) Stone reveals, was trained in medicine, partly in Germany. "When Dickens founded *Household Words* [in 1850] he asked Morley to contribute ... and in July 1851, he became a salaried member of the staff" of the magazine. In 1865 Morley "was appointed professor of English language and literature at University College, and subsequently at Queen's College, London."

2.   The great but poor poet and painter William Blake (1757-1827) earned a portion of his meager living by making engravings of Wedgwood pottery and other industrial goods for manufacturers' catalogues. His witnessing of the new machines and new classes of factory workers gave us not only his Satanic Wheels, but also lasting testimony to the genius that great poets have always had to explain the changes of history.

3.   William Hallock Park and Anna W. Williams, *Pathogenic Micro-Organisms Including Bacteria and Protozoa. A Practical Manual for Students, Physicians and Health Officers,* 2nd ed. (New York and Philadelphia, 1905), pp. 18-19.

4.   Much of the materials on the early nineteenth-century history of how these red spots were proven to be caused by the bacte-

rium *Serratia marcescens* are taken from the brilliant paper "From Superstition to Science: The History of a Bacterium," presented before the New York Academy of Sciences by Dr. Eugene R. L. Gaughran on January 26, 1968, and subsequently published in the *Transactions of the New York Academy of Sciences,* series II, vol. 31, no. 1, January 1969, pp. 3–24.

5.   Charles Hall, *The Effects of Civilization on the People in European States. With: Observations on the Principal Conclusion in Mr. Malthus' Essay on Population* (London, 1805; New York: Kelley, facsimile edition, 1965), preface, pp. i, ii.

6.   E. Royston Pike, *"Hard Times," Human Documents of the Industrial Revolution* (London; New York: Praeger, 1966), pp. 92–95. This book and Pike's matching anthology, *"Golden Times," Human Documents of the Victorian Age* (London; New York: Praeger, 1967), are two of the most useful books available describing the full impact of the Industrial Revolution on the human condition. Both volumes are also well illustrated.

7.   Robert Owen, *A New View of Society,* 1831, cited in Pike, *Hard Times,* pp. 37–42.

8.   The best single source book on the subject is the classic by B. L. Hutchins and A. Harrison, *A History of Factory Legislation,* 2nd ed., revised (London, 1911). It covers the history of legislation concerning the protection of workers from occupational diseases and industrial accidents in England since 1802, as well as laws affecting working conditions, wages, hours, child labor, education, and factory inspections since the start of the Industrial Revolution.

9.   The testimony by Drs. Blane and Ure, and by the noted parliamentary investigator J. E. White, are cited in Pike, *Hard Times,* pp. 107, 214; and in Pike, *Golden Times,* pp. 133–134. Dr. Ure, a professor of chemistry at Glasgow and member of the Royal Society, was, as Pike notes, an outspoken "antagonist of factory legislation, and his almost lyrical descriptions of factory life aroused the ire of reformers." One of these accounts of the welfare of child factory workers is taken from Ure's book *The Philosophy of Manufactures,* published in 1835.

10.   In 1775 Sir Percival Pott (1713–1788), surgeon at St. Bartholomew's Hospital in London, published a study in which he showed that the epidemic of scrotal cancer then raging in boys and small men who worked as chimney sweeps was caused by coal soot. This epidemic occurred after the seventeenth- and eighteenth-century wood famine caused England to become the world's first coal-burning society. See Allan Chase, *The Biological Imperatives* (New York: Holt, Rinehart & Winston, 1971), pp. 178–179.

11.   Gillian Avery, *Victorian People in Life and Literature* (New York: Holt, Rinehart & Winston, 1970), pp. 166–169.

12.   William Buchan, *Domestic Medicine: Or a Treatise on the Prevention and Cure of Diseases,* 12th ed. (London, 1791), preface, pp. xi, xii.

13.   C. Turner Thackrah, *The Effects of the Principal Arts, Trades, and Professions, and of Civic States and Habits of Living, on Health and Longevity: With a Particular Reference to the Trades and Manufactures of Leeds: and Suggestions for the Removal of Many of the Agents Which Produce Disease, and Shorten the Duration of Life* (London, 1831).

14.   Samuel E. Finer, *The Life and Times of Sir Edwin Chadwick* (London: British Book Centre, 1952; New York: Barnes & Noble, 1970), p. 29.

15.   Ibid., p. 32.

16.   Thomas McKeown and C. R. Lewis, *An Introduction to Social Medicine,* 2nd ed. (Oxford, England, 1974), pp. 292–295.

17.   Peter B. Medawar, *Advice to a Young Scientist* (New York: Harper & Row, 1979), pp. 102–103.

18.   R. J. Mitchell and M. D. R. Leys, "Edwin Chadwick's London," *A History of London Life* (London: Longmans, 1958; Baltimore: Penguin, 1963), chapter XIII, pp. 272–273.

19.   R. A. Lewis, *Edwin Chadwick and the Public Health Movement* (London: Longmans, 1952), pp. 230–233. See also Finer, op. cit., pp. 347–348.

20.   Edwin H. Kass, "Infectious Diseases and Social Change," *Journal of Infectious Diseases,* 123, 1:113, January 1971.

21.   See Allan Chase, *The Legacy of Malthus* (New York: Alfred A. Knopf, 1977), pp. 429, 403–405.

CHAPTER 4

1.   Norman Howard-Jones, *The Scientific Background of the International Sanitary Conferences, 1851–1938,* World Health Organization, Geneva, 1975, pp. 17, 20, and others, including page 28 for a portrait of Pacini.

2.   Ibid., pp. 17, 27.

3.   René Vallery-Radot, *The Life of Pasteur* (Paris, 1901), p. 227.

4.   Hubert A. Lechevalier and Morris Solotorovsky, *Three Centuries of Microbiology* (New York: Dover Publications, 1974), p. 69. Probably the best modern history of microbiology and particularly useful because the authors included long excerpts from the original journal papers of the people who made modern microbiology.

5.   Ibid.

6.   Ibid., p. 84.

7.   Vallery-Radot, op. cit., p. 289.

8.   Ibid., p. 291.
9.   Ibid., p. 274.
10.   Ibid., p. 413.

CHAPTER 5

1.   Norman Howard-Jones, *The Scientific Background of the International Sanitary Conferences 1851-1938,* World Health Organization, Geneva, 1975.

2.   Hans Zinsser, "Biographical Memoir of Theobald Smith, 1859-1934," *National Academy of Sciences, Biographical Memoirs,* vol. XII, 1936, pp. 261-303. See also Charles R. Stockard, "Obituary," *Science,* December 21, 1934, pp. 579-580; E. E. Tyzzer, "Theobald Smith," *New England Journal of Medicine,* January 24, 1935, pp. 168-171; and William Bulloch, "Obituary Notice of Deceased Member, Theobald Smith," *Journal of Pathology,* XL:621-635, 1940.

3.   R. M. Allen, *The Microscope,* 5th ed. (New York: D. Van Nostrand, 1947), p. 8.

4.   Joseph Lister, "On the Antiseptic Principle of the Practice of Surgery," *British Medical Journal,* II:246-248, 1867, cited in C. N. B. Camac, *Classics of Medicine and Surgery* (New York, 1909; reprinted, Dover Publications, 1959).

5.   Lister was as generous in giving credit for scientific discoveries to their originators as he was ready to admit his own scientific errors. In a letter to Louis Pasteur dated February 13, 1874, Lister wrote: "I do not know whether the records of British *Surgery* ever meet your eye. If so, you will have seen from time to time notices of the antiseptic system of treatment, which I have been labouring for the last nine years to bring to perfection. Allow me to take this opportunity to tender to you my most cordial thanks for having, by your brilliant researches, demonstrated to me the truth of the germ theory of putrefaction, and thus furnished me with the principle upon which alone the antiseptic system can be carried out."

William Bulloch, in an article in the Lister Centenary Celebrations issue of the *British Medical Journal,* April 9, 1927, pp. 664-666, wrote of how when Pasteur corrected one of his errors, Lister observed that "next to the promulgation of truth, the best thing I can conceive that a man can do is the recantation of a published error."

6.   From a letter on Semmelweis Centenary by L. Iffy, M.D. (Budapest), in the *Journal of the Canadian Medical Association,* August 14, 1965, p. 327. These words might not be found in this form in Lister's writings, since they sound as if they were translated from Hungarian to English.

7.   Howard-Jones, op. cit., pp. 67-68.

8. Olga Metchnikoff, *Life of Elie Metchnikoff* (Boston, 1921), pp. 154–157. The materials on this and other episodes in Metchnikoff's career derive in large part from his wife's biography of him.

9. Hubert A. Lechevalier and Morris Solotorovsky, *Three Centuries of Microbiology* (New York: Dover Publications, 1974), pp. 214–215.

10. Martha Marquardt, *Paul Ehrlich* (New York: Henry Schuman, 1950). This memoir by Ehrlich's secretary is the source of these accounts of his work.

11. See note 10.

12. R. L. Simmons and R. J. Howard, eds., *Surgical Infectious Diseases* (New York: Appleton-Century-Crofts, 1981).

CHAPTER 6

1. Not every American doctor, President, and intellectual accepted the phrenology fad as a science. The scholar-statesman Caleb Cushing wrote that "phrenology is the perversion of physiology, as alchemy is of chemistry, astrology of astronomy, and mesmerism of electromagnetism." Oliver Wendell Holmes, Sr., professor of medicine at Harvard, dismissed phrenology as a "pseudo-science." The most underrated President in American history, John Quincy Adams, "felt, as did Cicero about the Roman augurs, he could not see how two phrenologists could look each other in the face without bursting into laughter," cited in John D. Davies, *Phrenology, Fad and Science* (New Haven: Yale University Press, 1955).

2. Gerald B. Webb and Desmond Powell, *Henry Sewall, Physiologist and Physician* (Baltimore: Johns Hopkins University Press, 1946), pp. 74–78. See also Henry Sewall, "Experiments on the Preventive Inoculation of Rattlesnake Venom," *Journal of Physiology* (England), 8:203–210, 1887; and A. McGehee Harvey, "Snake Venom and Medical Research—Some Contributions Related to the Johns Hopkins University School of Medicine," *Johns Hopkins Medical Journal,* February 1978, pp. 47–60.

3. René Vallery-Radot, *The Life of Pasteur* (Paris, 1901), p. 453.

4. Ralph H. Major, *Classic Descriptions of Disease* (Springfield, Ill.: C. C. Thomas, 1947), pp. 136–137; see also pp. 137–161 for descriptions of diphtheria by Baillou, Bretonneau, and other physicians.

5. Ibid. For Hippocrates and Aretaeus on tetanus, see pp. 134–135. Wesley W. Spink in *Infectious Diseases* has an informative subchapter on tetanus before and after World War I, pp. 299–302.

The tetanus bacilli were for many years common contaminants of smallpox vaccine preparations, and killed so many children that it helped the antivaccination movements slow the enactment and administration of compulsory vaccination laws in the nineteenth and twentieth centuries. The same tragedies followed the uses of diphtheria antisera that had been contaminated with tetanus organisms. In a recent book Dr. Joel M. Solomon wrote of one such "medical disaster that shocked the American people. Beginning in 1894, the City of St. Louis employed a bacteriologist to prepare diphtheria antitoxin from the blood of immunized horses and to distribute it free to physicians. During 1901, 14 children who had received diphtheria antitoxin died of tetanus. An investigation established that the blood of one of the horses used in the manufacture of the antitoxin contained live tetanus organisms that were the source of the infection. These deaths spurred the introduction in Congress of two bills, both of which were enacted on July, 1902. One established the Public Health and Marine Hospital Service [now the U.S. Public Health Service], the second authorized the new service to regulate the sale and transportation of any virus, therapeutic serum, toxin or analogous product in interstate commerce or from any foreign country." Morris Schaeffer, *Federal Legislation and the Clinical Laboratory,* (Boston: G. K. Hall Medical Publishers, 1981), pp. 145–146.

6.   Lewis Thomas, *The Lives of a Cell* (New York: Viking Press, 1974), p. 76.

7.   Simon Flexner and James Thomas Flexner, *William Henry Welch and the Heroic Age of American Medicine* (New York: Viking Press, 1941). While studying under Weigert in Leipzig in 1885, Welch in a letter to his father wrote that Weigert had just been denied an appointment as a professor. Welch wrote, "It is a terrible outrage as Weigert is unquestionably one of the leading pathologists living, but he is a Jew and it seems that no Jew is likely to get an appointment in a German university," p. 140.

8.   Hubert A. Lechevalier and Morris Solotorovsky, *Three Centuries of Microbiology* (New York: Dover Publications, 1974), p. 439.

9.   Wade Oliver, *The Man Who Lived for Tomorrow: A Biography of William Hallock Park* (New York: E. P. Dutton, 1941). Many of the biographical notes on Park in this book are derived from Oliver's biography.

10.   Theobald Smith, "Active Immunity Produced by So-called Balanced or Neutral Mixtures of Diphtheria Toxin and Antitoxin," *Journal of Experimental Medicine,* 11:241–256, 1909; and "Degree and Duration of Passive Immunity to Diphtheria Toxin Transmitted by Immunized Female Guinea-pigs to Their Immediate Offspring," *Journal of Medical Research,* 16:259–379, 1907.

11.   W. H. Park, "The History of Diphtheria in New York

City," *American Journal of Diseases of Children,* 42:1439–1445, 1931; "Active Immunization in Diphtheria by Toxin-Antitoxin Mixture," *American Journal of Obstetrics,* 68:1213–1215, 1913; William H. Park and Eugene Famulener, "Toxin-Antitoxin Mixtures as Immunizing Agents," *Proceedings of the Society for Experimental Biology and Medicine,* 33rd meeting, April 21, 1909, pp. 98–99; and William H. Park and Abraham Zingher, "Active Immunization in Diphtheria and Treatment by Toxin-Antitoxin," *Journal of the American Medical Association* (*JAMA*), September 1914, pp. 859–863; December 25, 1915, pp. 2216–2220, [Two articles].

12. William H. Park, "Toxin-Antitoxin Immunization Against Diphtheria," *JAMA,* November 4, 1922, pp. 1584–1591.

13. Julius Blum, "Active Immunization Against Diphtheria in a Large Child-Caring Institution," *American Journal of Diseases of Children,* 1920, pp. 22–28.

CHAPTER 7

1. Simon Flexner and James Thomas Flexner, *William Henry Welch and the Heroic Age of American Medicine* (New York: Viking Press, 1941), pp. 376–377.

2. W. I. B. Beveridge, *Influenza, the Last Great Plague* (London: Heinemann Ed., 1977), p. 32.

3. Major Greenwood, *Epidemics and Crowd-Diseases: An Introduction to the Study of Epidemiology* (London, 1935).

4. Alison Glover, "The Incidence of Rheumatic Diseases," *Lancet,* March 8, 1930, pp. 499–505. See fig. 5, p. 503.

5. John M. Gibson, *Physician to the World: The Life of General William C. Gorgas* (Durham, N.C.: Duke University Press, 1950), pp. 237–244.

6. The literature on infectious diseases and the outcomes of wars throughout history is vast. To cite only four books, as done below, slights dozens of other fine volumes. Any such list must include the now classic book by Hans Zinsser, *Rats, Lice and History,* (Boston: Little, Brown, 1934), and the recent book by the University of Chicago historian William H. McNeill, *Plagues and Peoples,* (Garden City, N.Y.: Doubleday, 1976). Paul E. Steiner's *Disease in the Civil War, Natural Biological Warfare in 1861–1865* (Springfield, Ill.: C. C. Thomas, 1968) is invaluable for a mature understanding of the many roles of common contagions in that seminal conflict. Alfred W. Crosby, Jr., like McNeill a professor of history, gave us *Epidemic and Peace, 1918* (Westport, Conn.: Greenwood Press, 1976), which draws extensively on the annals of military medicine as well as on the records of the impact of the great influenza pandemic on the home front.

7. Crosby, op. cit., p. 27.

8. May C. Schroeder, "The Duration of the Immunity Conferred by the Use of Diphtheria Toxin-Antitoxin," *Archives of Pediatrics,* June 1921, pp. 368–378.

9.   Abraham Zingher, "Diphtheria Preventive Work in the Public Schools of New York City," ibid., pp. 336–359. On June 5, 1927, six years after this historic report appeared, Zingher, who held doctorates in medicine and public health, was asphyxiated in his laboratory at the old Willard Parker Hospital for Infectious Diseases. The Roumanian-born professor of bacteriology and pediatrics, and director of the Bureau of Laboratories of the New York City Department of Health, was forty-two years old at the time of his death.

10.   See note 9.

11.   Wade Oliver, *The Man Who Lived for Tomorrow: A Biography of William Hallock Park* (New York: E. P. Dutton, 1941).

CHAPTER 8

1.   Surgeon General William C. Gorgas and Professor Lewis J. Johnson, *Two Papers on Sanitation and the Single Tax,* Walter Mendelson, ed., Joseph Fels Fund of America, Cincinnati, Ohio, 1915.

2.   Quoted in S. Adolphus Knopf, "Major General William C. Gorgas, M. C., U.S.A., 1854–1920," *American Review of Tuberculosis,* IV:10, December 1920, p. 730. W. C. Gorgas, presidential address to the American Medical Association, *Journal of the American Medical Association (JAMA),* 1909. Gorgas also wrote a book, *Sanitation in Panama* (New York, 1915). Michael H. Ellman, in a commentary on Gorgas on the 125th anniversary of his birth, writes how the work of Gorgas made the death rate for Americans living in Panama "lower than in most parts of the United States," *JAMA,* February 15, 1980, pp. 659–660.

3.   Ibid.

4.   David McCullough, *The Path Between the Seas* (New York: Simon & Schuster, 1977), pp. 443–444. See also "The Imperturbable Dr. Gorgas," chapter 15, pp. 405–437.

5.   Ibid., pp. 473–474.

6.   Ibid.

7.   Ibid., pp. 477–478.

8.   W. C. Gorgas, "Recommendation as to Sanitation Concerning Employees of the Mines on the Rand Made to the Transvaal Chamber of Mines," *JAMA,* 62:1855–1865, 1914.

9.   John M. Gibson, *Physician to the World: The Life of General William C. Gorgas* (Durham, N.C.: Duke University Press, 1950), p. 198.

10.   Ibid., p. 93.

11.   While Gorgas was late in accepting Nott's concept of malaria and yellow fever as mosquito-vectored infections, Gorgas

never accepted the pseudoscience for which Nott was much more famous—what Nott himself termed "niggerology." This was a blend of cranial measurements, pop history, and ultimately even a perversion of Darwinian evolution to prove that black people were biologically inferior to whites, and that therefore slavery was morally justified. After the American Civil War ended chattel black slavery, Nott was in the forefront of many American intellectuals and statesmen who fought the federal Freedmen's Bureau and all other programs to educate and train and provide adequate medical care for the newly enfranchised blacks. See Stephen Jay Gould, *The Mismeasure of Man,* (New York, 1981), chapter 2, subsection "The American School and Slavery"; also John S. Haller, Jr., *Outcasts From Evolution: Scientific Attitudes of Racial Inferiority, 1859-1900* (Urbana: University of Illinois Press, 1971), chapter 3, subsection "Josiah C. Nott," p. 86.

12. Gorgas and Johnson, Mendelson, ed., op. cit., pp. 9–10.

13. Robert Austrian, "Of Gold and Pneumococci: A History of Pneumococcal Vaccines in South Africa," *Transactions of the American Clinical and Climatological Association,* 89:141–161, 1977.

14. William Osler, *Man's Redemption of Man. A Lay Sermon* (London, 1910).

15. Austrian, op. cit., p. 141.

16. Gibson, op. cit.

17. Sir Almroth Wright et al., "Pharmaco-therapy of Pneumococcus Infections," *Lancet,* December 14, 1912, pp. 1633–1637 (part I), and December 21, 1912, pp. 1701–1705.

18. Sir Almroth Wright et al., "Prophylactic Inoculation Against Pneumococcus Infections and on the Results Which Have Been Achieved by It," *Lancet,* January 3, 1914; January 10, 1914, pp. 1–10, 87–95.

19. Wright et al., op. cit., December 21, 1912, p. 1703.

20. Austrian, op. cit., p. 147.

21. W. C. Gorgas, op. cit., *JAMA,* 1914.

22. Mendelson, op. cit., p. 9.

23. Franz Neufeld and Ludwig Händel, "Weitere Untersuchen über Pneumokokken-Heilsera. III. Über Vorkommen und Bedeutung atypischer Vareitäten der Pneumokokkus," *Arbeiten aus dem Kaiserlichen Gesundheitsamte* (Berlin), 34:293–304, 1910.

24. René J. Dubos, *The Professor, the Institute and DNA* (New York: Rockefeller University Press, 1976), pp. 101–102. The "Professor" was Oswald Avery, and this book is in part a biography.

25. Ibid., p. 63.

26. A. G. Auld, "Remarks on the Morphology and Chemical Products of the Diplococcus pneumoniae, and Some Results of Vaccination," *British Medical Journal,* March 27, 1897, pp. 775–777.

27. A. R. Dochez and O. T. Avery, "The Elaboration of Specific Soluble Substance by Pneumococcus During Growth," *Journal of Experimental Medicine,* 26:477, 1917. See also *Transactions of the Association of American Physicians,* 32:281, 1917.

28. Ibid.

29. Michael Heidelberger, "A 'Pure' Organic Chemist's Downward Path," *Annual Review of Microbiology,* 1977, pp. 1–12.

30. Ibid., p. 1.

31. Ibid., p. 8.

32. M. Heidelberger and O. T. Avery, "The Soluble Specific Substance of the Pneumococcus," *Journal of Experimental Medicine,* 38:73–79, 1923.

33. Wolfgang A. Casper, "Abraham Buschke 1868–1943. Centennial of His Birth," *Archives of Dermatology,* December 1968, p. 662.

34. Felton wrote a number of detailed reports on his capsular polysaccharide pneumococcal vaccines, including one in the *Journal of Immunology* in 1932, p. 45, and a detailed account of his Civilian Conservation Camp mass trials in the *Public Health Reports,* 53:1855, 1938. The fine science writer J. D. Ratcliff wrote an informative, detailed account of Felton's work on these vaccines, "Bully-Boy Microbe," in the January 27, 1940, issue of *Collier's* magazine, pp. 19–63. Ratcliff brought the pneumococcal vaccine story up to date after the war in a shorter article, "You Can Be Immune to Pneumonia," in the February 1948 issue of *McCall's* magazine, p. 2.

35. Michael Heidelberger, "A 'Pure' Organic Chemist's Downward Path: Chapter 2—The Years at P. and S.," *Annual Review of Biochemistry,* 48:1–21, 1979. See also Colin M. MacLeod et al., "Prevention of Pneumococcal Pneumonia by Immunization With Specific Capsular Polysaccharides," *Journal of Experimental Medicine,* December, 1945, pp. 445–465. Heidelberger was one of the three coauthors.

36. Oswald T. Avery, Colin M. MacLeod, and Maclyn McCarty, "Studies on the Chemical Nature of the Substance Inducing Transformation of Pneumococcal Types," *Journal of Experimental Medicine,* 79:1944, pp. 137–158.

CHAPTER 9

1. The four article excerpts in the epigraph are all from Lechevalier's and Solotorovsky's beautifully documented *Three Centuries of Microbiology* (New York: Dover Publications, 1974): Beijerinck, p. 287; Loeffler and Frosch, p. 286; Reed and Carroll, p. 299; Ellerman and Bang, p. 301.

2. A very condensed and selective list of published references would have to include John N. Mackenzie, "The Massacre of the Tonsil," *Maryland Medical Journal*, June 1912, pp. 138-150, Kenelm H. Digby, "The Functions of the Tonsils and the Appendix," *Lancet*, January 20, 1912, pp. 160-161; and *Immunity in Health: The Function of the Tonsils and Other Subepithelial Lymphatic Glands in the Bodily Economy* (London, 1919). See also Albert D. Kaiser, "Effect of Tonsillectomy on General Health in Five Thousand Children," *Journal of the American Medical Association (JAMA)*, 1922, pp. 1869-1873, and "Significance of the Tonsils in the Development of the Child," *JAMA*, 1940, pp. 1151-1156; Selwyn D. Collins, "An Epidemiological and Statistical Study of Tonsillitis," *Public Health Bulletin No. 175, July 1927*, Washington, D.C., 1928, pp. 1-159; J. Alison Glover and Fred Griffith, "Acute Tonsillitis and Some of Its Sequels," *British Medical Journal*, September 19, 1931, pp. 521-527. J. Alison Glover and Joyce Wilson, "The End-results of the Tonsil and Adenoid Operation in Childhood and Adolescence," *British Medical Journal*, September 10, 1932, pp. 506-512; J. Alison Glover, "The Incidence of Tonsillectomy in School Children," *Proceedings of the Royal Society of Medicine*, 31:1219-1236, 1938; T. B. Layton, "What Can We Do to Diminish the Number of Tonsil Operations?" *Lancet*, January 20, 1934, pp. 117-119; Maxwell Finland, William H. Robey, et al., "The Effect of Tonsillectomy on the Occurrence and Course of Acute Polyarthritis," *American Heart Journal*, 8:343-356, 1933; J. Alison Glover, "Tonsillectomy in the School Medical Service. IV. Increased Incidence Since 1948," *Monthly Bulletin of the Ministry of Health and the Public Health Laboratory Service* (London), 9:62-68, 1950; Lois P. McCorkle et al., "Relation of Tonsillectomy to Incidence of Common Respiratory Diseases in Children," *New England Journal of Medicine*, June 23, 1955, pp. 1066-1069; John Fry, "Are All 'T's and A's' Really Necessary?" *British Medical Journal*, January 19, 1957, pp. 124-129; Harry Bakwin, "The Tonsil-Adenoidectomy Enigma," *Journal of Pediatrics*, March 1958, pp. 339-361; R. S. Illingsworth, "Is the Removal of Tonsils and Adenoids Necessary?" *Proceedings of the Royal Society of Medicine*, May 1961, pp. 393-402; and Macfarlane Burnet and David O. White, *Natural History of Infectious Disease*, 3rd ed. (Cambridge, England, 1962).

3.   R. Chamovitz, C. H. Rammelkamp, Jr., et al., "The Effect of Tonsillectomy on the Incidence of Streptococcal Respiratory Disease and Its Complications," *Pediatrics*, September 1960, pp. 355-367.

4.   John V. Bennett, "Human Infections: Economic Implications and Prevention," *Annals of Internal Medicine*, part 2, 89:761-763, 1978.

5.   S. Monckton Copeman, "Pathology of Vaccinia and Variola," British Medical Journal, January 7, 1896, p. 9. See also Copeman, *Vaccination: Its Natural History and Pathology* (Milroy

Lectures, 1898), London, 1899, and Copeman, "Bacteriology of Vaccinia and Variola," *British Medical Journal,* May 23, 1896, pp. 1277-1279.

In the same article which first described how Copeman successfully vaccinated children with lymph from calves which had previously been inoculated with the products of these egg cultures of variola "germs," he also wrote of his concurrent experiments with the production of a possible "antitoxic serum which might be useful in the treatment of small-pox, it being well known that vaccination is of practically no avail when once the disease has developed." Copeman hoped that such an antitoxin "would form a fitting complement to the Jennerian process of preventive vaccination." Other doctors in England and elsewhere, in this centennial year of Jenner's vaccine, were also working on antisera to cure smallpox, and many of them reported achieving cures, while others reported failures to cure the disease with their antismallpox sera.

6.   Hubert A. Lechevalier and Morris Solotorovsky, *Three Centuries of Microbiology* (New York: Dover Publications, 1974), pp. 286-289.

7.   Ibid.

8.   Ibid., p. 283. See also T. D. Brock, *Milestones in Microbiology,* Washington, D.C., 1975, pp. 149-153, for excerpt from Loeffler-Frosch report.

9.   Walter Reed and James Carroll, "Experimental Yellow Fever," *Transactions of the Association of American Physicians,* 16, 1901, p. 45. Less than one year after this was published, Walter Reed died, at the age of fifty-two, of peritonitis following an appendectomy. Peritonitis, once a common inflammation of the peritoneum secondary to bacterial infection acquired during appendectomies, became rare after the introduction of systemic antibiotic drugs during World War II.

10.   F. W. Twort, "The Discovery of the Bacteriophage," *Science News,* Hammondsworth, England, 14:33-43, 1949.

11.   Felix d'Herrelle, "The Bacteriophage," *Science News,* 14:44-59, 1949.

12.   Wolfhard Weidel, *Virus* (Ann Arbor, University of Michigan Press, 1959), pp. 39-40.

13.   Alfred Mirsky, "the Discovery of DNA," *Scientific American,* June 1968, p. 78.

14.   W. A. Dorland, *Dorland's Illustrated Dictionary,* 24th ed. (Philadelphia: Saunders, 1968), p. 906.

15.   W. Barry Wood, Jr., *From Miasmas to Molecules* (New York: Columbia University Press, 1961), pp. 52-73. See also V. J. Freeman, "Studies on the Virulence of Bacteriophage-Infected Strains of Corynebacterium diphtheriae," *Journal of Bacteriology,* 1951, p. 675; and Alwin M. Pappenheimer, Jr., "The Diphtheria Toxin," *Scientific American,* October 1952, p. 32.

16.   Lewis Thomas, *The Lives of a Cell* (New York: Viking Press, 1974), p. 76. See also Roger Y. Stanier, Michael Doudoroff, and Edward A. Adelberg, *The Microbial World,* 3rd ed., (Englewood Cliffs, N.J.: Prentice-Hall, 1970), p. 788.

17.   See, for example, William Bulloch's *History of Bacteriology* (London: Oxford University Press, 1938; reprinted, 1960). Bulloch, a close friend of Twort's, made no mention of bacteriophages or d'Herrelle in his text, but in his biographical notices of outstanding bacteriologists, he describes Twort as "the original discoverer of the bacteriophagic phenomena," p. 400.

18.   A. P. Waterson and Lise Wilkinson, *An Introduction to the History of Virology* (Cambridge, England, 1978), pp. 95–99, 110–113. See also Gunther Stent, *Molecular Biology of the Bacterial Viruses* (San Francisco: Freeman, 1963), pp. 308–312.

19.   D. Carleton Gajdusek, Clarence J. Gibbs, Jr., and Michael Alpers, eds., *Slow, Latent, and Temperate Virus Infections,* Washington, D.C., 1965, pp. 3–12.

20.   James D. Watson, *Molecular Biology of the Gene,* 2nd ed. (New York: W. A Benjamin, 1970), p. 199

21.   Jill M. Forrest, in Allan Chase, *The Legacy of Malthus* (New York: Alfred A. Knopf, 1977), p. 545. See also Ji-Won Yoon et al., "Virus-Induced Diabetes," *New England Journal of Medicine,* 1974, p. 1173.

22.   George E. Burch and Thomas D. Giles, "The Role of Viruses in the Production of Heart Disease," *American Journal of Cardiology,* February 1972, pp. 231–240. See also Burch, Giles, and H. L. Colcolough, "Pathogenesis of 'Rheumatic' Heart Disease: Critique and Theory," *American Heart Journal,* October 1970, pp. 556–561.

23.   D. A. J. Tyrrell et al., "Possible Virus in Schizophrenia and Some Neurological Disorders," *Lancet,* April 21, 1979, pp. 839–844.

24.   Wilson Smith, C. H. Andrewes, and P. P. Laidlaw, "A Virus Obtained From Influenza Patients," *Lancet,* July 3, 1933, pp. 66–68. See also Sir Christopher Andrewes, *In Pursuit of the Common Cold* (London: Heinemann Ed., 1973).

25.   Nathaniel Bowditch Potter and Oswald T. Avery, "Opsonins and Vaccine Therapy," in Hare and Landis, *Modern Treatment* (Philadelphia and New York, 1910), pp. 515–550. See also Sir Almroth Wright et al., "Pharmaco-therapy of Pneumococcus Infections," *Lancet,* December 21, 1912, p. 1703.

26.   Anna I. Von Sholly and William H. Park, "Report on the Prophylactic Vaccination of 1536 Persons Against Acute Respiratory Disease, 1919-1920," *Journal of Immunology,* 6:103–115, 1921.

27.   H. J. Parish, *A History of Immunization* (London: William & Wilkins, 1965), p. 304.

28.   F. W. Henderson, A. M. Collier, W. A. Clyde, Jr., et al., "The Epidemiology of Acute Otitis Media in Childhood," *Abstract 188,* 16th Interscience Conference on Antimicrobial Agents and Chemotherapy, American Society for Microbiology, Washington, D.C., 1976.

29.   Victor Fainstein, Daniel M. Musher, and Thomas R. Cate, "Bacterial Adherence to Pharyngeal Cells During Viral Infection," *Journal of Infectious Diseases,* February 1980, pp. 172–176.

30.   Harry Rubin, "Carcinogenic Interactions Between Virus, Cell, and Organism," *JAMA,* 1964, pp. 727–731; and Rubin, "Virus-Host Interactions of Avian Tumors," in W. J. Burdette, *Viruses Inducing Cancer* (Salt Lake City: University of Utah Press, 1966), pp. 100–106.

31.   Kari Cantell, "Why Is Interferon Not in Clinical Use Today?" in vol. 1, *Interferon 1979,* Ion Gresser, ed. (New York: Academic Press, 1979), p. 23.

32.   Ibid.

33.   Personal communication, Dr. Rauscher, November 9, 1981.

34.   Cantell, op. cit., p. 17.

CHAPTER 10

1.   John R. Paul, *A History of Poliomyelitis* (New Haven, Conn.: Yale University Press, 1971), p. 132. Paul was a professor of preventive medicine and epidemiology at Yale University, and a member of its Poliomyelitis Unit established in 1931. Paul's over thirty years' experience as a leading polio investigator makes his book one of the most useful and readable yet written on a single disease. Chapter 10 owes much to this book.

2.   Maurice Brodie and William H. Park, "Active Immunization Against Poliomyelitis," and William H. Park, "The Prevention of Poliomyelitis," *New York State Journal of Medicine,* August 15, 1935, pp. 815–818, 818–820. See also Brodie and Park, "Active Immunization Against Poliomyelitis," *Journal of the American Medical Association (JAMA),* October 5, 1935, pp. 1089–1093.

3.   Brodie and Park, op. cit., *JAMA,* 1935.

4.   Ibid.

5.   J. P. Leake, "Poliomyelitis Following Vaccination Against This Disease," ibid., p. 2152.

6.   F. M. Burnet and J. Macnamara, "Immunological Differences Between Strains of Poliomyelitic [sic] Virus," *British Journal of Experimental Pathology,* 12:57–61, 1931.

7.   Theiler's father, Sir Arnold Theiler (1867–1936), a Swiss-born and Swiss-trained doctor of veterinary medicine, settled in South Africa in 1891 and became South Africa's chief veterinarian during the rinderpest epidemic of 1896. He developed new methods to control infectious diseases of animals, and encouraged research in his adopted country.

8.　　Hans Zinsser, *As I Remember Him, The Biography of R. S.* (Boston: Little, Brown, 1940), pp. 47–48.

9.　　Ibid.

10.　　John F. Enders, Thomas H. Weller, and Frederick C. Robbins, "Cultivation of the Lansing Strain of Poliomyelitis Virus in Cultures of Various Human Embryonic Tissues," *Science,* January 28, 1949, pp. 85–87.

CHAPTER 11

1.　　Howard A. Howe, "Antibody Response of Chimpanzees and Human Beings to Formalin-Inactivated Trivalent Poliomyelitis Vaccine," *American Journal of Hygiene,* 1952, pp. 265–279.

2.　　Jonas S. Salk et al., "Studies in Human Subjects on Active Immunization Against Poliomyelitis," *Journal of the American Medical Association (JAMA),* 151:1081–1098, 1953.

3.　　John R. Paul, *A History of Poliomyelitis* (New Haven, Conn.: Yale University Press, 1971), pp. 419–420.

4.　　Ibid.

5.　　Ibid.

6.　　Albert Sabin, "Oral Poliovirus Vaccine. History of Its Development and Prospects for Eradication of Poliomyelitis," *JAMA,* November 22, 1965, p. 873.

7.　　K. Lapinleimu and M. Stenvik, "The Efficacy of Polio Vaccination in Finland," *Developments in Biological Standardization* (Basel), 41:137–139, 1978.

8.　　In health statistics dealing with vaccine-preventable diseases, one must always examine the data before and after the vaccines were developed. In 1952, for example, two years before the Salk vaccine was licensed and put into wide use in 1954, there were 57,872 cases of paralytic poliomyelitis, for an attack rate of 12.8 per 100,000 population. In 1970, 1972, and 1979 when thirty-one, twenty-nine, and twenty-six cases of postvaccine paralytic polio were reported, the attack rate for each year stood at 0.01. The year 1952 happened to be a polio epidemic year. However, 1953 was a more or less average prevaccine polio year: 35,592 cases of acute or paralytic polio were reported, for an attack rate of 22.5 per 100,000 population. Five years later—1958—the acute poliomyelitis attack rate was down to a rapidly shrinking 3.3 per 100,000 population.

9.　　Sabin, op. cit., pp. 872–876.

10.　　Paul, op. cit., pp. 449–450.

CHAPTER 12

1.   Nancy Rosenberg and Louis Z. Cooper, *Vaccines and Viruses*, (New York: Grosset & Dunlap, 1971), pp. 52–53.

2.   Alan R. Hinman, A. David Brandling-Bennett, and Philip I. Neiburg, "The Opportunity and Obligation to Eliminate Measles From the United States," *Journal of American Medical Association,* September 14, 1979, pp. 1157–1162.

3.   Macfarlane Burnet and David O. White, *Natural History of Infectious Disease,* 4th ed. (Cambridge, England, 1972), pp. 115–116.

4.   Ibid.

5.   Thomas H. Weller and Franklin A. Neva, "Propagation in Tissue Culture of Cytopathic Agents From Patients With Rubella-like Illness"; and P. D. Parkman, E. L. Buescher, and M. S. Artenstein, "Recovery of Rubella Virus From Army Recruits," both articles in *Proceedings of the Society for Experimental Biology and Medicine,* vol. VIII, 1962, pp. 215–225, 225–230.

6.   Louis Z. Cooper, in Allan Chase, *The Biological Imperatives* (New York: Holt, Rinehart & Winston, 1971), p. 153.

7.   Paul D. Parkman, Harry M. Meyer, Ruth L. Kirschstein, and Hope E. Hopps, "Attenuated Rubella Virus. I. Development and Laboratory Characterization," *New England Journal of Medicine,* September 15, 1966, pp. 569–574. See also Harry M. Meyer, Paul D. Parkman, and Theodore C. Panos, "II. Production of an Experimental Live-Virus Vaccine and Clinical Trial," ibid., pp. 575–580.

8.   R. E. Weibel et al., "Live Attenuated Mumps-Virus Vaccine. 3. Clinical and Serologic Aspects in a Field Evaluation," *New England Journal of Medicine,* 1967, pp. 245–251; R. E. Weibel et al., "Long-term Follow-up for Immunity After Monovalent or Combined Live Measles, Mumps, and Rubella Virus Vaccines," *Pediatrics,* 56:380, 1975; and Robert E. Weibel, "What You Should Know About New and Current Viral Vaccines," *Modern Medicine,* November 30, 1977, pp. 36–41.

CHAPTER 13

1.   Margaret G. Smith, "Propagation of Salivary Gland Virus of the Mouse in Tissue Cultures," *Proceedings of the Society for Experimental Biology and Medicine,* 1954, pp. 435–440.

2.   Margaret G. Smith, "Propagation in Tissue Cultures of a Cytopathogenic Virus From Human Salivary Gland Virus (SGV) Disease," *Proceedings of the Society for Experimental Biology and Medicine,* 1956, pp. 424–430; and Wallace P. Rowe, Janet W. Hartley,

et al., "Cytopathogenic Agent Resembling Human Salivary Gland Virus Recovered From Tissue Cultures of Human Adenoids," ibid., pp. 418–424.

3. J. B. Hanshaw, "Congenital Cytomegalovirus Infections: A Fifteen Year Perspective," *Journal of Infectious Diseases*, 1971, pp. 555–561; and Thomas H. Weller, "The Cytomegaloviruses: Ubiquitous Agents With Protean Clinical Manifestations," *New England Journal of Medicine*, 1971, pp. 203–214, 267–274, (two parts); S. D. Elek and H. Stern, "Development of a Vaccine Against Mental Retardation Caused by Cytomegalovirus Infection *in utero*," *Lancet*, January 5, 1974, pp. 1–5. S. A. Plotkin, T. Furukawa, N. Zygraich, and C. Huygelen, "Candidate Cytomegalovirus Strain for Human Vaccination," *Infection and Immunity*, September 1975, pp. 521–527; Stanley A. Plotkin, John Farquhar, and Elizabeth Hornberger, "Clinical Trials of Immunization With the Towne 125 Strain of Human Cytomegalovirus," *Journal of Infectious Diseases*, November 1976, pp. 470–475; and Sergio Stagno et al., "Congenital Cytomegalovirus Infection; Occurrence in an Immune Population," *New England Journal of Medicine*, June 2, 1977, pp. 1254–1258.

4. Eli Gold and George A. Nankervis, "Cytomegalovirus," *Viral Infections of Humans*, Alfred S. Evans, ed., (New York and London, 1976), chapter 7, p. 143.

5. S. D. Elek, "Cytomegalovirus Vaccine: Justification and Problems," *Recent Advances in Clinical Virology, No. 1*, A. P. Waterston, ed. (Edinburgh: Churchill & Livingstone, 1977), Chapter 7, pp. 117–134.

6. H. Stern, S. D. Elek, et al., "Microbial Causes of Mental Retardation: The Role of Prenatal Infections with Cytomegalovirus, Rubella Virus, and Toxoplasma," *Lancet*, August 30, 1969, p. 7618; and James B. Hanshaw, Albert P. Scheiner, et al., "School Failure and Deafness After 'Silent' Congenital Cytomegalovirus Infection," *New England Journal of Medicine*, August 26, 1977, pp. 468–470.

7. Sergio Stagno, David W. Reynolds, et al., "Auditory and Visual Defects Resulting From Symptomatic and Subclinical Congenital Cytomegaloviral and Toxoplasma Infections," *Pediatrics*, May 5, 1977, pp. 669–677.

8. A. E. Churchill and R. C. Chubb, "Immunisation Against Marek's Disease Using a Live Attenuated Virus," *Nature*, 1969, pp. 744–747.

9. Elek, 1977, op. cit., p. 128.

10. Personal Communication, Dr. Gordon R. B. Skinner. Maurice R. Hilleman, "New Developments with New Vaccines," *New Developments With Human and Veterinary Vaccines. Proceedings of the Oholo Biological Conference, Israel, March 24–27, 1980* (New York: Alan R. Liss, Inc., 1980), pp. 21–49.

11.   Werner Henle, Gertrude Henle, and Evelyne T. Lennette, "The Epstein-Barr Virus," *Scientific American,* July, 1979, pp. 48–59.

        As a young physician in Germany, Werner Henle became an instant candidate for extermination in 1932 when the Nazis came to power, because he had one Jewish grandfather. The fact that this ancestor happened to have been Jakob Henle, teacher of Robert Koch and author of what since became known as the "Koch postulates" of microbiology, cut no ice with the New Order. Henle was forced to flee for his life to the United States, where he became a clinical investigator.

12.   See note 11.

13.   See note 11.

14.   See note 11.

15.   L. J. Old et al., "Precipitation Antibody in Human Serum to an Antigen Present in Cultured Burkitt's Lymphoma Cells," *Proceedings of the National Academy of Sciences,* 1966, pp. 1699–1704.

16.   Henle et al., op cit. See also Werner Henle and Gertrude Henle, "Epstein-Barr Virus and Infectious Mononucleosis," *New England Journal of Medicine,* 1973, pp. 263–264.

17.   D. Kufe and S. Spiegelman, "RNA Related to That of Murine Leukemia Virus and Nasopharyngeal Carcinoma," *Proceedings of the National Academy of Sciences, USA,* 70:5–9, 1973. See also D. Kufe, R. Hehlmann, and S. Spiegelman, "Human Sarcomas Containing RNA Related to the RNA of a Mouse Leukemia Virus," *Science,* January 14, 1972, pp. 182–185.

18.   G. F. Smith and J. M. Berg, *Down's Anomaly,* 2nd ed. (Edinburgh: Churchill & Livingston, 1976), pp. 223–224, 263–264.

19.   Henle et al., op. cit.

20.   M. A. Epstein, "Epstein-Barr Virus as the Cause of a Human Cancer," *Nature,* August 24, 1978. See also R. Hehlmann et al., *Lancet,* September 20, 1980, for communication on two patients "in whom serologically confirmed mononucleosis is associated with definite and probable acute monocytic leukemia," pp. 652–653.

21.   Wolf D. Szmuness et al., "Hepatitis B. Vaccine; Demonstration of Efficacy in a Controlled Clinical Trial," *New England Journal of Medicine,* October 9, 1980, pp. 833–841.

22.   Ibid.

23.   Ibid.

24.   See Richard A. Lerner, Nicola Green, et al., "Chemically Synthesized Peptides Predicted From the Nucleotide Sequence of the Hepatitis B Virus Genome Elicit Antibodies Reactive With the Native Envelope Protein of Dane Particles," *Proceedings of the National Academy of Sciences, USA,* June 1981, pp. 3403–3407.

These authors reported that they had synthesized chemically thirteen peptides (or compounds formed of two or more amino acids) corresponding to amino acid sequences "predicted from the nucleotide sequence of the hepatitis B surface antigen." These synthetic peptides reacted antigenically with native or natural hepatitis B virus molecules. This suggested to them that "peptides such as these could prove to be ideal vaccines." They wrote that "synthetic peptides prepared by using nucleotide sequences as patterns should be ideal for use in vaccination. For example, a combination of polypeptides (such as 1, 3, 4 and 6) might provide broad protection against hepatitis B virus, thereby obviating biological variables such as serotypic diversity, antigenic drift of the infectious agent, and the individuality of the host immune response." This not only raised the possibility of a very inexpensive vaccine against serum hepatitis, but also of a much more useful vaccine against the virus of influenza, a pathogen highly subject to antigenic drift.

25. Stephen M. Feinstone, Albert Z. Kapakian, and Robert H. Purcell, "Hepatitis A: Detection by Immune Electron Electronmicroscopy of a Viruslike Antigen Associated with Acute Illness," *Science,* December 7, 1973. See also Daniel W. Bradley et al., "Isolation and Characterization of Hepatitis A Virus," *American Journal of Clinical Pathology,* 65:876-889, 1976; Carmine C. Mascoli et al., "Recovery of Hepatitis Agents in the Marmoset from Human Cases Occurring in Costa Rica," *Proceedings of the Society for Experimental Biology and Medicine,* January 1973, pp. 276-282; M. R. Hilleman et al., "Immune Adherence and Complement-Fixation Tests for Human Hepatitis A. Diagnostic and Epidemiologic Investigations," *Developments in Biological Standardization* (Basel), 1975, pp. 383-389. See also Hilleman et al., "Characterization of CR326 Human Hepatitis A Virus, a Probable Enterovirus," ibid., pp. 418-424, and Philip J. Provost and Maurice R. Hilleman, "Propagation of Hepatitis A Virus in Cell Culture *in vitro,*" *Proceedings of the Society for Experimental Biology and Medicine,* 160:213-221, 1979.

26. Stephen C. Hadler, Hannah M. Webster, et al., "Hepatitis A in Day-Care Centers: A Community-wide Assessment," *New England Journal of Medicine,* May 29, 1980, pp. 1222-1227; *Morbidity and Mortality Weekly Report* (*MMWR*), Centers for Disease Control, November 28, 1980, pp. 555-557; *Hospital Surveillance Report No. 45,* Centers for Disease Control, May 1980; and G. Storch, et al., "Viral Hepatitis Associated With Day-Care Centers," *Journal of American Medical Association,* 1979, pp. 1514-1518.

27. See note 26.

CHAPTER 14

1.   Victor Fainstein, Daniel M. Musher, and Thomas R. Cate, "Bacterial Adherence to Pharyngeal Cells During Viral Infections," *Journal of Infectious Diseases,* February 1980, pp. 172–176.
2.   Anonymous, "Spanish Influenza Much Like Grippe," *New York Times,* September 22, 1918.
3.   Cited in Greer Williams, *Virus Hunters* (New York: Alfred A. Knopf, 1959), pp. 204–205.
4.   Wilson Smith, C. H. Andrews, and P. P. Laidlaw, "A Virus Obtained From Influenza Patients," *The Lancet,* July 3, 1933.
5.   H. W. Kim et al., "Epidemiology of Respiratory Syncitial Virus Infection in Washington, D.C.," *American Journal of Epidemiology,* 1973, pp. 216–225. See also Robert M. Chanock, Hyun Wha Kim, Carl Brandt, and Robert H. Parrott, "Respiratory Syncitial Virus," *Viral Infections of Humans,* Alfred S. Evans, ed., 1976, Chapter 17, pp. 365–382.
6.   Maurice R. Hilleman, "New Developments With New Vaccines," *New Developments With Human and Veterinary Vaccines. Proceedings of the Oholo Biological Conference, Israel, March 24–25, 1980* (New York: Alan R. Liss, 1980), p. 14.
7.   Hjordis M. Foy and J. Thomas Grayston, "Adenoviruses," in Evans, op. cit., Chapter 3, p. 59.
8.   Maurice R. Hilleman, in W. J. Burdette, *Viruses Inducing Cancer* (Salt Lake City: University of Utah Press, 1966), p. 377.
9.   *Federal Register,* April 15, 1980, p. 25729.
10.   News release, Walter Reed Army Medical Center, Washington, D.C., July 30, 1980.
11.   Ibid.
12.   Hilleman, in Burdette, op. cit, p. 378.
13.   John J. Trentin, Yoshiro Yabe, and Grant Taylor, "The Quest for Human Cancer Viruses. A New Approach to an Old Problem Reveals Cancer Induction in Hamsters by Human Adenovirus," *Science,* September 14, 1962, pp. 835–841. See also Harvey M. Shein and John F. Enders, "Transformation Induced by Simian Virus 40 in Human Renal Cell Cultures," *Proceedings of the National Academy of Sciences,* 1962, pp. 1164–1171.
14.   R. M. McAllister, R. V. Gilden, and M. Green, "Adenoviruses in Human Cancer," *Lancet,* April 15, 1972, pp. 831–833.
15.   "Human Viruses in Water, Wastewater and Soil," *WHO Technical Report Series No. 639,* 1980.
16.   Peter B. Collis et al., "Adenovirus Vaccines in Military Recruit Populations: A Cost-Benefit Analysis," *Journal of Infectious Diseases,* December 1973, pp. 745–752.
17.   Cited by Jack Merrit Gwaltney, Jr., "Rhinoviruses,"

Virus Infections of Humans, Alfred S. Evans, ed., (New York and London: Plenum, 1976), chapter 18, p. 383.

18.	See Sir Christopher Andrewes, *In Pursuit of the Common Cold* (London: Heinemann Ed., 1973).

19.	William J. Mogabgab, "Upper Respiratory Illness Vaccines—Perspectives and Trials," *Annals of Internal Medicine,* October 1962, p. 526.

20.	Cesar Milstein, "Monoclonal Antibodies," *Scientific American,* October 1980, pp. 66–74.

21.	Ibid.

22.	Ibid.

23.	P. Potocnjak, N. Yoshida, R. S. Nussenzweig, and V. Nussenzweig, "Monovalent Fragments (Fab) of Monoclonal Antibodies to a Sporozoite Surface Antigen (Pb44) Protect Mice Against Malarial Infection," *Journal of Experimental Medicine,* June 1980, pp. 1504–1513.

24.	J. Gregor Sutcliffe et al., "Nucleotide Sequence of Moloney Murine Leukemia Virus," *Nature,* October 1981, pp. 543–548. See also Richard A. Lerner, Gregor Sutcliffe, and Thomas M. Shinnick, "Antibodies to Chemically Synthesized Peptides Predicted From DNA Sequences as Probes of Gene Expression," *Cell,* February 1981, pp. 309–310; Sutcliffe et al., "Chemical Synthesis of Polypeptide Predicted From Nucleotide Sequence Allows Detection of a New Retroviral Gene Product," *Nature,* October 30, 1980, pp. 801–805; and Richard A. Lerner et al., "Nucleotide Sequence of a Cloned Murine Leukemia Virus DNA Fragment," *Cold Spring Harbor Symposium in Quantitative Biology, 1980,* 44:2, pp. 1275–1279.

CHAPTER 15

1.	Charles Hall, *The Effects of Civilization* (London: 1805; New York: Kelley facsimile edition, 1965).

2.	Allan Chase, *The Legacy of Malthus* (New York: Alfred A. Knopf, 1977), p. 208.

3.	Michael Heidelberger, "A 'Pure' Organic Chemist's Downward Path: Chapter 2—The Years at P. and S.," *Annual Review of Biochemistry,* 1979, p. 9.

4.	René J. Dubos, *The Professor, the Institute and DNA* (New York: Rockefeller University Press, 1976), pp. 102–103.

5.	Robert M. Chanock, Leonard Hayflick, and Michael F. Barile, "Growth on Artificial Medium of an Agent Associated With Atypical Pneumonia and Its Identification as a PPLO," *Proceedings of the National Academy of Sciences,* January 1962, pp. 41–49.

6.	Ibid.

7.	Heidelberger, op. cit., pp. 12–13.

8.	Robert Austrian, "The Current Status of Bacteremic Pneumococcal Pneumonia. Re-evaluation of an Underemphasized

Clinical Problem," *Transactions of the Association of American Physicians,* 76:117-125, 1963.

9.   Maxwell Finland, "Occurrence of Serious Bacterial Infections Since the Introduction of Antibacterial Agents," *Journal of the American Medical Association,* 170:2188-2197, 1965. See also Finland, "Changing Ecology of Bacterial Infections as Related to Antibacterial Therapy," *Journal of Infectious Diseases,* November 1970, pp. 419-431.

10.   Robert Austrian and Jerome Gold, "Pneumococcal Bacteremia with Especial Reference to Bacteremic Pneumococcal Pneumonia," *Annals of Internal Medicine,* May 1964, pp. 759-776.

11.   Paul Kaufman et al., "Pneumonia in Old Age. Active Immunization Against Pneumonia With Pneumococcus Polysaccharide; Results of a Six Year Study," *Archives of Internal Medicine,* 79:518-531, 1947.

12.   Robert Austrian, "Random Gleanings From a Life With the Pneumococcus," *Journal of Infectious Diseases,* April 1975, pp. 474-484.

13.   Robert Austrian, "Of Gold and Pneumococci: A History of Pneumococcal Vaccines in South Africa," *Transactions of the American Clinical and Climatological Association,* vol. 89, 1977.

14.   Ibid.

15.   Ibid.

16.   Unpublished paper delivered in Copenhagan, Denmark, in 1977. Courtesy of Dr. Robbins.

17.   E. C. Gotschlich, I. Goldschneider, M. S. Artenstein, and T. Y. Liu, "Human Immunity to the Meningococcus," *Journal of Experimental Medicine,* 129:1307-1385, 1969; E. C. Gotschlich, M. Rey, J. Etienne, et al., "The Immunological Response Observed in Field Studies in Africa with Group A Meningococcal Vaccines," *Progress in Immunobiological Standards,* 5:485-491, 1972; and R. Gold, M. L. Lepow, I. Goldschneider, T. S. Draper, and E. L. Gotschlich, "Clinical Evaluation of Group A and Group C Meningococcal Polysaccharide Vaccines in Infants," *Journal of Clinical Investigation,* 51:89-96, 1972.

18.   P. H. Makela et al., "Effect of Group A Meningococcal Vaccine in Army Recruits in Finland," *Lancet,* II:883-886, 1975; Heikki Peltola, Helena Makela, Helena Kayhty, et al., "Clinical Efficacy of Meningococcus Group A Capsular Polysaccharide Vaccine in Children Three Months to Five Years of Age," *New England Journal of Medicine,* September 29, 1977, pp. 686-691; P. H. Makela, H. Peltola, and H. Kayhty, "Polysaccharide Vaccines of Group A Neisseria meningitidis and Haemophilus influenzae type b: A Field Trial in Finland," *Journal of Infectious Diseases,* 136: suppl. S-43-S-550, 1977; and Martha L. Lepow and Ronald Gold, "Further Conquest of the Meningococcus," *New England Journal of Medicine,* September 29, 1977, pp. 721-722.

19.   Ibid.

20. Personal communication, Dr. E. C. Gotschlich, 1978.

21. Finland, op. cit.

22. Sarah H. W. Sell et al., "Long-Term Sequellae of Hemophilus [sic] influenzae Meningitis," *Pediatrics,* 49:206–211, February 1972. See also the analogous Swedish study by Johan Lindberg et al., "Long-term Outcome of Hemophilus [sic] influenzae type b Meningitis Related to Antibiotic Treatment," *Pediatrics,* 60:1–6, 1977; and Joel I. Ward, David W. Fraser, et al., "Haemophilus influenzae Meningitis. A New National Study of Secondary Spread in Household Contacts," *New England Journal of Medicine,* July 19, 1979, pp. 122–126.

CHAPTER 16

1. Carol J. Baker, Dennis L. Kasper, and Charles E. Davis, "Immunochemical Characterization of the 'Native' Type III Polysaccharide of Group B Streptococcus," *Journal of Experimental Medicine,* 143:258, 1976.

2. *Health in America: 1776–1976,* Publication No. (HRA) 76-616, U.S. Department of Health, Education & Welfare, Washington, D.C., 1976.

3. Carol J. Baker, "Summary of the Workshop on Perinatal Infections Due to Group B Streptococcus," *Journal of Infectious Diseases,* 136:137, 1977.

4. Ibid.

5. Carol J. Baker, Diana K. Goroff, et al., "Vaginal Colonization With Group B Streptococcus: A Study in College Women," *Journal of Infectious Diseases,* March 1977, pp. 392–397. See also C. J. Baker and F. F. Barrett, "Transmission of Group B Streptococci Among Parturient Women and Their Neonates," *Journal of Pediatrics,* 83:919–925, 1973; Ralph D. Feigin, "The Perinatal Group B Streptococcal Problem: More Questions Than Answers," *New England Journal of Medicine,* January 8, 1976, pp. 106–107; Carol J. Baker and Dennis L. Kasper, "Microcapsule of Type III Strains of Group B Streptococcus: Production and Morphology," *Infection and Immunity,* January 1976, pp. 189–194; and Baker and Kasper, "Correlation of Maternal Antibody Deficiency With Susceptibility to Neonatal Group B Streptococcal Infection," *New England Journal of Medicine,* April 1, 1976, pp. 753–756.

6. See note 5.

7. Edward B. Fiske, "New Cuts in U.S. School Aid Will Be Both Deep and Wide," *The New York Times,* July 11, 1982, p. 1 and p. 30.

8. Louis Sauer, "Whooping Cough Vaccine as an Immunizing Agent," *New York State Journal of Medicine,* 16:821–824. A valuable clinical report and review of the literature since 1913.

9. C. E. Frasch, L. Parkes, R. M. McNelis, and E. C. Gotschlich, "Protection Against Group B Meningococcal Disease," *Journal of Experimental Medicine,* August 1, 1976, pp. 319–329; and Carl E. Frasch, "Noncapsular Surface Antigens of Neisseria meningitidis," *Seminars in Infectious Disease,* vol. II, Louis Weinstein and Bernard N. Fields, eds. (New York: Stratton Intercontinental Medical Book Corp., 1979), chapter 10, pp. 304–337.

10.   W. D. Zollinger, R. E. Mandrell, et al., "Complex of Meningococcal Group B Polysaccharide and Type 2 Outer Membrane Protein Immunogenic in Man," *Journal of Clinical Investigation,* May 1979, pp. 836–848. See also Zollinger et al., "Safety and Immunogenicity of a Neisseria meningitidis Type 2 Protein Vaccine in Animals and Humans," *Journal of Infectious Diseases,* June 1978, pp. 728–739; and Wendell D. Zollinger and Robert E. Mandrell, "Type-Specific Antigens of Group A Neisseria meningitidis Lipopolysaccharide and Heat-Modifiable Outer Membrane Proteins," *Infection and Immunity,* May 1980, pp. 451–458.

11.   Carl E. Frasch, Mark S. Peppler, Thomas R. Cate, and John M. Zahradnik, "Immunogenicity and Clinical Evaluation of Group B Neisseria meningitidis Outer Membrane Protein Vaccines." Courtesy of Dr. Frasch.

12.   Zollinger and Mandrell, op. cit, 1979.

CHAPTER 17

1.   Wesley W. Spink, *Infectious Diseases* (Minneapolis: University of Minnesota Press, 1978), pp. 311–312.

2.   Wolfgang A. Casper, *Medical Bulletin,* New York University College of Medicine, 1939, p. 100.

3.   King J. Holmes, "Sexually Transmitted Diseases," *University of Washington Bulletin,* 3:1, Winter 1976, pp. 17–24.

4.   "Low Birth Rate in Central Africa Causes Concern," *New York Times* (Reuters), January 22, 1978, p. 8.

5.   *Sexual Medicine Today,* July 1979, p. 10.

6.   The late Willie Sutton was an American bank robber who was as adept at escaping from prison as he was inept at robbing banks. When asked why he persisted in robbing banks, he replied: "Because that's where the money is." This became known as Sutton's Law.

7.   Personal communication, Dr. John Swanson, 1979.

8.   Theodor Rosebury, *Microbes and Morals: The Strange Story of Venereal Disease* (New York: Viking Press, 1973), pp. 15–16.

9.   Spink, op. cit., p. 308.

10.   Ralph H. Major, *Classic Descriptions of Disease* (Springfield, Ill.: C. C. Thomas, 1948), pp. 45–46.

11.   William B. Ober, "Boswell's Gonorrhea," *Bulletin of the New York Academy of Medicine,* June 1969, pp. 587–636.

12. Ibid.

13. Norman E. Himes, *Medical History of Contraception* (New York: Gamut Press, 1936, 1963).

14. *Boswell's London Journal 1762–1763*, Frederick A. Pottle, ed. (New York: McGraw-Hill, 1950), p. 139. Boswell's entire affair with "Louisa" and its pathological and clinical consequences are covered in pp. 83–212.

15. S. M. Laird and R. B. Roy, "How Infectious Is Gonorrhea?" *British Medical Journal*, December 23, 1972, p. 733.

16. Edward B. Shaw, "Gonorrheal Ophthalmia neonatorum," *Pediatrics*, 52:281, 1973. See also Shaw, "Questions Need for Prophylaxis With Silver Nitrate," Letters to the Editor, *Pediatrics*, 59:792, 1977.

17. Frank Billings, "Chronic Focal Infections and Their Etiologic Relation to Arthritis and Nephritis," *Archives of Internal Medicine*, 9:484, 1912. Also Billings, "Chronic Focal Infection as a Causative Factor in Chronic Arthritis," *Journal of the American Medical Association*, (*JAMA*), 61:818, 1913; *Focal Infection, the Lane Medical Lectures 1915* (New York and London: D. Appleton & Co., 1916); and "Focal Infection" in *Oxford Medicine*, vol. 1, 1919, p. 319. For a review of the reasons for the abandonment of the concept of focal infection, see Hobart A. Reimann and W. Paul Havens, "Focal Infection and Systemic Disease: A Critical Appraisal," *JAMA*, vol. 114, 1940, pp. 1–6. See also Paul B. Beeson, "Focal Infection and Systemic Disease," *Advances in American Medicine: Essays at the Bicentennial*, vol. 1, John Z. Bowers and Elizabeth F. Purcell, eds. (New York: Josiah Macy, Jr., Foundation, 1976).

18. Beeson, op. cit., pp. 151–152.

19. Ibid.

20. Nathaniel B. Potter and Oswald T. Avery, "Opsonins and Vaccine Therapy," in *Modern Treatment*, ed. A. Hare, Vol. 1, 1910, p. 515.

21. A. P. Ohlmacher, "A Series of Medical and Surgical Affections Treated by Artificial Autoinoculation According to Wright's Theory of Opsonins," *Journal of the American Medical Association* (*JAMA*), February 16, 1907.

22. Benjamin A. Thomas, *JAMA*, January 22, 1919, pp. 258–260.

23. *British Medical Journal*, December 20, 1913, p. 1609. See also R. Tanner Hewlett, *A Manual of Bacteriology, Clinical and Applied*, 5th ed., (St. Louis, Mo.: C. V. Mosby, 1915). Pages 246–247 deal with recommended toxin, antiserum, and vaccine treatments of gonorrhea. The "vaccine may be prepared by sterilising cultures with heat, and has proved of service in chronic gonorrhoeal infections."

24. See note 22.

25. L. Greenberg, B. B. Diena, et al., "Preliminary Studies on the Development of a Gonococcal Vaccine," *Bulletin of the World Health Organization*, 45:531–535, 1971. See also Greenberg, Diena, et al., "Gonococcal Vaccine Study in Inuvik," *Canadian Journal of Public Health*, January–February 1974, pp. 29–33.

CHAPTER 18

1. The question of whether or not the capsule or capsule-like structure seen on the gonococci is really one that is equivalent to the polysaccharide capsules of the virulent pneumococci and meningococci is still being debated by equally competent bacteriologists, immunochemists, and research physicians. In 1921 Clara Israeli, pathologist-in-chief of the New Hampshire State Laboratory of Hygiene, published in the May 21 issue of *JAMA* (pp. 1497–1498) two micrographs of what she believed to be gonococcal capsules. In this article, "Demonstration of a Capsule-like Appearance in Staining Gonococci," Dr. Israeli opened by saying, "It has been a question whether or not the gonococcus possesses a capsule. Some hold that it does possess a capsule, some question its presence, and some flatly deny this organism has a capsule." She herself felt that while the stain she developed "brings out the capsule-like periphery around the gonococcus distinctly, it is perhaps a little too soon to claim that it is the capsule of the gonococci until more work has been done on it."
2. Wolfgang A. Casper, "The Preparation of the Type-Specific Carbohydrates of Gonococci," *Journal of Immunology*, June 1937, pp. 421–439.
3. Wolfgang Casper, "Spezifische Cutireaktionen an Gonorrhoikern mit Spezifischen, Eiwess-Freien Substanzen aus Gonokokken," *Klinische Wochenschrift* (Berlin), November 15, 1930, p. 2154.
4. Wolfgang A. Casper, "Abraham Buschke 1868–1943. Centennial of His Birth," *Archives of Dermatology*, December 1968.
5. W. A. Casper, "Degeneration and Variation of Gonococci," *Journal of Bacteriology*, 36:111, 1938. See also Casper, "Morphologic and Cultural Behavior of the Gonococcus in the 'Carrier,'" *American Journal of Syphilis, Gonorrhea and Venereal Diseases*, September 1942, pp. 614–628.
6. Wolfgang A. Casper, "The Biochemistry of the Gonococcus and Its Practical Importance," *Venereal Disease Information*, vol. 22, April 1941, pp. 119–123.
7. See note 1.
8. Andrew G. Plaut, Joanne V. Gilbert, Malcolm S. Artenstein, and J. Donald Capra, "Neisseria gonorrhoeae and Neisseria meningitidis: Extracellular Enzyme Cleaves Human Immunoglob-

ulin A," *Science,* December 12, 1975. See also Gilbert Plaut and Richard Wistar, Jr., "Loss of Antibody Activity in Human Immunoglobulin A Exposed to Extracellular Immunoglobulin A Proteases of Neisseria gonorrhoeae and Streptococcus sanguis," *Infection and Immunity,* July 1977, pp. 130–135; and Milan Blake, King K. Holmes, and John Swanson, "Studies on Gonococcus Infection. XVII. IgA₁-Cleaving Protease in Vaginal Washings from Women With Gonorrhea," *Journal of Infectious Diseases,* January 1979, pp. 89–92.

9.   Malcolm B. Perry, Benito B. Diena, and Fraser Ashton, "Lipopolysaccharides of Neisseria gonorrhoeae," *The Gonococcus,* Richard B. Roberts, ed. (New York: Wiley, 1977), chapter 13, pp. 286–301. See also J. E. Heckels, "The Surface Properties of Neisseria gonorrhoeae: Isolation of the Major Components of the Outer Membrane," *Journal of General Microbiology* (England), 99:333–341, 1977; B. B. Diena, F. E. Ashton, A. Ryan, and R. Wallace, "The Lipopolysaccharide (*R* type) as a Common Antigen of Neisseria gonorrhoeae. I: Immunizing Properties," *Canadian Journal of Microbiology,* February 1978, pp. 117–123; and C. R. Gregg, M. A. Melly, and Z. A. McGee, "Mechanisms of Gonococcal Pathogenicity: Role of Gonococcal Lipopolysaccharide in Toxic Damage to Human Fallopian Tube Mucosa," *Clinical Research 26,* December 1978, p. 799A.

10.   C. C. Brinton, Jr., A. Buzzell, and M. A. Lauffer, "Electrophoresis and Phage Susceptibility Studies on a Filament-Producing Variant of the E. coli B Bacterium," *Biochem. Biophys. Acta 15,* 1954, p. 533; C. C. Brinton, Jr., "Non-Flagellar Appendages of Bacteria," *Nature,* 183:782, 1959; and Charles C. Brinton, Jr., "The Piliation Phase Syndrome and the Uses of Purified Pili in Disease Control," *Proceedings of the 13th U.S. Conference on Cholera,* D. C. Miller, ed., Atlanta, September 1977; Washington, D.C., 1978, preprint ms., p. 44.

11.   See note 10. J. van Houte, and W. F. Liljemark, "Parameters that Affect the Adherence of Streptococcus Salivarius to Oral Epithelial Surfaces," *Journal of Dental Research,* March–April 1972, pp. 424–435.

12.   Brinton, op. cit., *Proceedings,* preprint ms., 1977, p. 59. See also Charles C. Brinton et al., "Uses of Pili in Gonorrhea Control: Role of Bacterial Pili in Disease, Purification and Properties of Gonococcal Pili, and Progress in the Development of a Gonococcal Pilus Vaccine for Gonorrhea," *Immunobiology of Neisseria gonorrhoeae: Proceedings of a Conference Held in San Francisco, January 18–20, 1978,* Geo. F. Brooks, Emil C. Gotschlich, King K. Holmes, William D. Sawyer, and Frank E. Young, eds., American Society for Microbiology, Washington, D.C., pp. 155–178; Zell A. McGee, M. Ann Melly, and Clark R. Gregg, "Role of Attachment in the Pathogenesis of Gonococcal Infections: Implications for the Development of a Gonococcal Vaccine," *Proceedings of the In-*

ternational Symposium on Bacterial Vaccines, September 15–18, 1980, National Institutes of Health, Washington, D.C., 1981; and Charles C. Brinton, Jr., et al., "Gonococcal Pili as Vaccines in Volunteers," ibid.

13. Zell A. McGee, M. Ann Melly, et al., "Virulence Factors of Gonococci: Studies Using Human Fallopian Tube Organ Cultures," *Immunobiology of Neisseria gonorrhoeae,* 1978, pp. 258–262.

14. Stephen J. Kraus, "Complications of Gonococcal Infections," *Medical Clinics of North America,* vol. 56, 1972, pp. 1115–1125.

15. King K. Holmes, in *Harrison's Textbook of Medicine,* 9th ed. (New York: 1980), p. 624.

16. Ibid.

17. *Sexual Medicine Today,* July 1979, p. 10. See also E. Stolz and J. Schuller, "Gonococcal Oro- and Nasopharyngeal Infection," *British Journal of Venereal Diseases,* 50:104, 1974; F. E. Willmott, "Transfer of Gonococcal Pharyngitis by Kissing?" *British Journal of Venereal Diseases,* 50:317, 1974; and Paul J. Wiesner, "Gonococcal Pharyngeal Infection," *Clinical Obstetrics & Gynecology,* 18:121, 1975.

18. Morris Schaeffer, *Federal Legislation and the Clinical Laboratory,* Morris Schaeffer, ed. (Boston: G. K. Hall Medical Publishers, 1981), pp. xv–xxv (introduction), 173–184.

19. "Charity," editorial in *New York Times,* March 29, 1981.

20. Richard E. Neustadt and Harvey V. Fineberg, *The Swine Flu Affair; Decision-Making on a Slippery Disease,* GPO stock no. 017-000-00210-4, U.S. Department of Health, Education, and Welfare, Washington, D.C., 1978.

21. James Howie, "Gonorrhea—A Question of Tactics," *British Medical Journal,* December 22–29, 1979, pp. 1631–1633.

22. King K. Holmes, "Sexually Transmitted Diseases: An Overview and Perspectives on the Next Decade," guest editorial, *Infectious Diseases,* April 1980, pp. 1–18, 24–28.

23. Ibid.

24. See, for example, Ivan Illich, *Medical Nemesis* (New York: Pantheon, 1976), and Bernard Dixon, *Beyond the Magic Bullet; The Real Story of Medicine* (New York: Harper & Row, 1978).

25. *Advance Data,* No. 78, National Center for Health Statistics, May 12, 1982.

CHAPTER 19

1. Victor C. Vaughan, *Infection and Immunity* (Chicago: American Medical Association, 1915), p. 120.

2. "Charity," editorial in *New York Times,* March 29, 1981, p. 20E.

3.   John B. Robbins, Rachel Schneerson, Carl E. Frasch, et al., "Immunization Against Diseases Caused by Encapsulated Bacteria," unpublished paper presented at meeting in Copenhagen, Denmark.

4.   John Herbers, "Alarm Rises Over Decay in U.S. Public Works," *The New York Times,* July 18, 1982, p. 1 and p. 24. See also David W. Fraser, "What Are Our Bacterial Infectious Disease Problems?" *Proceedings of the International Symposium on Bacterial Vaccines,* September 15–18, 1980, National Institutes of Health, Washington, D.C.

5.   M. B. Skirrow, "Campylobacter Enteritis: A 'New' Disease," *British Medical Journal,* ii:9–11, 1977; Martin J. Blaser, F. Marc LaForce, Nancy A. Wilson, and Wen Lan Lou Wang, "Reservoirs for Human Campylobacteriosis," *Journal of Infectious Diseases,* May 1980, pp. 665–669.

Campylobacter fetus was originally called Vibrio fetus. See also Wesley W. Spink, "Human Vibriosis caused by Vibrio Fetus," *Journal of the American Medical Association* (*JAMA*), January 19, 1957; T. A. Reyman and B. Silberberg, "Vibrio Fetus Septicemia," *American Journal of Clinical Pathology,* May 1969, pp. 578–583; Marion Hood and James M. Hood, "Vibrio-Fetus—a Cause of Human Abortion," *American Journal of Obstetrics & Gynecology,* September 1960, pp. 506–511; Henry Loeb et al., "Vibrio Fetus Endocarditis," *American Heart Journal,* March 1966, pp. 381–386; V. Bokkenheuser and T. Dunston in *Microorganisms and Infectious Diseases,* Vol. 1, A. von Gravenitz and T. Sall, eds. (New York: Marcel Dekker, Inc., 1975), p. 25. Bokkenheuser reveals that "the first case of V. fetus infection in man was recorded in 1947."

6.   See note 5.

7.   J. H. Bryner, J. W. Foley, W. T. Hubbert, and P. J. Matthews, "Pregnant Guinea Pig Model for Testing Efficacy of Campylobacter Fetus Vaccines," *American Journal of Veterinary Research,* January 1978, pp. 119–121.

8.   See Allan Chase, *The Legacy of Malthus* (New York: Alfred A. Knopf, 1977), pp. 389–391.

9.   *Report of the Committee on Infectious Diseases* ("The Redbook"), 17th ed. (Evanston, Ill.: American Academy of Pediatrics, 1974), pp. 2–4.

10.   The late Louis E. Siltzbach, head of the division of thoracic diseases in Mt. Sinai Hospital, New York, was a ranking expert in sarcoidosis, a disease in which sarcoids, nonmalignant tumors resembling sarcomas, spread through the lungs, lymph nodes, skin, spleen, liver and other sites, including the optic nerves, where they caused blindness. When confronted with the reigning dogma that sarcoidosis is rare in the arctic regions and in the tropics, he observed that "this is not unanticipated when one remembers that there are very few people living above the Arctic

Circle and that in the tropics there are very few physicians. *A minimal requirement for the diagnosis of sarcoidosis is a patient and a physician.*" The italics are mine in honor of the author of what I have since always called Siltzbach's law, here stated for the first time, in the *Transactions of the New York Academy of Sciences,* February 1967, p. 369. The word "sarcoidosis" can, of course, be replaced by the names of any and all diseases.

11.   J. Alison Glover, "Milroy Lectures on the Incidence of Rheumatic Diseases," *Lancet,* March 8, 1930, p. 503; Lewis Wannamaker, "The Chain That Links the Heart to the Throat," T. Duckett Jones Memorial Lecture, *Circulation,* July 1973, pp. 9–18; and Katherine Dodge Brownell and Frances Bailen-Rose, "Acute Rheumatic Fever in Children; Incidence in a Borough of New York City," *JAMA,* June 18, 1973, pp. 1593–1597. See also Milton Markowitz, "Eradication of Rheumatic Fever; an Unfilled Hope," T. Duckett Jones Memorial Lecture, *Circulation,* June 1970, pp. 1077–1084.

12.   See note 11.

13.   Rebecca C. Lancefield, "Current Knowledge of Type-Specific M Antigens of Group A Streptococcus," *Journal of Immunology,* 87:303–313, 1962.

14.   Philip A. Cavelti, "Autoantibodies in Rheumatic Fever," *Proceedings of the Society for Experimental Biology and Medicine,* 60:379–381, 1945.

15.   Melvin H. Kaplan and Mary Meyeserian, "An Immunological Cross-reaction Between Group-A Streptococcal Cells and Human Heart Tissue," *Lancet,* April 7, 1962, pp. 706–710; John B. Zabriskie and Earl H. Freimer, "An Immunological Relationship Between the Group A Streptococcus and Mammalian Muscle," *Journal of Experimental Medicine,* 124:661–678, 1966; I. van de Rijn, J. B. Zabriskie, and M. McCarty, "Group A Streptococcal Antigens Cross-reactive With Myocardium. Purification of Heart-Reactive Antibody and Isolation and Characterization of the Streptococcal Antigen," *Journal of Experimental Medicine,* 146:579–597, 1977; and Lily C. Yang, Pandu R. Soprey, Masako K. Wittner, and Eugene N. Fox, "Streptococcal-Induced Cell-Mediated Immune Destruction of Cardiac Myofibers *in vitro,*" *Journal of Experimental Medicine,* 146:344–360, 1977.

16.   See note 15.

17.   Various authors, "Community Control of Rheumatic Heart Disease in Developing Countries: 1. A Major Public Health Problem"; "2. Strategies for Prevention and Control," *WHO Chronicle,* 34:336–345, 389–395, 1980.

18.   See note 17.

19.   O. B. Nesbit, "Dick Test and Immunization Against Scarlet Fever," *JAMA,* March 15, 1925, pp. 805–807.

20.   Benedict F. Massell, Larry H. Honikman, and Jacqueline Amecuza, "Rheumatic Fever Following Streptococcal Vaccina-

tion. Report of Three Cases," *JAMA*, February 10, 1969, pp. 1115–1119. See also earlier paper: Massell, J. Gabriel Michael, Amecuza, and Myron Siner, *Applied Microbiology*, March 1968, pp. 509–518.

21.   V. A. Fischetti and B. N. Manjula. "The Close Structural Relationship Between Streptococcal M Protein and Mammalian Tropomyosin and Its Possible Role in the Biology of the Group A Streptococcus," *Proceedings of the International Symposium on Bacterial Vaccines*, 1980. See also earlier paper: Barbara Hosein, Maclyn McCarty, and Vincent A. Fischetti, "Amino Acid Sequence and Physicochemical Similarities Between Streptococcal M Protein and Mammalian Tropomyosin," *Proceedings of the National Academy of Sciences, U.S.A.*, August 1979, pp. 3765–3768.

22.   Jack L. Paradise, "Otitis Media in Infants and Children," *Pediatrics*, May 1980, pp. 917–943.

23.   Jerome O. Klein, in *Briefing for Medical Editors*, New York, April 24, 1979.

24.   Robert Austrian, Virgil M. Howie, and John H. Ploussard, "The Bacteriology of Pneumococcal Otitis Media," *Johns Hopkins Medical Journal*, September 1977, pp. 104–111.

25.   Vanja A. Holm and LuVern H. Kunze, "Effect of Chronic Otitis Media on Language and Speech Development," *Pediatrics*, May 1969, pp. 833–839.

26.   M. P. Downs, "Hearing Loss: Definition, Epidemiology and Prevention," *Public Health Reviews* (Israel), 4:225–280, 1975.

27.   David M. Kessner, Carolyn Kalk Snow, and James Singer, *Assessment of Medical Care for Children: Contrasts in Health Status*, Institute of Medicine, National Academy of Sciences, Washington, D.C., vol. 2, pp. 29–66, vol. 3, pp. 38–54, 1974.

28.   John Fry et al., "The Outcome of Acute Otitis Media. A Report to the Medical Research Council," *British Journal of Preventive and Social Medicine*, 23:205–209, 1969; John Fry, "Acute Otitis Media in General Practice," *Proceedings of the Royal Society of Medicine*, July 1970, pp. 741–742; and Gary J. Kaplan et al., "Long-term Effects of Otitis Media. A Ten-Year Cohort Study of Alaskan Eskimo Children," *Pediatrics*, October 1973, pp. 577–585.

29.   C. D. Bluestone and P. A. Shurin, "Middle Ear Disease in Children: Pathogenesis, Diagnosis, and Management," *Pediatric Clinics of North America*, May 1974.

30.   Paradise, op. cit.

31.   Klein, op. cit.

32.   Paul A. Shurin, Stephen I. Pelton, Allen Donner, and Jerome O. Klein, "Persistence of Middle-Ear Effusion After Acute Otitis Media in Children," *New England Journal of Medicine*, May 17, 1979, pp. 1121–1123.

33.   David D. Beal, "Prevention of Otitis Media in the Alaskan Native," *Otitis Media*, A. Glorig and K. S. Kerwin, eds.

(Springfield, Ill.: Charles C. Thomas, 1972).

34. Charles D. Bluestone, Jerome O. Klein, and John D. Nelson, "The Changing Challenge of Otitis Media. Fact File and Literature Review," 1979, p. 14.

35. V. M. Howie, John H. Ploussard, and John L. Sloyer, "Immunization Against Recurrent Otitis Media," *Annals of Otology, Rhinology and Laryngology,* March–April 1976, suppl. 25, part 2, pp. 254–258.

36. F. W. Henderson, A. M. Collier, W. A. Clyde, Jr., and F. W. Denny, "The Epidemiology of Acute Otitis Media in Childhood," *Abstract 188,* 16th Interscience Conference on Antimicrobial Agents and Chemotherapy, American Society for Microbiology, Washington, D.C., 1976; Margaret A. Sanyal, Frederick W. Henderson, Eileen C. Stempel, Albert M. Collier, and Floyd W. Denny, "Effect of Upper Respiratory Tract Infection on Eustachian Tube Ventilatory Function in the Preschool Child," *Journal of Pediatrics,* July 1980, pp. 11–15, and C. T. Ramey, A. M. Collier, J. J. Sparling, et al., "The Carolina Abecedarian Project, a Longitudinal and Multidisciplinary Approach to the Prevention of Developmental Retardation," in *Intervention Strategies for High-Risk Children,* T. Tjossen, ed. (Baltimore: University Park Press, 1976), p. 629.

37. See note 36.

38. "Cholera" was a misnomer. What they had actually discovered was one of the agents of the cholera-like salmonellosis, a diarrheal disease of swine, people, and other mammals.

39. *Morbidity and Mortality Weekly Report (MMWR), Annual Summary 1979,* Centers for Disease Control, September 1980, vol. 28, no. 54, p. 65.

40. Ibid.

41. René Germanier, "Development of a New Oral Attenuated Typhoid Vaccine," *Proceedings of the International Symposium on Bacterial Vaccines,* 1980; R. Germanier, "Immunity in Experimental Salmonellosis. I. Protection Induced by Rough Mutants of Salmonella typhimurium," *Infection and Immunity,* 2:309–315, 1970; R. Germanier and E. Furer, "Immunity in Experimental Salmonellosis. II. Basis for the Avirulence and Protective Capacity of gal E Mutants of Salmonella typhimurium," ibid. 4:663–673, 1971; Germanier and Furer, "Isolation and Characterization of gal E Mutant Ty 21a of Salmonella tyhpi: A Candidate Strain for a Live, Oral Typhoid Vaccine," *Journal of Infectious Diseases,* 131:553–558, 1975; and M. H. Wahdan et al., "Controlled Field Trial of Live Oral Typhoid Vaccine Ty 21a," *Bulletin of the World Health Organization,* 58:469–474, 1980.

42. Vincent R. Racaniello and David Baltimore, "Molecular Cloning of Poliovirus DNA and Determination of the Complete Nucleotide Sequence of the Viral Genome," *Proceedings of the National Academy of Sciences U.S.A.,* August 1981, pp. 4887–4891.

43.   Paul Berg, Konrad Bloch, George Dunlop, Mahlon Hoagland, et al., "Notes on the Status of Science," May 6, 1981. Within a year, this delegation of biomedical investigators would be followed by investigators and clinicians concerned about the health effects of huge cuts in federal programs for social and preventive medicine, such as the 30 percent cut in the WIC (women, infants, children) program and in the federal immunization program for children—from funds sufficient to immunize 6.3 million children in 1981 to only 3.8 million in the 1983 budget.

The Nobel laureate Dr. Frederick C. Robbins, whose work helped make polio vaccines feasible, testifying as president of the Institute of Medicine at the National Academy of Sciences, told a congressional committee that "most of the disease agents are still present in the population, just waiting for the number of susceptible children to become large enough that a wave of disease can sweep through them." He asked the federal government to reexamine its announced cutbacks in the childhood immunization program against polio, measles, rubella, and other once major killing and crippling infectious diseases.

At the same House Energy and Commerce Subcommittee on Health and the Environment hearings, Dr. Samuel Katz, chairman of pediatrics at the Duke University Medical Center—another important former collaborator with vaccine pioneer John F. Enders—reminded the nation's legislators that from its inception, the federal childhood immunization program had saved ten dollars in medical costs for every single dollar of tax monies spent on the vaccines recommended by the American Academy of Pediatrics for use in all children between the ages of two months and four years.

According to the *New York Times*'s account of the doctors' testimony. "Dr. James Chin, chief of the infectious diseases section of the California Department of Health, said that as many as half of the state's children received at least some of their vaccines from public programs. He warned that the [federal] cutbacks imposed this year alone were making it increasingly difficult to reach the 400,000 infants born every year." Robert Reinhold, "Experts Warn Cutbacks May Revive Serious Childhood Epidemics," *New York Times*, February 5, 1982, p. 19A. See also "The Safety Net and 1977," editorial *New York Times*, March 31, 1982.

44.   John A. D. Cooper, "Manpower Resources for Research," *Annals of Internal Medicine*, part 2, November 1978, pp. 806–808.

45.   Craig R. Johnson, "Genetic Engineering. Why the Microbe Makers Got Stung," *New York Times*, March 14, 1982, p. 2F.

46.   See note 43.

47.   See note 43.

48.   Joseph A. Califano, Jr., *Governing America. An Insider's Report From the White House and the Cabinet* (New York: Simon & Schuster, 1981).

Institutional Abbreviations

American Academy of Pediatrics	**AAP**
American Cancer Society	**ACS**
American Medical Association	**AMA**
Centers for Disease Control	**CDC**
(originally Center for Communicable Diseases, later Center for Disease Control, now Centers)	
Civilian Conservation Corps	**CCC**
Food and Drug Administration	**FDA**
National Academy of Sciences	**NAS**
National Cancer Institute	**NCI**
National Center for Health Statistics	**NCHS**
National Foundation for Infantile Paralysis	**NFIP**
National Institute for Allergy and Infectious Diseases	**NIAID**
National Institutes of Health	
(formerly National Institute of Health)	**NIH**
National Science Foundation	**NSF**
United States Public Health Service	**USPHS**
(usually shortened to Public Health Service)	**PHS**
Walter Reed Army Institute of Research	**WRAIR**
World Health Organization	**WHO**

Glossary of Medical and Scientific Terms

A

abscess: A localized collection of pus in a cavity of tissues disintegrated by bacterial infection.

adjuvant (in vaccines):   Any single material, or combination of biological, mineral, chemical or other materials, that increases the immunogenicity of a vaccine.

agglutination (in microbiology):   The clumping together of bacteria when exposed to some antibodies, as when bacterial cells are added to blood serum containing specific antibodies.

antibody: Proteins formed in the lymphocytes, mucosal cells, and other bodily tissues in response to the presence of foreign antigens, which include cell-surface proteins, and carbohydrates, as well as toxins of bacteria. The antibodies combine or interact with the foreign antigens or microbial cells and neutralize them. (See also *immunoglobulins.*)

antigens: Any substances—usually of exogenous, or foreign, origin—that trigger the synthesis of antibodies against themselves.

antiserum: A blood serum containing one or more antibodies against one or more microbial antigens. (See *immune serum.*)

antitoxin: Antibody against specific microbial toxin. (See *serotherapy.*)

attenuation (in immunity):   The loss of virulence in microbial pathogens such as bacteria and viruses. Heat, aging, and chemicals are used to attenuate microbes without reducing their immunogenicity, or ability to induce the production of antibodies.

autogenous (vaccines):   Vaccines made from bacteria that are found in the patients themselves, in contrast to regular or stock vaccines, which are made from bacteria of the same but not autogenous types and strains of bacteria that cause the patients' infections.

B

bacillus (pl.: bacilli)   A rod-shaped bacterium.

bacteremia: The presence of bacteria in the blood.

bacteria (sing.: bacterium):   Various groups of prokaryotic microorganisms, invisible to the human eye but can be seen under the light and electron microscopes. They are distantly related to plants and blue-green algae. Some species of bacteria cause infectious diseases in people; other bacterial species, harmless to people, produce antibiotics, cause fermentation, help dispose of sewage, and fix nitrogen in the soil. (See *prokaryotic cells.*)

bactericidal: Substances, such as antibiotics, or processes that kill bacteria.

bacteriolysis: The disintegration or bursting of bacterial cells.

bacteriophages: Viruses that attack and kill bacteria. Usually called phages.

bacteriostatic: Substances, such as the sulfa drugs, which slow the growth of bacteria but do not kill them.

BCG: *Bacillus Calmette-Guérin.* Attenuated tubercle bacilli employed as a vaccine against tuberculosis.

C

capsid: The protein outer coat around the nucleic acid core of a virus.

capsular polysaccharides: Carbohydrates consisting of ten or more monosaccharides or simple sugars found in the outer capsules of virulent types or groups of pneumococci, meningococci and other bacteria.

carbohydrates: Compounds in which oxygen and hydrogen are present in the same proportions found in water. Sugars, starches, celluloses, and vegetable gums are major carbohydrates. They are essential in the metabolism of all living organisms.

cerebrospinal meningitis: Inflammation of the meninges, or membranes, of both the brain and the spinal cord.

Chlamydia: Bacteria that proliferate in the cytoplasms of living cells, related to the *Rickettsia.* They include the agents of trachoma, psittacosis, and lymphogranuloma venereum, and can be killed by some but not all antibiotic drugs.

chromatin: A structure consisting of proteins and DNA, found in the nucleus of living cells. The chromatins are carriers of the genes.

chromosome: A thread-shaped structure, containing DNA and—in higher organisms—protein, found in nucleus of all living cells. In people the chromosomes consist of twenty-three matched and linear pairs; in bacteria they consist of a single filament of DNA. Before every nuclear division, the matched pairs of chromosomes double, and the duplicates separate to form the nuclei of the two daughter cells.

chronic: Referring to a disease or disorder that persists for a long time.

clinical: Relating to human diseases or disorders.

coliphages: Bacteriophages that attack *Escherichia coli* (*E. coli*).

commensal (in medical microbiology): Referring to a microorganism living in or on human cells without causing any injury to the host.

complement: One of a group of substances in blood serum that combines with antigen-antibody complex and lyses, or destroys, the complex when the antigen is a bacterial or other virulent microbial cell.

congenital: Associated with birth but not necessarily hereditary.

contagion: The transmission of infectious disease from one person to another, by exhalation droplets, or by bodily (such as venereal) contact.

convalescent serum: Blood serum from patients convalescing from infectious diseases that is proven or presumed to contain antibodies against the agents of these diseases.

cross-protecting antigens: Antigens of one type or species of microorganism which protect people or animals against infections caused by another type or species.

cross-reacting antigens: Antigens of one species or type of microbial pathogen which react with antibodies of another type or species but do not necessarily protect against the other organisms.

culture (in medical microbiology): Bacteria and viruses are cultured or grown in broths and agar plates containing bacterial nutrients, or in tissue cultures of living cells in which viruses replicate.

cytoplasm: Everything inside of a living cell except the nucleus.

D

diploid cells: Cells possessing twice the number of chromosomes normally found in a germ cell (a cell whose function is the reproduction of the kind).

DNA: Deoxyribonucleic acid. The nucleic acid that comprises the genetic or hereditary material, found in the nucleus or the chromosomes of the cell of nearly all forms of life. (Some viruses contain only RNA.)

droplet infections: Infections transmitted by virulent bacteria or viruses present in drops of moisture expelled from the mouth in exhaling, coughing, sneezing, or speaking.

dysuria: Painful or difficult urination; an early symptom of gonorrhea or nongonococcal urethritis.

E

E. coli: *Escherichia coli.* Gram-negative bacilli found in the human and animal gut. Harmless in the intestine, but highly pathogenic when they get into and colonize the lungs, urinary tract, and other abnormal body sites. With the discovery of bacterial viruses, *E. coli* became the "guinea pigs" of modern virology. For over a generation, *E. coli* have been one of the leading causes of American hospital-acquired (nosocomial) infections.

electron microscope: A microscope that uses electrons instead of light rays, and electromagnetic fields instead of glass lenses. It is a hundred times more powerful than the best optical microscope. Viruses invisible under the light or optical microscope can be seen using the electron microscope. Bacterial structures such as the pili, the attachment organelles of bacteria, first became visible under the electron microscope.

encapsulated bacteria: Bacteria surrounded by a slimy outer capsule, generally composed of polysaccharides that interfere with phagocytosis and thus protect the encapsulated organisms.

encephalitis: Inflammation of the brain, often caused by measles, coxsackie virus, cytomegalovirus, and other viral infections.

endemic: Prevalent in a region or nation. An endemic disease is one that is always present, but not at epidemic levels.

enteric: Relating to the intestines. Water-borne infections, such as cholera, typhoid, and bacterial dysentery, comprise one group of enteric diseases.

enzymes: Proteins produced in living cells that act as catalysts or promoters of chemical changes. Enzymes produced by people are essential to many life processes, such as metabolism and digestion.

epidemic: A disease that spreads widely after being introduced into a region or country, and/or an endemic disease that suddenly spreads to much greater numbers of people. Epidemic diseases usually subside to low endemic levels between outbreaks.

epidemiology: The science dealing with the causes and distributions of infectious and noninfectious diseases.

erysipelas: An extremely severe and often fatal streptococcal infection of the skin and subcutaneous tissue. Now a rare disease, it was very common before the development of sulfa drugs and antibiotic drugs.

eugenics: A scientistic (pseudoscientific) cult started in Victorian England by Francis Galton, who described all good and bad human physical and mental traits as being due to either superior (eugenic) or inferior (dysgenic) blood, and preached that most people were, by inescapable biological inheritance, "ineffectives" and "mediocrities." In experimental medicine, as recently as the 1950s, such eugenical dogmas served to rationalize the testing of new drugs and vaccines in children institutionalized as "feebleminded" or as "low-grade idiots or imbeciles."

eukaryotic cells: Cells with the nuclear material contained in a number of linear chromosomes, and with the nucleus separated from the cytoplasms by a nuclear membrane. (See also *prokaryotic cells.*)

F

fecal contamination: Water or other matter containing the feces of people or other animals, which often carry microbial and protozoan disease agents such as bacteria, viruses, amoebas, and *Giardia lamblia.*

fermentation: Decomposition of sugars and other nonprotein organic materials by bacteria, yeasts, and other organisms. (See *putrefaction; zymotic.*)

fibroblast (fibrocyte): A connective-tissue cell found in vertebrate connective tissue.

filtrate: A liquid that has passed through a filter. In medical microbiology a fluid from which bacteria and other organisms have been filtered out, leaving viruses and other filterable particles in the liquid.

folic acid: One of the constituents of the vitamin B complex. Folic acid is essential in the synthesis of the nucleic acids and is therefore essential to the continuation of life.

formalin: A solution of formaldehyde in water. Formaldehyde is a powerful antiseptic and disinfectant used to sterilize surgical instruments in hospitals. Formalin is used to activate (or kill) polioviruses used in Salk-type polio vaccines.

G

gangrene: The death of bodily tissues or organs following loss of blood to affected sites due to injury or arterial disease. Gas gangrene, caused by bacteria (*Clostridia*) that proliferate in military or accident wounds, was a major cause of deaths in the western world until antibacterial drugs like the sulfas and antibiotics came into general use.

gene: Unit of the material of biological inheritance. In most organisms this material is deoxyribonucleic acid (DNA). Certain tumor viruses or retroviruses contain only ribonucleic acid (RNA) replicate with the aid of a newly discovered enzyme, reverse transcriptase, that uses RNA as a template to synthesize DNA.

genetics: The science dealing with the observed biological, chemical, and physical realities of heredity and variation in living organisms. Genetics is the opposite of eugenics.

germicidal: Bactericidal.

globulins: Proteins found in the blood serum and other tissues. Antibodies are globulins. (See *immunoglobulins.*)

glycoproteins: Protein-carbohydrate compounds, including antigens found in some virus capsids, or coats.

gonococcus: A Gram-negative bacterium, *Neisseria gonorrhoeae*, that causes gonorrhea.

gonorrhea: A sexually transmitted infection and inflammation of the mucous membrane, generally but not always in the sexual organs. Curable by antibiotics. Also known as clap. (See *nongonococcal urethritis.*)

H

Haemophilus influenzae (originally Pfeiffer's bacillus):   Gram-negative bacterium, usually found in the form of a small rod. An important cause of bacterial pneumonia secondary to influenza and other respiratory virus infections. During great flu pandemic of 1918–1919, was erroneously believed to be the cause of influenza itself. *H. influenzae type b* is now a major cause of meningitis in infants, as well as of acquired mental retardation due to brain damage caused by bacterial meningitis in infancy and early childhood.

hapten: An incomplete antigen which, combined with proteins, can become a complete antigen capable of reacting with specific antibodies.

hematology: The medical specialty that deals with blood and blood-forming tissues, and the treatment of diseases of the blood.

hemolytic (in microbiology):   Pertaining to bacteria and other agents that lyse, or burst, blood cells.

hereditary: Relating to biological traits and disorders chromosomally transmitted from parents to their offspring. Most common diseases are not hereditary, nor are any behavior traits, such as intelligence, honesty, business ability, and other social characteristics. (See *congenital.*)

host defense system (in immunology):   The wide array of circulating and cellular antibodies, complements, opsonins, properdins, interferons, and phagocytes that combine to defend people and other animals against exogenous, or foreign, proteins and microbial and protozoan pathogens.

I

iatrogenic: Medically induced.

immune serum: Serum containing antibodies against specific antigens, such as measles virus and pertussis bacteria antigens or tetanus toxins.

immunity (in infectious diseases):   An inborn, congenital, postinfection or artificially acquired (through vaccination) resistance to an infectious disease agent. *Active immunity,* a long-lasting form acquired after a natural infection or induced by vaccination, causes the body to synthesize specific antibodies. *Passive immunity* is a short-lived form transmitted by maternal antibodies *in utero* or in colostrum in mother's milk to infants, as well as in sera of animals hyperimmunized with inoculations of specific causal agents.

immunogen: An antigen that stimulates the production of antibodies and active immunity. All immunogens are antigens, but not all antigens are immunogenic.

immunoglobulins: Antibodies or immunoproteins produced in living cells and tissues. Abbreviated Ig.

immunology: The science and medical specialty dealing with immunity and allergy.

infection: The multiplication or proliferation of microbial disease agents in the body proper. Infections are usually caused by exogenous, or foreign, microbes, but can also be caused by normally benign enteric bacteria, such as *E. coli,* when they get into the urinary tract, the lungs, and other abnormal sites.

in vitro: In laboratory glassware, such as test tubes and culture plates.

in vivo: In living bodies.

leukocytes: White blood cells.

lipopolysaccharides: Endotoxins, or toxic molecules found on certain bacteria. The lipid (fat) component is toxic; the saccharide (sugar) portion is nontoxic and immunogenic.

lymph nodes: Nodules throughout the body that store lymph, the clear circulating fluid that carries the lymphocytes.

lymphocytes: White blood corpuscles whose functions include the production and delivery of specific antibodies in response to stimulation by their antigens.

lysis: The act of lysing, or bursting.

lysogenic (in microbiology):   Pertaining to bacteria that carry dormant bacteriophages for generations before chemical agents, radiations, or other factors cause the phage genes to become active or vegetative, induce the replication of hundreds of mature phage particles, and thus lyse (burst) the host bacterial cells.

lysogenic conversion: Phage-mediated acquisition of new metabolic functions by bacteria after dormant phages become vegetative and start replicating in lysogenic bacteria. Lysogenic strains of *Corynebacterium diphtheriae* and *Streptococcus pyogenes,* for example, start producing the toxins of diphtheria and scarlet fever following their lysogenic conversion. Nonlysogenic strains of *C. diphtheriae* and *S. pyogenes* never produce either toxin.

M

Magic Bullets: The name Paul Ehrlich gave to antibodies and chemicals that attacked only specific pathogens and harmed no other body tissues.

meningitis: Inflammation of the membranes of the brain or spinal cord from infection by bacteria or viruses. Many different viruses and bacteria can cause meningitis, but most cases of bacterial meningitis are caused by the meningococci, the pneumococci, and Group B streptococci.

meningococcal meningitis: Cerebrospinal and other forms of meningitis caused by specific groups of *Neisseria meningitidis,* one of the leading causes of bacterial meningitis.

metabolism: The sum of all the physical and chemical bodily processes by which organisms are formed, kept alive, and supplied with energy.

metabolite: A substance that takes part in a metabolic process. Most metabolites are produced by the body; others, essential to metabolism, must be taken in from the environment. The latter group of essential metabolites includes certain vitamins, amino acids, and carbohydrates present in many common foodstuffs.

microbe: .   A microorganism, such as the bacteria, protozoa, and fungi, too small to be visible to the human eye. Although not living organisms, viruses are generally included among the microbes.

morphology: The study of form.

mucosa: Mucous membrane.

mutation: An alteration in an organism's characteristics, caused by a sudden change in that organism's DNA.

N

nasopharynx: The nose and throat.

natural selection: The primary mechanism of evolution.

nephritis: An inflammation of the kidney. Has many causes, including alcohol, lead poisoning, beestings, and the complications of such bacterial infections as pneumococcal pneumonia and syphilis. One of the most common causes of nephritis before the antibiotic era was post-streptococcal inflammation, the aftereffect of an ordinary "strep throat."

nongonococcal urethritis: A disease with all the clinical signs and symptoms of gonorrhea, but is caused by *Chlamydia* and other nongonococcal organisms.

notifiable diseases: Any diseases that by local or state laws must be reported to local health departments by the doctors who treat them.

nucleic acids: See *DNA* and *RNA.*

O

opsonins: A class of circulating antibodies that help phagocytes (white blood cells) destroy invading bacteria. Not all antibodies are opsonic. (See *phagocytosis.*)

organelles: Structures in living cells analogous to organs in a mammalian body.

otitis media: An inflammation of the middle ear caused by bacterial infections secondary to upper respiratory viral infections, such as the common cold.

P

pandemic: A disease that grows from a regional or a national epidemic to attack many nations or even the entire world, such as the eighteenth- and twentieth-century pandemics of smallpox and influenza.

pathogen: A disease-causing microbe or material.

pathology: All aspects of a disease or disorder.

phage: See *bacteriophages.*

phagocytosis (in bacteriology):   The engulfment and digestion of bacteria and other foreign cells by leukocytes (white blood cells) circulating in the blood serum. It is usually mediated by opsonic antibodies that combine with the surface antigens of microbes to make them much more susceptible to phagocytosis. The protective actions of phagocytosis are further enhanced by the presence of complement.

placebo: An inert compound, such as chalk or distilled water, used in experimental medical research to mimic drugs or vaccines being tested.

pneumococcus: *Streptococcus pneumoniae.* The agent of pneumococcal pneumonia. Also major cause of otitis media, bacterial meningitis, sinus infections, and osteomyelitis. Formerly known as *Diplococcus pneumoniae.*

prokaryotic cells: Cells without separate nuclei or linear chromosomes, as in cells of all higher orders of life. Bacteria are prokaryotes. Their nuclear materials are contained in simple filaments of DNA, often in circular form. The rigid cell walls of bacteria contain amino acids and carbohydrates in the form of mureins. (See *eukaryotic cells.*)

properdin: A serum globulin which, in the presence of both complement and magnesium ions, combines with and kills invading bacteria. One of the components of the human inborn host defense systems against microbes.

prophylaxis: The prevention of disease (as in vaccination or immunization against infectious diseases).

proteins: Proteins of infinite varieties comprise three quarters of the mass of all living cells. All living species have proteins peculiar to themselves. They are made of thousands of amino acid molecules, and are synthesized in the cells. The sequences of amino acids in all proteins are determined by information carried from the DNA in the cells' nuclei to the ribosomes and other organelles by RNA, which is made on the DNA templates, or molds for the synthesis of other nucleic acids.

prototype: An original type species or example. An ancestral form.

pus: A viscous liquid, containing leukocytes and liquor puris, found in inflammation sites.

pustule: A small skin eruption filled with pus, as in both smallpox and cowpox.

putrefaction: Bacterial decomposition of proteins, with the production of foul-smelling compounds, such as hydrogen sulfide, ammonia, and mercaptans. (See *fermentation; zymotic.*)

R

respiratory system: All the air passages from the nose to the lungs.

revaccination (booster shots):   Secondary and tertiary vaccinations subsequent to primary vaccinations for smallpox, diphtheria, tetanus, polio, and other diseases for which more than one dose is or was required.

rheumatic fever: A disease marked by high fevers, chills, and arthritic pains following infection of the throat by Group A streptococci ("strep throat"). Cardiac side effects include valvular heart disease and endocarditis, both serious and often fatal disorders. Sydenham's chorea (St. Vitus' dance) is another common side effect of rheumatic fever.

RNA: Ribonucleic acid, the nucleic acid synthesized by DNA in the cell nucleus. RNA carries the genetic information in DNA from the nucleus to the cytoplasm of living cells.

S

sepsis: The poisoning caused by products of putrefaction, such as contaminated food. Puerperal sepsis (childbed fever) occurs after childbirth as a result of putrefactive matter in the birth canal.

septicemia: Proliferating or multiplying bacteria and bacterial toxins disseminated in the blood

serotherapy: The treatment of infectious diseases by the injection of serum antitoxins or specific serum antibodies, as in pre-antibiotic-era treatments of diphtheria and tetanus, and of some types of pneumococcal pneumonia.

Serratia marcescens: Enteric, Gram-negative bacteria. The pigmented types produce bloodlike red colonies, and are not pathogenic to people. The nonpigmented types found in mixed cultures, however, are a serious cause of hospital-acquired septicemias, pneumonias, and other infections.

serum: A fluid component of blood; blood plasma minus fibrinogen and other clotting factors.

species: A group of individuals or microorganisms able to breed among themselves but not with organisms of other groups. Members of a genus of similar organisms.

spirochete: A spiral-shaped bacterium, such as *Treponema pallidum,* the agent of syphilis.

Staphylococcus: Gram-positive spherical bacterium, a very common cause of human infections, ranging from boils and carbuncles to septicemia, endocarditis, meningitis, puerperal sepsis, pneumonia, and brain abscess.

strep throat: Pharyngitis caused by Group A streptococci.

Streptococcus: A genus of ubiquitous Gram-positive lancet-shaped or spherical bacteria that form chains, and include the pneumococci; the Group A hemolytic streptococci that cause septic sore throat, endocarditis, poststreptococcal nephritis, rheumatic fever, and rheumatic heart disease; and the agents of Group B streptococcal infection and neonatal meningitis.

subcutaneous: Immediately beneath the skin.

subunit vaccines: Vaccines made of surface and structural antigens found on or in microbial pathogens, but not of whole live, or attenuated, or dead bacteria, viruses, mycoplasma, or protozoa.

synergism: The joint action of drugs, antigens, and other agents so that their combined effect is greater than the sum of their parts.

T

tissue (biological):   An organization or region of living cells; the fundamental structure of which plant and animal organs are composed.

tissue cultures: Living tissue fragments, or their individual cells, grown in a liquid nutrient medium that keeps them alive. Viruses, which can replicate only in living cells, are reared and their cytopathogenic effects (CPE) studied in whole tissue or separated cell cultures.

toxic: Poisonous.

toxins (in bacteriology):   Poisons synthesized by certain bacteria, such as the tetanus, clostridial (gas gangrene), and diphtheria toxins.

toxoids: Bacterial toxins altered chemically so that they become nonpoisonous but remain antigenic, and used as vaccines to protect against such toxin-induced diseases as diphtheria and tetanus.

tubercle bacillus: The bacterium of tuberculosis.

types (in microbiology):   Bacteria, viruses, and other microbial pathogens that differ from other organisms of the same species by sharing very specific serological, capsular, and other characteristics, including their susceptibility or resistance to specific phages.

U

urethritis: Inflammation of the urethra; one of the first symptoms of gonorrhea. Also called urethritis venerea. (See also *nongonococcal urethritis.*)

V

vaccination: The induction of long-term or lifelong immunity against infectious diseases by the injection or oral ingestion of whole live, altered, or inactivated microbial pathogens; or antigens removed from the structures of microbes; or toxoids made by chemically altering bacterial toxins.

vaccinia: The cowpox virus.

variola: The smallpox virus.

variolation: A method of protecting people against smallpox by the inoculation of materials from smallpox pustules that carry variolae. Often caused serious outbreaks of smallpox and was abandoned and even made illegal in some countries both before and after vaccination proved much safer than variolation.

vector: An insect or other live carrier that carries microbial pathogens to people, like mosquitoes that carry malaria parasites from birds to human beings, and the lysogenic strains of *Corynebacterium diphtheriae* that transmit the toxin of diphtheria to children and adults. (See *lysogenic conversion.*)

vesicle: (1) A small serum-containing elevation on the skin, such as a blister, or an encephalitic vesicle of the brain. (2) Any small membranous cyst, cavity, or sac.

virulence: The condition of being extremely poisonous; the ability of a microbe to induce disease in people, plants, and other hosts.

virus: Submicroscopic particle consisting of a protein or glycoprotein coat and core of either DNA or RNA but never—as in all living cells—both nucleic acids. Viruses lack metabolisms but can replicate by invading specific living cells of animals, plants, and even microorganisms, and converting the metabolic or chemical systems of virus-parasitized cells to produce hundreds of new mature virus particles. Mature viral particles are called virions.

viscera: The internal organs of the body, including the stomach, liver, kidney, heart, and lung, but excluding the muscles, nerves, and bones.

W

whole-organism vaccine: A vaccine made of a whole bacterial organism or viral particle that is used live and unaltered; or live but attenuated or otherwise altered; or killed (inactivated) by heat, chemicals, or other means. (See *subunit vaccines.*)

Wonder Drugs: The popular name bestowed upon antibiotic drugs when they were originally introduced during World War II.

Z

zymotic: Literally, caused by fermentation (from the Greek word for "causing fermentation," *zymotikos*). During pregerm theory generations of the nineteenth century, and until well into the twentieth century, infectious diseases were classified as zymotic diseases by European and American health agencies. (See *fermentation; putrefaction.*)

Index

Fleming, Alexander, 26, 33, 194
Flexner, Simon, 191, 226, 227, 228, 278, 279, 301, 302
Florence Nightingale Architecture hospitals, 106
Flügge, Carl, 157
Focal infection concept for treatment of gonorrhea, 423–425
Folic acid, 26
Folic acid vitamin, 241
Foot-and-mouth disease, 244–245
Formaldehyde, 294
Formalin, 204–205
Formalin-inactivated polio vaccine, see Salk vaccine
Four-virus vaccine (multivalent vaccine) for the common cold, 353
Fowl cholera
  Pasteur and, 131–133
  vaccine against, 121, 124, 129, 131–133, 136, 141, 142, 153
Fowl pox virus, 243
Fracastoro, Girolamo, 85
Fraenkel, Albert, 218, 360
Fraenkel, Carl, 173, 174
Francis, Thomas, Jr., 23, 24, 232, 290, 295, 301, 343, 438
Franco-Prussian War (1870–1871), 62–63, 125, 151
Frasch, Carl, 375, 392–395, 446
Fraser, David W., 474
Freimer, Earl, 481
Freund, Jules, 501
Freund incomplete adjuvant, 501
Fried, Martin A., 370
Friedlander, Carl, 360
Frosch, Paul, 237, 244

Galton, Sir Francis, 67
Gamma globulin, rubella and, 315
Gangrene, 105, 111, 148, 149
Gaskell, Peter, 100–101
Gear, James H. S., 372
General Virology (Luria), 250
Genetic diseases, 329–330
Gengou, Octave, 391
Genital herpes, 325–326
Georgia Warm Springs Foundation, 276, 277
Gerlough, T. D., 30, 31, 441, 442
Germanier, René, 495–499
German measles, see Rubella
Germ Theory and Its Applications to Medicine and Surgery, The (Pasteur), 121, 502

Germ theory of infectious diseases, 75, 85, 86, 88, 99, 113, 118–125, 129–139, 143–144, 161
  development of, 241–245
Gilbert, Walter, 268
Gilden, R. V., 348
Gillespie, L. J., 219–220
GL 2060 (rhinovirus), 352, 353
Glaxo (drug company), 351
Gloucester Anti-Vaccination Society, 73
Gold, Jerome, 369
Gold, Ronald, 37
Goldberger, Joseph, 311, 362
Goldschneider, Irving, 37, 394
Goldwater Memorial Hospital (New York City), 370
Gonococcal capsular polysaccharide vaccines, 434–439, 441–445
Gonococcal ophthalmia neonatorum, 419–420
Gonococcal pili vaccine, 448–454
  trial tests with, 452–454
Gonorrhea, 26, 111, 142, 229, 331, 397–466
  Bell and, 414, 415, 421, 445
  Boswell and, 415–419, 422
  Buchan and, 410–414, 415
  Buchanan and, 421–422
  Cockburn and, 414–415
  cost of treatment, 32, 404
  discovery of gonococci, 419–420, 445
  early history of disease and its treatments, 408–410
  early 20th-century treatment for, 422–426
  Hunter and, 410, 414
  incidence rate in U.S., 458–459, 461
  Korean War and, 400
  NIAID funded research and, 406–407, 450–451
  pelvic inflammatory disease and, 403–406
  penicillin and, 31, 32, 398–399, 440–441
    resistance to, 402, 442
  post-World War II increase in, 31–32, 399–400
  putative vaccines against, 192
  reinfection rates of, 460
  social factors contributing to increase of, 400–403
  sulfa drugs and, 26, 398–399, 440
    resistance to, 399–400
  syphilis and, 445–446
  underreporting by medical profession of, 404–405, 461
  upward social mobility of, 405–406
  vaccines against, 22–32, 231, 406–408, 420–421, 439–441

566

Rhazes, 310, 408–409, 413
Rheumatic fever, 35, 88, 105, 169, 194, 218, 221, 240, 479, 482
Rheumatic heart disease, 218, 226
Rhinolaryngology, 180
Rhinoviruses, 352, 354
Rickettsia, 248, 249
Rifampin, 33
Rivers, Thomas, 283–284
RNA (ribonucleic acid), 253, 255, 256, 268, 289
Robbins, Frederick, 287, 291, 292, 294, 315
Robbins, John, 375, 395
Robbins, John B., 21, 470
Robert Koch Institute for Infectious Diseases, 219, 229, 230, 364, 436, 437
Roberts, Richard B., 32, 404, 459
Robinson, Victor, 408–409
Rockefeller Institute, 22, 23, 197, 217, 219, 221, 223, 226, 228, 231, 232, 266, 274–275, 280, 284, 301–302, 312, 341, 363, 380, 393, 437
Römer, Paul Heinrich, 294
Roosevelt, Franklin Delano, 276–277
Roosevelt, Theodore, 210–211
Roosevelt Hospital (New York City), 181
Rosenbach, Julius, 141
Rosenow, Edward C., 423, 424
Rosewood Training School (Owings Mills, Md.), 295
Rous, Peyton, 266
Rous sarcoma virus (RSV), 266–267
Rous sarcoma virus—Rous helper virus (RSV-RHV), 329
Roux, Émile, 129, 130, 167, 168, 171–172, 179, 183, 223, 249, 250, 365
Rowe, Wallace, 322, 345
Roy, R. M., 418–419
Royal Baking Powder Company, 223
Royal Colleges of Physicians and Surgeons, 61, 224, 410
Royal Victoria Hospital (Bournemouth), 418
Rubella (German measles), 35, 262, 309, 313–317, 322
    vaccine against, 40, 317, 469
Rubin, Harry, 266–267, 329
Rudolph Virchow Hospital (Berlin), 22, 229, 434, 435, 436, 440, 456
Russell, Lord John, 68

Sabin, Albert, 281, 285, 299, 300, 303–304, 306

Sabin vaccine, 259, 299–300, 301–304, 306, 477, 496–497
Sadler, Michael Thomas, 94, 97
Sadoff, Jerry, 444, 454
St. Bartholomew's Hospital (London), 351, 415
St. Mary's Hospital (London), 159
St. Thomas's Hospital (London), 41, 65, 105
Salk, Jonas, 281–282, 285, 290, 294–301, 306, 343
Salk vaccine, 259, 294–301
Salmon, Daniel E., 142, 143, 496
Salmonella, 160
    pili and, 449, 450
Salvarsan (arsphenamine), 179, 226, 267, 398
San Francisco Medical Center, 454–455
Scanning electron microscope, 254
Scarlet fever, 35, 88, 109, 138, 169, 257
    Dick test for, 481
    putative vaccines against, 192
Schaudinn, Fritz, 445
Schering Corp., 24
Schering-Kahlbaum (drug company), 436–437
Schick, Béla, 179, 188, 200
Schick test for diphtheria, 188–189, 200–201, 290
Schiemann, Oscar, 23, 28, 38, 229–231, 232
Schroeder, May, 189, 200, 202
Schwann, Theodor, 115, 123
Scripps Clinic, 356
Scurvy, 96
Sela, Michael, 500
Sell, Sarah W., 36, 383–384
Semmelweis, Ignaz Philipp, 100, 145–148, 149, 152
Septicemia, 138, 145, 147–149
Serotherapy, 50, 165, 166, 175, 187, 193, 245
    for pneumonia, 219–221, 363, 364–365
Serrati, Serafino, 87
Serratia marcescens, 87, 88, 119
Serum and Vaccine Institute (Switzerland), 495
Serum hepatitis, *see* Hepatitis B
Sette, Vicenzo, 85, 87, 88, 119
Sewall, Henry, 163, 164–168, 171, 175, 209, 219
Sewall, Samuel, 164
Sewall, Thomas, 164
Sex pili, 448
Sexual revolution, increase in gonorrhea rate and, 401–402